Pain

A textbook for health professionals

Pain
A textbook for health professionals
Third Edition

Edited by

Hubert van Griensven
Institute of Medical and Biomedical Education
St George's, University of London
Cranmer Terrace
London

Jenny Strong
Emeritus Professor
Division of Occupational Therapy
School of Health and Rehabilitation Sciences
The University of Queensland
Brisbane, Australia

ELSEVIER

First edition 2002
Second edition 2014

Notices

Practitioners and researchers must always rely on their own experience and knowledge in evaluating and using any information, methods, compounds or experiments described herein. Because of rapid advances in the medical sciences, in particular, independent verification of diagnoses and drug dosages should be made. To the fullest extent of the law, no responsibility is assumed by Elsevier, authors, editors or contributors for any injury and/or damage to persons or property as a matter of products liability, negligence or otherwise, or from any use or operation of any methods, products, instructions, or ideas contained in the material herein.

ISBN: 978-0-323-87033-7

Content Strategist: Trinity Hutton
Content Project Manager: Taranpreet Kaur
Design: Miles Hitchen
Marketing Manager: Deborah Watkins
Illustration Manager: Akshaya Mohan

Printed in India

Last digit is the print number: 9   8   7   6   5   4   3   2   1

Working together
to grow libraries in
developing countries

www.elsevier.com • www.bookaid.org

Contents

Foreword
to the first edition

I am convinced that physiotherapy and occupational therapy are sleeping giants. This book is one of the welcome signs that the long sleep is over. For well over 2000 years classical physiotherapy was practised in every culture as a folk tradition. It was all there: heat, cold, massage, manipulation, acupuncture, reflexology, aromatherapy, etc. Since it was deeply embedded in every society and therefore attracted little intellectual attention, it was simply accepted as an empirical fact of life without the mechanisms being questioned. Occupational therapy is a newer profession: it emerged in response to the many veterans of the 20th century world wars who returned home traumatized, often disabled and in need of occupational rehabilitation. Still, a central tenet of occupational therapy, that humans have a need for meaningful occupation to cope and live with health problems, has been with us for centuries.

In the 18th century, a disaster hit the subsequent development of rehabilitative professions: it was the Age of Reason and the time when academic medicine was developing. This powerful and hugely successful movement was based on two essentials: diagnosis based on pathology and an obsessional search for cures based on rational therapy. Rehabilitation interventions lost out on both counts. The conditions treated often had a vague or non-existent pathology. Only the wildest who exhibited both charisma and the confidence of the charlatan claimed to effect permanent cure. The vast honest majority were proud of the ability to ameliorate the condition. Physiotherapists and occupational therapists were not the only professionals to be demoted by academic medicine. Palliative care, for example, had to wait for two centuries before regaining respectability, since it made no claim to cure. It climbed back to acceptance, once 'proper' doctors said, 'there is nothing more to be done'.

Physiotherapy and occupational therapy survived at the very bottom of the academic hierarchy. From the more-honest doctors, physiotherapists won a certain respect because it was clear that they were indeed helping some patients. For the less-honest doctors, physiotherapy represented a polite dumping ground for patients who had been labelled as unfit for appropriate rational medical or surgical therapy. Occupational therapy was considered useful to keep patients busy and diverted from their problems.

In the spirit of the times in the twentieth century, there was a partial move away from the traditional apprenticeship in which skills were taught by a senior physiotherapist who looked back with cosy pride to the traditional art. Bright younger physiotherapists and occupational therapists began to seek education to learn the rationale for what they were doing.

But what education? The answer seemed to be obvious: an abbreviated and dumbed-down version of what medical students were taught. This was a particularly unfortunate approach to the crucial subject of pain. Classical medicine had deliberately downgraded the study of symptoms, such as pain. Symptoms were regarded as no more than signposts that should not direct exploration of the only true road which led from diagnosis to cure. The phrase 'symptomatic medicine' became offensive, designating a low-grade practice that failed to face the deep professional problem of fundamental cure. This attitude condemned physiotherapists and occupational therapists to stick to the bottom of the academic ladder. It is symbolic that the physiotherapy and occupational therapy departments are often found in the windowless basement of most hospitals.

Medical school gave short shrift to an explanation of symptoms. Pain was inevitably caused by the pressure of damaged tissue which excited special nociceptor nerve fibres. These fibres fed a system in the central nervous system which was hard wired and modality dedicated, which triggered activity in a specific pain centre. This plan was completely accepted, and naturally directed the attention of the new academic physiotherapy entirely to the periphery. This resulted in a gaudy flowering of plausible but unlisted hypotheses to explain the aim and effect of the therapy. Since it was accepted that pain could be produced only by clearly pathological tissue and since physiotherapy was directed at that tissue, the hypotheses proposed tissue changes. Changes of arterial or venous or lymphatic flow, speeding the resolution of the inflammation by heating or cooling, release of trapped nerves by breaking adhesions or readjusting bones, relaxation of cramped muscles all make up the canon of courses in the intent and rationale of physiotherapy.

Four new areas of discovery have moved the emphasis from an entirely peripheral explanation for the source of pain and have opened up the field of debate to include the central nervous system. The first was the recognition of the crucial significance of referred pain. The site of the perceived pain and target therapy is not necessarily the site of causative pathology. For example, angina is undoubtedly caused by ischaemia in the heart and yet the arm may be the area of the troublesome disorders in spite of the fact that no pathology resides in the arm. The recognition of the phenomenon forced a conclusion that convergences occur within the central nervous system. Therapy may be directed successfully at both the primary and the secondary site.

Next, it was shown that widespread tenderness and muscle contraction associated with the peripheral damage can be caused by a rising secondary excitability in the spinal cord. This shows that the use of crippling pain may migrate from its original area in the periphery into central areas. This is one of the clear signs that the pain mechanism is not rigid, dedicated and hard wired, but plastic and changes with time.

The third change was the discovery that the pain producing messages reaching the brain are controlled descending symptoms originating in the brain. This opened the entire field to psychology, with the understanding that pain is not simply a mechanical response to the presence of tissue damage but is affected by the mood and the attitude of the one who suffers. The most obvious example is the role of attention, which must be directed to that area, if pain is to be felt. It also offers a rationale for the use of distraction and counter-stimulation, by cognitive therapies, which seize the opportunity to direct attention to some event other than pain. This advance shatters the old dualism in favour of an integrated whole, where mind and body or sensation and perception cannot be divided. This change had tremendous implication for occupational therapy in the area of pain: it provided a conceptual rationale for understanding how participating in activities that are meaningful to the patient might influence perception of pain and in turn decrease disability and improve function in daily life. For perhaps the first time, occupational therapy had a respected role in the management of pain particularly for the patient with chronic pain.

The last change comes from the new techniques of brain imaging, where we must now question the traditional separation of sensory and motor mechanisms. It becomes reasonable to propose that sensory events are analysed in terms of what might be the appropriate action. If this turns out to be reasonable, then therapies directed at active movement planning, posture and active participation in daily life may well influence perceived sensation. The chapter headings of this book show how the thinking of the editors and authors has expanded to incorporate this fundamentally new thinking about the origins of pain and the direction of new therapies.

Patrick D. Wall

Foreword
to the second edition

Pain research has made revolutionary advances in the past half-century. The traditional concept of pain as a specific sensation has evolved into a broader concept of pain as comprising sensory, affective and cognitive dimensions. Many people suffer severe chronic pain that is out of proportion to any detectable physical cause, which forces us to explore neural programs in the brain, where subjective experience occurs. Research on the language of pain has produced questionnaires that allow us to evaluate subjective pain experience.

The revolution in pain management has taken us from surgical section of a "pain pathway" to multiple interacting approaches. Countless drugs, ranging from aspirin to morphine, are used to produce relief of severe acute pains, postoperative pain, and even persistent pain from cancer and arthritis that destroy body tissue. Cancer pain, for example, can be greatly diminished, sometimes abolished entirely, by appropriate doses of morphine or other opioid drugs. Yet despite the best efforts in hospitals with outstanding facilities, 5-10% of patients with cancer continue to have moderate to high levels of pain.

Chronic pain is the most challenging type of pain. When it follows an earlier injury, it is out of proportion to the injury or other pathology, and persists long after healing is complete. The traditional assumption that a spinal pathway must be causing the pain has led to the use of spinal anaesthetic blocks to stop the pain. Sometimes severe chronic pains are diminished or even abolished. More often, however, the pain returns to its former intensity.

Forty-plus years of active research based on the traditional "bottom-up" theory of pain has yet to discover any major new classes of drugs. Aspirin, acetaminophen and morphine are still the first line of attack on all pains and many variants of these drugs with fewer undesirable side-effects have been produced. Most remarkable, however, is the discovery of two new classes of drugs that were originally developed for other purposes. Drugs that were prescribed to control depression were unexpectedly found to produce significant relief of several forms of chronic pain. Similarly, drugs developed to control epilepsy were found to relieve severe chronic pains associated with diseases of nerves. Recently developed variants of both classes of drugs are more effective and have fewer side-effects. These drugs, which evolved from the "top-down" approach based on patients' subjective descriptions of their pain, opened the gate to a new pharmacology of chronic pain focussed on the brain. Both classes of drugs are now major sources of relief for many severe, previously intractable chronic pains.

Despite the advances, chronic pains remain difficult to treat. For example, backaches and pelvic pains may be relieved in some patients by spinal blocks or some combination of drugs, but no widely effective treatment has yet been found. Similarly, excellent new drugs are effective for some kinds of chronic headache, but not for all. The most terrible chronic pains that are rarely relieved are "central pains" due to strokes or other neurological diseases.

The recognition that pain is a multidimensional experience determined by psychological as well as physical factors has broadened the scope of pain therapies. Patients with chronic pain as well as terminally ill cancer patients with intense pain need every bit of the armamentarium to battle the pain. John Bonica, a brilliant American anaesthesiologist, played a huge role in these developments. The gate control theory, published in 1965, provided a scientific foundation for Bonica's contention that chronic pain is not a "symptom" but a syndrome in its own right, and requires a pain clinic that includes therapists from a wide range of disciplines. At the same time, Cicely Saunders in England recognized the importance of psychological approaches as part of palliative care for dying patients in addition to effective levels of morphine. Bonica and Saunders argued that unrelenting pain is an evil to be abolished by every available means.

The rapid rise of non-drug therapies is a major result of the new concept of pain. Psychological therapies, which were once used as a last resort when drugs or neurosurgery failed to control pain, are now an integral part of pain management strategies. The recognition that pain is the result of multiple contributions gave rise to a variety of psychological approaches such as relaxation, hypnosis, and cognitive therapies. So too, transcutaneous electrical nerve stimulation (TENS) and physical therapy procedures evolved rapidly, bringing substantial pain relief to large numbers of people.

The pain revolution has taken us from a direct-line pain pathway to an open biological system that comprises multiple sensory inputs, memories of past experiences, personal and social expectations, genetic contributions, gender, aging, and stress patterns involving the endocrine, autonomic and immune systems. Pain is now universally recognized as a major challenge for medicine, psychology, physical therapy, occupational therapy and all other health sciences and professions. Every aspect of life, from birth to dying, has characteristic pain problems. Genetics, until recently, was rarely considered relevant to understanding pain, but sophisticated epidemiological and laboratory studies have established genetic predispositions related to pain as an essential component of the field. The study of pain, therefore, has broadened and now incorporates research in epidemiology and medical genetics as well as sociological and cultural studies.

The authors of this book are highly respected practitioners as well as university and hospital teachers and scientists. They have the knowledge and wisdom of years of practice. I commend them for the excellent organization and valuable information they provide in this volume.

Ronald Melzack
McGill University

Foreword
to the third edition

This textbook is both a welcome update on familiar areas and more inclusive than its predecessors. It represents and aims to be used by a wide range of healthcare professionals working in pain, not just physiotherapists and occupational therapists, and it now includes the voices of people with pain, experts by experience, and voices from less well-resourced countries and healthcare systems. This integration of viewpoints, of interests, and of research targets is characteristic of the pain field, in which it is highly valued, and evident in multidisciplinary journal and academic meetings.

What is new? We seem still to be trying to tackle the enduring problem of engaging colleagues inside and outside the pain field, and patients and the public, in an integrated biopsychosocial understanding of pain, against what the two editors, in their introductory chapter, aptly describe as the "deeply embedded" assumption that pain corresponds with pathology. However, there are imaginative additions to the ways of informing people with pain about their situation, with much better evidence accruing from which we can select the best for our purposes, and here a critical appraisal of some of the accepted wisdom about 'patient education' that has not been supported by research findings. Patients' voices now help to guide the scientific information into more acceptable and respectful language, and at best, the understanding of pain is co-produced between each patient and her or his clinician (who in turn draws on the research literature), to serve as a solid and long-standing basis for treatment and rehabilitation initiatives.

There is more attention than before to social aspects of the lives of people with pain, resonating with patient voices and concerns about stigma and stereotyping, but now moving beyond models of influence to clinically applicable frameworks. The increased interest in social factors also appears in chapters on psychological and cultural influences in pain.

Another new area is a chapter on opioids, necessitated by the crisis of overuse and overdose in North America, and the now clear evidence on the lack of long-term benefit and on the risks of prolonged use of opioids. Treatment pathways are more comprehensible, organised as guidelines, referred to in multiple chapters, reflecting the growth in methods of synthesising evidence. Notably, there are no particularly new treatments, but the existing mainstream methods delivered by physiotherapists, occupational therapists and psychologists, alongside other clinicians, are judiciously appraised, including in their application in previously neglected groups of people with pain, including older adults, children and teenagers, and minoritised populations.

Thus this textbook represents well what has and what has not changed in the 10 years since the previous edition. Pain as a medical problem is in the unusual position of being so ubiquitous that specialist understanding is unrecognised, as are many forms of treatment and alleviation, within and outside health services. It is also so universal an experience, thankfully most often as a temporary acute pain, that the many more dimensions of difficulty that accompany persistent pain are often overlooked, or even denied, by those close to people in pain as much as by those responsible for their health care. Pain comes with moral values attached by which people in pain are judged, often unkindly, to be at fault in having a pain problem or in failing to overcome it. Only by deepening our awareness of these difficulties, eloquently articulated by people with persistent pain, and incorporating them into our theoretical models and practical interventions, will we be able to provide better treatment for more of the millions of people who live with pain. The editors have produced a forward-looking and optimistic account of what the field has to offer now, and some of the improvements we can anticipate in the coming decade.

Amanda C de C Williams

Preface

The first edition of this textbook was written in response to the first IASP pain curriculum for physiotherapists and occupational therapists, published in the mid-1990s. There were books, such as Melzack and Wall 's seminal Textbook of Pain, but none covered all topics considered essential in the new curriculum. What was missing was a textbook dedicated to allied health professionals, nurses and other healthcare practitioners wanting to build on current neuroscience and psychology, and translate these into clinical interventions.

The second edition continued to cover a broad range of subjects relevant for the understanding, assessment, treatment and management of persistent pain. It was written with the intention to equip health professionals to more effectively understand pain and enable people living with chronic pain to live their best lives. In line with this, it provided a greater patient-centred focus by starting with chapters presenting patients' perspectives on living with pain and the social aspects of pain.

When we started to prepare plans for the third edition, we decided to give the person in pain centre stage to an even greater degree. We felt that the personal perspective of the patient was still missing from books and curricula, as was advice for clinicians about connecting with the individual to establish a meaningful therapeutic alliance. This led to the inclusion of new chapters on the language of pain, communication and pain education. The topic of social aspects was expanded in a much-needed chapter about indigenous and vulnerable people, and those living in countries with limited resources. Sadly, Anita Unruh, who had been a driving force behind the first and second edition, passed away before the current edition was proposed.

This book is aimed at a wide range of healthcare professionals who work with people in pain. In our view, this means that it is relevant for all clinicians, but especially those who have an interest in pain that persists over a long time. In addition to the subjects mentioned before, the book covers basic sciences such as neuroanatomy, neurophysiology and psychology. It also addresses specific approaches such as exercise therapy, acupuncture, work rehabilitation and TENS, particular conditions such as neuropathic pain, CRPS, psychiatric disorders and acute pain, and specific populations such as children and older people. We encourage readers to begin reading about topics of interest and then allow themselves to explore less familiar subjects. We have aimed to broaden horizons and deepen practice through this text. Ultimately, we hope that this will lead to improved services for patients who live with pain.

Hubert van Griensven and Jenny Strong

Contributors

The editors would like to acknowledge and offer grateful thanks for the input of all contributors from previous editions.

Awais Aftab
Clinical Assistant Professor of Psychiatry
Case Western Reserve University
Cleveland, Ohio, USA

Nicole E. Andrews
Research Fellow
RECOVER Injury Research Centre
The University of Queensland
Queensland, Australia

Cheryl Barnabe
Professor
Departments of Medicine and
Community Health Sciences
University of Calgary
Calgary, Canada

Joletta Belton
Independent pain advocate
Fraser Colorado
Co-chair, Global Alliance of Partners for
Pain Advocacy
International Association for the study
of Pain
Washington DC, USA

Sally Bennett
Professor
Occupational Therapy
School of Health and Rehabilitation
Sciences
The University of Queensland
Brisbane, Australia

Jonathan Bullen
Associate Professor
Faculty of Health Sciences
Curtin University
Perth, Australia

Nicola U. Cook
Cape Byron Medical Centre
Byron Bay
NSW, Australia

Kenneth D. Craig
Emeritus Professor of Psychology
Department of Psychology
University of British Columbia
Vancouver, Canada

Mike Cummings
Medical Director
British Medical Acupuncture Society
Royal London Hospital for Integrated
Medicine
London, UK

Samantha R. Fashler,
Ph.D., R. Psych.
Vancouver Coast Health
Vancouver, Canada

Nadine E. Foster
Director
STARS Education and Research Alliance
Surgical Treatment and Rehabilitation
Service (STARS)
The University of Queensland and Metro
North Health

Mary P. Galea
Professorial Fellow
Department of Medicine
Royal Melbourne Hospital
The University of Melbourne
Victoria, Australia

Roger Goucke
Clinical Associate Professor
Medical School
University of Western Australia
Perth, Australia

Janet Hardy
Director of Palliative and Supportive
Care
Mater Health Services, SE Queensland
Head of Palliative Care Research
Mater Research – University
Queensland
South Brisbane, Queensland, Australia

Adrienne Ruth Harvey
Senior Research Fellow
Neurodisability and Rehabilitation
Murdoch Children's Research Institute
Victoria, Australia

Melanie A. Holden
Research Fellow in Applied
Osteoarthritis,
NIHR Research Professor of
Musculoskeletal Health in Primary Care
Arthritis Research UK Primary Care
Research Centre
Keele University
Keele, UK

George Ikkos
Professor
Consultant Liaison Psychiatrist
Royal National Orthopaedic Hospital NHS
Trust
Stanmore, UK

Tom Jesson
Independent writer and clinician
Physiotherapist
Houston, Texas
USA

Paul St John-Smith
Retired Consultant Psychiatrist and
Independent Scholar
Chair of The Evolutionary Psychiatry
Special Interest Group
Royal college of Psychiatrists
London, UK

Mark I. Johnson
Professor of Pain and Analgesia
Director of the Centre for Pain
Research
School of Health
Leeds Beckett University
Leeds, UK

Ivan Lin
Senior Lecturer/Specialist Musculoskeletal
Physiotherapist
Western Australian Centre for Rural
Health
University of Western Australia
Geraldton Regional Aboriginal Medical
Service
Geraldton, Australia

Chris McCarthy
Associate Professor
Manchester School of Physiotherapy
Faculty of Health and Education
Manchester Metropolitan University
Manchester, UK

Geoffrey Mitchell
Emeritus Professor
School of Medicine
The University of Queensland

Arjun Muralidharan
Group Leader
Neurobiology of Chronic Pain
Charles Perkins Centre
The University of Sydney
NSW, Australia

Michael Nicholas
Professor and Director of Pain Education
Unit Sydney Medical School-Northern
Faculty of Medicine and Health
University of Sydney
NSW, Australia

Mandy Nielsen
Research and Development Officer
Division of Rehabilitation
Princess Alexandra Hospital
Metro South Hospital and Health
Service
Queensland, Australia

Maria O'Reilly
Senior Lecturer and Head of Course
Occupational Therapy
Central Queensland University
Queensland, Australia

Susan E. Peters
Harvard T.H. Chan School of Public
Health
Center for Work, Health, and Well-
being
Department of Social and Behavioral
Sciences
Boston, MA, USA

Parashar Ramanuj
Royal National Orthopaedic Hospital
Brockley Hill
Stanmore, UK

Lewis Rawson
Head of Clinical Services & Advanced
Practice Physiotherapist
Circle Integrated Care
Circle Health Group
London, UK

Stephan A. Schug
Emeritus Professor and Honorary Senior
Research Fellow
Discipline of Anaesthesiology and Pain
Medicine
Medical School
University of Western Australia
Perth, Australia

Saurab Sharma
Department of Exercise Physiology
School of Health Sciences
Faculty of Medicine and Health
University of New South Wales
Sydney, Australia

Cate Sinclair
Occupational Therapist
Murdoch Childrens Research institute
Victoria, Australia

Maree T. Smith
Emeritus Professor
Director, CIPDD
School of Biomedical Sciences
The University of Queensland
Brisbane, Australia

Mike Stewart
Physiotherapist & Know Pain Course Tutor
Know Pain Ltd.
Westgate-on-sea
Kent, UK

Jenny Strong
Emeritus Professor
Division of Occupational Therapy
School of Health and Rehabilitation
Sciences
The University of Queensland
Brisbane, Australia

Bronwyn Lennox Thompson
Academic Lead
Postgraduate Programmes in Pain & Pain
Management
Department of Orthopaedic Surgery &
Musculoskeletal Medicine
University of Otago
Christchurch, New Zealand

Teodora Trendafilova
Postdoctoral Neuroscientist
Nuffield Department of Clinical
Neurosciences John Radcliffe Hospital
Oxford, UK

Hubert van Griensven
Institute of Medical and Biomedical
Education
St George's, University of London
Cranmer Terrace
London, UK

Joost van Wijchen
Head of Bachelor Physiotherapy Program
Western Norway University of Applied
Sciences
Bergen, Norway

Marc Walden
Senior Pain Medicine Physician
Tess Cramond Pain and Research Centre
Royal Brisbane and Women's Hospital
Queensland, Australia

Chapter | 1 |

Introduction to pain

Hubert van Griensven and Jenny Strong

Globally, many people, and in fact *too many people*, continue to live with and suffer from pain. Pain remains a serious and often debilitating problem for people who live with it, for their families and for our societies. Epidemiological and economic research has helped to quantify the extent and cost of the pain problem in many countries. In Australia, 3.24 million people are living with persistent pain, with the cost to the country reaching a staggering $73.2 billion Australian dollars (Deloitte Access Economics 2019). In the United States, the total financial cost of pain was found to range from $560 to $635 billion dollars (Gaskin & Richard 2011). One in five Americans currently live with chronic pain (Kuehn 2018). In Canada, one in four Canadians live with chronic pain, with the total costs of such pain estimated to be between $38.3 and $40.4 billion in 2019 (Canadian Pain Task Force Report 2020). Meanwhile, in the United Kingdom, it has been estimated that between one-third and half of the population live with chronic pain (Fayaz et al. 2016). One in six New Zealanders report chronic pain (Dominick et al. 2011). In Japan, a survey of 6000 adults found 39.3% had chronic pain (Inoue et al. 2015), while a recent study from China found 31.5% of the population were afflicted with chronic pain (Yongjun et al. 2020).

Pain is often seen as an early warning system of possible harm. It alerts the person experiencing it to danger and the need to withdraw from a situation. Pain may be associated with the bumps and bruises of childhood, health procedures, injuries, illnesses and diseases that may occur over a normal lifespan. It helps the sufferer to avoid actions and situations that may worsen the problem and is a strong motivator to take remedial action and seek help. Despite its association with injury and disease, pain is a subjective experience that cannot be measured objectively in the way that temperature can be measured with a thermometer. That subjectivity is part of its presenting challenge. Many factors aside from

pain such as age, gender, underlying disability, and social or cultural contexts shape how we experience pain and communicate pain to others. The relationship between pain and the experience of suffering is complex. Moreover, pain may no longer serve its protective function when it persists for months or years, thus becoming a problem in its own right. For all these reasons, pain is an intensely personal experience with biological, psychological and social components, existing as a person experiences it (http://www.iasp-pain.org/).

This book was initially written in 2002 as a textbook for occupational therapists and physiotherapists involved in caring for and treating people who live with pain, and helping them, their carers and their families to deal with that pain. It has since become an interprofessional text on pain for students and practitioners in any health profession. In this chapter, we will briefly examine what pain is before discussing how the many aspects of pain are dealt with in this book. To prepare, please turn to the Box 1.1 and complete the questions.

BOX 1.1 Reflective practice

Gather some blank white paper and a set of coloured markers. Think about a pain experience that you have had in the past 3 weeks. The pain can be intense or minor, troublesome or not.
- What caused the pain?
- Was it familiar or something unexpected?
- Were you alone or with others?
- How have you communicate your pain to others? What was their response?
- What factors affected whether you were concerned about the pain or saw it as of no great consequence?
- Did you change your behaviour in response to the pain?
- What did you do to ease the pain? Was it effective?
  On the paper, draw a picture of your pain. It does not have to be realistic.
  Having drawn the picture, do you think that others would know that this is how you experienced it?

What is pain?

In 2020, the International Association for the Study of Pain (IASP) updated its definition of pain to 'an unpleasant sensory and emotional experience associated with, or resembling that associated with, actual or potential tissue damage' (www.iasp-pain.org). This definition highlights the duality of pain as both a physiological and psychological experience. It is a physiological event within the body that is dependent on subjective recognition, that is, the psychological aspect is part of the essence of pain. The definition also highlights several other important aspects of the pain experience. Pain is usually interpreted as a warning signal of actual or potential tissue damage, i.e. it is viewed and experienced as an indication of a physical threat. As such, pain is part of a protective mechanism, a perception that is ingrained biologically, psychologically and socially in human nature. Nevertheless, pain can occur in the absence of tissue damage, even though the experience is likely to be described by the individual as if damage had occurred. The assumption that pain corresponds with pathology is strongly held and deeply embedded, both in patients and healthcare professionals. It is an assumption that can be difficult to break, but which is challenged when pain develops and persists in the absence of identifiable tissue pathology.

The term *acute pain* is used for the initial pain associated with trauma or the onset of pathology. After 1 or 2 weeks it may be called *subacute*. If it persists, it may be referred to as *chronic* or *persistent*, but there are different approaches to defining what chronic pain is. A common but somewhat arbitrary description is that pain is chronic when it has been present for more than 3 to 6 months; 3 months for clinicians and 6 for researchers (Merskey et al. 1994). Turk & Okifuji (2019) on the other hand suggest that chronicity should not be determined by time alone, but rather by the balance of the duration of the pain and the level of tissue pathology.

Another approach to defining pain persistence, based on tissue healing, applies the term chronic to pain that persists beyond the expected healing time (Loeser & Melzack 1999). At that point the pain no longer has its protective function and becomes increasingly associated with additional psychological, social and physical problems (Bonica 1990). These problems may be more important in the conceptualisation of chronicity than the mere duration of the pain (Larner 2014). Some authors have therefore suggested that the term *problematic pain* may be more appropriate (Barker et al. 2014).

Despite its importance for patients, clinicians and researchers, chronic pain was not represented systematically in the International Classification of Diseases (ICD) until its most recent inception (Treede et al. 2019). ICD-11 divides chronic pain into a number of types of chronic *secondary* pain which is the consequence of, for instance, cancer, trauma or musculoskeletal conditions, and chronic primary pain (Treede et al. 2019). The latter is pain present for longer than 3 months, associated with significant emotional distress or functional ability, and not better accounted for by another chronic pain condition (ibid). This definition acknowledges the importance of the wider aspects of the persistent pain experience. Among chronic primary pain conditions are chronic widespread pain, complex regional pain disorder and chronic primary musculoskeletal pain.

Issues in pain—about this book

This book is aimed at practitioners and students from a range of healthcare professions. We feel strongly that it is important for clinicians to be aware what it means for a person to suffer with pain, especially when this pain is persistent. Pain can be associated with a range of interconnected emotional, mental, physical and social experiences. It is therefore not sufficient to simply provide medical treatment to relieve pain. A holistic and person-centred approach is often required, and this demands that the clinician understands what their pain patient may be experiencing. To this end, we set the scene with the patient's perspective in Chapter 2, The patient's voice. This is followed by a chapter about communication, which is new to this edition. Open and effective communication is essential if clinicians are to understand the personal pain experience of their patients. Conversely, it is equally important that information, advice and assistance are provided in ways that connect with the patient. Communication is therefore an adaptive two-way process that optimises connection and exchange of information.

Although pain is a personal experience, this experience, how people respond to it and how they manage it is strongly influenced by social factors. It follows that ongoing pain also influences a patient's behaviour, activities and social connections. Clinicians often see patients in the restricted setting of a clinic or perhaps a small group, but they should have an appreciation of the wider context of the person in pain and consider this when devising pain management strategies. The chapter on the social determinants of pain therefore concludes the introductory section of this book.

In Section 1, we move from personal and social aspects to the basic sciences that underpin our understanding of pain. Patients turn to clinicians not only for treatment but also to gain an understanding of their pain. The pain experience is influenced by thoughts, emotions and activities, in ways that often contradict expectation. Without understanding, patients have no good basis for self-management strategies and may suffer with uncertainty, anxiety and depression. Moreover, strategies that seem to make sense, such as resting, can make their pain experience worse. Pain clinicians must therefore have a grasp of the psychology and neurobiology of persistent pain. These topics are covered in the chapters about psychology, neuroanatomy of the nociceptive system and the neurophysiology of pain. The reader is reminded about how the Gate Control Theory of pain, conceived in 1965 by Ronald Melzack and Patrick Wall, opened the door to understanding the importance of central mechanisms in the experience of pain. We are also indebted to these pioneers of pain research for kindly writing the forewords for the first two editions of this textbook.

Topics relating to the assessment and management of pain are the subject of Section 2. It will be clear, even from the brief discussion earlier, that pain is a multifaceted issue. Assessing it by asking a patient to rate the intensity of their pain by giving it a figure out of 10 is an oversimplification that is neither realistic nor helpful. Ideally, clinicians assess all aspects that are relevant to their patient. Chapter 8, Assessing pain, discusses how physically this may include the location, quality and behaviour of the pain, but ideally goes further by assessing the impact of the pain on, for example, physical and psychological function, as well as quality of life.

Having listened to their patient and completed an initial assessment, the clinician's first task is to help the patient understand their pain. The aforementioned importance of pain as a personal experience and communication means that pain education should be more than the simple provision of information. The chapter about pain education (Chapter 9), which is new to this edition and links directly with Chapters 2–4, explores what challenges may be encountered when helping the patient learn about pain. It also proposes new and collaborative ways to deal with these challenges, which promise to develop pain education in ways that may be fulfilling for patient and clinician alike. Effective education can form the basis for effective self-management strategies, which are the subject of another new chapter (Chapter 10, Participating in life roles through self management). This includes activities that focus on the individual, but also those that relate to their social environment, including family and friends, work and leisure activities. The chapter provides strategies to put into practice the knowledge gained in Chapter 4. One such strategy is exercise, which is a cornerstone of many approaches to pain management. Chapter 11, Exercise therapy, discusses the application of exercise therapy, as well as some of the potential difficulties. For example, clinicians should consider not only what the most appropriate forms of exercise may be for the individual, but also how to maximise adherence and continuation.

Interestingly, the most important determinants may be patient preference and what fits into the patient's life, thus linking exercise prescription with patient voice, communication and social aspects of pain.

The importance of understanding and applying psychologically informed approaches to treatment when working with patients with chronic pain is expounded in Chapter 12, Psychological management of pain. The need for an individually relevant, targeted multimodal approach is proposed, with the case-formulation approach providing a clear framework to guide practice with patients.

Next, the section moves on to more specific conditions and approaches, starting with a chapter on neuropathic pain and complex regional pain disorder (Chapter 13). These pain conditions present challenges to clinicians and patients alike. They are not always well understood, which has consequences for their treatment and management. The chapter therefore provides insight into the pathobiology and provides strategies for thorough assessment and therapy.

A specific approach in the management of pain is manual therapy, which is the subject of Chapter 14, Manual therapy and the influence on pain perception. Since the introduction of psychological approaches to pain management, clinicians have wondered whether to continue with hands-on approaches. In some cases, these approaches have been abandoned altogether, even when patients have experienced benefits from them. The chapter makes it clear that manual therapy can have a role to play and provides information for those who wish to incorporate it within the overall management of pain.

Approaches to provide direct control of pain include medication, transcutaneous electrical nerve stimulation (TENS) and acupuncture. Chapter 15 provides a detailed discussion of the wide range of pharmacological approaches that are currently available. These include opioid and nonopioid analgesics, as well as adjuvants used for specific types of pain such as neuropathic pain. The chapter links with information about pain physiology in order to explain the pharmacological actions of medication and issues relating to prescription. This is followed by Chapter 16 which is about the nonpharmacological approaches of TENS and acupuncture. These techniques have different origins, but both are seen as sophisticated ways of influencing the way the nervous system processes nociceptive signals. They are accessible and relatively safe, if sometimes controversial. For example, current UK guidelines for low back pain advise against the use of acupuncture for low back pain but includes it in its recommendations for patients with chronic pain (NICE 2021a, b).

In Chapter 17, the importance of work in people's lives is acknowledged. It discusses how healthcare professionals can assist patients with pain to stay at work, to return to work or to seek work. This can be guided by conceptual models of work disability prevention and work rehabilitation. Like much of pain management, the role of the person with pain and their partnership with the healthcare professional is pivotal for successful outcomes, along with engagement with other critical players such as employers, other workers, unions and workers' compensation systems.

Our final section covers a wide range of special issues associated with persistent pain. These issues are not always acknowledged in professional literature, let alone discussed in detail. We are therefore pleased to introduce several new and rather unique topics in this edition, starting with multidisciplinary and interdisciplinary working. To deal effectively with the multidimensional nature of pain, a number of professionals may need to be involved. This incurs a risk of fragmented and contradictory approaches, even in established pain management teams. These risks can be mitigated against if the issues relating to collaboration and teamwork are understood, in the context of pain management.

Next, the section turns to issues relevant for specific age groups: children and older adults. Individuals have different capacities and needs at different life-stages, so clinical approach of *one size fits all* will provide less than ideal outcomes for children, adolescents and older people who have pain. In Chapter 19, readers are alerted to the importance of family and carers of children and adolescence with chronic pain. When working with an adult patient, clinicians may focus solely on that individual patient, but young patients are nested within parental and family systems and must not be managed in isolation. An awareness of developmental factors is critical. Chapter 20 is concerned with the other end of the developmental spectrum, i.e. older adults who may suffer chronic pain. Given the current and projected growth in the numbers of older people in our societies, clinicians need to understand the pain issues many older people face. Specifically, they need to be sensitive to pain problems faced by those who develop dementia and are unable to communicate verbally about their pain experience.

In Chapter 21, Cancer pain, readers' attention is drawn to differences between the management of patients with cancer pain compared with noncancer pain. Opioid medications are a mainstay for patients with cancer pain, but therapeutic management does not stop with analgesic prescription. Attention needs to be given to the overall pain which the patient may be experiencing.

Although anyone can develop persistent pain, its impact on the individual, their environment and society is subject to inequities. Chapter 22 addresses issues associated with pain and its management in low- and middle-income countries, as well as pain in Indigenous peoples. We are proud to have this unique chapter in this edition of our book. While resources are tailored for and available to those with a certain amount of wealth and education, many people are marginalised and find it difficult to access care. Clinicians may struggle to communicate with patients with a different cultural background and not be certain how to devise strategies that help the person within their community, which are exactly the issues which this book opens with. The chapter provides essential insight of the difficulties, as well as examples of remarkable developments that have led to improved engagement and healthcare provision.

Another group of patients who may not receive the most appropriate care are those with psychiatric issues. Specifically, psychiatric disorders are not always recognised. Chapter 23 provides a clear discussion of types of psychiatric disorders and how they relate to persistent pain. This provides the clinician with indications of when involvement of a psychiatrist may be beneficial or even essential.

Persistent pain is different from acute pain, for instance due to adaptations in the central nervous system, as well as psychological and social factors. However, there is acknowledgement in the literature that persistent pain often starts as acute pain. Understanding acute pain and managing it effectively is therefore important for the prevention of persistent pain, as well as in its own right. Chapter 24 focuses on how acute pain can be managed most effectively, specifically in a hospital setting. Finally, legal matters pertinent to pain management are discussed in Chapter 25. The legal frameworks that govern health practitioners provide an important system to ensure patient safety. These include public health law, therapeutic goods laws and common law. Clinicians should be cognisant of standards of consent and standards of care that must be afforded patients in their care. The chapter also discusses the expectations of a health practitioner when providing expert witness testimony.

We finish the book with our review of the historical developments of our time. Important developments have led to an improved understanding of the mechanisms underlying persistent pain. However, while these have generated novel treatments, sometimes with greater efficacy and at other times with fewer negative consequences, genuine breakthrough developments and different approaches to pain management are yet to be harnessed. Worse still, the relatively recent opioid crisis has revealed that our most potent approach to treating pain has come at great personal and societal cost. We discuss difficulties and achievements, but also what may lie ahead. We see education as an essential tool to improve the provision of effective treatment and management of persistent pain. We hope that this book will play a role in this. We are grateful for the contributions of many experienced, knowledgeable and talented authors, who have helped to make this text a comprehensive learning resource.

References

Barker, C., Taylor, A., Johnson, M., 2014. Problematic pain – redefining how we view pain? Br. J. Pain 8, 9–15.

Bonica, J., 1990. Definitions and taxonomy of pain. In: Bonica, J. (Ed.), The Management of Pain, second ed. Lea & Febiger, Philadelphia.

Canadian Pain Task Force Report, 2020. Working together to better understand, prevent and manage chronic pain: what we heard. October https://www.canada.ca/content/dam/hc-sc/documents/corporate/about-health-canada/public-engagement/external-advisory-bodies/canadian-pain-task-force/report-2020-rapport/report-2020.pdf.

Deloitte Access Economics, 2019. The cost of pain in Australia: Painaustralia. https://www2.deloitte.com/au/en/pages/economics/articles/cost-pain-australia.html.

Dominick, C., Blyth, F., Nicholas, M., 2011. Patterns of chronic pain in the New Zealand population. N. Z. Med. J. 124 (1337), 63–76.

Fayaz, A., Croft, P., Langford, R.M., Donaldson, L.J., Jones, G.T., 2016. Prevalence of chronic pain in the UK: a systematic review and meta-analysis of population studies. BMJ Open 6 (6), e010364.

Gaskin, D.J., Richard, P., 2011. The economic costs of pain in the United States. In: Institute of Medicine (US) Committee on Advancing Pain Research, Care and education. Relieving pain in America: a blueprint for transforming prevention, care, education and research. Appendix C. National Academies Press (US), Washington, DC.

Inoue, S., Kobayashi, F., Nishihara, M., Arai, Y.-C.P., Ikemoto, T., Kawai, T., et al., 2015. Chronic pain in Japanese community – prevalence, characteristics and impact on quality of life. PLoS. One 10 (6), e0129262.

Kuehn, B., 2018. Chronic pain prevalence. J. Am. Med. Assoc 320 (16), 1632.

Larner, D., 2014. Chronic pain transition: a concept analysis. Pain. Manag. Nurs 15, 707–717.

Loeser, J., Melzack, R., 1999. Pain: an overview. Lancet 353, 1607–1609.

Merskey, H., Lindblom, U., Mumford, J., Nathan, P., Sunderland, S., 1994. Pain terms, a current list with definitions and notes on usage. In: Merskey, H., Bogduk, N. (Eds.), Classification of Chronic Pain. IASP Press, Seattle.

NICE (National Institute for Health and Clinical Excellence), 2021a. Chronic pain (primary and secondary) in over 16s: assessment of all chronic pain and management of chronic primary pain (NG193). https://www.nice.org.uk/guidance/ng193.

NICE (National Institute for Health and Clinical Excellence), 2021b. Managing low back pain and sciatica. http://pathways.nice.org.uk/pathways/low-back-pain-and-sciatica (NG59). <https://www.nice.org.uk/guidance/ng59>.

Treede, R., Rief, W., Barke, A., Aziz, Q., Bennett, M., Benoliel, R., et al., 2019. Chronic pain as a symptom or a disease: the IASP Classification of Chronic Pain for the International Classification of Diseases (ICD-11). Pain 160, 19–27.

Turk, D., Okifuji, A., 2019. Pain terms and taxonomies of pain. In: Ballantyne, J., Fishman, S., Rathmell, J. (Eds.), Bonica's Management of Pain. Wolters Kluwer, Philadelphia.

Yongjun, Z., Tingjie, Z., Xiaoqiu, Y., Zhiying, F., Feng, Q., Guangke, X., et al., 2020. A survey of chronic pain in China. Libyan. J. Med 15 (1), 1730550.

Chapter |2|

The patient's voice

Mandy Nielsen

LEARNING OBJECTIVES

At the end of this chapter, readers will understand the:
1. Importance of listening to the patient's story.
2. Impact that chronic pain can have across varied life domains.
3. Link between the individual experience of pain and the social environment.
4. Association between healthcare provider–patient communication and health outcomes.

Overview

This chapter is concerned with the importance and value of listening to the patient's voice in our practice with people in pain. Living with pain involves so much more than managing the pain sensation. Pain has the potential to affect every domain of an individual's life, as well as that of their family and others close to them. Listening and responding to a patient's story must therefore be more than a sympathetic gesture. It can have direct consequences for the relevance and quality of health delivery and may influence postconsultation outcomes. This chapter will explore the experience of living with chronic pain

to establish why listening to the patient's voice is important (also see Chapter 3). To facilitate this, we will be hearing from four patients with different pain conditions throughout the chapter: Ron, Catherine, Beth and Mat.

The experience of living with chronic pain

Understanding illness begins with an understanding of illness as it is lived (Johansson et al. 1999, p. 1800).

The excerpt from the interview with Ron (Box 2.1) clearly demonstrates that living with pain involves much more than managing the sensation of pain. It shows that the experience of persistent pain has had a significant impact on several aspects of Ron's life, including his sense of self, career, family relationships, and social and recreational activities. Honkasalo aptly described chronic pain as 'an intruder or thief that takes away the most precious things in life. Pain discontinues stories, interrupts life projects, it messes up life plans' (Honkasalo 2001).

One of the difficulties associated with pain is that each individual's experience is unique. Ron's experience of living with fibromyalgia will not mirror the experience of someone else. It is important therefore to acknowledge the heterogeneity of people living with pain, recognising that it is not possible to apply a 'one-size-fits-all' treatment or management framework, however tempting this may be. The full impact that pain has on a person's life can only begin to be understood by talking with them about what they are experiencing, and what pain means to them. As practitioners, we need to give patients the time and the permission to 'tell their story' (Nielsen et al. 2009).

Adopting the practice of listening as the departure point for our work with people in pain may create a sense of uncertainty. Is this a completely unmapped journey we are embarking on, or are there some signposts to provide

BOX 2.1 **One patient's voice: Ron**

'I still continue with regular bouts of chronic fatigue and very, very defined muscle, joint and, I would say, bone pain. My career has ground to a halt, I've been to lots of specialists, and now I reside at home. I'm pretty stuffed I suppose, stuffed in many ways. The consequences of it are, I've lost my career, I'm a lousy father in the sense of my ability to handle the kids for more than an hour at a time, there's no football, running on beaches, the ability to socialise, all those sorts of things I can't do because movement aggravates pain, any movement aggravates muscle and joint pain. The fatigue denies me any ability to keep my brain alive, so going out to dinner and talking to someone is generally just not on. By about three in the afternoon I start winding down, by five I'm pretty uncomfortable, by seven I'm asleep on the sofa or very quiet watching TV somewhere. Life has ground to a halt. So my circumstances are aggravated beyond my physical symptoms to now include emotional and psychological ones, because my relationship with life in the context of a family and career is distorted from I suppose expectations, or what you try to achieve or what you dream for. So now I'm an invalid, I don't leave the house much, I drive the kids to school occasionally, go to the shops and get some milk and bread and those sorts of things, go to doctors, but I've become socially isolated, and it's difficult. I'm in my 40s, but it's like I'm living a life in my 80s, and my mind and emotions aren't prepared for it or still comfortable with it, so a natural depression comes out of that, a difficulty relating to life, trying to find your place in it. My mindset has always been, be useful, or in other words, don't be a nuisance in life, so relying on a partner to do a lot of the domestic work, and not being able to step forward and take an equal, or even a lead role is very difficult. The kids are, as kids are, very accommodating. It's great that Dad gets up, helps them with a bit of breakfast and goes back to bed. Dad doesn't join them at the beach or on social occasions, and they seem to adjust. But from my point of view, there's a disconnection and missing out, and I suppose a degree of deficiency as a parent. I've been a hard worker for the last 25 odd years, and so not working is…I was built for working, I spent 25 years training and skilling myself up, and so what do you do with your mind? Life becomes very internalised and contemplative. It is very difficult, and you become disconnected from a degree of reality … you're socially removed. I do try to socially join in, but I find that I'm brain dead or very uncomfortable in my body pain wise or fatigue wise, that I'm not a very good conversationalist. So that sort of gives a viewpoint of where I am.'

Excerpt from narrative interview with Ron, 3 years after the onset of a chronic condition diagnosed as chronic fatigue syndrome and/or fibromyalgia.

a bit more direction for improved practice with this patient? Fortunately, phenomenological research in this area can help to identify similarities of experience, knowledge of which will help when listening to patients' stories. Three relevant themes within this literature are the search for restoration, the experience of loss and the stigma that is encountered.

The search for restoration

'I said is it in my head or is there something wrong? Because it doesn't show anything on the CAT scan. And he said, "Well it's definitely not in your head." But nobody can tell me what it is!'

Mat

Not surprisingly, when people first experience pain they try to relieve or stop it. For most of us, there is an expectation of what Hilbert (1984) described as 'normal' pain, reflecting the sociocultural expectation that, with the exception of particular identifiable conditions, pain is temporary and treatable, and normal life will soon be restored. This expectation is continually reinforced, for example through the advertising of medications and other products purported to quickly eliminate pain.

If pain does not resolve as expected, many people will embark on an often long and convoluted search for a diagnosis and cure for their pain. In contemporary, industrialised societies this search typically focuses on resources within the biomedical healthcare system, involving frequent consultations with multiple medical practitioners and allied health professionals. The search can sometimes stretch over years, and it is not uncommon for people to list 10 or more health professionals they have consulted in the quest to eradicate pain from their lives. This journey can be not only time-consuming and expensive, but also the process of retelling their story multiple times may be overwhelming and demoralising, particularly when it does not result in a cure for the pain. In addition, patients may receive as many different diagnoses as consultations they have attended. As one participant in a research study said, 'It takes a lot to have to keep repeating your story over and over again…all these medical people come from their own little sides of the fence and put their take on things. And they still don't really even get the whole picture of what's going on' (Nielsen 2009). It is therefore important that clinicians acknowledge to patients that they are aware of their frustrating journey searching for pain relief. While it may not be possible to avoid a retelling of the story, demonstrating an awareness of the journey they have been on is an important part of developing a therapeutic relationship with the patient.

It is not uncommon for people who have consulted numerous healthcare professionals to become frustrated and angry when this process has not resulted in a diagnosis or effective treatment. Healthcare professionals may experience what on the surface appears to be undeserved anger being directed at them. Often much of a patient's anger is the emotional consequence of previous treatment experiences, experiences related to legal or compensation processes associated with an injury or accident, or the impact that their pain is having on their family and social relationships. It is important to allow patients to talk about these experiences and associated emotions. Avoid 'individualising' the anger and attributing it to particular individual characteristics. Listening to the patient's story and considering the individual within their social context can avoid 'blaming the victim' and develop a more constructive relationship with the patient.

Research suggests that an additional trigger of patients' frustration and anger can be the way people are dealt with during the healthcare encounter (Hambraeus et al. 2020; McGowan et al. 2007; Nicola et al. 2021; Nielsen 2009). This can be particularly so in cases where an identifiable cause of ongoing pain cannot be found, as the reality of the pain may be implicitly or explicitly questioned, resulting in feelings of de-legitimation. The term *de-legitimation* describes the experience when an individual's perceptions and knowledge of their pain are systematically disconfirmed or discounted (Garro 1994, p. 788). De-legitimation is a recurring theme in phenomenological research with chronic pain sufferers and can have wide-ranging effects. These include people becoming reluctant to disclose their chronic pain condition due to concern that others will not understand and will label them as 'malingerers', the possibility that disclosure could have a negative impact on a work situation, or the perception that stigmatisation will affect access to, or the quality of, medical treatment. A similar concept developing in recent literature is *pain invalidation*, where the lack of validation of a person's pain experience in various life domains can result in denial of social support and resources that can assist the person with pain (Nicola et al. 2021). People may disengage from a healthcare system that they feel is not only unable to ameliorate their pain, but also doubting of the veracity of their pain.

An important starting point in practice with patients with chronic pain is to confirm the legitimacy of their pain, to validate it and to normalise their experiences. Therapists should clearly state their belief in the reality of the pain that patients are experiencing. It is also important to let patients know that they are not alone in this experience—what they are feeling and thinking is commonly reported by other people with chronic pain conditions.

Loss

> '…there are all sorts of big deal things that I feel like I've lost, that while they're not exactly about my pain, they're all sort of linked…There's so many things to grieve about.'
>
> Catherine

Chronic pain, particularly when combined with impairment, often results in a series of losses across numerous life domains, including employment and income, family and social relationships, lifestyle and interests, social status, and future life plans (Hadi et al. 2019; Johnston-Devin et al. 2021; Munday et al. 2021; Wallace et al. 2014). In their research with people with chronic back pain, Walker and colleagues identified 'a catalogue of socioeconomic and other material and psychological losses' (Walker et al. 2006, p. 204), including loss of abilities and roles, employment, finances, relationships, and identity and hope.

Loss of employment

Loss of or reduced employment is frequently identified as a consequence of chronic pain (Antao et al. 2013; Deloitte Access Economics 2019; Grant et al. 2019; Liedberg et al. 2021). People often describe a long process of trying to return to work after an accident or illness. Mat, for example, was seriously injured in a car accident. After 9 months of rehabilitation he returned to his job driving a sugar cane harvester:

> 'It was hard. Like I used to ache and I couldn't jump up and down off the machines anymore. Eventually it got that way I couldn't drive a harvester or bin out anymore, it was too rough, just the shakin…'

When he could no longer deal with the physical demands of cane harvesting, Mat started driving taxis for a living. He described this as '…alright for a couple of years, but you work such long hours. And from the constant driving I got to the point I was up at the doctor's more times than I was actually working'. He gave up the job due to his pain again. Despite this, Mat managed to earn a living for a further 10 years, until he reached a point when he had to admit he could no longer work and applied for 'the thing', as he called the government disability pension. Mat was so ashamed of having to do this that he had difficulty saying what 'the thing' was, let alone discussing it further.

Catherine, a healthcare professional, was told she could not come back to work until she was '100% fit'. Although she tried to return to work on two occasions, she said lack of support and understanding by supervising staff and consequent legal proceedings led her to eventually resign from her valued work role (see Chapter 10).

These examples point to the enabling or constraining potential of the workplace to affect the lives of people with chronic pain. Research has identified several social environmental factors that can contribute to loss of employment, including attitudes of employers and lack of flexibility in employment arrangements (Gulseren and Kelloway 2021). Additionally, people with chronic pain may have complex and interacting needs which can impact on their capacity to successfully return to work, regardless of their motivation to do so (Holmes et al. 2020). For example, the fluctuating levels of pain and incapacity that are often a feature of chronic pain can make work capacity difficult to predict and manage (Oakman et al. 2017). Ideally, employment policies and programmes should enable people with chronic pain to negotiate employment arrangements in ways that meet their changing needs and abilities (Gulseren and Kelloway 2021). Initiatives such as increased flexibility within the workplace and individualised return to work support (Holmes et al. 2020) could improve this situation and contribute to a reduction in the social and economic suffering experienced by people with chronic pain.

The broader individual and social outcomes resulting from loss of employment are evident when the associated loss of income is considered. The financial impact of unemployment is frequently articulated by people with chronic pain (Mukhida et al. 2020; Nielsen 2009). Recent research estimates that in the year 2018, productivity losses for people with chronic pain in Australia, in terms of reduced employment, absenteeism and presenteeism, were $48.34 billion, or $21,830 per working age person with chronic pain (Deloitte Access Economics 2019). The ongoing financial cost of having chronic pain, in terms of visits to health practitioners and accessing services or equipment which provide relief and aid functioning, can be an additional financial burden. For example, in 2018, Australians living with chronic pain paid $2.7 million in out-of-pocket expenses to manage their chronic pain, including costs for medical services, pharmaceuticals and aids and appliances (Deloitte Access Economics 2019). For some people, loss of income due to unemployment means that they cannot afford treatment or therapies which alleviate their pain. Catherine, for example, felt that she was in a Catch-22 situation: she was advised by her GP

and physiotherapist to stop working, but she needed an income to continue to afford services such as physiotherapy, which she believed decreased her pain and increased her functional capacity.

Having a disability increases the risk of poverty and hardship (Saunders 2019), with a link identified between chronic pain and lower socioeconomic status (Deloitte Access Economics 2019). While loss of employment due to chronic pain may be seen as an individual crisis, lack of flexibility in employment arrangements and inadequate financial support for those receiving a government pension demonstrates the broader social aspect of the suffering that job loss can engender.

Loss of social and family roles

Living with chronic pain can also limit social activities, with a subsequent loss of valued roles in this domain. On one level, people with chronic pain may not feel physically able or comfortable to participate in social activities due to difficulty walking or sitting for any length of time, associated fatigue and medication side effects, or the all-consuming effort of managing their pain. This is illustrated in the excerpt in Box 2.1, in the interview with Ron, when he described himself as 'brain dead' and 'not a very good conversationalist'. Similarly, Beth described life in general as becoming 'sort of non-existent' after the onset of her pain:

> *'For the last almost two years it's just been working full time and managing my pain, seeing medical people. So I haven't had a lot of social life. And even, like with the pain, it's hard to drive sometimes. And because of my back I haven't been able to go to the movies until recently because I haven't been able to sit for two hours. So the pleasurable things in life sort of became non-pleasurable because of the pain that was involved.'*

Lack of involvement in social activities can contribute to people becoming socially isolated. While in part this can be due to the mechanics of being in pain, it can also be related to what Hilbert (1984) has described as *the acultural aspect of chronic pain*. When the search for restoration does not result in a cure for their pain, people find themselves experiencing pain they cannot understand, and which others in society do not understand or talk about. Chronic pain is not a problem that can be put aside to be dealt with later; it is, as Hilbert described, an ongoing, ever present somatic reminder that 'things are not as they should be:

> *'At home, at work, and in their social life generally, sufferers are saddled with an insoluble dilemma, of*

paramount concern to them, in the presence of others for whom no such priority exists. This preoccupation further documents in sufferers' minds their isolation and estrangement from the society around them.'

(Hilbert 1984, p. 370).

While a common way of dealing with a problem in our society is to talk it over with others, the acultural nature of chronic pain may serve to isolate sufferers even further due to a lack of understanding and the prospect of delegitimation mentioned earlier. Social isolation is compounded by an inability to communicate what is a major issue in sufferers' lives. Beth described pain as 'a lonely thing': 'If somebody says "How are you going?" or "How are you?", they don't really want to know. This is a perfect opportunity to whinge about all your aches and pains. But normally you don't burden other people with that sort of thing … You just keep it to yourself.'

People with chronic pain therefore can experience not only loss of physical participation in social activities, but also the loss of a previously taken-for-granted social membership. Hilbert identified this as a form of suffering 'which transcends physical pain' and can result in what he describes as *falling out of culture*:

'… sufferers, though living within a society and within a culture, are precariously and continuously approaching the amorphous frontier of non-membership'

(Hilbert 1984, p. 375).

In addition to the impact on social relationships, living with chronic pain can also have a significant impact on family relationships. People with children will often talk about their guilt about not being able to play with and do things with their children. Ron described himself as 'a lousy father', while Mat talked of being 'stuffed for a week' if he spent half an hour playing cricket in the backyard with his kids. While Beth said she had been very involved in her children's activities, she identified 'the one big downer' of her life with pain as being the impact it had had on her experience as a parent:

'The saddest part of having a bad back is when your children are little and they're sick, they don't call for Mum, because they know Mum can't come and pick them up … Dad was the one they called for when they were sick.'

People with chronic pain also talk about the impact pain has had on relationships with their partners. Ron described his partner as a wonderful person who had passionately stood by him. However, he felt his pain experience had done a lot of damage to this relationship:

'Needless to say, being personal, sexuality is a no-go area, as much on my part, as much on her part. It's just when you're dealing with such [pain related] issues all the time, it's not an easy comfortable dynamic.'

Beth described her partner as 'really really good' but her pain had changed their relationship, as he did the majority of the household activities, which she found very frustrating. She also identified the importance of having a loving family: '…it was a dreadful thought but it was quite often, if I didn't have a loving family I wouldn't want to go on. Knowing it [the pain] is going to be there forever.'

Not all people with chronic pain will experience such support from their partners. Living with someone with chronic pain in the family can have a detrimental impact on the partners and families of those with pain. Strunin & Boden (2004), for example, found that partners and children took over the family responsibilities previously undertaken by the person with pain, and that this led to stress within family relationships. These findings are reflected in other qualitative studies (Ostlund et al. 2001; Richardson et al. 2007; Smith et al. 2021; West et al. 2012). This suggests consideration of a family-centred focus in our chronic pain work, rather than a focus limited to the individual living with pain.

As well as identifying numerous functional limitations as a consequence of pain, people will often express regret and distress at these losses. It may be beneficial, therefore, to explore these individual experiences of loss with clients. Walker and colleagues have suggested that the experience of loss may have implications for existing cognitive-based therapies for pain, such as relaxation techniques, changing negative pain beliefs, and problem-solving strategies (for example, see Nielsen et al. 2014), which are based on the premise that pessimistic beliefs are a result of cognitive distortion and/or a preexisting psychological vulnerability (Walker et al. 2006, p. 204). They propose an alternative perspective: that negative cognitive beliefs may represent *realistic* appraisals of tangible losses and negative social consequences, rather than some form of latent personal vulnerability that preexisted in the individual prior to the development of chronic pain. Helping people come to terms with tangible losses may therefore be an important precursor to pain management strategies aimed at cognitive change and functional improvement. Forms of cognitive behavioural approaches that focus on acknowledgement and acceptance of psychological processes such as acceptance and commitment therapy (ACT) are also worth exploring (Kaiser et al. 2015).

Loss of 'self'

Long-term interference with social roles, combined with changing perceptions of personal attributes, has been shown to have an impact on a person's identity or *sense of self* (Harris et al. 2003). From a sociological perspective, the self is developed and maintained through social relations; that is, one's identity is essentially social in nature (Charmaz 1983, p. 170). Charmaz (1983) identified loss of self as a fundamental form of suffering experienced by people who are chronically ill. She contended that serious chronic illness 'results in spiraling consequences such as loss of productive function, financial crises, family strain, stigma and a restricted existence' and that 'suffering such losses results in a diminished self':

> '*Chronically ill persons frequently experience a crumbling away of their former self-images without simultaneous development of equally valued new ones. The experiences and meanings upon which these ill persons had built former positive self-images are no longer available to them … Over time, accumulated loss of formerly sustaining self-images without new ones results in a diminished self-concept.*'

(Charmaz 1983, p. 168)

The previous discussion regarding the impact of chronic pain on social and family roles illustrates that people with chronic pain can experience the spiraling consequences that Charmaz described. Living with pain and associated restrictions of quality of life can challenge prepain self-identities; people experience the *crumbling away* of their former self, without developing an acceptable alternative identity. This sense of loss of identity will often become apparent when people with chronic pain talk about their before-pain self and their after-pain self. The before-pain self is usually physically, intellectually and/or socially active. Mat and Ron described energetic before-pain selves, involved in sport or other physical activities. For example, Mat said he used to do whatever he liked before the accident: 'Did everything. Rode motorbikes. Now I couldn't. Last time I rode a bike, which was about 20 minutes, I was in bed for three days. So I don't ride bikes anymore … now I can barely walk from here to the shop.' Mat described his postpain self as 'useless'. Similarly, Ron described himself as 'pretty stuffed in many ways … there's no football or running on beaches.'

Patients also commonly identify a loss of identity and purpose associated with no longer being able to work. Catherine described the loss of her health professional position as being more than the loss of a job; it was more a loss of who she was:

> '…*when I'm trying to sleep at night I think about so many things that I've lost; it's not just I've lost a fully functioning arm, I've lost my career, I've lost the other thing that was probably the thing that*

gave me joy in life, music and playing the piano, and I did that as a semi-professional, which I can't do anymore. So you know, there are all sorts of big deal things that I feel like I've lost …'

Beth also talked about a loss of identity, although for her the cognitive impact of living with pain had more salience: 'You feel as if you're brain dead. I used to consider myself as reasonably intelligent, now I have to really think about everything I'm doing.' Ron described himself as going from being 'rather successful' to 'stuffed'; living like an invalid and trying to find his 'place in life.'

Chronic pain can therefore have an impact on people's identities in varying ways—their physical, intellectual, social and emotional selves. Charmaz (1983) identified the loss of self suffered by people with chronic illness generally as leading to a continued struggle to lead valued lives and maintain or develop positive and worthwhile definitions of self.

Stigma

In the previous section, the crumbling away of the former self through loss of social roles and personal attributes was discussed in terms of the impact this has on the individual with pain and their family. For therapists it is also important to look beyond the individual in pain and consider their social environment, as this can have a powerful influence on how they experience their chronic pain; the social environment is described more fully in Box 2.2. As with the development of self-identity via social relations, individual understanding and experience of pain is formed within a social environment, making pain an

---

BOX 2.2 **What is the 'social environment'?**

'*Human social environments encompass the immediate physical surroundings, social relationships, and cultural milieus within which defined groups of people function and interact. Components of the social environment include built infrastructure; industrial and occupational structure; labour markets; social and economic processes; wealth; social, human and health services; power relations; government; race relations; social inequality; cultural practices, the arts; religious institutions and practices; and beliefs about place and community…Embedded within contemporary social environments are historical social and power relations that have become institutionalised over time.*'

(Barnett & Casper 2001, p. 465)

intrinsically interpersonal and social phenomenon (Mardian et al. 2020).

When telling the story of their pain, patients often spend relatively little time describing the location and bodily sensation of the pain per se. Rather, their focus will be on the process of trying to cope with the pain on a daily basis and the impact of the pain on their life as a whole. As the previous discussion on loss illustrates, clients can experience a form of suffering which, while experienced by the individual, is partly a consequence of political, economic and institutional structures outside their control. Kleinman and colleagues refer to this as *social suffering*, where the focus widens from the individual experience to include 'what political, economic and institutional power does to people, and, reciprocally…how these forms of power themselves influence responses to social problems' (Kleinman et al. 1996, p. XI). Emerging evidence for shared neurobiological mechanisms between physical pain and social pain, that is, painful feelings related to social rejection, exclusion or loss (Eisenberger 2015), suggests that social suffering is more than a sociological construct—it may be felt somatically and is therefore part of the sociopsychobiological experience of pain.

While there may be many aspects of social suffering that are not in our power as therapists to address, social suffering is an important concept to be aware of when listening to clients' stories, as it will help us consider the experience of living with chronic pain as a whole, rather than focusing on an individual body part or functional activity. One aspect of social suffering which may be in the therapist's capacity to effect is the experience of stigma.

The relationship between stigma and chronic pain has been well established (De Ruddere and Craig 2016; Holloway et al. 2007; Nicola et al. 2021; Nielsen 2012). The annual Chronic Pain Australia National Pain Survey consistently identifies stigma as a key concern of people living with chronic pain, with over 50% of the 2233 respondents to the 2021 survey indicating they felt stigmatised on account of their chronic pain (Chronic Pain Australia 2021). Stigmatisation of people with chronic pain is a cumulative and social process that can have serious consequences for the person with pain and their family, with some evidence that invalidating responses from others is associated with poorer physical and psychological well-being (Ghavidel-Parsa et al. 2015; Kool et al. 2013). It is therefore important that therapists understand how the stigmatising process occurs so that they can avoid it in their own practice *and* challenge it in the practice of other health professionals when they see it occurring.

For many people with chronic pain, the lack of diagnosis and a clear treatment path leads them to acquire a label of *different* or *difficult*. This, combined with the open-ended nature of chronic pain, means that they cannot perform the role of the socially acceptable sick person, that is,

actively participate in the recommended treatment regime and then return to normal duties (Parsons 1958). Additionally, as Bodwell (2010) has pointed out, people with chronic pain cannot tell the preferred 'restitution story of illness', where they become sick, receive treatment and recover. Clients may find themselves negatively stereotyped because of their chronic pain. A 'heart sink patient' (Mengshoel et al. 2021) and 'malingerer' (Zajacova et al. 2021) are two not uncommon stereotypes used to describe people with chronic pain who present for treatment. Research indicates that many people with chronic pain believe that health professionals, and society more generally, question the reality of their pain in the absence of an identifiable cause or an observable manifestation of disability. As Beth said: 'If it's not explained by a blood test or an X-ray or whatever, it doesn't exist.' Stereotyping of the client with chronic pain in this way may indeed result in more than stigmatisation; Chibnall and Tait's body of work suggests that biomedical evidence has an 'inordinate amount of influence' on physician pain judgements and may contribute to the under-treatment of pain (Chibnall et al. 1997, 2000, 2018; Chibnall & Tait 1999; Tait & Chibnall 1997).

Stereotyping people with chronic pain as somehow different from us constructs a rationale for devaluing and excluding people within society. This process, which Link & Phelan (2001, 2006) termed *separation*, may mean that the reactions of others produce a sense of being devalued or disrespected, or in some way different in a negative way to others in society. Many people with chronic pain will describe this process of separation as they talk about their gradual recognition that their pain was somehow atypical, as it did not conform to the previously discussed expectation of 'normal' pain. The omnipresent nature of chronic pain, which cannot be left at home for a good night out, can create and continually reinforce a sense of isolation and estrangement from society.

This experience of separation can be greatly exacerbated if patients feel they are being negatively stereotyped by healthcare professionals. In telling the story of his pain, Ron deliberately structured his narrative to include a section which he introduced as 'how the medical profession has dealt with me'. He described being treated with cynicism and suspicion, particularly when requesting pain-relieving medication. Catherine said she believed she had been considered 'a liar and a cheat' in her dealings with some healthcare professionals and with her employer. Without a socially condoned diagnosis for their pain, it is easy for chronic pain sufferers to be positioned in a negative stereotype that separates them not only from society as a whole, but also from more 'deserving' people with legitimate health problems. This can be related to what Holloway and colleagues (2007) termed *moral stigma*; that is, chronic pain sufferers are labelled as *morally weak* when there is a lack of congruity between their pain report and biomedical findings.

An emerging area of stigmatisation of people living with chronic pain is related to what is colloquially termed the *opioid epidemic*. Increasing evidence of detrimental effects associated with long-term prescription opioid use has focused attention on reduction and cessation of these medications in the management of chronic pain (Benintendi et al. 2021). An unintended consequence of health policy and practice changes in this area has been an extension of the historical social stigma related to illicit substance abuse to people who use prescribed opioids (Dassieu et al. 2021), in addition to the existing stigma of having chronic pain.

It is critically important that therapists do not fall into the trap of labelling and stereotyping clients with chronic pain. Not only might it compromise the strength of the relationship and the trust between the therapist and their client, there is also evidence of an association between healthcare provider–patient communication and patient health outcomes (Lie et al. 2022). The value of listening and responding to the client's story, therefore, goes beyond the immediate consultation period.

The value of the patient's voice

'I really think doctors need to learn to listen to people who know their own body. You know when it's not quite right, you know when things aren't working properly, and you try to explain it to them and they just, it seems to go in one ear and out the other, or they just totally dismiss it.'

Beth

Research has demonstrated an association between healthcare provider–patient communication and patient health outcomes (Street et al. 2009). In a review of literature concerned with doctor–patient communication and patient health outcomes, Stewart (1995) concluded that patient health outcomes can be improved with good doctor–patient communication (see Chapter 3). He suggested that good communication can have a positive influence on the emotional health of patients, as well as symptom resolution, functional and physiological status, and pain control. Other research has suggested that interpersonal communication processes between patients and healthcare providers can influence patient satisfaction with the care provided, adherence to treatment recommendations, retention of information and understanding of health conditions, and improvement in health (Duggan 2006; Ong et al. 1995; Street 2001; Vranceanu et al. 2009).

> ### BOX 2.3 Features of the 'good back consultation' (Laerum et al. 2006)
>
> - To be taken seriously (be seen, heard and believed).
> - To be given an understandable explanation of what is wrong.
> - To have patient-centred communication (seeking patients' perspectives and/or preferences).
> - To receive reassurance and, if possible, be given a favourable prognosis.
> - To be told what can be done (by the patient themselves and by the healthcare provider).

What aspect of communication between healthcare practitioners and their patients improves healthcare outcomes? More specifically, what makes for good communication? Communication is integral to nearly every aspect of pain management, including assessing pain and the impact on function, deciding on pain management goals, and implementing treatment plans and assessing their effectiveness (Henry and Matthias 2018). The importance of practitioners and patients talking with each other is obvious at a basic level, in the sense that patients tell the practitioner what their symptoms are and the practitioner applies their knowledge and experience to identify a correct diagnosis and appropriate treatment or management regime. However, effective communication between practitioners and their patients is more complex, particularly in situations where there is no clear diagnosis, as is the case in many instances of chronic pain.

In a study by Laerum and colleagues (2006), patients with chronic low back pain were asked what they considered were the most important characteristics of a good back consultation. The results, ranked according to the frequency, emphasis and stated importance by patients, are presented in Box 2.3. The findings of this study emphasise that one of the most important aspects of effectively communicating with people with chronic pain is listening and valuing what they say about their experience, which continues to be a consistent theme in qualitative research in this area (see, for example, Evers et al. 2017; Gordon et al. 2017; Hadi et al. 2019).

It is also important to integrate client beliefs and knowledge into a pain management partnership between the therapist and the client. This practice will contribute to improved congruency between the patient and the healthcare provider. Lack of congruency, particularly about beliefs about the causes of pain, treatment preferences and desired outcomes, may have a negative effect on the therapeutic relationship and health outcomes (Brown 2003). Patient beliefs and expectations have been identified as being at the core of the therapeutic consultation process, particularly in terms of having the potential to influence adherence to recommended management regimes and as mediators of outcomes (Main et al. 2010).

It is therefore critical to explicitly discuss with clients, at an early stage of the therapeutic relationship, why they think they have pain and what they want to achieve from their involvement with the therapist. Be aware that what the client wants out of a therapeutic programme may differ from what the therapist wants, but it is necessary to privilege the client's desired outcomes to ensure that the interventions are individually meaningful, appropriate and acceptable (Brown 2003).

The patient may hold beliefs about the reason for their ongoing pain which are not supported by the current scientific knowledge. Alternatively, clients may have no idea why they have persistent pain and be frustrated and distressed by this. By identifying these issues early, it is possible for the therapist to address specific concerns expressed by the client, and to explore and clarify beliefs that are not supported by the available evidence. Main et al. (2010) suggest that all patients should be given a credible but simple explanation of differences between acute and chronic pain, the role of central pain mechanisms and the development of disability. As a therapist, it is necessary to provide such an explanation using language that the client will understand. It is possible for patients to understand the neurophysiology of pain if it is explained appropriately, but healthcare professionals often underestimate patients' ability to understand and may therefore not include appropriate explanations in their practice with chronic pain patients (Moseley 2003). On the other hand, patients may misunderstand or forget 40%–80% of information provided by healthcare professionals (Lie et al. 2022). It is therefore also important to integrate checking mechanisms into your practice, such as asking patients to recall and restate what they have been told, to monitor their comprehension of the information you are providing.

Shared voices: the value of peer support

'There is a great need for somewhere where you can be recognised and supported, and it's not psychology services, it's a step back from that…All the [internet] blogs I am on, probably the most outstanding thing people are saying is "I have lost all my family, I have lost all my social network, I have lost all my employment, I have lost all that and mostly I can't deal with x, y, and z aspects of my life because they still don't believe or recognise that this is not just me making it up".'

Ron

As discussed earlier in this chapter, living with chronic pain often results in feelings of social isolation and estrangement. The acultural nature of chronic pain can result in people feeling that they have what Hilbert (1984) described as *an extreme personal idiosyncrasy* that cannot be shared with others in society. It can be expected that social isolation will result in reduced social support, and this is supported by research. For example, Fernandez-Pena et al. found people with chronic pain reported 'reduced participation in social leisure activities' and 'weakened social ties' (Fernandez-Pena et al. 2018). Kotarba's (1983) early work with professional athletes and blue-collar manual labourers suggests that where pain is an inherent part of a particular profession or group, a shared language and understanding may develop, providing sufferers with a sense of belonging and strategies for managing and living with pain. In this final section of the chapter, the potential benefits of creating networks of *shared voices* for people living with chronic pain will be discussed.

Peer support is one avenue for people with chronic pain to share knowledge and experience, and reduce feelings of social isolation. While there is no universally agreed upon definition of peer support, it generally refers to processes 'through which people who share common experiences or face similar challenges come together as equals to give and receive help based on the knowledge that comes through shared experience' (Riessman 1989 cited in Penney 2018). Peer support can take a variety of forms, including one-on-one or a group; face-to-face, on the phone or online; and through workshops or social activities (Farr et al. 2021; Penney 2018).

Pain patients form and join peer support groups for different reasons. One reason may be to meet with and obtain support from other people living with chronic pain. In an online survey of people living with chronic pain in Australia, 66% of the 587 participants indicated that they would be interested in joining a support group of some kind (Nielsen 2009). While there is limited research on peer support for chronic pain, a recent pilot study of a peer support intervention for people with chronic musculoskeletal pain found improvements in perceived social support, self-efficacy, pain cognitions, patient activation, and pain intensity and interference (Matthias et al. 2015). A related qualitative study identified elements of peer support groups valued by participants (Box 2.4). Other potential benefits of participating in a peer-led support group include legitimisation of the chronic pain condition, feeling understood by others (Friedberg et al. 2005), decreased physical and emotional isolation, and feelings of belonging and acceptance (Finlay et al. 2018).

Not everyone with chronic pain will want to or be able to attend a face-to-face support group. One of the potential problems with peer-led pain support groups is the difficulty actively participating in such groups

> **BOX 2.4 Valued elements of peer support groups for chronic pain (Matthias et al. 2016a)**
>
> - Making interpersonal connections
> - Providing/receiving encouragement and support
>   - Listening
>   - Changes in attitude toward and acceptance of pain
> - Facilitating use of pain management strategies
>   - Helping to navigate healthcare resources
>   - Discussing exercises and activity
>   - Sharing ideas about pain self-management strategies
>   - Challenging and motivating

> **BOX 2.5 Advocacy and chronic pain**
>
> Advocacy is about supporting another person's cause. There are a number of ways of doing this, including:
> - individual advocacy
> - systems advocacy.
>
> **Individual advocacy** involves supporting people to exercise their rights by providing personal support to voice their concerns, access information, satisfy any issues of concern and/or identify available options. An example could be assisting someone with chronic pain negotiate reasonable accommodation in the workplace.
>
> **Systems advocacy** is primarily concerned with influencing and changing the system in ways that will benefit people with chronic pain as a group within society. This can include legislative, policy and practice aspects of systems. Lobbying politicians for increased funding for community-based pain management resources is an example of systems advocacy.
>
> Adapted from https://www.justice.qld.gov.au/public-advocate/about-the-public-advocate/what-is-systemic-advocacy.

can present for people with ongoing pain and limited resources. In a study involving active and inactive members of chronic fatigue syndrome and fibromyalgia support groups, nearly 30% of the 135 members who had become inactive or dropped out of a group cited being too sick as the reason for their nonattendance (Friedberg et al. 2005). Additional frequently reported reasons for nonattendance were inconvenient location (37.8%) or time (37.0%) (ibid). Other studies have identified similar barriers to support group participation (Cooper et al. 2017; Finlay and Elander 2016; Matthias et al. 2015, 2016b). Therapists should therefore not automatically assume that a person with chronic pain will be interested in attending a support group. It may be useful to consider alternative social networking and support options, for example websites, blogs and other virtual social media platforms that enable people living with chronic pain to create, document and share their lived experiences (Tsai et al. 2018). Most importantly, talk with people to identify if they would like more support and, if so, what form such support should take.

Consumers may also form or join a group with the aim of improving the lives of people with chronic pain through healthcare policy and practice change. This type of consumer group is more focused on individual, group and/or systems advocacy, rather than individual support (Box 2.5).

Of course, it is possible for a consumer group to have both a support and advocacy focus. Whether or not people with chronic pain are involved in support and/or advocacy groups, they may appreciate assistance from healthcare professionals. This could be in the form of helping with transport to and from group meetings, providing administrative support, or talking about specific topics at meetings. It is important, however, to talk with patients to determine whether assistance is required and, if so, what form this could take. It would be a mistake to assume that consumer groups will always want or need

healthcare professional involvement or that therapists know what sort of assistance will be helpful.

Conclusion

Listening and responding to the patient's story is integral to the successful management of chronic pain. Actively listening to their story validates the patient's experience and provides the basis for a trusting and effective healthcare partnership. It is only by listening to the patient's voice that the therapist will develop a true understanding of what living with pain means to individual clients, how it has affected their lives and the lives of their family members, and what they hope to achieve from their involvement with the therapist.

Respecting and incorporating the patient's voice into practice requires a shift in the balance of power between the healthcare provider and the patient. The client is the expert in their pain; the therapist's role is to provide resources and facilitate appropriate and relevant pain management practices. This can be challenging, but to neglect or devalue the patient's voice will affect the potential for successful health outcomes. It is not so difficult. To give Mat the final word:

'Don't call people liars. Look and talk to them like they're people, not an X-ray walking through the door. And listen to what they have to say.'

Review questions
Q

1. What aspects of a person's life can be affected by chronic pain?
2. Why is it important to allow the patient to tell their story?
3. What is meant by the term 'de-legitimatise' and why is it important?
4. List some losses that a person may experience as a consequence of chronic pain.
5. How can health outcomes be affected by patient–provider communication?

References

Antao, L., Shaw, L., Ollson, K., Reen, K., To, F., Bossers, A., et al., 2013. Chronic pain in episodic illness and its influence on work occupations: a scoping review. Work 44, 11–36.

Barnett, E., Casper, M., 2001. A definition of 'social environment. Am. J. Public Health 91 (3), 465.

Benintendi, A., Kosakowski, S., Lagisetty, P., Larochelle, M., Bohnert, A.S.B., Bazzi, A.R., 2021. I felt like I had a scarlet letter": recurring experiences of structural stigma surrounding opioid tapers among people with chronic, non-cancer pain. Drug Alcohol. Depend. 222.

Bodwell, M.B., 2010. How to listen in chronic pain narratives. In: Fernandez, J. (Ed.), Making Sense of Pain: Critical and Interdisciplinary Perspectives. Proceedings of the First Global Conference on Making Sense of Pain. Inter-disciplinary Press, Oxford. Available from: http://www.inter-disciplinary.net/wp-content/uploads/2010/10/pain2010ever11007102.pdf.

Brown, C.A., 2003. Service users' and occupational therapists' beliefs about effective treatments for chronic pain: a meeting of the minds or the great divide? Disabil. Rehabil. 25 (19), 1115–1125.

Charmaz, K., 1983. Loss of self: a fundamental form of suffering in the chronically ill. Sociol. Health. Illn. 5 (2), 168–195.

Chibnall, J.T., Tait, R.C., 1999. Social and medical influences on attributions and evaluations of chronic pain. Psychol. Health 14, 719–729.

Chibnall, J.T., Tait, R.C., Ross, L.R., 1997. The effects of medical evidence and pain intensity on medical student judgements of chronic pain patients. J. Behav. Med. 20, 257–271.

Chibnall, J.T., Tait, R.C., Gammack, J.K., 2018. Physician judgements and the burden of chronic pain. Pain. Med. 19, 1961–1971.

Chibnall, J.T., Dabney, A., Tait, R.C., 2000. Internist judgements of chronic low back pain. Pain Med. 1 (3), 231–237.

Chronic Pain Australia National Pain Survey, 2021. Available from: https://static1.squarespace.com/static/60c09e36d6b6dd3bebc eda16/t/60fe6cb2f96f69368a2c65c8/1627286709536/Nation al+Pain+Survey+2021.pdf.

Cooper, K., Schofield, P., Klein, S., Smith, B.H., Jehu, L.M., 2017. Exploring peer-mentoring for community dwelling older adults with chronic low back pain: a qualitative study. Physiotherapy 103 (2), 138–145.

Dassieu, L., Heino, A., Develay, E., Kabore, J., Page, M.G., Moor, G., et al., 2021. They think you're trying to get the drug": qualitative investigation of chronic pain patients' health care experiences during the opioid overdose epidemic in Canada. Can. J. Pain 5 (1), 66–80.

Deloitte Access Economics, 2019. The Cost of Pain in Australia. Deloitte Access Economics, Sydney.

De Ruddere, L., Craig, K.D., 2016. Understanding stigma and chronic pain: a-state-of-the-art review. Pain 157 (8), 1607–1610.

Duggan, A., 2006. Understanding interpersonal communication processes across health contexts: advances in the last decade and challenges for the next decade. J. Health. Commun. 11, 93–108.

Eisenberger, N.I., 2015. Social pain and the brain: controversies, questions, and where to go from here. Annu. Rev. Psychol. 66 (1), 609–629.

Evers, S., Hsu, C., Sherman, K.J., Balderson, B., Hawkes, R., Brewer, G., et al., 2017. Patient perspectives on communication with primary care physicians about chronic low back pain. Perm. J. 21, 16–177.

Farr, M., Brant, H., Patel, R., Linton, M., Ambler, N., Vyas, S., et al., 2021. Experiences of patient-led chronic pain peer support groups after pain management programs: a qualitative study. Pain Med. 22 (12), 2884–2895.

Fernandez-Pena, R., Molina, J.L., Valero, O., 2018. Personal network analysis in the study of social support: the case of chronic pain. Int. J. Environ. Res. Publ. Health 15, 2695.

Finlay, K.A., Elander, J., 2016. Reflecting the transition from pain management services to chronic pain support group attendance: an interpretative phenomenological analysis. Br. J. Health. Psychol. 21 (3), 660–676.

Finlay, K.A., Peacock, S., Elander, J., 2018. Developing successful social support: an interpretive phenomenological analysis of mechanisms and processes in a chronic pain support group. Psychol. Health 33 (7), 846–871.

Friedberg, F., Leung, D.W., Quick, J., 2005. Do support groups help people with chronic fatigue syndrome and fibromyalgia? A comparison of active and inactive members. J. Rheumatol. 32 (12), 2416–2420.

Garro, L.C., 1994. Narrative representations of chronic illness experience: cultural models of illness, mind, and body in stories concerning the Temporomandibular Joint (TMJ). Soc. Sci. Med. 38 (6), 775–788.

Ghavidel-Parsa, B., Maafi, A.A., Aarabi, Y., et al., 2015. Correlation of invalidation with symptom severity and health status in fibromyalgia. Rheumatology 54, 482–486.

Gordon, K., Rice, H., Allcock, N., Bell, P., Dunbar, M., Gilbert, S., et al., 2017. Barriers to self-management of chronic pain in primary care: a qualitative focus group study. Br. J. Gen. Pract. e209.

Grant, M., O-Beirne-Elliman, J., Froud, R., Underwood, M., Seers, K., 2019. The work of return to work. Challenges of returning to work when you have chronic pain: a meta-ethnography. BMJ. Open 9, e025743. https://doi.org/10.1136/bmjopen-2018-025743.

Gulseren, D., Kelloway, E.K., 2021. Working through the pain: the chronic pain experience of full-time employees. Occup. Health Sci. 5, 69–93.

Hadi, M.A., McHugh, G.A., Closs, S.J., 2019. Impact of chronic pain on patients' quality of life: a comparative mixed methods study. J. Pat. Exp 6 (2), 133–141.

Hambraeus, J., Hambraeus, K.S., Sahlen, K., 2020. Patient perspectives on interventional pain management: thematic analysis of a qualitative interview study. BMC. Health. Serv. Res. 20, 604.

Harris, S., Morley, S., Barton, S.B., 2003. Role loss and emotional adjustment in chronic pain. Pain 105, 363–370.

Henry, S.G., Matthias, M.S., 2018. Patient-clinician communication about pain: a conceptual model and narrative review. Pain. Med. 19 (11), 2154–2165.

Hilbert, R.A., 1984. The acultural dimensions of chronic pain: flawed reality construction and the problem of meaning. Soc. Probl. 31 (4), 365–378.

Holloway, I., Sofaer-Bennett, B., Walker, J., 2007. The stigmatisation of people with chronic back pain. Disabil. Rehabil. 29 (18), 1456–1464.

Holmes, M.M., Stanescu, S.C., Linaker, C., Price, C., Maguire, N., Fraser, S., et al., 2020. Individualised placement support as an employment intervention for individuals with chronic pain: a qualitative exploration of stakeholder views. BJGP. Open 4 (3). https://doi.org/10.3399/bjgpopen20X101036. bjgpopen20X101036.

Honkasalo, M., 2001. Pain, self and the body. Am. J. Semiotic 17 (4), 9–31.

Johansson, E.E., Hamberg, K., Westman, G., Lindgren, G., 1999. The meanings of pain: an exploration of women's descriptions of symptoms. Soc. Sci. Med. 48, 1791–1802.

Johnston-Devin, C., Oprescu, F., Gray, M., Wallis, M., 2021. Patients describe their lived experience of battling to live with complex regional pain syndrome. J. Pain 22, 1111–1128.

Kaiser, R.S., Mooreville, M., Kannan, K., 2015. Psychological interventions for the management of chronic pain: a review of current evidence. Curr. Pain. Headache. Rep. 19, 43.

Kleinman, A., Das, V., Lock, M., 1996. Introduction. Daedalus 125 (1), XI–XX.

Kool, M.B., van Middendorp, H., Lumley, M.A., Bijisma, J.W.J., Geenen, R., 2013. Social support and invalidation by others contribute uniquely to the understanding of physical and mental health of patients with rheumatic diseases. J. Health. Psychol. 18, 86–95.

Kotarba, J.A., 1983. Chronic Pain: Its Social Dimensions. Sage, Beverly Hills, CA.

Laerum, E., Indahl, A., Skouen, J.S., 2006. What is 'the good back consultation'? A combined qualitative and quantitative study of chronic low back pain patients' interaction with and perceptions of consultations with specialists. J. Rehabil. Med. 38, 255–262.

Lie, H.C., Juvet, L.K., Street Jr., R.L., Gulbrandsen, P., Mellblom, A.V., Brembo, E.A., et al., 2022. Effects of physicians' information giving on patient outcomes: a systematic review. J. Gen. Intern. Med. 37, 651–663.

Liedberg, G.M., Bjork, M., Dragioti, E., Turesson, C., 2021. Qualitative evidence from studies of interventions aimed at

return to work and staying at work for persons with chronic musculoskeletal pain. J. Clin. Med. 10 (6), 1247.

Link, B.G., Phelan, J.C., 2001. Conceptualizing stigma. Annu. Rev. Sociol. 27, 363–385.

Link, B.G., Phelan, J.C., 2006. Stigma and its public health implications. Lancet 367, 528–529.

Main, C.J., Buchbinder, R., Porcheret, M., Foster, N., 2010. Addressing patient beliefs and expectations in the consultation. Best. Pract. Res. Clin. Rheumatol. 24, 219–225.

McGowan, L., Luker, K.A., Creed, F., Chew-Graham, C., 2007. 'How do you explain a pain that can't be seen?': the narratives of women with chronic pelvic pain and their disengagement with the diagnostic cycle. Br. J. Health. Psychol. 12, 261–274.

Mardian, A.S., Hanson, E.R., Villarroel, L., Karnik, A.D., Sollenberger, J.G., Okvat, H.A., et al., 2020. Flipping the pain care model: a sociopsychobiological approach to high-value chronic pain care. Pain. Med. 21 (6), 1168–1180.

Matthias, M.S., McGuire, A.B., Kukla, M., Daggy, J., Myers, L.J., Bair, M.J., 2015. A brief peer support intervention for veterans with chronic musculskeletal pain: a pilot study for feasibility and effectiveness. Pain. Med. 16 (1), 81–87.

Matthias, M.S., Kukla, M., McGuire, A.B., Bair, M.J., 2016a. How do patients with chronic pain benefit from a peer-supported pain self-management intervention? A qualitative investigation. Pain. Med. 17, 2247–2255.

Matthias, M.S., Kukla, M., McGuire, A.B., Damush, T.M., Gill, N., Bair, M.J., 2016b. Facilitators and barriers to participation in a peer support intervention for veterans with chronic pain. Clin. J. Pain 32 (6), 534–540.

Mengshoel, A.M., Bjorbækmo, W.B., Merja, S., Wahl, A.K., 2021. 'It takes time, but recovering makes it worthwhile'- a qualitative study of long-term users' experiences of physiotherapy in primary health care. Physiother. Theory. Pract. 37 (1), 6–16.

Moseley, L., 2003. Unraveling the barriers to reconceptualisation of the problem in chronic pain: the actual and perceived ability of patients and health professionals to understand neurophysiology. J. Pain 4 (4), 184–189.

Mukhida, K., Carroll, W., Arseneault, R., 2020. Does work have to be so painful? A review of the literature examining the effects of fibromyalgia on the working experience from the patient perspective. Can. J. Pain 4 (1), 268–286.

Munday, I., Kneebone, I., Newton-John, T., 2021. The language of chronic pain. Disabil. Rehabil. 43 (3), 354–361.

Nicola, M., Correia, H., Ditchburn, G., Drummond, P., 2021. Invalidation of chronic pain: a thematic analysis of pain narratives. Disabil. Rehabil. 43 (6), 861–869.

Nielsen, A., 2009. 'It's a Whole Lot More than Just about My Pain': Understanding and Responding to the Social Dimension of Living with Chronic Pain. University of Queensland, Brisbane.

Nielsen, A., 2012. Journeys with chronic pain: acquiring stigma along the way. In: McKenzie, H., Quintner, J., Bendelow, G. (Eds.), At the Edge of Being the Aporia of Pain. Inter-Disciplinary Press, Oxford.

Nielsen, M., Keefe, F.J., Bennell, K., Jull, G.A., 2014. Physical therapist–delivered cognitive-behavioral therapy: a qualitative study of physical therapists' perceptions and experiences. Phys. Ther. 94 (2), 197–209.

Nielsen, A., Copleston, P., Wales, C., 2009. Pain Is Not Invisible Project Interim Report: Chronic Pain. Unpublished.

Oakman, J., Kinsman, N., Briggs, A.M., 2017. Working with persistent pain: an exploration of strategies utilized to stay productive at work. J. Occup. Rehabil. 27, 4–14.

Ong, L.M.L., Haes, C.J.M., Hoos, A.M., Lammes, F.B., 1995. Doctor–patient communication: a review of the literature. Soc. Sci. Med. 40 (7), 903–918.

Ostlund, G., Cedersund, E., Alexanderson, K., Hensing, G., 2001. 'It was really nice to have someone' – lay people with musculoskeletal disorders request supportive relationships in rehabilitation. Scand. J. Public Health. 29, 285–291.

Parsons, T., 1958. Definitions of health and illness in the light of American values and social structure. In: Gartly Jaco, E. (Ed.), Patients, Physicians and Illness. Free Press, Glencoe, IL.

Penney, D., 2018. Defining "peer support": implications for policy, practice and research. Advocates for Human Potential Available from: http://ahpnet.com/AHPNet/media/AHPNetMediaLibrary/White%20Papers/DPenney_Defining_peer_support_2018_Final.pdf.

Richardson, J.C., Ong, B.N., Sim, J., 2007. Experiencing chronic widespread pain in a family context: giving and receiving practical and emotional support. Sociol. Health. Illn. 29 (3), 347–365.

Saunders, P., 2019. Revisiting Henderson: Poverty, Social Security and Basic Income. Melbourne University Publishing, Melbourne.

Smith, T., Fletcher, J., Lister, S., 2021. Lived experiences of informal caregivers of people with chronic musculoskeletal pain: a systematic review and meta-ethnography. Br. J. Pain 15 (2), 187–198.

Stewart, M.A., 1995. Effective physician-patient communication and health outcomes: a review. Can. Med. Assoc. J. 152 (9), 1423–1433.

Lie, H.C., Juvet, L.K., Street, R.L., Gulbrandsen, P., Mellblom, A.V., Brembo, E.A., Eide, H., Heyn, L., Saltveit, K.H., Stromme, H., Sundling, V., Turk, E., Menichetti, 2021. Effects of physicians' information giving on patient outcomes: a systematic review. J. Gen. Intern. Med. 37, 651–663.

Street, R.L., Makoul, G., Arora, N.K., Epstein, R.M., 2009. How does communication heal? Pathways linking clinician-patient communication to health outcomes. Patient. Educ. Couns. 74, 295–301.

Strunin, L., Boden, L.I., 2004. Family consequences of chronic back pain. Soc. Sci. Med. 58, 1385–1393.

Tait, R.C., Chibnall, J.T., 1997. Physician judgments of chronic pain patients. Soc. Sci. Med. 45 (8), 1199–1205.

Tsai, S., Crawford, E., Strong, J., 2018. Seeking virtual social support through blogging: a content analysis of published blog posts written by people with chronic pain. Digital. Health 4, 1–10.

Vranceanu, A., Cooper, C., Ring, D., 2009. Integrating patient values into evidence-based practice: effective communication for shared decision-making. Hand. Clin. 25, 83–96.

Walker, J., Sofaer, B., Holloway, I., 2006. The experience of chronic back pain: accounts of loss in those seeking help from pain clinic. Eur. J. Pain 10, 199–207.

Wallace, L.S., Wexler, R.K., McDougie, L., Miser, W.F., Haddox, J.D., 2014. Voices that may not otherwise be heard: a qualitative exploration into the perspectives of primary care patients living with chronic pain. J. Pain Res. 7, 291–299.

West, C., Usher, K., Foster, K., Stewart, L., 2012. Chronic pain and the family: the experience of the partners of people living with chronic pain. J. Clin. Nur 21, 3352–3360.

Zajacova, A., Grol-Prokopczyk, H., Zimmer, Z., 2021. Sociology of chronic pain. J. Health. Soc. Behav. 62 (3), 302–317.

Chapter |3|

Developing your communication toolkit: a practical guide for healthcare professionals

Mike Stewart

LEARNING OBJECTIVES

At the end of this chapter, readers will be able to:
1. Explore the current evidence relating to healthcare communication.
2. Reflect upon common communication challenges in clinical practice.
3. Develop communication skills by exploring potential evidence based solutions to overcome communication challenges in clinical practice.

Introduction

'Pain cannot easily be divided from the emotions surrounding it. Apprehension sharpens it, hopelessness intensifies it, loneliness protracts it by making hours seem like days. The worst pain is unexplained pain.'

Hilary Mantel (2013)

The ability to communicate effectively, both as a healthcare professional and as somebody who is living with pain, cannot be understated. Kourkouta & Papathanasiou (2014) define communication as 'the exchange of information, thoughts and feelings among people using speech and other means'. Meaningful communication requires a collaborative, synchronised understanding between two equals. Although this sounds simple enough, the shared understanding, which so frequently forms a critical foundation for beneficial therapeutic alliances, has been found lacking, with healthcare communication described as customarily didactic, paternalistic and clinician-led throughout the literature (Dierckx et al. 2013; Jones et al. 2014; Stenner et al. 2015). Rather than feeling like equals, evidence shows that people in pain are often cast as passive recipients of information, leaving them feeling unheard, disconnected and isolated in what should be a therapeutic opportunity to share their experiences (Dow et al. 2012).

Our clinical knowledge and expertise count for very little if we are unable to communicate what we know to patients in a way that makes sense to them (Gardner & Winner 1982). The formation of a collaborative partnership and the subsequent pivotal therapeutic alliance are at risk if people experiencing pain feel unable to openly express how it feels and how it impacts on their lives (Barker et al. 2009; Biro 2010; Linton 2005). The desire to understand and the need to be understood form the basis of any caring human interaction.

Living with pain can be a distressing and isolating experience (Eccleston & Crombez 2007; Linton 2005). On the surface, pain seems to be a simple term. However, if we dig a little deeper, we reveal a myriad of subjective human beliefs and emotions which lie beneath. The widespread distress that frequently accompanies persistent pain can be compounded with feelings of depression, anxiety, isolation, uncertainty and chaos (Bullington et al. 2003; Linton 2005). From this chaotic blend of emotions comes not only a desire to seek meaning but also a need to 'get it out'. To express what lies beneath the surface may in itself be therapeutic (Bullington et al. 2003).

Despite this desire for meaning and expression, Biro (2010) suggests that pain forms an isolating barrier which blocks meaningful communication. It can create a linguistic brick wall, which not only prevents people in pain from communicating their experience to others but also restricts others (family, friends, colleagues, clinicians) from entering (ibid). It is perhaps this challenging 'unshareability' of pain (Scarry 1985) that makes the development of communication skills in healthcare so important. If clinicians are to get better at understanding patients and making them feel understood, they need practical, chisel-like tools which enable them, and the people they are trying to help, to gradually chip away at Biro's linguistic brick wall. Biro (2010) also suggests that pain is 'an all-consuming interior experience that threatens to destroy everything except itself and can only be described through metaphor'. Shinebourne & Smith (2010) suggest that metaphors provide people in pain with a linguistic 'safe bridge' through which they feel able to express emotions that may be too distressing to communicate literally. This chapter therefore explores the important role of metaphors in healthcare communication.

As Hilary Mantel's opening quote suggests, all pain demands an explanation. The challenge facing clinicians when attempting to help people make sense of their pain is how best to communicate current science-informed understanding of pain in a tailored, nonformulaic and meaningful way that mirrors the individual's lived pain experience. After all, 'to encounter another human is to encounter another world' (Bullington et al. 2003). It is easy to assume that all clinicians understand this simple truth and regard their 8:30 patient as completely different from their 9:00 patient. However, in a time-pressured clinical environment, it is often easy to forget the idiosyncratic nature of communication and the need to remain adaptable to differing individual needs. It may take two to tango, but when it comes to healthcare communication, our dance partners, steps, rhythm and timings are in constant flux.

The need for a shared understanding formed a central theme of the previous chapter, which highlighted the need for people to rediscover a sense of who they were prior to the onset of their pain. It considered how the overwhelming sense of loss, so commonly described by people living with pain, can impact on their feelings of self-worth and perceived value as a functioning member of society. This chapter develops these concepts further by providing the reader with a practical, clinically relevant guide to help expand their communication toolkit.

This chapter is divided into two sections. It starts by reflecting on the challenges and problems that may impede effective communication. Then, it explores a range of practical, evidence-based solutions for use in clinic. Throughout the chapter we shall aim for a solution-focused approach because, as can so easily be forgotten in the challenging muddle of practice, the problem is not the problem, finding the solution is the problem. Finally, a case study (Case Study 3.1) is added so that the reader can test their learning and consider how they might use their knowledge and skills in practice.

Reflecting on communication problems: why might we sometimes get it wrong?

The educationalist Dewey (1933) suggests that we do not learn purely from experience, but that we learn and adapt by reflecting on experiences that have challenged us. Therefore in order for the reader to develop their communication skills, they must be willing to reflect upon moments throughout their careers when perhaps their communication skills were lacking, resulting in a less than satisfactory outcome for themselves and their patients. These moments may produce worry and frustration for all involved, but it is important to remember that they are entirely normal. There is no such thing as perfect communication. Everyone gets it wrong from time to time, so it is important to bear this in mind in order to maintain perspective. This is especially important when considering the disconcerting rise in burnout among frontline healthcare professionals (Reith 2018). The late astrophysicist Stephen Hawking once said that he did not become a medical doctor like his father because healthcare was far too chaotic, uncertain and unpredictable. Moreover, surgeon Atul Gawande (2002) observes that healthcare communication consists of 'constantly changing knowledge, uncertain information, fallible individuals, and at the same time lives on the line'.

Following several years of interviewing clinicians, researchers and people in pain, healthcare journalist Judy Foreman (2014) concluded that 'There is an appalling mismatch between what people in pain need and what healthcare professionals know'. The following statement illustrates how this may manifest in clinical practice:

'She told me that the high point of her life was playing the organ for her church choir. She lived for the twice-a-week practices and Sunday performances. Now, with pain immobilising her elbow, she could no longer manage the keyboard. Her days held nothing that she looked forward to. The constant aching had robbed her of any hope. Life seemed empty of everything except pain. When I asked her if she had explained this to the staff in the clinic, she replied that they had not asked. Her medical history, as one might expect, read exactly like the history of an elbow.'

D. B. Morris (1991)

Let's take a moment to reflect on this statement and consider possible reasons as to perhaps why such unfortunate, disconnected human experiences appear frequently in literature about healthcare communication (Sharon et al. 2015). Are healthcare professionals receiving training that equips them with the necessary communication skills to meet the needs of people living with pain? Bolton (2010) suggests that communication skills are often merely assumed in both practice and research. Indeed, Briggs et al. (2011) found that in many healthcare disciplines, pain education and communication skills accounted for less than 1% of undergraduate programme hours in the United Kingdom. In Canada, only a third of universities could identify dedicated pain content in the curriculum (Watt-Watson et al. 2009).

Padfield et al. (2010) suggest that an inherent dilemma exists in many clinical consultations, with clinicians and patients searching for separate goals with separate meanings. Jones et al. (2014) found that the main obstacle to achieving a more collaborative, empowering therapeutic relationship through effective communication skills seemed to be the clinician's compelling desire to treat and advise the patient. This problem is illustrated in the following reflective exercise (Box 3.1). As mentioned in the previous chapter, it is not just the body that is threatened during a pain experience, it is the person's whole identity (Loftus 2011). Therefore healthcare professionals must do all they can to ensure a collaborative, narrative approach that is intrinsically linked to individual values (Parsons et al. 2012; Schoeb et al. 2014).

Stenner et al. (2015) used semi-structured interviews to explore how physiotherapists collaborate with patients when prescribing exercises. They revealed a lack of patient-centred practice, with participating physiotherapists making assumptions about what was best for the patients. On examination of the rationale and language used by these clinicians and with a supportive arm rather than a pointed judgemental finger, we may begin to identify possible areas for development. Most strikingly, the word which appears most is 'I'. This suggests a paternalistic, clinician-led approach to communication, which is at odds with best practice, shared-decision making and patient empowerment (Elwyn et al. 2005). Empowering others involves an acknowledgement that clinicians must be prepared to relinquish some power when communicating with people in pain.

The ability to enable people in pain to share their narratives openly, rather than to impose our own knowledge and beliefs, begins with an understanding that the answers to people's problems often lie in *their* words, thoughts and metaphors, not ours. Effective communication requires an understanding of when to lead or walk ahead of patients by talking, when to walk beside them by collaborating and sharing decisions as equals, and when to listen and follow their lead (Daloz 1999). Communication is an essential component of education. The Latin word for education is 'educare', to draw out that which lies within. Many healthcare professionals unfortunately appear to try pouring knowledge into the patient rather than drawing out the patient's understanding, beliefs and wishes (Dierckx et al. 2013, Jones et al. 2014). Communication is unlikely to be effective if it is not continually an active and constructive process of expression and shared understanding.

Fig. 3.1 illustrates three approaches to healthcare communication. It provides a simplified visual framework to consider when communicating with people in pain and offers an understanding why the patient's motivations and narrative in Morris' (1991) study went unheard. Furthermore, we may better understand how the didactic, clinician-led rationales in Box 3.1 might leave the patient feeling frustrated and disengaged.

Effective healthcare communication involves two people coming together, with each person openly sharing their knowledge and experience. While the clinician may have vast medical knowledge, the process of healthcare is incomplete if clinicians fail to recognise the *patient's* knowledge and expertise regarding their values, preferences, attitude to risk, social circumstances and experience of illness (Coulter & Collins 2011).

In their study examining why some clinician–patient relationships break down while others flourish, Frankel & Levinson (2014) used audio recordings of 125 doctors communicating with their patients. They found correlations between communication style and malpractice claims, with a perceived lack of respect for their narratives

BOX 3.1 **Reflective practice**

Read and reflect on the following statements. What are your thoughts? Do you recognise these rationales when caring for people with pain? Have you overheard similar ideas in clinics? What do you notice about the words that are used?
1. 'I don't ask the patient what they want. Giving them choice can confuse them. It can be too much for them.' *Clinician*
2. 'I will give exercise to almost every patient. I don't think about it too much, it's just part of the package that I like to give.' *Physiotherapist*
3. 'Overall, the physical assessment is the main influence on the choice of exercises. I tend to work out what I think is best for the patient.' *Physiotherapist*

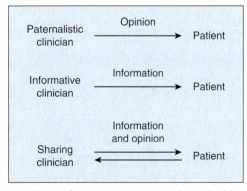

Fig. 3.1 Types of communication approaches in healthcare.

the main cause of patients' complaints. They also found that consultation times were only a mean 3.3-minute longer for doctors who did not receive malpractice claims from patients. This contradicts the widely held belief among clinicians that there is no time for a more narrative approach to communication (Padfield et al. 2010; Stenner et al. 2015). Interestingly, no differences were found between the amount and quality of information provided by clinicians (Frankel & Levinson 2014). The main difference was the clinicians' ability to relate to the patient's narrative (ibid). This illustrates the benefits of active listening and responding to the patient's idiosyncratic story, skills which have been found to be undervalued and underused in clinical practice (Cooper et al. 2008; Dierckx et al. 2013; Jones et al. 2014; Stenner et al. 2015).

Without listening, we cannot hope to meet patients' needs. As a rule of thumb, there is something wrong when clinicians are talking more than their patients. Linton (2005) suggests that there are three steps to good communication: listen, listen and listen. Listening begins with an active acknowledgement that the other person needs to be heard. The following rules can facilitate collaborative partnerships with people in pain:

1. Listen to their story.
2. Find out what they need (this cannot be achieved without listening).
3. Guide and signpost patients towards what they need.

Table 3.1 shows an evidence-based list of things to avoid when attempting to develop therapeutic relationships.

Much of the power that is held by clinicians lies in the words they use and their knowledge. Vignette 3.1 shows how healthcare communication can be ambiguous, lending itself to misinterpretation and confusion (Clarke

---

Table 3.1 Communication: what to avoid in clinic

Providing opportunities for misinterpretations (see Vignette 3.1).

Giving in to the pressure of communicating a structural diagnosis.

Asking directed (yes/no) questions.

Interrupting during the first 2 minutes.

Missing opportunities to capture issues that require perceptual change (see Fig. 3.2 and Box 3.4).

Judging the patient, i.e. not acknowledging that it is their story.

Going it alone, i.e. not seeking clinical companionship and feedback from peers on your communication.

Assuming that you are on the same page. Check, clarify and confirm meanings (see Vignette 3.2).

---

et al. 2012; Linton 2005). The more comfortable clinicians become with what they know, the more they may be at risk of losing sight of the fact that other people may not share their views. Pinker (2014) terms this *the curse of knowledge*. This issue is illustrated in Vignette 3.1.

Vignette 3.1 illustrates a common communication problem. It shows how the clinician's thinking influences their choice of words. Furthermore, not creating opportunities to clarify meaning through two-way collaboration (see Fig. 3.1) reinforces the clinician's misconception that they are on the same page as their patient. The clinician in the vignette correctly identifies the patient's misinterpretation of degenerative changes as 'worn out' and seeks to reduce the potential for harm by saying 'wear and tear'. Unfortunately this reinforced the patient's belief that their foot has worn out as a consequence of lifting at work, thus consolidating their unhelpful pain beliefs and behaviours. Evidence shows that people in pain often misinterpret medical terminology (Barker et al. 2009) with terms such as 'wear and tear' perceived as 'something rotting away'. Indeed, one participant in Padfield et al. (2010) depicted 'wear and tear' as a piece of rotten fruit when they explored how people in pain chose to communicate their experience through photography.

Communication decisions we make can have a lasting impact, for better or for worse. What we say or do not say is as important as what we do or do not do. In a speech to The Royal College of Surgeons in 1923, Rudyard Kipling stated: 'Words are, of course, the most powerful drug used by mankind.' Words have the potential to either heal or cause devastating and lasting harm (Biro 2010). Like drugs, words have an ability to change the way another person thinks and feels. Words are capable of influencing thoughts, emotions and actions that can lead towards beneficial or detrimental changes. Clinicians play a pivotal role in patient's lives. Their words can either make or break a positive clinical outcome (Darlow et al. 2013).

The following reflective exercise in Box 3.2 provides an opportunity to consider a variety of ways in which communication may either help or hinder a shared understanding between patients and clinicians.

Exploring communication solutions: what can happen when we get it right?

Having reflected on common problems and challenges when communicating with people in pain, this chapter now turns towards practical solutions. In the previous section, two themes emerged as considerations for the development of communication skills in clinical practice:

Vignette 3.1 The curse of knowledge

A vignette showing excerpts from a healthcare consultation. Unspoken thoughts, beliefs and actions are shown in bold parentheses.

Patient	Clinician
'So, now you've assessed my foot, what do you think is causing my pain?'	'Well, there is nothing to worry about. Although, your X-ray does show some degenerative changes and I have found some mechanical malalignments or overpronation here in your foot that are causing your pain.' **(The clinician shows the patient an anatomical model of the foot.)**
'Oh I see, that doesn't sound good. So, my foot is knackered and out of place! What do you need to do now?' **(The patient is finding it hard to listen as they are now worried about 'degeneration', 'malalignment' and 'overpronation'.)**	'As I've said, it really is nothing to worry about. Lots of people your age have degenerative changes. Think of it as normal wear and tear to your body.' **(This will hopefully reassure the patient.)**
'So, the degenerative wear and tear has knocked my bone out of place? No wonder it hurts so much!' **(Now I am really worried, but there must be a fix?)**	'Yes. This problem can cause a lot of pain, but we can fix that with some simple orthotic corrections and exercises.' **(Hoping to validate the patient's pain experience while again pointing to the foot model.)**
'Great! This makes sense now. I told my boss that all the standing I've been doing at work has been wearing me out. What should I do about it now?' **(Stop work, avoid standing, surgery?)**	'Well, it's best to try and stay active as much as you can. Let your pain guide how much you do. It's your body's way of warning you.' **(The clinician does not want the patient to stop work.)**
'Ok. I understand now. Thank you.' **(My pain is causing more damage. I must protect and rest. Stop if it hurts.)**	'Great. I'll see you again next time. Let's get you booked back in again. Do you have any more questions before you leave?'
'Yes. Can you please write down those words for me? "Degenerative wear and tear," Also, how do you spell "malalignment" and "overpronation"?' **(I need to look at these problems on the internet and then show them to my wife, and to my boss.)**	'Sure. No problems. Here you go. I'll see you next time.' **(I think that went really well. The patient has a good understanding and is motivated to get better.)**

BOX 3.2 Reflective practice

1. List any potential barriers and/or facilitators in Vignette 3.1 that could help or hinder communication.
2. Think back to communication experiences you've had in clinic. Can you identify any moments of potential ambiguity that may have resulted in similar misinterpretations between you and the patient?

1. Listen, listen, listen. The answers to other people's problems often lie in their own words and thoughts, so clinicians need practical tools to shift communication towards listening and drawing out peoples' experiences, rather than a clinician-led dynamic.

2. Empowerment. To empower patients, clinicians must be prepared to relinquish some of their power. This chapter will explore strategies to put the patient in the communication driving seat.

'The history-taking was so structured, so searching, so thorough, that I felt that, for the first time, my pain was being listened to. The consultation was, in itself, therapeutic.'

(Hilary Mantel 2013).

This positive experience illustrates not only the importance of listening, but also the need for people in pain to feel believed and validated. In their study exploring talk of frustration by people living with pain, Dow et al. (2012) found that ongoing pain can cause people to feel unseen, unheard and socially isolated. They concluded that communication may improve if the frustration of living with persistent pain is explicitly (and perhaps repeatedly) acknowledged by the health professional (ibid). By listening and validating Mantel's pain experience, the clinician turned a frustrating, invisible and hard-to-share ordeal into a liberating therapeutic alliance with a tangible sense of connection.

Unfortunately, despite the importance of explicitly communicating that we understand a patient's thoughts and concerns, evidence points towards a worrying lack of validation in healthcare consultations (Edmond & Keefe 2015). This may reflect a contrast between how clinicians might display empathy and validation when communicating with a distressed friend or family member, while withholding this innate human response when communicating professionally. When listening to a friend's distress, many of us might say, 'I'm so sorry to hear that. That sounds really hard. No wonder you're upset. How have you been coping?' Yet clinicians may either avoid or forget to validate their patient's experience, for instance by moving quickly to the next question in the subjective examination format (Padfield et al. 2010). They may even respond to their patient's distress by asking them to rate it on a numerical scale between 0 and10.

Edmond & Keefe (2015) suggest that many healthcare professionals are hesitant to display empathy and validation because of a concern that this may reinforce their patient's unhelpful pain behaviours. However, validation has been shown to result in a reduction in pain, worry and pain behaviours (Edlund et al. 2017; Linton et al. 2012). Furthermore, as Mantel suggests, empathetic validation has the potential to increase trust and strengthen the therapeutic alliance.

The key to any meaningful therapeutic alliance is collaboration. This requires a genuine desire and active interest between two equals to identify and solve problems together (Cross et al. 2006). Vignette 3.2 shows a more collaborative and solution-focused alternative to the conversation from Vignette 3.1.

By comparing and contrasting the consultation dialogues in Vignettes 3.1 and 3.2, we may begin to note important differences. The clinician in Vignette 3.2 facilitates a collaborative approach by communicating an active interest in both identifying and solving problems jointly with the patient. Rather than casting the patient as a passive recipient of information, the clinician in Vignette 3.2 engages the patient by drawing out their understanding and beliefs ('I'm interested to hear why you think your foot hurts'). Readers are invited to explore the implications for their own practice (Box 3.3).

Clinician may worry that asking patients to share their thoughts and beliefs might result in patients becoming frustrated: 'I don't know! I thought you were the expert so I expect you to tell me why it hurts.' This may happen, but moments like these should be embraced rather than

avoided, as they provide useful opportunities to work with the patient. Coulter & Collins (2011) suggest that any therapeutic alliance must be based on a negotiation between equals. A healthcare consultation is the coming together of two experts who share their knowledge and understanding. No matter how much clinical knowledge and expertise a clinician may have, they will never reach the level of knowledge and expertise that their patient has about themselves.

Socrates reminds us of our facilitatory responsibilities as healthcare communicators by suggesting that in order to find yourself, you must first think for yourself. Encouraging active participation in the communication process, as in Vignette 3.2, reduces the risk of merely teaching people in pain the shape of the spoon that we use to feed them. Rather than patients remaining as passive recipients of information from clinicians, a two-way Socratic approach to communication is based on an understanding that people discover more about themselves through their own words and thoughts. It consists of asking a series of focused, open-ended questions that encourage reflection (Clark & Egan 2015).

Colameco (2012) suggests that by resisting the urge to give advice and applying Socratic questioning, people may be guided towards their own conclusions. It may help to see patients as learners and help them to question their own experiences. This requires that the clinician remains nonjudgemental, resists giving advice and somewhat naive (Hinchliff 2004).

Colameco (2012) considers the following three types of Socratic enquiry:

Three types of Socratic question:
1. Information seeking questions: What happened?
2. Analysis questions: Why do you think this happened?
3. Synthesis questions: Based on our discussion how do you see this now?

Vignette 3.2 shows the use of Socratic questioning to facilitate dialogue and check a patient's understanding. By asking, 'Can you walk me through what you now understand about your foot pain? Imagine I'm your boss asking "what did they say to you at the hospital?"', the clinician is gently eliciting the patient's understanding as a critical friend. In doing so they are providing an opportunity for the patient to learn through their own words and thoughts, as well as gaining important feedback regarding the effectiveness of their own communication. The importance of clarifying meaning cannot be understated.

Another key difference between the communication styles in Vignettes 3.1 and 3.2 is a noticeable shift in the clinician's focus from fixing, treating and advising, to a communication style that focuses on observing, reflecting and challenging by listening. Scott-Dempster et al. (2014) used

Vignette 3.2 An example of collaborative communication	
Patient	**Clinician**
'So, now you've assessed my foot, what do you think is causing my pain?'	'Well, everything looks good, with some normal age-related changes on your X-ray and small changes to the posture of your foot. I'm interested to hear why you think your foot hurts?' **(An active interest in exploring the patient's understanding and beliefs).**
'It's been painful for a couple of years now, and it's stopping me from doing things, so I suppose there must be some damage inside there causing the pain?' **(Feeling able to express beliefs, worries and concerns).**	'I can certainly reassure you that there is no damage, but your foot has become sensitive and stiff over the past couple of years, which sounds like it has led to you being less able to do things physically?' **(Listening to the patient's story and reconfirming what they have heard).**
'Yes. I am getting more pain and I am really struggling to stand for long when I'm working and when playing with my kids. Should I keep doing these things or stop and rest?' **(This is nice. I don't usually get to ask these questions when visiting the hospital).**	'I'm sorry to hear that. That sounds really frustrating. What do you think? What might happen if you stop going to work and stop playing with your kids?' **(Validation followed by an active attempt to draw out thoughts and beliefs rather than pouring in knowledge and advice).**
'Thanks. Yeah, it can be really frustrating at times. Well, I suppose it will probably become more stiff and more painful, and then I won't be able to earn money or be a good parent?' **(It is probably best to keep moving).**	'Yes, stopping is not a good idea. Not because of harm, but because, as you've said, your foot will get stiffer and sorer. You are safe to keep active.' **(Confirmation of patient's own deduction).**
'That is great news thanks! So, besides keeping active, what else can we do to make it better?' **(What can I do? What can the clinician do? How long will it take to get better?).**	'Okay. We have some choices that we can explore together. But before we chat about these, can you walk me through what you now understand about why your foot hurts? Imagine I'm your boss asking "what did they say to you at the hospital?"' **(Essential to check the patient's interpretation rather than to assume they have understood what I've said).**
'Erm. Well, the good news is that there is no damage. However, my foot has become more sensitive and stiffer over the past couple of years. To make this better I need to keep moving.' **(Reconfirmation of reassuring safety information).**	'That's great! Now you've got it. So, let's start exploring what we can both do to make things better.' **(An invitation to continue collaborating and foster a therapeutic alliance through shared-decision making).**

BOX 3.3 Reflective practice

1. Read the dialogues in Vignettes 1 & 2.
2. Create a list of differences between the two dialogues. What are the most important communication changes?
3. Consider how you might begin to introduce some of these changes when communicating with people in pain. Which changes in communication style do you feel most confident to try in clinic?
4. You may find it helpful to practice this new communication style by role playing different patient scenarios with colleagues.
5. It may be helpful to audio record your role play (and your conversations with patients if they give you permission), to help you reflect on aspects of your communication that have improved, as well as aspects requiring further development.

interpretative phenomenological analysis (IPA) to explore the communication styles of physiotherapists when prescribing exercises for people in pain. They concluded that phsiotherapists' mindsets need to shift from 'fix it' to 'sit with it'. Refer back to Fig. 3.1 to reconsider the impact of clinician-led, 'fix it' mindsets when communicating with people in pain. Jevne (2015) reminds us that, as clinicians, 'We are not mechanics and we are not dealing with motorcars.'

Evidence-based communication strategies

As Vignette 3.2 shows, reconceptualisation of clinical communication requires active listening and attention to what patients are saying. Crucially, this involves actively listening to the metaphors that people in pain use to express their experience. Furthermore, it involves using the patient's own metaphors to facilitate behaviour change (Stewart & Ryan 2020).

Metaphorical thinking is essential to how we communicate, learn, discover and create meaning (Geary 2011). Metaphors enable us to link the abstract to the known (Loftus 2011; Semino 2011). We use metaphors most when attempting to convey experiences that are resistant to expression (Lakoff & Johnson 1980). Pain is such an experience.

Clinicians should capture moments that require perceptual change when communicating with people in pain. Fig. 3.2 shows a typical metaphor used by people in pain—'It's gone again.' On the surface, this expression seems simple enough. However, taking time to collaborate and seeking to guide and discover a deeper meaning through Socratic questioning may reveal therapeutic opportunities. If we ask the patient what they mean by 'it's gone again', a typical answer based on traditional biomedical thinking might be 'my back muscle/joint/disc has gone' (Darlow et al. 2015). This provides an opportunity for further exploration of unhelpful beliefs of mechanical vulnerability, e.g. 'Why do think your disc has "gone"? Where did you discover this? Shall we discuss the relevance and irrelevance of back disc injuries relating to pain?' However, as Fig. 3.2 shows, the patient's metaphor also provides a window through which we can communicate and make sense of the wider complexities of the biopsychosocial impact of pain. By continuing to ask, 'Would you mind if we explore what else has "gone" from your life since your back pain has worsened?', both clinician and the patient may find it easier to talk about their broader difficulties, worries and concerns. This can then lead to an exploration of potential solutions.

Evidence suggests that visualising the metaphors that people in pain use has therapeutic value. Padfield et al. (2010) suggest that, 'Verbal metaphors remain formulaic, offering the individual little opportunity to express how they feel, or to contextualise the symptoms within a personal narrative. Furthermore, a well-documented stasis exists in many pain consultations as a result of physicians and patients searching for different meanings.' In an attempt to address this issue, the authors used a set of 64 photographic representations of the pain experience, developed in collaboration with people living with pain. Participants in the study were asked to choose any image which best represented their pain experience. Eight-six percent of participants related at least one image to their pain, 67% felt the images had facilitated dialogue, while 82% of the healthcare professionals reported improved communication and a greater understanding of the patient's experience (ibid). This suggests that patient-generated metaphors may provide healthcare professionals and people living with pain with a chisel to break through Biro's (2010) communication brick wall. Padfield et al. (2010) concluded that the metaphoric images offered 'a narrative space for people to step into, the possibility of some kind of identification and empathy with the other … some kind of slippery surface for further narrative'.

In psychotherapy, the use of patient-generated metaphors is recognised as an effective method for eliciting change (Kopp 1995; Tompkins & Lawley 2002). Box 3.4 provides an example of the way clinicians can use patients' metaphors to facilitate dialogue and foster a therapeutic alliance.

Clinician:

'Last time we met I showed you a few exercises for your back pain. Have they helped?'

Patient:

'Sadly not. I have not had time to do them as I've got so much on my plate.'

Clinician:

'I'm sorry to hear that. I'm interested in what you've just said. Do you mind if we try something a bit different?'

Patient:

'Yes that's fine. Different sounds good as I've already tried lots of things which haven't worked.'

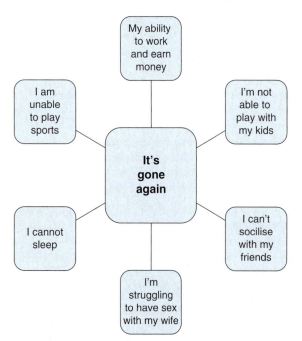

Fig. 3.2 Highlighting problems and finding solutions through patient-generated metaphors.

BOX 3.4 **A therapeutic application of patient-generated metaphors**

This approach requires a degree of flexibility, creativity and serious playfulness as discussed. Clinicians are therefore encouraged to practice it by considering how they might adapt their communication when responding to patient metaphors such as 'Every time I get back on track, things just keep going off the rails', 'It's an absolute mess. Everything feels so tangled up these days' or 'It's so frustrating. I feel like I'm going around in circles with no answers.' They could also use these and other metaphors for role play with colleagues. Here are more tips provided by a wide range of healthcare professionals trained in this communication approach:

1. Build your confidence by breaking the process into manageable steps. First, simply listen out for the metaphors that people in pain use, make a note of them and consider how they might be used next time.
2. There is no right and wrong way to use this communication tool. For example, sometimes the clinician will draw the metaphor, sometimes the patient will. Sometimes, patient and clinician will collaborate by drawing the metaphor together. At other times, it may be less appropriate to draw the metaphor. There is no set formula or recipe so clinicians need to adapt.
3. Avoid the urge to advise and fix the patient's metaphoric problem. Instead, provide the patient with an opportunity to consider how they might advise a friend in this situation. Tompkins & Lawley (2002) suggest that human beings are often much better at advising others than they are at advising themselves.
4. Remember that the aim of this communication approach is to sow cognitive seeds of behaviour change, which may take time to germinate. It is therefore best to allow time for people to reflect on their own advice in between visits to the clinic.

Clinician:
'That's great. You've just said that you feel like you've got too much on your plate. If I were to try drawing what that might look like, would it look like this? A plate that is so full with food that some of it is falling onto the floor?'

Patient:
'Yes. I suppose so. I feel like I can't cope with the amount of things I need to do, which means I cannot do my exercises.'

Clinician:
'If a friend of yours said that they had too much food on their plate, how would you advise your friend? What things might you suggest that they could do to change or improve the situation?'

Patient:
'Well, I suppose I would advise them to take something off the plate, or to eat something perhaps, or maybe they could get a bigger plate.'

Clinician:
'They sound like some helpful solutions for your friend. Now, let's keep these in mind and think about how we can work together to find some solutions too.'

Patient:
'Thanks. That sounds like a great idea!'

Table 3.2 shows an evidence-based list of ideas to consider using in practice when seeking to develop your communication skills:

Table 3.2 Communication: evidence-based ideas to consider using when communicating with patients

See communication as a fundamental skill in your toolkit.

Set the tone to 'join' with your patient as a person, e.g. start by talking about the weather or their kids. Remember: hairdressers often make excellent communicators. They don't begin conversations by asking 'How has your hair been?' unlike in healthcare consultations where people are typically asked 'How has your pain been?'

Attend to what you say and how you say it. Think about your nonverbal communication, e.g. make eye contact and nod your head to show you understand.

Follow the patient's lead and be flexible. Remember: the art of effective communication is knowing when to walk ahead, when to walk behind and when to walk together (Daloz 1999).

Active listening. 'Go on. Tell me more about that.'

Prompt sensitive information 'Pain is hard to deal with. Tell me about how you're coping.'

Display empathy and validation (see Vignette 3.2).

Follow the three rules of facilitation: Listen, find out what they need, then tailor how you guide.

Conclusion

This chapter has provided ways for clinicians to develop their communication skills, so that they feel better equipped to help people living with pain. Communication is a key foundation of effective healthcare. Without the development of communication skills, people in pain are likely to feel disconnected from their clinicians and the therapeutic process, but also feel isolated from their friends, family, work colleagues and society (Dow et al. 2012). Elaine Scarry (1985) suggests, 'Whatever pain achieves, it achieves in part through its unshareability, and it ensures this unshareability through its resistance to language. To have great pain is to have certainty; to hear that another person has pain is to have doubt.' Clinicians should therefore seek to help people in pain feel validated and believed. Throughout their careers, clinicians develop a variety of technical skills. Communication should be one such skill, a unique key which needs to be polished, refined and reflected upon to unlock its potential therapeutic value.

CASE STUDY 3.1

The referral from GP

Dear Colleague,

Please see this 48-year-old lady who has recently had an L4/5 decompression and is still complaining of low back pain. I would be grateful if you could arrange to see her at home as she is struggling to leave the house.

Marilyn's story

My pain journey began on Christmas day 2 years ago. I had lots of family staying over and had to lift a heavy chair to make some room. I immediately felt a hot, lightning shock type pain in my lower back, which made me drop to the floor. It was the most frightening thing that I've ever experienced.

An ambulance was called and I was rushed to the hospital. They moved me around and did an X-ray but said there was nothing to worry about. They diagnosed a possible torn ligament and I was told that I would have physiotherapy.

The physiotherapist saw me 2 weeks later. By this point, the pain had got worse and I couldn't do simple day-to-day things. The physio did more tests and thought my pain was coming from a trapped nerve in my back, probably due to a disc prolapse. He explained that the 'jelly' in the disc would repair itself within a few more weeks and I'd be fine again. He pushed on my back, which was excruciating and I was given exercises to do at home. I was also told not to bend or lift.

My pain did not get better and when I went back to see the physio 1 week later I was very upset. He too was worried that my pain kept getting worse. He had never seen someone with so much pain and was concerned, as his treatment should have helped. It didn't. I was advised to stop the exercises and was sent back to my doctor for an urgent referral to a spinal surgeon.

I eventually saw the surgeon (2 months later!!!) who explained that I might need surgery. He ordered an MRI scan and told me to come back once it had been done. The MRI took another 6 weeks and by now I had stopped everything. My boss was worried and told me to not come back to work until I was fully better. Before the pain started, I was very happy and active. I had a lovely home life with 3 kids and a loving husband. I also worked full time in a local school for disabled children. This has all changed now.

When I saw the surgeon again, he told me that I needed an operation to remove some of my disc at L4/5. I was told that this would get rid of my pain and that I would be back to normal in no time. This was excellent news!

That operation was almost a year ago and my pain has continued to get worse. The surgeon could not understand why my pain had not improved with the operation and thought I had something called failed back surgery syndrome.

I am really angry and wish that I had never had that operation. I wanted to see another surgeon for a second opinion so I arranged this privately. He told me that I would need further surgery called a Coflex and an epidural. I was relieved to hear that this problem could be fixed and I had this operation 6 weeks ago. I cannot believe that my pain has not gone away and, once again, nor can my surgeon who has now discharged me.

I now feel like I've been thrown on the scrapheap. I spend all my time in the house. I tried to go to the shop around the corner last week but couldn't do it. I didn't even make it past my front door! Everything now hurts and everything I do causes more pain and more damage. My teeth even hurt when I brush them!!

As if to add insult to injury, all my other problems have also got worse. My irritable bowel syndrome has been more noticeable and I've developed an alarming shortness of breath when I do anything. The doctor thinks that I might have COPD. I've had eczema since I was a child. This was always really easy to manage but now it's worse than ever.

I stay in bed all day as I can't sit or stand. I read an article on the internet, which told me that lying down helps to repair prolapsed discs. I'm doing everything I can to get rid of this but nothing is working.

I get very upset when I think of how I can't do what I was put here to do. I used to love my job—caring for all those sick children. I also have an elderly mother who needs my help. I tried to keep helping her for as long as I could but I've been forced to give in. Who is going to look after my mum now? I feel like a failure. I can't see how you can help me but thank you for coming.

CASE STUDY 3.1—Cont'd

Case study questions

1. Refer back to Fig. 3.2. What type of communication approach best describes Marilyn's healthcare experience?
2. Marilyn says she feels like she's been 'thrown on the scrapheap'. Using Box 3.4 as a guide, think about how

you might use Marilyn's scrapheap metaphor to help her explore some possible solutions.
3. Choose two more ideas that you have learnt from this chapter which you might consider using in clinic to help Marilyn. Why did you choose these particular ideas for this particular person?

References

Barker, K., Reid, M., Minns Lowe, C., 2009. Divided by a lack of common language? A qualitative study exploring the use of language by health professionals treating back pain. BMC. Musculoskelet. Disord. 10, 123.

Biro, D., 2010. The Language of Pain. W.W Norton & Company, New York.

Bolton, G., 2010. Reflective Practice, Writing and Professional Development, third ed. Sage Publications, London.

Briggs, E., Carr, E., Whittaker, M., 2011. Survey of undergraduate pain curricula for healthcare professionals in the United Kingdom. Eur. J. Pain. 15 (8), 789–795.

Bullington, J., Nordemar, R., Nordemar, K., 2003. Meaning out of chaos: a way to understand chronic pain. Scand. J. Caring. Sci. 12 (4), 17–21.

Clark, G.I., Egan, S.J., 2015. The Socratic method in cognitive behavioural therapy: a narrative review. Cogn. Ther. Res 39, 863–879.

Clarke, A., Anthony, G., Gray, D., Jones, D., Mcnamee, P., Schofield, P., et al., 2012. "I feel so stupid because I can't give a proper answer..." How older adults describe chronic pain: a qualitative study. BMC. Geriatr. 12 (1), 1–8.

Colameco, S., 2012. Chronic Pain: A Way Out. Createspace Publishing, Charleston.

Cooper, K., Smith, B., Hancock, E., 2008. Patient-centredness in physiotherapy from the perspective of the chronic low back pain patient. Physiotherapy 94, 244–252.

Coulter, A., Collins, A., 2011. Making Shared Decision Making a Reality. No Decision About Me, Without Me. The Kings Fund, London.

Cross, V., Moore, A., Morris, J., Caladine, L., Hilton, R., Bristow, H., 2006. The Practice-Based Educator: A Reflective Tool for CPD & Accreditation. John Wiley & Sons, Chichester.

Daloz, L., 1999. Mentor: Guiding the Journey of Adult Learners. Jossey-Bass, San Francisco.

Darlow, B., Dowell, A., Baxter, G., Mathieson, F., Perry, M., Dean, S., 2013. The enduring impact of what clinicians say to people with low back pain. Ann. Fam. Med. 11 (6), 527–534.

Darlow, B., Dean, S., Meredith, P., Mathieson, F., Baxter, G., David, D., et al., 2015. Easy to harm, hard to heal: patient views about the back. Spine 40 (11), 842–850.

Dewey, J., 1933. How We Think. A Restatement of the Relation of Reflective Thinking to the Educative Process. D. C. Heath, Boston.

Dierckx, K., Devugele, M., Roosen, P., Devisch, I., 2013. Implementation of shared decision making in physical therapy: observed level of involvement and patient preference. Phys. Ther (10), 1321–1330.

Dow, C., Roche, P., Ziebland, S., 2012. Talk of frustration in the narratives of people with chronic pain. Chronic. Illn 8 (3), 134–145.

Eccleston, C., Crombez, G., 2007. Worry and chronic pain: a misdirected problem solving model. Pain. 132 (3), 233–236.

Edlund, S.M., Wurm, M., Holländare, F., Linton, S.J., Fruzzetti, A.E., Tillfors, M., 2017. Pain patients' experiences of validation and invalidation from physicians before and after multimodal pain rehabilitation: associations with pain, negative affectivity, and treatment outcome. Scand. J. Pain. 17, 77–86.

Edmond, S.N., Keefe, F.J., 2015. Validating pain communication: current state of the science. Pain 156 (2), 215–219.

Elwyn, G., Hutchings, H., Edwards, A., Rapport, F., Wensing, M., Cheung, W.Y., et al., 2005. The OPTION scale: measuring the extent that clinicians involve patients in decision-making tasks. Health Expect. 8, 34–42.

Foreman, J., 2014. A Nation in Pain. Healing Our Biggest Health Problem. Oxford University Press, London.

Frankel, R., Levinson, W., 2014. Back to the future: can conversation analysis be used to judge physicians' malpractice history? Commun. Med. 11 (1), 27–39.

Gardner, H., Winner, E., 1982. U-Shaped Behavioural Growth. Academic Press Inc., New York.

Gawande, A., 2002. Complications: A Surgeon's Notes on an Imperfect Science. Metropolitan Books, New York, NY.

Geary, J., 2011. I Is An Other. The Secret Life of Metaphor and How it Shapes the Way We See the World. Harper Collins, London.

Hinchliff, S., 2004. The Practitioner as Teacher, third ed. Churchill Livingstone, London.

Jevne, J., 2015. Stabbed in the back: moving the knife out of back pain. Br. J. Sports Med Blog. Accessed on Friday 24 March 2017.

Jones, L., Roberts, L., Little, P., Mullee, M., Cleland, J., Cooper, C., 2014. Shared decision making in back pain consultations: an illusion or reality? Eur. Spine. J. 23, 13–19.

Kopp, R., 1995. Metaphor Therapy: Using Client-Generated Metaphors in Psychotherapy. Brunner, New York.

Kourkouta, L., Papathanasiou, I., 2014. Communication in nursing practice. Mater Sociomed. 26 (1), 65–67.

Lakoff, G., Johnson, M., 1980. Metaphors We Live By. University of Chicago Press, Chicago.

Linton, S., 2005. Understanding Pain for Better Clinical Practice. A Psychological Perspective. Elsevier, London.

Linton, S.J., Boersma, K., Vangronsveld, K., Fruzzetti, A., 2012. Painfully reassuring? The effects of validation on emotions and adherence in a pain test. Eur. J. Pain. 16 (4), 592–599.

Loftus, S., 2011. Pain and its metaphors: a dialogical approach. J. Med. Hum. 32, 213–230.

Mantel, H., 2013. How much pain is too much pain? IASP Insight Magazine 2 (1): 8-12.

Morris, D.B., 1991. The Culture of Pain. University of California Press, Berkeley.

Padfield, D., Janmohamed, F., Zakrzewska, J., Pither, C., Hurwitz, B., 2010. A slippery surface: can photographic images of pain improve communication in pain consultations? Int. J. Surg. 8 (2), 144–150.

Parsons, S., Harding, G., Breen, A., Foster, N., Pincus, T., Vogel, S., 2012. Will shared decision making between patients with chronic musculoskeletal pain and physiotherapists, osteopaths and chiropractors improve patient care? Fam. Pract 29 (2), 203–212.

Pinker, S., 2014. The sense of style: the thinking person's guide to writing in the 21st Century. Penguin, New York, NY.

Reith, T.P., 2018. Burnout in United States healthcare professionals: a narrative review. Cureus. 10 (12), e3681.

Scarry, E., 1985. The Body in Pain: The Making & Unmaking of the World. Oxford University Press, New York.

Schoeb, V., Staffoni, L., Parry, R., Pilnick, A., 2014. "What do you expect from physiotherapy?": a detailed analysis of goal setting within physiotherapy. Disabil. Rehabil. 36 (20), 1679–1686.

Scott-Dempster, C., Toye, F., Truman, J., et al., 2014. Physiotherapists' experiences of activity pacing with people with chronic musculoskeletal pain: an interpretative phenomenological analysis. Physiother. Theory. Pract. 30 (5), 319–328.

Semino, E., 2011. The adaptation of metaphors across genres. Rev. Cogn. Linguist. 9 (1), 130–152.

Sharon, L., Delany, T., Sweet, L., Battersby, M., Skinner, T., 2015. Barriers and enablers to good communication and information-sharing practices in care planning for chronic condition management. J. Prim. Health. 21 (1), 84–89.

Shinebourne, P., Smith, J., 2010. The communicative power of metaphors: an analysis and interpretation of metaphors in accounts of the experience of addiction. Psychol. Psychother. 83, 59–73.

Stenner, R., Swinkels, A., Mitchell, T., Palmer, S., 2015. Exercise prescription for non-specific chronic low back pain (NSCLBP): a qualitative study of patients' experiences of involvement in decision making. Physiotherapy 102 (4), 339–344.

Stewart, M., Ryan, S.-J., 2020. Do metaphors have therapeutic value for people in pain? A systematic review. J. Physiother. Pain. Assoc. 48, 10–22.

Tompkins P, Lawley J (2002) The mind, metaphor & health. Positive Health 78. 2-9.

Watt-Watson, J, J., McGillion, M., Hunter, J., Choiniere, M., Clark, A.J., Dewar, A., et al., 2009. A survey of prelicensure pain curricula in health science faculties in Canadian universities. Pain. Res. Manag. 14 (6), 439–444.

Chapter | 4 |

Social determinants of pain

Kenneth D. Craig and Samantha R. Fashler

LEARNING OBJECTIVES

At the end of this chapter, readers will have:
1. An understanding of the causal role of social determinants in the experience and expression of pain.
2. An evidence-based theoretical framework encompassing these social determinants, the social communication model of pain.
3. An understanding of how modifying social risk factors can be applied to prevent and control pain.

Overview

The social contexts of people's lives, past and present, are powerful determinants of the pain they experience. Social factors govern whether people will experience pain, what they think, feel and sense during the experience, how they behave and communicate their distress to others, and whether others will provide care to the person in pain. Thus presence, perception, expression, maintenance, exacerbation and respite from pain all are influenced by social factors. In this chapter, we provide a theoretical framework with supporting evidence to argue that social events have a strong causal impact on pain experience. By examining social determinants of pain, we redress the narrow, yet overwhelming, emphasis on biological processes and direct attention to the importance of the social environment in understanding and controlling pain.

Focus on social causes of pain provides a relatively novel perspective on understanding pain and pain management. It contributes to understanding how pain experience and expression are shaped by the familial and ethnocultural factors specific to each person's background. Furthermore, it encourages recognition that all efforts to prevent and control pain, whether biomedical or psychosocial, are inherently social in nature. Attending to how social systems structure delivery of care for people in pain in medical, occupational, familial and other environments has the potential to mitigate pervasive, inadequate and unsuccessful treatment of pain. This provides a basis for transforming and enhancing interventions, thereby extending the armamentarium beyond the sometimes inefficacious and at times harmful standard medical applications of drugs, surgery and other biologically oriented approaches.

There is considerable evidence supporting the importance of the biopsychosocial model as it applies to pain (Engel 1977; Gatchel et al. 2007; Ng et al. 2021; Turk & Okifuji 2002), but attention to biological features overwhelms the field. Pain should be appreciated as a complex perceptual experience with emotional, cognitive and social features, in addition to sensory features (Williams & Craig 2016). Social determinants of pain receive little attention, despite their importance in understanding inter- and intraindividual differences in pain experience and expression (Blyth et al. 2007; Morris 2010; Skevington & Matson 2004). Fortunately, pain research and management are shifting towards greater recognition of the importance of social factors and their impact on psychological features of the pain experience (Craig & MacKenzie 2021). This is reflected in a note accompanying the latest definition of pain developed by the International Association for the Study of Pain: 'Pain is always a personal experience that is influenced to varying degrees by biological, psychological, and social factors' (Raja et al. 2020, p. 1997).

Any incident of pain must be recognised as having multiple determinants. Proximate and distal causes often can be described when attempting to prioritise causal factors to manage intervention (Schwebel 2019). The pain of a workplace accident typically is attributed to injury, but the physical and social structure of the workplace may have made important contributions and must be considered in efforts to improve safety, prevent further painful injury, ease the resulting discomfort and reduce the personal and institutional costs of accidents. Distal interventions, including those that are preventive, may be the most cost-effective.

The position advocated here acknowledges the fundamental biological nature of pain. The dominant mechanistic theories of pain (specificity theory, pattern theory, the neuromatrix perspective, neural plasticity and central sensitisation, etc.) focus on biological phenomena (Cope 2010), but typically fail to place the role of pain in the context of personal and social lives of people. Increasingly, neurobiological variation in the response to painful events is attributed to social and cultural factors (Anderson & Losin 2017; Belfer 2013; Losin et al. 2020). Identifying the social causes of pain therefore supports a more comprehensive understanding of the nature of pain.

A focus on social processes is particularly important in understanding human pain. Diverse patterns of adaptive behaviour supporting survival are evident across species, with their complexity reflecting evolution of biological systems that sustain functioning in remarkably diverse environments. In all animals, including the simplest of organisms, pain serves to warn about tissue damage and motivates escape or avoidance behaviour. These specific adaptations designed to protect against physical insult have been conserved across species. Unique behavioural phenotypes can be understood as adaptations to specific ecological niches. Early in the evolutionary history of complex organisms, a capacity to utilise the social environment to provide protective care emerged. Organisms became social and interactions with other members of the species provided means for recognising and avoiding danger and providing protective care (de Waal 2009). In this context, pain also came to acquire social functions and roles.

Human capacities for social engagement extend the possibilities for protection from pain. Whether the human brain evolved because of the challenges of life in complex social environments or whether an evolved brain permitted the complex adaptations of human attachment, cooperation and communal living, these adaptations are integral features of human experience and living (DeSilva et al. 2021). They enhance opportunities for prevention and reduction of pain. The provision of care incorporating technological and healthcare system arrangements perhaps epitomises social engineering in the interests of minimising pain and suffering. It is not surprising that these unique human social capacities should be integrated with pain experience and its expression, and one would expect the human pain system to incorporate advanced capacities for cognitive and social functioning.

The social communication model of pain

The social communication model of pain provides a comprehensive and detailed framework for understanding biological and psychological features of pain, within a broad social context that recognises how humans engage with the world around them (Craig 2009) (Fig. 4.1). The following features of the model are examined as they unfold during an episode of pain in sequence: sources of pain, the experience of pain, how pain is communicated to others and how others recognise, interpret and respond to information about a person's pain. This process is dynamic and recursive. Each stage has an impact on whether the individual or others come to control the pain and whether the pain persists. Intrapersonal (biological and psychological) and interpersonal (social) factors interact at each stage. Unlike most models of pain, the social communication model of pain explicitly includes the reactions of caregivers and others as potentially implicated in the person's pain. It also acknowledges the impact of policies and organisational practices that determine whether care is made available to the person in pain.

Sources of pain: opportunities for prevention

Social circumstances often dictate whether people will be exposed to injury or disease. Therein lie opportunities for engaging in primary prevention, precluding the likelihood of pain before it happens. Epidemiological approaches to studying the distribution and determinants of pain have identified sociodemographic variations, social risk factors and population health trends in the prevalence and care of diverse painful conditions (Mansfield et al. 2016; von Korff & LeResche 2005). In establishing the complex web of causation, opportunities for prevention emerge. For example, oestrogen therapy for postmenopausal adult women is associated with increased risk of

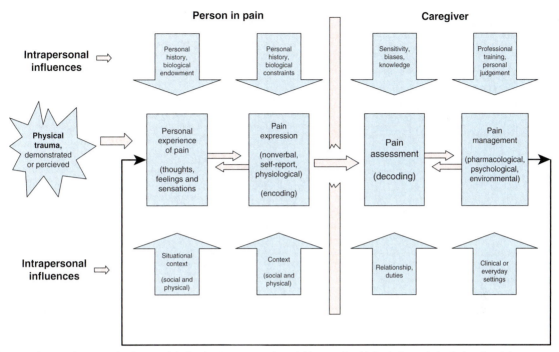

Fig. 4.1 The social communication model of pain. A conceptual model integrating biological, psychological and social perspectives at the level of interaction between the person in pain and persons present. (Adapted from Craig, K.D., Korol, C.T., 2008. Developmental issues in understanding, assessing, and managing pediatric pain. In: Walco, G., Goldschnieder, K. (Eds.), Pain in Children: A Practical Guide for Primary Care. Humana Press Inc., pp. 9–20, fig 2.1, with kind permission of Springer Science + Business Media.)

temporomandibular disorder (LeResche et al. 1997). Awareness of this relationship contributes to cost–benefit analysis of hormone-replacement therapy, perhaps decreasing the incidence of this painful condition. In this manner, public awareness of social factors may have an impact on use of a biomedical intervention strategy for chronic pain.

Characterisation of social origins as risk factors has received minimal attention, despite interests of epidemiologists in risk and ecological factors (Dworkin et al. 1992). Major categories of social risk factors can be conceptualised (Box 4.1). The illustrations are not exhaustive; they are designed to highlight potential social causes of pain across the major social contexts of people's lives. The balance between interpersonal and intrapersonal control of these sources of pain is not always evident. Some events may be the consequence of personal decisions of the person in pain, such as risk taking in dangerous sports, but social pressures and constraints influence such decisions. Pain imposed by others in the interests of the person's wellbeing, albeit accepted voluntarily, is perhaps best typified by medical procedures, including medical prophylaxis, diagnosis and treatment (including surgery). Medical

pain usually is construed as an undesirable, but inevitable, event. Nevertheless, recent interpretations characterise pain as an adverse event and argue that more should be done to preclude or mitigate pain (Chorney et al. 2010). Without special consideration, the experience of medical pain can be a reason to avoid seeking medical attention, such as pain resulting from needle injections (McMurtry et al. 2015). Fear of needles and associated pain can have far-reaching and public health consequences, as evidenced by avoidance of vaccination during the COVID-19 pandemic (Nazlı et al. 2021). Pain during childhood warrants special consideration for many reasons including the reality that pain conditions in childhood often continue into adulthood (Palermo 2020). For example, substantial neonatal exposure to pain is often characterised as the inevitable consequence of risk factors associated with preterm delivery, very low birth weight or congenital conditions. Nevertheless, there is reason to believe that early exposure to pain is often unnecessarily excessive and disposes infants to adverse pain experience and behaviour later in life (Grunau & Tu 2007). Similarly, early life experience of dental pain predisposes children and adults to dental fears and avoidance of treatment (Versloot & Craig 2009).

Many sources of pain encountered outside the healthcare system are shaped by social factors. Pain may be a consequence of intentional, aggressive acts, such as domestic violence, criminal behaviour, police enforcement or military action. Painful harm can also be a consequence of unintentional or voluntary exposure to risky settings in work, domestic, recreational or community environments, particularly when protective procedures, equipment or training are not provided or utilised. For example, workplace safety standards depend on policies and procedures and subsequent compliance by employers and employees. Similarly, major risks associated with driving a motor vehicle have been diminished by programs designed to enhance vehicular safety, such as use of seatbelts, child restraints, highway engineering, improved signage and markings, and reducing driving under the influence of drugs and alcohol. Social interventions have important roles in pain prevention. Similar consideration should be given to prevention of pain that is socially sanctioned in the absence of malicious intent and conducted with or without the full consent of the individual, as seen with male circumcision and female genital mutilation. The interaction between social events and the experience of pain is further complicated by consensual painful actions in which people undergo severe discomfort for cosmetic purposes (e.g. body piercing, tattoos, branding, scarification or plastic surgery) or for the sensation derived from the painful experience itself, as seen in masochism or self-inflicted injury. Similarly, neglecting to treat or assuage painful conditions with available resources represents another form of socially derived pain. Undertreatment of pain is widely reported in the elderly, among infants and children, with cancer pain, in emergency care, and during postoperative care (Hopp et al. 2014; Resnik and Rehm 2001).

Painful experiences may be maintained or exacerbated by social events. Stress accompanies both daily life and periods of major social adjustment and can contribute directly to psychophysiological disorders, lower immune functioning and promote tumour growth. This may compromise healing, thereby contributing to the manifestation, exacerbations and preservation of pain diseases and injuries (Antoni et al. 2006). Stressful family, employer or other relationships tend to have a negative impact on coping and result in increased healthcare utilisation. Under this strain, there is potential for vicious circles of family conflict, dysfunctional relationships, unemployment and social isolation that in turn perpetuate stress and pain. For example, parental physical and mental health contribute to interpersonal fear avoidance in children suffering from chronic pain (Birnie et al. 2020). Alleviating circumstances creating stress for the individual can have an impact on the experience and expression of pain. Pain associated with social injustices is experienced as more severe and debilitating (Miller et al. 2018; Scott et al. 2013).

The experience of pain

Sensory, affective and cognitive features of the experience of pain are shaped over the lifespan by familial/cultural influences and the social contexts of people's lives. Substantial and sometimes dramatic variations in how people react to and describe apparently comparable disease and injuries are well documented (Craig 2020; Fillingim 2010; Mogil 1999; Waller et al. 2021). This variability is usually represented as unidimensional: some people respond with considerable stoicism whereas others react with hysterical distress. This unidimensional perspective, however, fails to capture the richness and complexity of the cognitive, emotional and sensory features of painful experience (Williams et al. 2010). Complex thoughts reflecting prior episodes of pain, including the social contexts in which they are experienced, as well as the current context invariably accompany all painful experiences, including, 'What's happening to me?', 'How serious is this?', 'Will it last long?' and 'What can I do?'. Memories of painful events are shaped by how mothers and fathers reminisce about children's pain experiences (Noel et al. 2019). The pain experienced by children can be diminished through social engagement, including telling them stories (Brockington et al. 2021). In addition, emotional distress, such as anxiety and depression, greatly varies among patients. Of particular importance are maladaptive patterns of thinking, such as catastrophising (Sullivan et al. 2004) and hypervigilance (Van Damme et al. 2010), or emotional reactions, such as anxiety and fear avoidance (Vlaeyen & Linton 2000). These exacerbate and maintain dysfunctional pain and pain-related disability and influence the ability to benefit from treatment.

Although individual variations are conventionally described in terms of intrapersonal factors (e.g. the person is 'anxious' or 'catastrophising'), these emotions and thought patterns have origins in biological inheritance and life experience, with the latter including interpersonal events. The biological features of pain are of unquestioned importance (Mogil 1999). They can be 'hardwired', as exemplified by the capacity of even the prematurely born neonate to signal pain (Craig et al. 1993; Grunau & Craig 1987). In turn, such biologically endowed signalling patterns probably have social origins because of the success of cry, facial expression and other nonverbal behaviour in capturing parental attention and interventions, thereby enhancing the likelihood of survival. In humans, the biological systems reflect remarkable flexibility and transform with maturity and life experience.

Humans have adapted to remarkably different physical environments, as well as to social environments that vary dramatically in cultural customs and practices, socioeconomic opportunity, discrimination and prejudice, and access to healthcare (Keefe et al. 2005). Cultural variation includes differences in beliefs and practices concerning pain, reflecting unique histories in adapting to ecosystems and discovery of solutions to the challenges of physical danger (Craig & Pillai 2003). Culture-specific practices in the way we appraise and react emotionally to pain dominate people's lives from birth to death (Bates 1987; McCracken et al. 2001; Nayak et al. 2000; Zborowski 1969). In Western societies 40 plus years ago, infants were deemed to be insensitive to pain, and doctors responded in a culturally specific manner by not using anaesthetics during surgical procedures. But there has been a substantial shift in analgesic use in infants and young children; today, using less anaesthetic would be deemed primitive and inhuman, even though it was considered appropriate in the near past (American Academy of Pediatrics/Canadian Pediatric Society 2006). Similarly, at the opposite end of the life span, elderly people, particularly those with cognitive impairment, used to be deemed insensitive to pain (Hadjistavropoulos et al. 2007). Recent development of pain measures independent of self-report capability now indicate the capacity to experience pain is not impaired even though the ability to self-report is diminished by dementias and other impairments (Hadjistavropoulos et al. 2000; Kunz et al. 2007).

Human adaptive capabilities support adjustment to those family, ethnic and cultural environments in which the individual is born and raised. Maternal factors contribute to individual differences in infant behaviour very early in life (Pillai Riddell et al. 2007). Culture and family-specific dispositions to the challenges of pain are transferred through social learning to children, thereby determining the dynamics and structure of the painful experiences of succeeding generations. The intergenerational transfer of acquired meanings of pain has a strong basis in social experience (Goubert et al. 2011; Wilson et al. 2020). Pain cannot be experienced without

meanings; they become an integral feature of the experience.

Life experience provides ample opportunities for children to learn ways of experiencing and expressing pain through direct and vicarious experience (Van Lierde et al. 2020). The inevitable physical trauma of early childhood includes frequent opportunities for minor pain as a result of falls, sprains, cuts, burns and pain inflicted by age peers and adults (Fearon et al. 1996; von Baeyer et al. 1998). Direct experience vigorously instructs about hazards for painful experience and the consequences of exposure, including strategies for avoiding and minimising painful distress. The reactions of others to the child at risk or in pain also represent a major source of sociocultural influence as parents and significant others endeavour to shape the child's reactions in accordance with familial and cultural expectations (Campbell et al. 2018; Chambers et al. 2002; McMurtry et al. 2010). Concern for children's safety motivates parents to impose strong protective controls (Vervoort et al. 2019). Parental preoccupation with danger and safety lead to instruction on personal safety through physical guidance, warnings, verbal instruction, reinforcement of behaviour conforming to parental expectations and reprimands, criticism and other forms of punishment for failure to conform to strict demands. These parental appraisals and expectancies can be enforced by constructing safe environments, providing physical guidance, and supervising infants and younger children, progressively reducing scrutiny and supervision as children mature and acquire personal skills.

Observational learning greatly expands occasions for this type of learning without direct exposure to pain (Craig 1986; Goubert et al. 2011; Van Lierde et al. 2020). Most human skills are acquired through social modelling experiences (Bandura 1977). The benefits of this form of instruction are easily observed in nonhuman mammals (Mineka & Zinbarg 2006). In humans, social modelling represents a foundation for intergenerational transfer of cultural knowledge and emotional learning. Observational learning provides opportunities to learn with diminished personal threat in dangerous circumstances. Observers may note what happens to others when they are not prudent or protected by others, how the person in pain behaves (effectively and ineffectively) and the physical, psychological and social consequences of injury. Also noted is how others react to the person's distress and injuries. What is demonstrated and what is perceived reflects beliefs, expectancies, illness role models and accepted practices for expressing pain and providing for those in pain based on familial, community and cultural circumstances. Children exposed to atypical pain in the family, including excessive, recurrent or persistent pain, become vulnerable to atypical patterns of pain display (Beveridge et al. 2018; Craig 1986; Hermann 2006). Similarly, peer relationships can be expected to influence reactions to painful events with exclusion/inclusion in social groupings potentially leading to more severe or diminished pain (Fales & Noel 2020; Karos 2020). Persistent pain can also have long-lasting impacts on relationships with others leading to changes in social support patterns, depression and loneliness (Forgeron et al. 2018).

Successful socialisation includes acquisition of skills needed for self-management of pain. People may learn realistic ways of interpreting pain, acquire a sense of self-efficacy when confronting pain and develop emotional control appropriate to the situation. They come to understand social norms for various patterns of coping response and learn effective coping skills. In many ways, therapeutic instruction in pain self-management skills mimics this process. Experiences within the family, in contact with peers, or broader socialisation through use of media can also convey misinformation, maladaptive beliefs, misinterpretation of pain symptoms, adverse ways of thinking and coping with pain, emotional distress, fear and hypervigilance. Sullivan et al. (2004) have proposed a communal coping model of pain catastrophising, demonstrating that intrapersonal traits should be interpreted from an interpersonal perspective. The cognitive pattern (pain magnification, rumination and feelings of helplessness) serves social communication functions in that overt expressions solicit empathic responses and social support. Goubert et al. (2011) have similarly proposed a primarily observational learning account of the origins of destructive fear of pain.

How pain is communicated to others

Pain is often characterised as a private experience unknowable to others (Bustan 2016; Illich 1976), but this fails to acknowledge important social features. While detailed knowledge of sensory, affective and cognitive features of another's pain would not correspond to the reality of the experience, sources of information in behavioural reactions are very difficult to inhibit entirely (Craig et al. 1991). Public manifestations of pain that provide access to the subjective experience can be of great value to others, whether for purposes of self-interest, e.g. recognising danger, or providing care. Relatively stereotyped patterns of protective and communicative behaviour are observable in people in pain (Hadjistavropoulos & Craig 2002; Revicki et al. 2009). Some reactions indirectly communicate pain, for example, efforts to protect against pain by disengaging from contact with the noxious event. This withdrawal may be unconscious, such as in the case of nociceptive flexion reflexes that pull one's hand away from a red-hot object,

or more deliberate, such as limping as a more complex, integrated response typically used to control pain. Other actions directly communicate distress (and protect indirectly by engaging the assistance of others) through behaviours such as crying, facial grimaces, gestures (Rowbotham et al. 2013) and pleas for help (Sullivan 2008). Facial expressions that convey specific information about the subjective experience of the person during painful events are of particular importance, especially when the individual in pain is unable to communicate their discomfort verbally, as with infants and elderly people with cognitive impairment (Craig et al. 2011; Kappesser 2019; Kunz et al. 2019; Prkachin 1992). Especially with these populations, there is increasing interest in capturing behavioural and physiological reactions of painful events using computer vision, psychophysiological recording and machine learning to generate algorithms for pain severity to improve pain management (e.g. Susam et al. 2022).

Behavioural reactions reflect underlying neuroregulatory systems that can be characterised as automatic or controlled. Automatic reactions tend to be reflexive, unintentional and unconscious, whereas controlled reactions are voluntary, conscious and goal-oriented (Hadjistavropoulos & Craig 2002; McCrystal et al. 2011). Automatic reactions can be either immediately protective (e.g. defensive reflexes permitting escape from a source of pain) or communicative (e.g. facial grimaces of pain or certain vocalisations). Controlled reactions similarly include protective actions (e.g. using analgesic medication) and communicative behaviour (e.g. verbal report of pain). Controlled reactions are more likely to reflect socialisation experiences and to reflect their functional value (Akbari et al. 2020).

Some features of pain expression are biologically inherited reflexes, whereas others are acquired during socialisation in familial and cultural contexts. Newborn infants readily communicate painful distress through facial action, bodily movement and crying. These reflexive responses may have ancient social origins in genetic histories because of their functional value to the infant (Darwin 1871). As a child matures and acquires life experience, facial actions become increasingly amenable to voluntary control, although the basic structure of the facial expression remains consistent through the life span (Craig et al. 2011; Kunz et al. 2019). Vocalisations are similar: newborns cry reflexively in response to painful events (Grunau & Craig 1987). The cry subsequently acquires linguistic overtones as the capacity for language emerges (Lilley et al. 1997). Reflexive crying thereby transforms to become a speech act.

The use of language to convey painful distress to others is acquired slowly during the first years of life (Franck et al. 2010; Stanford et al. 2005). Language is culture specific, modelled within the child's family and community, and gradually refined as an effective communication tool. Developmental processes are important in understanding the expression of pain, with maturation of motor, cognitive, emotional and social capabilities subjected to the influence of life experience, social and otherwise (Craig & Korol 2008). It is noteworthy that automatic expression comprises both inherited reflexes and over-learned automatic behaviour that no longer requires purposeful or conscious decision making (Craig et al. 2010). Automatic manifestations appear to be most often observed during moderate to severe acute pain and exacerbations of chronic pain. Chronic pain patients not experiencing paroxysmal pain utilise controlled expression, including self-report and convincing depictions of pain distress, when interviewed about their current symptomatic status (Werner & Malerud 2003).

Both verbal and nonverbal behaviours have automatic and voluntary features. While verbal behaviour typically requires social skills and conscious deliberation, nonlinguistic features of verbalisations (e.g. pitch, amplitude, hesitancies, overtones) are less subject to purposeful control. Self-report of pain is often described as the gold standard for pain assessment, but it cannot be interpreted as a mirror of subjective experience. People do not always 'speak their mind' and when they do it seems notable—they are characterised as 'forthright', 'outspoken' or 'honest'. In particular, verbal behaviour is moderated because of its influence on others and consequently people vary in their report of symptoms (Mechanic 1986; Pennebaker 1982). Although nonverbal behaviour tends to be seen by others as less subject to personal control, a competent adult can effectively feign persuasive nonverbal expression (Hadjistavropoulos et al. 1996; Poole & Craig 1992) with skills acquired during childhood (Boerner et al. 2013; Larochette et al. 2006). Thus people use both verbal and nonverbal expression to achieve personal objectives. Incentives for faked or exaggerated pain may be financial (long-term disability payments, the outcome of litigation), access to potent drugs, avoidance of work or domestic duties, or manipulation of others through use of the sick role. Conversely, people can suppress pain expression to avoid social disapprobation (appearing weak or complaining), denial of usual roles (e.g. parent, worker, athlete), conformity to social demands and fearing sick role imposition (and its stigma), diagnoses, drugs, needles or other invasive procedures. Although numerous complex strategies have been devised for the detection of pain malingering, there is currently no reliable method for doing so (Tuck et al. 2019). Unfortunately, we lack a satisfactory understanding of pain misrepresentations; it is conceivable that the incidence of representing oneself as in pain or efforts to prevent others from knowing one is in pain is so low that the risk of false positives is not warranted as it can do harm to patients (Craig et al. 1999).

Acquisition of linguistic and social skills in pain expression is imperative if the individual is to be successful in persuading others to provide the best pain relief possible. The importance of this skill is perhaps most conspicuous in its absence, in people who have diminished capacity to elicit care from others (Hadjistavropoulos et al. 2010). This large group includes those who are critically ill, infants and young children, and people with cognitive and motor impairments. They frequently lack skills to effectively access healthcare and are handicapped further by current emphasis on self-report as the gold standard of pain assessment (Schiavenato & Craig 2010). Consequently, substantial evidence indicates that seniors with dementia are significantly under-treated for their pain compared to other seniors (Tsai & Chang 2004; van Herk et al. 2007; Zwakhalen et al. 2006), even though they do not differ in prevalence of chronic health conditions that lead to pain (Hadjistavropoulos et al. 2007; Herr et al. 2006; Smith 2005). Please refer to Chapters 8 and 20 for further consideration of understanding pain in a nonverbal individual. Achieving access to healthcare systems can be a greater challenge than is commonly acknowledged.

Pain expression is also contingent on the audience, reflecting the evolutionary benefit of different responses in the presence of different audiences, predators, enemies, or friends and kin. Disclosing vulnerability can be dangerous in the presence of predators and enemies, leading to at least the pretence of strength and resilience when in pain. Evidence suggests that stoical presentation is more common in the presence of others, particularly strangers, with people more expressive when alone (Badali 2008), yet social threat can provoke greater efforts to seek care (Karos et al. 2020). Culture influences whether people share or conceal their pain from their families and healthcare providers (Latimer et al. 2018; Tung & Li 2015). The presence of people of the same ethnicity leads to more intense pain expressions (Hsieh et al. 2011), whereas being around someone of high status diminishes expressions of painful distress (Campbell et al. 2017; Kállai et al. 2004). Depending on the cultural context and group, pain may be ignored (Dean et al. 2011), considered an indication of a fragile body (Rogers & Allison 2004), or perceived as a naturally occurring process (Lin et al. 2013). In the clinic, patients must present in a convincing manner if a physician is to provide access to medical care, including analgesics, psychotropics or surgery, as well as the diagnoses necessary to justify time off work or domestic duties, disability income, workers' compensation, insurance settlements and so forth. The challenge is perhaps greatest for patients with chronic pain who present without physical pathology to legitimate their needs (Werner & Malerud 2003). Diagnostic uncertainty associated with a lack of pathophysiology typically provokes a search for other causal factors, pain-related fear and purposive or unwitting avoidance of pain-related activities (Tanna et al. 2020).

How others recognise, interpret and respond to the person's pain

A major social determinant of pain is access to provision of care. Providing care requires recognition of pain, skills in assessment and treatment, and the physical resources necessary to accomplish required tasks. Successful recognition that a person is suffering from pain can be difficult to accomplish. In many cases, all the requisite cues are present, especially in the case of acute pain: the person reacts vigorously verbally and nonverbally, attempts are made to escape the noxious event, the source can be identified and tissue damage is evident. However, often one or more of these sources of information may be absent or there are suspicions of suppressing, exaggerating or faking pain (Poole & Craig 1992), with issues of trust then becoming important (e.g. Dassieu et al. 2021). The absence of tissue pathology is perceived as especially suspicious and is a common barrier for receiving proper treatment in patients with chronic, nonmalignant pain.

The neuroregulatory systems responsible for automatic and controlled pain expression also play a role in observer reactions (Craig et al. 2010). Witnessing others displaying pain provokes major peripheral and central nervous system activity, as demonstrated by studies of autonomic arousal (Craig & Prkachin 1978) and brain imaging (Jackson et al. 2006; Ochsner et al. 2008; Simon et al. 2006), often with lasting impact on the observer (Simons et al. 2016). These studies indicate that personal and vicarious experiences can be differentiated physiologically, findings consistent with engagement of higher-level processes when observers seek to understand another person's distress. The observer typically is not beset by painful distress to the same extreme and can benefit from learning about the other's experiences. This provides an opportunity to learn about what constitutes potentially painful circumstances based on another individual's display of pain (e.g. a grimace and groan), how other people respond to the display of pain and how other observers react to the person's distress, behaviour and circumstances. Substantial variation characterises the reactions of observers to the pain expression of others (Akbari et al. 2020) with personal characteristics (Bartley et al. 2015) and contextual variables (Twigg & Byrne 2015) often determining decisions about providing care. Observer reactions are likely to depend on the relationship between the person in pain and the observer. Kin and friend motivation reflect inherent biological dispositions to provide care, enemies to

exacerbate or exploit distress, and healthcare practitioners may or may not be motivated to intervene, depending on professional duties and financial incentives.

A model of empathic reactions to others in pain (Goubert et al. 2005) distinguishes 'bottom-up' input to the observer's reactions (the expressive behaviour of the person in pain, as well as salient situational events, including the source of pain and evidence of tissue damage) from 'top-down' processing of this information, whereby the observer appraises and comes to understand the person's predicament. The observer brings to the situation not only ancient, intuitive dispositions to react emotionally, but also capacities to arrive at a considered judgement as to what is happening. This may reflect rational and probabilistic understanding, perhaps a consequence of professional education and training. However, understanding is also vulnerable to personal biases because of personal experience, idiosyncratic belief and attitudinal systems, and subculture myths. In consequence, the observer may overreact (Goubert et al. 2009) or underreact, as is evident in widespread tendencies to underestimate pain in others (Chambers et al. 1999; Kappesser et al. 2006; Prkachin et al. 2007). Both response patterns have immediate and long-term consequences (Brandao et al. 2019), with a potentially detrimental effect on the person in pain (Fales et al. 2014).

Social policy and healthcare delivery

The likelihood that appropriate care for pain is made available is determined by broad social policies concerning healthcare and the social and cultural environments (Rashiq et al. 2008). Systems factors representing standards of care, public policy and access to resources are important determinants of care for people in pain. Healthcare politics and ideologies (e.g. universal public healthcare vs private healthcare), socioeconomic resources (national and regional economic disparities; Bonham 2001), dominant beliefs concerning various forms of treatment (e.g. use of opioids, requirements for empirically supported interventions) and ethical principles (Craig & Shriver 2021) determine provision of care. The determinants are informed to the extent that research has been available to establish innovative and superior practices. It is increasingly recognised that access to care is governed by racial, ethnic and socioeconomic demographic factors (Morales & Yong 2021; Summers et al. 2021; Wallace et al. 2021; also see Chapter 22). Given the large number of people for whom pain research and pain management have failed to relieve pain (Resnik & Rehm 2001), it is evident that current healthcare policies are ineffective for many patients. This can be described as widespread discrimination against these patients. The Canadian Pain

Task Force Report (2020) noted systems barriers leading to shortages of healthcare professionals and multidisciplinary care, long waitlists and financial barriers, particularly for people with low incomes or those without private or public insurance. There is a clear shortfall of multidisciplinary pain treatment facilities in Canada (Choinière et al. 2020). Patients, their families and significant others often become angry and frustrated about the inadequacies of public policies, compensation and insurance programs, and healthcare providers regarding unresolved chronic pain (Walker et al. 2007).

Conclusion

Pain is suffered by the individual, but it always occurs in complex social contexts driven by family, vocational, community, political, and cultural factors. These factors influence the extent to which pain is suffered, how it is experienced and expressed, how it is interpreted by others, and whether or not care will be provided. Dissatisfaction with care has led to pressures for change in the current system of delivery of health services. Social determinants of pain must receive attention in examining the nature and quality of services for people in pain to ensure optimal care for everyone. Recognition of the contributions of social factors to the experience of pain supports a multidimensional model of pain, advances interdisciplinary care and supports use of nonmedical interventions, such as cognitive behavioural therapy and instruction in self-management. There are many opportunities for improvement, including introducing preventive interventions, teaching people to self-regulate and accurately communicate their painful experiences, improving the decision-making capacities of healthcare providers, and revising public and institutional policies, standards and practices for the delivery of care.

Review Questions

1. Why is it important to consider social processes in understanding human pain?
2. How might the greater recognition of social factors provide opportunities to prevent pain?
3. What are some social risk factors for the development of pain?
4. In what ways are the experience and display of pain a social interaction?
5. Other than self-report, what are other ways that pain can be communicated and assessed?

References

Akbari, F., Dehgamani, M., Mohammadi, S., Goubert, L., Sanderman, R., Hagedoorn, M., 2020. Why do patients engage in pain behaviors? A qualitative study examining the perspective of patients and partners. Clin. J. Pain 36 (10), 750–756.

American Academy of Pediatrics/Canadian Pediatric Society, 2006. Prevention and management of pain in the neonate. Pediatrics 118 (5), 2231–2241.

Anderson, S.R., Losin, E.A.R., 2017. A sociocultural neuroscience approach to pain. Culture Brain 5, 14–35.

Antoni, M.H., Lutgendorf, S.K., Cole, S.W., Dhabhar, F.S., Sephton, S.E., McDonald, P.G., 2006. The influence of bio-behavioural factors on tumour biology: pathways and mechanisms. Nat. Rev. Cancer 6 (3), 240–248.

Badali, M.A., 2008. Experimenter Audience Effects on Young Adults' Facial Expressions during Pain [Unpublished Doctoral Dissertation]. University of British Columbia.

Bandura, A., 1977. Social Learning Theory. General Learning Press.

Bartley, E.J., Boissoneault, J., Vargovich, A.M., Wandner, L.D., Hirsh, A.T., Lok, B.C., et al., 2015. The influence of health care professional characteristics on pain management decisions. Pain Med. 16 (1), 99–111.

Bates, A.M.S., 1987. Ethnicity and pain: a biocultural model. Soc. Sci. Med. 24 (1), 47–50.

Belfer, I., 2013. Nature and Nurture of Human Pain. Scientifica. https://doi.org/10.101155/2013/415279. Epublish 415279.

Beveridge, J.K., Neville, A., Wilson, A.C., Noel, M., 2018. Intergenerational examination of pain and posttraumatic stress disorder symptoms among youth with chronic pain and their parents. Pain. Rep. 11, e667.

Birnie, K.A., Heathcote, L.C., Bhandari, R.P., Feinstein, A., Yoon, I.A., Simons, L.E., 2020. Parent physical and mental health contributions to interpersonal fear avoidance processes in pediatric chronic pain. Pain 161 (6), 1202–1211.

Blyth, F.M., Macfarlane, G.J., Nicholas, M.K., 2007. The contribution of psychosocial factors to the development of chronic pain: the key to better outcomes for patients? Pain 129 (1–2), 8–11.

Boerner, K.E., Chambers, C.T., Craig, K.D., Pillai Riddell, R.R., Parker, J.A., 2013. Caregiver accuracy in detecting deception in facial expressions of pain in children. Pain 154 (4), 525–533.

Bonham, V.L., 2001. Race, ethnicity, and pain treatment: striving to understand the causes and solutions to the disparities in pain treatment. J. Law Med. Ethics 29 (1), 52–68.

Brandao, T., Campos, L., de Ruddere, L., Goubert, L., Bernardes, S.F., 2019. Classism in pain care: the role of socioeconomic status on nurses' pain assessment and management practice. Pain Med. 20 (11), 2094–2105.

Brockington, G., Moreira, A.P.G., Buso, M.S., da Silva, S.G., Altszyler, E., Fischer, R., et al., 2021. Storytelling increases oxytocin and positive emotions and decreases cortisol and pain in hospitalized children. Proc. Natl. Acad. Sci. 118 (22) e2018409118.

Bustan, S., 2016. Voicing pain and suffering through linguistic agents: nuancing Elaine Scarry's view on the inability to express pain. Subjectivity 9 (4), 363–380.

Campbell, P., Hope, K., Dunn, K.M., 2017. The pain, depression, disability pathway in those with low back pain: a moderation analysis of health locus of control. J. Pain Res. 10, 2331–2339.

Campbell, L., Pillai Riddell, R., Cribbie, R., Garfield, H., Greenberg, S., 2018. Preschool children's coping responses and outcomes in the vaccination context: child and caregiver transactional and longitudinal relationships. Pain 159 (2), 314–330.

Canadian Pain Task Force, 2020. Working Together to Better Understand, Prevent and Manage Chronic Pain: What We Heard. https://publications.gc.ca/collections/collection_2020/sc-hc/H134-17-2020-eng.pdf.

Chambers, C.T., Reid, G.J., Craig, K.D., McGrath, P.J., Finley, G.A., 1999. Agreement between child and parent reports of pain. Clin. J. Pain 14 (4), 336–342.

Chambers, C.T., Craig, K.D., Bennett, S.M., 2002. The impact of maternal behavior on children's pain experiences: an experimental analysis. J. Pediatr. Psychol. 27 (3), 293–301.

Choinière, M., Peng, P., Gilron, I., Buckley, N., Williamson, O., Janelle-Montcalm, A., et al., 2020. Accessing care in multidisciplinary pain treatment facilities continues to be a challenge in Canada. Reg. Anesth. Pain Med. 45 (12), 943–948.

Chorney, J.M., McGrath, P., Finley, G.A., 2010. Pain as the neglected adverse event. CMAJ (Can. Med. Assoc. J.) 182 (7), 732.

Cope, D.K., 2010. Intellectual milestones in our understanding and treatment of pain. In: Fishman, S.M., Ballantyne, J.C., Rathnell, J.P. (Eds.), Bonica's Management of Pain. Wolters Kluwer/Lippincott Williams & Wilkins, Philadelphia, pp. 1–12.

Craig, K.D., 1986. Social modeling influences: pain in context. In: Sternbach, R.A. (Ed.), The Psychology of Pain, second ed. Raven Press, New York, pp. 67–96.

Craig, K.D., 2009. The social communication model of pain. Can. Psychol/Psychol. Can 50 (1), 22–32.

Craig, K.D., 2020. A child in pain: a psychologist's perspective on changing priorities in scientific understanding and clinical care. Pediatric. & Neonatal. Pain 2 (2), 40–49.

Craig, K.D., Korol, C.T., 2008. Developmental issues in understanding, assessing, and managing pediatric pain. In: Walco, G., Goldschnieder, K. (Eds.), Pediatric Pain Management in Primary Care: A Practical Guide. Humana Press Inc., pp. 9–20.

Craig, K.D., MacKenzie, N.E., 2021. What is pain: are cognitive and social features core components? Paediatric. and. Neonatal. Pain 3, 106–118.

Craig, K.D., Pillai Riddell, R., 2003. Social influences, ethnicity, and culture. In: Finley, G.A., McGrath, P.J. (Eds.), The Context of Pediatric Pain: Biology, Family, Society, and Culture. IASP Press, pp. 159–182.

Craig, K.D., Prkachin, K.M., 1978. Social modeling influences on sensory decision theory and psychophysiological indexes of pain. J. Pers. Soc. Psychol. 36 (8), 805–815.

Craig, K.D., Shriver, A., 2021. Ethics of pain management in infants and children. In: Stevens, B., Hathway, G., Zempsky, W. (Eds.), Oxford Textbook of Pediatric Pain, second ed. Oxford University Press, pp. 649–659.

Craig, K.D., Hyde, S.A., Patrick, C.J., 1991. Genuine, suppressed, and faked facial behavior during exacerbation of chronic low back pain. Pain 46 (2), 161–172.

Craig, K.D., Whitfield, M.F., Grunau, R.V.E., Linton, J., Hadjistavropoulos, H.D., 1993. Pain in the pre-term neonate: behavioural and physiological indices. Pain 52 (3), 287–299.

Craig, K.D., Hill, M.L., McMurtry, B., 1999. Detecting deception and malingering. In: Block, A.R., Kramer, E.F., Fernandez, E. (Eds.), Handbook of Chronic Pain Syndromes: Biopsychosocial Perspectives. Lawrence Erlbaum, Mahwah, pp. 41–58.

Craig, K.D., Versloot, J., Goubert, L., Vervoort, T., Crombez, G., 2010. Perceiving others in pain: automatic and controlled mechanisms. J. Pain 11 (2), 101–108.

Craig, K.D., Prkachin, K.M., Grunau, R.V.E., 2011. The facial expression of pain. In: Turk, D., Melzack, R. (Eds.), Handbook of Pain Assessment, third ed. Guilford, pp. 117–133.

Darwin, C., 1871. The Descent of Man. Appleton and Company, New York.

Dassieu, L., Heino, A., Develay, E., Kaboré, J.L., Pagé, M.G., Moor, G., et al., 2021. "They think you're trying to get the drug": qualitative investigation of chronic pain patients' health care experiences during the opioid overdose epidemic in Canada. Can. J. Pain 5 (1), 66–80.

de Waal, F., 2009. The Age of Empathy. Harmony Books, New York.

Dean, S.G., Hudson, S., Hay-Smith, E.J.C., Milosavljevic, S., 2011. Rural workers' experience of low back pain: exploring why they continue to work. J. Occup. Rehabil. 21 (3), 395–409.

DeSilva, J.M., Traniello, J.F.A., Claxton, A.G., Fannin, L.D., 2021. When and why did human brains decrease in size: a new change-point analysis and insights from brain evolution in ants. Frontiers in Ecology and Evolution vol 9 Article 742639.

Dworkin, S.F., Von Korff, M., LeResche, L., 1992. Epidemiologic studies of chronic pain: a dynamic- ecologic perspective. Ann. Behav. Med. 14, 3–11.

Engel, G.L., 1977. The need for a new medical model: a challenge for biomedicine. Science 196 (4286), 129–136.

Fales, J.L., Noel, M., 2020. The effects of brief social exclusion on pain perception and pain memory in adolescents. J. Adolesc. Health 66 (5), 623–625.

Fales, J.L., Essner, B.S., Harris, M.A., Palermo, T.M., 2014. When helping hurts: miscarried helping in families of youth with chronic pain. J. Pediatr. Psychol. 39 (4), 427–437.

Fearon, I., McGrath, P.J., Achat, H., 1996. 'Booboos': the study of everyday pain among young children. Pain 68 (1), 55–62.

Fillingim, R.B., 2010. Individual differences in pain: the roles of gender, ethnicity and genetics. In: Fishman, S.M., Ballantyne, J.C., Rathnell, J.P. (Eds.), Bonica's Management of Pain. Wolters Kluwer/ Lippincott Williams & Wilkins, Philadelphia, pp. 86–97.

Forgeron, P.A., Chambers, C.T., Cohen, J., Dick, B.D., Finley, G.A., Lamontagne, C., 2018. Dyadic differences in friendship of adolescents with chronic pain compared with pain-free peers. Pain 159 (6), 1103–1111.

Franck, L., Noble, G., Liossi, C., 2010. From tears to words: the development of language to express pain in young children with everyday minor illnesses and injuries. Child Care Health Dev. 36 (4), 524–533.

Gatchel, R.J., Peng, Y.B., Peters, M.L., Fuchs, P.N., Turk, D.C., 2007. The biopsychosocial approach to chronic pain: scientific advances and future directions. Psychol. Bull. 133 (4), 581–624.

Goubert, L., Craig, K.D., Vervoort, T., Morley, S., Sullivan, M.J., de CAC, W., et al., 2005. Facing others in pain: the effects of empathy. Pain 118 (3), 286–288.

Goubert, L., Vervoort, T., Cano, A.M., Crombez, G., 2009. Catastrophizing about their children's pain is related to higher parent-child congruency in pain ratings: an experimental investigation. Eur. J. Pain 13 (2), 196–201.

Goubert, L., Vlaeyen, J.W.S., Crombez, G., Craig, K.D., 2011. Learning about pain from others: an observational learning account. J. Pain 12 (2), 167–174.

Grunau, R.V.E., Craig, K.D., 1987. Pain expression in neonates: facial action and cry. Pain 28 (3), 395–410.

Grunau, R.E., Tu, M.T., 2007. Long-term consequences of pain in human neonates. In: Anand, K.J.S., Stevens, B.J., McGrath, P.J. (Eds.), Pain in Neonates, third ed. Elsevier Science, pp. 45–55.

Hadjistavropoulos, T., Craig, K.D., 2002. A theoretical framework for understanding self-report and observational measures of pain: a communications model. Behav. Res. Ther. 40 (5), 551–570.

Hadjistavropoulos, H.D., Craig, K.D., Hadjistavropoulos, T., Poole, G.D., 1996. Subjective judgments of deception in pain expression: accuracy and errors. Pain 65 (2–3), 251–258.

Hadjistavropoulos, T., LaChapelle, D.L., MacLeod, F.K., Snider, B., Craig, K.D., 2000. Measuring movement-exacerbated pain in cognitively impaired frail elders. Clin. J. Pain 16 (1), 54–63.

Hadjistavropoulos, T., Herr, K., Turk, D.C., Fine, P.G., Dworkin, R.H., Helme, R., et al., 2007. An interdisciplinary expert consensus statement on assessment of pain in older persons. Clin. J. Pain 23 (Suppl. 1), 1–43.

Hadjistavropoulos, T., Breau, L., Craig, K.D., 2010. Pain assessment in adults and children with limited ability to communicate. In: Turk, D.C., Melzack, R. (Eds.), Handbook of Pain Assessment, third ed. Guilford Press, pp. 260–282.

Hermann, C., 2006. Modeling, social learning in pain. In: Schmidt, R.F., Willis, W.D. (Eds.), The Encyclopedia of Pain. Springer Publishing, pp. 1168–1170.

Herr, K., Bjoro, K., Decker, S., 2006. Tools for assessment of pain in nonverbal older adults with dementia: a state-of-the-science review. J. Pain. Symptom. Manage. 31 (2), 170–192.

Hopp, M., Bosse, B., Dunlop, W., 2014. The socioeconomic costs of the undertreatment of pain. Value Health 17 (7), A785.

Hsieh, A.Y., Tripp, D.A., Ji, L.J., 2011. The influence of ethnic concordance and discordance on verbal reports and nonverbal behaviours of pain. Pain 152 (9), 2016–2022.

Illich, I., 1976. Medical Nemesis: The Expropriation of Health. Random House, New York.

Jackson, P.L., Rainville, P., Decety, J., 2006. To what extent do we share the pain of others? Insight from the neural bases of pain empathy. Pain 125 (1), 5–9.

Kállai, I., Barke, A., Voss, U., 2004. The effects of experimenter characteristics on pain reports in women and men. Pain 112 (1–2), 142–147.

Kappesser, J., 2019. The facial expression of pain in humans considered from a social perspective. Philos. Trans. R. Soc. Lond. B Biol. Sci. 374 (1785), 1–7.

Kappesser, J., Williams, A.C.D.C., Prkachin, K.M., 2006. Testing two accounts of pain underestimation. Pain 124 (1–2), 109–116.

Karos, K., 2020. The enduring mystery of pain in a social context. J. Adolesc. Health 66 (5), 524–525.

Karos, K., Meulders, A., Goubert, L., Vlaeyen, J.W., 2020. Hide your pain: social threat increases pain reports and aggression, but reduces facial pain expression and empathy. J. Pain 21 (3–4), 334–346.

Keefe, F.J., Dixon, K.E., Pryor, R.W., 2005. Psychological contributions to the understanding and treatment of pain. In: Merskey, H., Loeser, J.D., Dubner, R. (Eds.), The Paths of Pain 1975–2005. IASP Press, pp. 403–420.

Kunz, M., Scharmann, S., Hemmeter, U., Schepelmann, K., Lautenbacher, S., 2007. The facial expression of pain in patients with dementia. Pain 133 (1–3), 221–228.

Kunz, M., Meixner, D., Lautenbacher, S., 2019. Facial muscle movements encoding pain—a systematic review. Pain 160 (3), 535–549.

Larochette, A.C., Chambers, C.T., Craig, K.D., 2006. Genuine, suppressed and faked facial expressions of pain in children. Pain 126 (1–3), 64–71.

Latimer, M., Sylliboy, J.R., MacLeod, E., Rudderham, S., Francis, J., Hutt-MacLeod, D., et al., 2018. Creating a safe space for First Nations youth to share their pain. Pain. Rep. 3 (Suppl. 1), e682.

LeResche, L., Saunders, K., Von Korff, M.R., Barlow, W., Dworkin, S.F., 1997. Use of exogenous hormones and risk of temporomandibular disorder pain. Pain 69 (1–2), 153–160.

Lilley, C.M., Craig, K.D., Grunau, R.E., 1997. The expression of pain in infants and toddlers: developmental changes in facial action. Pain 72 (1–2), 161–170.

Lin, I.B., O'Sullivan, P.B., Coffin, J.A., Mak, D.B., Toussaint, S., Straker, L.M., 2013. Disabling chronic low back pain as an iatrogenic disorder: a qualitative study in Aboriginal Australians. BMJ Open 3 (4), e002654.

Losin, E.A.R., Woo, C.W., Medina, N.A., Andrews-Hanna, J.R., Eisenbarth, H., Wager, T.D., 2020. Neural and sociocultural mediators of ethnic differences in pain. Nat. Human Behav. 4 (5), 517–530.

Mansfield, K.E., Sim, J., Jordan, J.L., Jordan, K.P., 2016. A systematic review and meta-analysis of the prevalence of chronic widespread pain in the general population. Pain 157 (1), 55–64.

McCracken, L.M., Matthews, A.K., Tang, T.S., Cuba, S.L., 2001. A comparison of blacks and whites seeking treatment for chronic pain. Clin. J. Pain 17 (3), 249–255.

McCrystal, K.N., Craig, K.D., Versloot, J., Fashler, S.R., Jones, D.N., 2011. Perceiving pain in others: validation of a dual processing model. Pain 152 (5), 1083–1089.

McMurtry, C.M., Chambers, C.T., McGrath, P.J., Asp, E., 2010. When "don't worry" communicates fear: children's perceptions of parental reassurance and distraction during a painful medical procedure. Pain 150 (1), 52–58.

McMurtry, C.M., Riddell, R.P., Taddio, A., Racine, N., Asmundson, G.J., Noel, M., et al., 2015. Far from "just a poke": common painful needle procedures and the development of needle fear. Clin. J. Pain 31, S3–S11.

Mechanic, D., 1986. The concept of illness behaviour: culture, situation and personal predisposition1. Psychol. Med. 16 (1), 1–7.

Miller, M.M., Wuest, D., Williams, A.E., Scott, E.L., Trost, Z., Hirsh, A.T., 2018. Injustice perceptions about pain: parent–child discordance is associated with worse functional outcomes. Pain 159 (6), 1083–1089.

Mineka, S., Zinbarg, R., 2006. A contemporary learning theory perspective on the etiology of anxiety disorders: it's not what you thought it was. Am. Psychol. 61 (1), 10–26.

Mogil, J.S., 1999. The genetic mediation of individual differences in sensitivity to pain and its inhibition. Pro. Natl. Acad. Sci. 96 (14), 7744–7751.

Morales, M.E., Yong, R.J., 2021. Racial and ethnic disparities in the treatment of chronic pain. Pain. Med. 22 (1), 75–90.

Morris, D.G., 2010. Sociocultural dimensions of pain management. In: Fishman, S.M., Ballantyne, J.C., Rathnell, J.P. (Eds.), Bonica's Management of Pain. Wolters Kluwer/Lippincott Williams & Wilkins, Philadelphia, pp. 133–144.

Nayak, S., Shiflett, S.C., Eshun, S., Levine, F.M., 2000. Culture and gender effects in pain beliefs and the prediction of pain tolerance. Cross Cult. Res. 34 (2), 135–151.

Nazlı, Ş.B., Yığman, F., Sevindik, M., Özturan, D.D., 2021. Psychological factors affecting COVID-19 vaccine hesitancy. Ir. J. Med. Sci. 1–10.

Ng, W., Slater, H., Starcevich, C., Wright, A., Mitchell, T., Beales, D., 2021. Barriers and enablers influencing healthcare professionals' adoption of a biopsychosocial approach to musculoskeletal pain: a systematic review and qualitative evidence synthesis. Pain 162, 2154–2185.

Noel, M., Pavlova, M., Lund, T., Jordan, A., Chorney, J., Rasic, N., et al., 2019. The role of narrative in the development of children's pain memories: influences of father–and mother–child reminiscing on children's recall of pain. Pain 160 (8), 1866–1875.

Ochsner, K.N., Zaki, J., Hanelin, J., Ludlow, D.H., Knierim, K., Ramachandran, T., et al., 2008. Your pain or mine? Common and distinct neural systems supporting the perception of pain in self and other. Soc. Cognit. Affect Neurosci. 3 (2), 144–160.

Palermo, T.M., 2020. Pain prevention and management must begin in childhood: the key role of psychological interventions. Pain 161 (Suppl. l), S114–S121.

Pennebaker, J.W., 1982. The Psychology of Physical Symptoms. Springer-Verlag.

Pillai Riddell, R.R., Stevens, B.J., Cohen, L.L., Flora, D.B., Greenberg, S., 2007. Predicting maternal and behavioral measures of infant pain: the relative contribution of maternal factors. Pain 133 (1–3), 138–149.

Poole, G.D., Craig, K.D., 1992. Judgments of genuine, suppressed, and faked facial expressions of pain. J. Pers. Soc. Psychol. 63 (5), 797–805.

Prkachin, K.M., 1992. The consistency of facial expressions of pain: a comparison across modalities. Pain 51 (3), 297–306.

Prkachin, K.M., Solomon, P.E., Ross, J., 2007. Underestimation of pain by health-care providers: towards a model of the process of inferring pain in others. Can. J. Nurs. Res. 39, 88–106.

Raja, S.N., Carr, D.B., Cohen, M., Finnerup, N.B., Flor, H., Gibson, S., et al., 2020. The revised International Association for the Study of Pain definition of pain: concepts, challenges, and compromises. Pain 161 (9), 1976–1982.

Rashiq, S., Schopflocher, D., Taenzer, P., Jonsson, E. (Eds.), 2008. Chronic Pain: A Health Policy Perspective. Wiley-VCH, Weinheim.

Resnik, D.B., Rehm, M., 2001. The undertreatment of pain: scientific, clinical, cultural, and philosophical factors. Med. Health. Care. Philos. 4 (3), 277–288.

Revicki, D.A., Chen, W.H., Harnam, N., Cook, K.F., Amtmann, D., Callahan, L.F., et al., 2009. Development and psychometric analysis of the PROMIS pain behavior item bank. Pain 146 (1–2), 158–169.

Rogers, A., Allison, T., 2004. What if my back breaks? Making sense of musculoskeletal pain among South Asian and African–Caribbean people in the North West of England. J. Psychosom. Res. 57 (1), 79–87.

Rowbotham, S., Wearden, A., Lloyd, D., Holler, J., 2013. A descriptive analysis of the role of co-speech gestures in the representation of information about pain quality. Health Psychology Update 22 (1), 19–25.

Schiavenato, M., Craig, K.D., 2010. Pain assessment as a social transaction: beyond the "gold standard". Clin. J. Pain 26 (8), 667–676.

Schwebel, D.C., 2019. Why "accidents" are not accidental: using psychological science to understand and prevent unintentional child injuries. Am. Psychol. 74 (9), 1137–1147.

Scott, W., Trost, Z., Bernier, E., Sullivan, M.J., 2013. Anger differentially mediates the relationship between perceived injustice and chronic pain outcomes. Pain 154 (9), 1691–1698.

Simon, D., Craig, K.D., Miltner, W.H., Rainville, P., 2006. Brain responses to dynamic facial expressions of pain. Pain 126 (1–3), 309–318.

Simons, L.E., Goubert, L., Vervoort, T., Borsook, D., 2016. Circles of engagement: childhood pain and parent brain. Neurosci. Biobehav. Rev. 68, 537–546.

Skevington, S.M., Mason, V.L., 2004. Social influences on individual differences in responding to pain. In: Hadjistavropoulos, T., Craig, K.D. (Eds.), Pain: Psychological Perspectives. Lawrence Erlbaum Associates, pp. 179–208.

Smith, M., 2005. Pain assessment in nonverbal older adults with advanced dementia. Perspect. Psychiatr. Care 41 (3), 99–113.

Stanford, E.A., Chambers, C.T., Craig, K.D., 2005. A normative analysis of the development of pain-related vocabulary in children. Pain 114 (1–2), 278–284.

Sullivan, M.J., 2008. Toward a biopsychomotor conceptualization of pain: implications for research and intervention. Clin. J. Pain 24 (4), 281–290.

Sullivan, M.J., Adams, H., Sullivan, M.E., 2004. Communicative dimensions of pain catastrophizing: social cueing effects on pain behaviour and coping. Pain 107 (3), 220–226.

Summers, K.M., Deska, J.C., Almaraz, S.M., Hugenberg, K., Lloyd, E.P., 2021. Poverty and pain: low-SES people are believed to be insensitive to pain. J. Exp. Soc. Psychol. 95, 104116.

Susam, B.T., Riek, N.T., Akcakaya, M., Xu, X., De Sa, V.R., Nezamfar, H., et al., 2022. Automated pain assessment in children using electrodermal activity and video data fusion via machine learning. IEEE Trans. Biomed. Eng. 69 (1), 422–431.

Tanna, V., Heathcote, L.C., Heirich, M.S., Rush, G., Neville, A., Noel, M., et al., 2020. Something else going on? Diagnostic uncertainty in children with chronic pain and their parents. Children 7 (10), 165.

Tsai, P.F., Chang, J.Y., 2004. Assessment of pain in elders with dementia. Medsurg Nurs. 13 (6), 364.

Tuck, N.L., Johnson, M.H., Bean, D.J., 2019. You'd better believe it: the conceptual and practical challenges of assessing malingering in patients with chronic pain. J. Pain 20 (2), 133–145.

Tung, W.C., Li, Z., 2015. Pain beliefs and behaviors among Chinese. Home Health Care Manag. Pract. 27 (2), 95–97.

Turk, D.C., Okifuji, A., 2002. Psychological factors in chronic pain: evolution and revolution. J. Consult. Clin. Psychol. 70 (3), 678.

Twigg, O.C., Byrne, D.G., 2015. The influence of contextual variables on judgments about patients and their pain. Pain Med. 16 (1), 88–98.

Van Damme, S., Legrain, V., Vogt, J., Crombez, G., 2010. Keeping pain in mind: a motivational account of attention to pain. Neurosci. Biobehav. Rev. 34 (2), 204–213.

Van Herk, R., Van Dijk, M., Baar, F.P., Tibboel, D., De Wit, R., 2007. Observation scales for pain assessment in older adults with cognitive impairments or communication difficulties. Nurs. Res. 56 (1), 34–43.

Van Lierde, E., Goubert, L., Vervoort, T., Hughes, G., Van den Bussche, E., 2020. Learning to fear pain after observing another's pain: an experimental study in schoolchildren. Eur. J. Pain 24 (4), 791–806.

Versloot, J., Craig, K.D., 2009. The communication of pain in paediatric dentistry. Eur. Arch. Paediatr. Dent. 10 (2), 61–66.

Vervoort, T., Karos, K., Johnson, D., Sütterlin, S., Van Ryckeghem, D., 2019. Parental emotion and pain control behaviour when faced with child's pain: the emotion regulatory role of parental pain-related attention-set shifting and heart rate variability. Pain 160 (2), 322–333.

Vlaeyen, J.W., Linton, S.J., 2000. Fear-avoidance and its consequences in chronic musculoskeletal pain: a state of the art. Pain 85 (3), 317–332.

von Baeyer, C.L., Baskerville, S., McGrath, P.J., 1998. Everyday pain in three-to five-year-old children in day care. Pain Res. Manag. 3 (2), 111–116.

von Korff, M., LeResche, L., 2005. Epidemiology of pain. In: Merskey, H., Loeser, J.D., Dubner, R. (Eds.), The Paths of Pain 1975–2005. IASP Press, pp. 339–352.

Walker, L.S., Smith, C.A., Garber, J., Claar, R.L., 2007. Appraisal and coping with daily stressors by pediatric patients with chronic abdominal pain. J. Pediatr. Psychol. 32 (2), 206–216.

Wallace, B., Varcoe, C., Holmes, C., Moosa-Mitha, M., Moor, G., Hudspith, M., et al., 2021. Towards health equity for people experiencing chronic pain and social marginalization. Int. J. Equity Health 20 (1), 1–13.

Waller, R., Melton, P.E., Kendell, M., Hellings, S., Hole, E., Slevin, A., et al., 2021. Heritability of musculoskeletal pain and pain sensitivity phenotypes: two generations of the Raine Study. Pain 163 (4), e580–e587.

Werner, A., Malterud, K., 2003. It is hard work behaving as a credible patient: encounters between women with chronic pain and their doctors. Soc. Sci. Med. 57 (8), 1409–1419.

Williams, A.C.D.C., Craig, K.D., 2016. Updating the definition of pain. Pain 157 (11), 2420–2423.

Williams, C.M., Maher, C.G., Hancock, M.J., McAuley, J.H., McLachlan, A.J., Britt, H., et al., 2010. Low back pain and best practice care: a survey of general practice physicians. Arch. Intern. Med. 170 (3), 271–277.

Wilson, A.C., Stone, A.L., Poppert Cordts, K.M., Holley, A.L., Mackey, S., Darnall, B.D., et al., 2020. Baseline characteristics of a dyadic cohort of mothers with chronic pain and their children. Clin. J. Pain 36 (10), 782–792.

Zborowski, M., 1969. People in Pain. Jossey-Bass, San Francisco.

Zwakhalen, S.M., Hamers, J.P., Abu-Saad, H.H., Berger, M.P., 2006. Pain in elderly people with severe dementia: a systematic review of behavioural pain assessment tools. BMC Geriatr. 6 (1), 1–15.

Section | 1 |

Overview: what is pain?

Chapter |5|

The psychology of pain: implications for the assessment and management of people in pain

Michael Nicholas

LEARNING OBJECTIVES

At the end of this chapter, readers will understand the:
1. Concept of mediating and modulating contributors to the experience and impact of chronic pain on an individual.
2. Most studied psychological constructs that mediate the experience and impact of chronic pain.
3. Concept of a clinical case formulation and how it differs from a diagnosis.

Overview

The chapter is focussed on the reader gaining an understanding of the psychological aspects of pain experience, which we know impact upon biological and neurophysiological aspects of the patient's pain experience, rather than directing the clinician as to what to assess or what assessment methods to use.

The ways in which researchers and clinicians have understood how psychological factors or processes might contribute to the experience of pain are central to interdisciplinary pain management. Not surprisingly, such understandings influence what psychological factors are assessed and managed by clinicians. Naturally, these perspectives have evolved considerably over the last 50 or so years. To appreciate the current status of psychological aspects of pain, it can help to briefly consider how these ideas have evolved in this period, starting with the description of the gate control theory (GCT) of pain (Melzack & Wall 1965).

Significance of the gate control theory of pain

A core message in the GCT was that pain was not an inevitable consequence of peripheral stimulation of nociceptors, but rather an end product of a series of dynamic, interacting processes. Although our understanding of these processes has developed considerably since 1965, that core message remains supported. It is widely accepted now that these processes involve the central nervous system (CNS), with ascending and descending influences playing an active role in determining the nature and degree of pain experienced following noxious stimulation at the periphery. Importantly, the gate theory provided a means of explaining pain that was not dependent upon the nature of the noxious stimulus alone—an advance later elaborated on by Woolf (2011), among others. Clinically, perhaps the key significance of the GCT was the realisation that the size or nature of an injury is a poor predictor of degree of pain experienced and its impact on the person concerned.

Woolf (2011) pointed out that 'nociceptive' pain reflects the perception of noxious stimuli and that, in the absence of such potentially damaging stimuli, a particular pain experience should not be considered as nociceptive. He went on to say that that does not mean such 'non-nociceptive' pain is not real, just that it is not activated by noxious stimuli. Unlike many earlier researchers (e.g. Merskey 2000), Woolf argued that rather than ascribing this category of pain to unspecified 'psychological' factors, there was evidence to indicate that CNS mechanisms (like central sensitisation) may amplify normal stimuli in inflammatory, neuropathic and (what he termed) 'dysfunctional pain disorders'. This does not mean that psychological factors are not involved, just that we should avoid assumptions that previously unexplained features of pain are due to amorphous 'psychological' factors, unless we have good evidence that specific psychological factors are involved. Of course, it has long been accepted that psychological and environmental factors can contribute to pain experience and impact but how this might happen has not always been clear.

Introduction of biopsychosocial models of illness and pain

Engel's (1977) original biopsychosocial model of illness posited that symptoms should be conceptualised as the result of a dynamic interaction between psychological, social and pathophysiological variables. Engel's model was subsequently adopted by leading pain clinicians and scholars, Loeser (1982) and Waddell et al. (1984), who described what became known as the 'onion ring' model of pain that comprised multiple interacting layers. In these accounts, there was an inner physiological layer level (e.g. nociception or neuropathy) involving changes initiated by trauma or pathology, but their impact on the person concerned depended also on outer layers of the onion, involving input by psychological variables (e.g. attention and appraisal of internal sensations, and emotional experiences, like suffering), as well as by behavioural, and social or environmental variables. The biopsychosocial model outlined by these, and other, authors also posited that psychological, behavioural and social variables can influence physiological responses, such as hormone production, activity in the autonomic nervous system and physical deconditioning (Turk & Flor 1999). For example, behavioural responses, such as avoidance of activities, due to fear of pain or expectation of further injury were thought to result in physical deconditioning and/or greater disability (e.g. Troup & Videman 1989; Vlaeyen & Linton 2002).

The 'onion ring' model of pain described by Loeser and Waddell also separated the suffering (or affective) aspects of pain from the sensory aspects of pain perception (typically described by words such as burning, sharp, throbbing). Whether this distinction is still justified is arguable, but it is true that the relationship between pain severity (as measured by intensity rating scales) and distress associated with pain is variable and can be influenced by factors such as the use of coping strategies, cognitions and environmental factors (Leeuw et al. 2007). Similarly, the relationship between pain severity, physical pathology findings and disability/pain behaviours is also variable. Many people with chronic pain seem to manage quite well, continue to work, do not become distressed and disabled, use few drugs and seek medical attention rarely (Blyth et al. 2005; Miedema et al. 1998). On the other hand, a large proportion of people with chronic pain do become distressed and disabled and seek medical care at levels at much higher rates than their numbers might suggest (Blyth et al. 2001; Frymoyer 1988; Miedema et al. 1998). More recently, for example, the Global Burden of Disease Study has reported that pain-related disorders, especially low back pain, are the leading cause globally of disability and disease burden (Vos et al. 2017). It is this latter group that typically present to health services for help.

Biopsychosocial model of pain in International Classification of Diseases—ICD-11 vs ICD-10

Reflecting this more comprehensive understanding of pain, the updated chronic pain classifications in the most recent version of the International Classification of Diseases, ICD-11 (Treede et al. 2019), have accepted that all chronic pain should be regarded as a multifactorial, biopsychosocial phenomenon. This means that biological, psychological and social factors are thought to contribute to the onset, maintenance or exacerbations of pain or are regarded as relevant consequences of the pain. But Treede and his colleagues were also careful to emphasise that clinicians should seek evidence for these contributions, and not just assume them. Accordingly, in ICD-11, it is recommended that clinicians should assess and report on their contributions in all chronic pain diagnoses.

It is important to realise that this approach is a marked departure from the perspectives of the widely used classifications of medical and mental health conditions, ICD-10 and Diagnostic and Statistical Manual (DSM)-V (Cosci & Fava 2016). In ICD-10 (until recently, the standard classification system for health data collected in most countries), for example, chronic pain has no specific diagnosis, and it refers to pain attributable exclusively to an underlying pathophysiological mechanism. In the absence of a clear (pathophysiological) aetiology (e.g. arthritic changes), and when a mix of biological, psychological and social factors seem to be contributing to a chronic pain presentation, ICD-10 offers only the option of 'somatoform pain disorder'. However, this classification cannot be used when pathophysiological factors are also considered to be contributing to the pain problem. Not only does this leave chronic pain somewhat adrift as a construct, but for patients with chronic pain diagnosed as 'somatoform pain disorder' this can be taken to mean they have a mental disorder—the very thing they typically describe as invalidating their condition and stigmatising.

Limitations of diagnostic and statistical manual (DSM) in classifying chronic pain

In the DSM published by the American Psychiatric Association (APA), diagnoses related to chronic pain have evolved from 'Psychogenic Pain Disorder' (DSM-III, APA, 1980), which required a lack of organic pathology or pain grossly in excess of what might be expected from 'physical findings' as well as evidence that psychological factors contributed to the development of the pain. This was followed by a new diagnostic term, 'Somatoform Pain Disorder' in DSM-IIIR (APA 1987), which removed the requirement for evidence of a psychological contribution but retained the reference to lack of organic pathology, or a pain report in excess of what might be expected. ICD-10, however, has continued to use this term. Subsequently, in DSM-IV (APA 1994), the term 'somatoform' was dropped, leaving just 'Pain Disorder' (DSM-IV). This diagnosis required that the pain must be related to one or more anatomical sites and be the main focus of the clinical presentation, as well as being the cause of significant distress and impairment in social, occupational or other areas of functioning, and that psychological factors must play an important role in the onset, severity, exacerbation or maintenance of the pain. In DSM-IV, three subtypes of pain disorder were described—Pain Disorder associated with psychological factors, Pain Disorder associated with a general medical condition only, or both.

In the most recent DSM iteration (DSM-V, APA 2013), 'pain disorders' have been deleted completely and replaced with 'Somatic Symptom Disorder', of which one subtype may be 'Somatic Symptom Disorder, with predominant pain'. The DSM-V manual notes this was previously called 'pain disorder' and is reserved for people 'whose somatic symptoms predominantly involve pain' (p. 311). The criteria for somatic symptom disorder include somatic symptoms that are distressing or causing significant disruption in daily life and reflected in 'excessive' thoughts, feelings or behaviours, and the state of being symptomatic must be present for at least 6 months. Unlike the previous versions in this diagnostic lineage, with Somatic Symptom Disorder, lack of a 'medical explanation' for the symptoms is not sufficient for the diagnosis and the symptoms may or may not be related to another medical condition (e.g. a myocardial infarction).

Each of these DSM diagnoses for persisting pain has had its supporters, but ultimately all have been found inadequate and not reflective of developments in the evolution of our understanding of chronic pain and associated contributors and mechanisms. For example, in relation to DSM-III, Turk & Rudy (1992) pointed out the problems of taking the position that pain was either physical or psychological, and they also questioned the assumption that it was currently possible to accurately determine all possible 'physical' findings. Fishbain (1995) criticised DSM-IIIR's reliance on what was essentially a value judgement in determining if a person's report of pain was 'excessive', quite apart from the problem of reliable assessment of 'lack of organic pathology'. In relation to the DSM-IV, Fishbain (1995) pointed to the over-inclusive nature of the condition that psychological factors could contribute to the onset, severity, exacerbation or maintenance of the pain, asserting that it would be hard to find a clinical case to which at least one of these did not pertain. In contrast to the earlier iterations, DSM-V is clearly agnostic about putative modes of causation and is limited to a more descriptive characterisation of the presentation of persisting pain. However, it provides no real justification for choosing 6 months as the criterion and again it refers to features such as thoughts, feelings or behaviours being 'excessive', which requires a clinician to make a value judgement about this, as in the earlier versions criticised by Fishbain. In addition, as with the earlier versions of DSM, the DSM-V definition does not include any reference to current knowledge about pain and pain mechanisms. Also, like the earlier versions of DSM, it leaves persisting pain within the realm of mental disorders and the appropriateness of this has been widely challenged (Rief & Isaac 2007).

In summary, it can be seen from the lines of enquiry into explaining pain phenomena stemming from the GCT and the more conceptual biopsychosocial models of pain, as well as the evolving classification/diagnostic perspectives, that psychological and environmental/contextual factors are generally accepted as likely contributors to pain experience and impact. However, it can also be seen that these accounts are more descriptive in nature rather than explanatory. That is, the studies of such factors do not identify and explain how psychological and environmental factors might influence the experience and impact of pain, especially in chronic pain conditions.

How might psychological and environmental factors influence pain outcomes?

Psychological mediators and modulators

Research that has explored the impact of psychological and environmental factors on patient outcomes has typically focussed on risk and prognostic factors for poor outcomes in groups such as injured workers and motorists, as well as for patients attending primary care with acute back pain, which is the most common pain site reported and the site most associated with long-term patient disability (Vos et al. 2017). Clinicians need to focus upon modifiable psychological risk factors (e.g. mood, beliefs, behaviours). These have also been called mediators or moderators (Vlaeyen & Morley 2005) and they should be amenable to change. On the other hand, factors like age, sex, work history, nature of the workplace etc., which might be predictive of outcomes following an injury, are not amenable to change by clinicians. These latter factors are often called modulators (Vlaeyen & Morley 2005). To see how these mediating and modulating factors might play a role in determining the outcomes for an injured worker, let us consider this example. If the injured worker was aged 55 years and had a physically demanding job and reported a history of persisting back pain, we might say (based on the modulators of his older age and physically demanding type of work) his chances of returning to work (RTW) are low. But if he was also distressed and preferred to avoid activities that aggravated his pain, we might see these as mediators or moderators and amenable to change. If this was achieved, then the chances of this injured worker RTW might be increased, despite his age and history. Of course, there would still need to be some adjustment to the type of work he performs, but without a change in the worker's mood and avoidance behaviours, any workplace changes would have little effect.

Using this mediator/modulator framework, we can examine the contribution of diverse factors, from a lesion in a peripheral nerve to a belief held by the patient about their pain. In other words, rather than thinking in terms of whether something is in one category or another (e.g. physical, or psychological), the Vlaeyen and Morley approach offers a more operational way of thinking about how different factors might combine to influence the experience and impact of pain.

Modifiable (mediating) psychological influencers and chronic, disabling pain

Reviews of multiple prospective studies have identified a degree of consistency in psychological risk factors for the development of chronic, disabling pain from acute pain (Chou & Shekelle 2010; Mallen et al. 2007). It should be noted that these are risks for chronic pain that is associated with disability, rather than just having chronic pain alone—as that may not be disabling. Indeed, many people with chronic pain conditions live with little or no disability (Blyth et al. 2001). The most commonly supported psychological mediating factors include depressed mood, anxiety, catastrophic beliefs about pain, fear-avoidance beliefs about pain and low pain self-efficacy beliefs, which are typically associated with behaviours aimed at avoiding or escaping pain, such as resting and taking opioids (Edwards et al. 2016; Fillingim et al. 2014; Jackson et al. 2014).

There is also evidence from treatment studies that changes in these psychological mediators are associated with improved outcomes for patients. Nicholas et al. (2014) reported significant improvements in self-reported pain-related disability, depression and anxiety severity were associated with significant reductions in pain catastrophising and fear-avoidance beliefs, as well as increased pain self-efficacy, following a 3-week cognitive-behavioural therapy (CBT)–based multidisciplinary pain management program with a heterogeneous chronic pain patient sample. These changes were maintained at 1-year follow-up. More recently, van Hoof et al. (2021) reported similar findings following a 2-week multidisciplinary pain management program with chronic low back pain patients. They also found that posttreatment pain self-efficacy levels, rather than the so-called 'dysfunctional' cognitions (catastrophising and fear of movement), were the best predictor of functional levels a year later.

Researchers studying exercise and weight loss in patients with osteoarthritis have also reported self-efficacy to be a significant mediator for adherence to exercise regimens and physical function. For example, Mihalko et al. (2019) reported that self-efficacy significantly mediated treatment effects on physical function and pain at 18-month follow-up. Another study with osteoarthritis (OA) patients also found high adherence to exercises in people with knee OA was associated with high self-determination and self-efficacy (Ledingham et al. 2020). These findings suggest that promoting self-efficacy for performing exercises should be targeted in interventions with OA patients, especially when pain may be an obstacle.

Pain catastrophising has been another focus of mediator research. Again, multiple treatment studies have found reductions in pain catastrophising to be associated with better patient outcomes in terms of severity of depressive symptoms, pain and disability (Racine et al. 2016). Interestingly, a recent systematic review of studies aimed at reducing pain catastrophising in patients with chronic pain found stronger effects when catastrophic styles of thinking were targeted specifically rather than more generic approaches (Schütze et al. 2018). Similar findings have been reported for fear-avoidance beliefs, although a systematic review of physiotherapist delivered psychological interventions (as part of a physiotherapy intervention) found reductions in fear of movement (commonly referred to as fear-avoidance beliefs) in patients presenting with mixed chronic pain conditions were small but statistically significant only in the short-term and not later (Guerrero et al. 2018).

In summary, prospective studies and treatment studies have generally found these commonly studied psychological mediators are predictive of future poor adjustment to chronic pain and that improvements in these variables after treatments in which these variables are targeted are usually associated with improvements in function, mood and pain.

While much of the evidence for the impact of these factors comes from patient samples, some community-based epidemiological evidence provides support for how different responses to pain are associated with different outcomes. For example, using a randomly selected community sample of people living with chronic pain, Blyth et al. (2005) found that relative to those who were not managing well, those who were coping seemed to find ways to remain generally active and occupied, with much less reliance on more passive coping strategies like activity avoidance (resting) and treatment provided by others (e.g. taking medication, hands-on therapies). Specifically, Blyth et al. found that the use of passive coping strategies was associated with an increased likelihood of having high levels of pain-related disability (odds ratio, 2.59) and more pain-related healthcare visits (odds ratio, 2.9), whereas using active strategies was associated with a substantially reduced likelihood of having high levels of pain-related disability (odds ratio, 0.2). Another population-based study (by Buchbinder & Jolley 2004) found that reduced endorsement of certain beliefs (about activity avoidance and treatment seeking being helpful in managing persisting low back pain) was associated with improved community-level outcomes in terms of reduced lost time from work and reduced treatment costs for back pain following a community-based education program (via public media).

Not surprisingly, psychological mediators for long-term disability associated with chronic pain do not have equal effects, and variations are found across studies, in part due to the measures employed as well as the populations studied. Supporting evidence for several psychological factors playing a mediating role in chronic pain that becomes disabling was reported in a systematic review by Lee et al. (2015). These researchers found 12 studies (N = 2961) that conducted mediation analyses to examine how pain might lead to disability. The review found evidence that self-efficacy, psychological distress and fear mediated

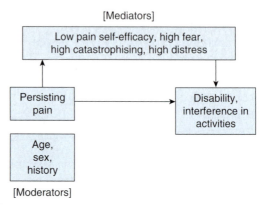

Fig. 5.1 Psychological factors mediating the impact of pain on disability.

the relationship between pain and disability, but catastrophising did not. However, other prospective studies have found catastrophising responses to pain predictive of emotional distress or severity of depressive symptoms (Sullivan et al. 2011).

The main significance of the findings from the studies of psychological mediators is the implications for treatment. Fig. 5.1 illustrates this point, which is important for clinicians to understand. When pain persists, there will usually be some interference in at least some of the patient's activities as a result (seen in the direct arrow from pain to disability), but if the patient also has low self-efficacy for functioning when in pain, or fear of pain, or is distressed and holds highly catastrophic beliefs about their pain, then the impact of pain on disability will be much greater than any disability due to pain alone. These were the types of relationships confirmed by Lee et al. (2015) in their systematic review.

The corollary of this mediating perspective is that when assessing patients experiencing chronic pain (and even in acute pain, for that matter), we must look for the presence of these types of psychological variables. If such variables are present and seem to be contributing to the patient's clinical presentation, such factors should be targeted in a treatment plan. If we can help the patient to minimise these sorts of mediators, their pain will have less effect on their level of disability in future and they may also have less severe pain. However, it should be remembered that there is considerable variation in these factors between patients (and within one patient over time), and we cannot assume that they are always present to the same degree. Hence, it is inadvisable to institute a standard treatment protocol for all patients with chronic pain. As Pincus & McCracken (2013) have pointed out, we need to determine this in each case and not assume it. For example, it would be incorrect to assume that everyone with chronic disabling pain holds high fear-avoidance beliefs. In one study, Nicholas et al. (2014) reported about 18% of their chronic pain patient cohort had low fear-avoidance scores (<33) on the Tampa Scale of Kinesiophobia (TSK) (Kori et al. 1990). In those with low fear-avoidance beliefs, an exposure task for fear-avoidance could therefore be unnecessary.

In case this sounds like an obvious point, it is important to add the caveat that a patient with chronic, disabling pain is likely to have many of these mediating, and moderating, variables in play, so these need to be assessed accordingly. The scenario illustrated in Fig. 5.1 is likely to be repeated several times over in the one case. This means it is very unlikely there will be a 'one-size-fits-all' treatment. Thus not every patient in pain requires 'reassurance about their pain' as they do not all have high fear of movement or catastrophic beliefs about their pain, so we need to assess for the presence of these and other likely drivers of anxiety and distress before we launch into a particular treatment paradigm.

In summary, by assessing if psychological variables are acting as mediators of a patients' disability, we may then be able to develop a treatment plan to target those mediators as well as other potentially modifiable contributors, such as the response of a patient's employer or spouse. This approach means we should avoid commencing treatment for a patient in chronic pain until we have a clear picture of the patient's problems and the contributing factors, especially those that may be amenable to intervention. This is termed a case-formulation approach, which comes from the CBT literature. It is widely used by CBT-trained psychologists but may be unfamiliar to other healthcare providers. This will be described next, but it is important to bear in mind that the approach comes from the concepts around mediators discussed in this section.

Case formulation, helping a patient understand their pain, its contributors and its impact on their lives

Case (or problem) formulation has long been an element of cognitive and behavioural therapies for mental disorders (Persons 1989; Turkat 1985) as a means of summarising assessment information in order to plan a treatment approach. It has also been a key element in psychological treatments for chronic pain (Turk et al. 1983).

A case-formulation approach provides a framework for utilising the assessment information obtained in a way that promotes both the patient's engagement as well as the development of a targeted treatment plan. Having identified the major presenting problems in the initial assessment, the next step is to consider how they might have developed over time and how they may be interacting, as

well as how they are being maintained. One way of providing a starting point to this process is to use a conceptual diagram like that shown in Fig. 5.2. This should be conducted with the involvement of the patient as it provides an opportunity for the clinician to confirm to the patient that they have been listening to them and it allows the clinician to check the accuracy of their understanding of the patient's problems. It also provides a simple means of fostering what Von Korff et al. (1997) described as a collaborative relationship with the patient, where there is a shared understanding of the patient's problems—something that will be critical if the patient is to be engaged in a self-management approach whereby many aspects identified in the case formulation are targeted (Nicholas & Blyth 2016).

The domains covered typically reflect the major elements in pain assessment. The arrows will often be bidirectional (to indicate interactions) and it needs to be tailored to the individual patient as some domains (boxes) will not apply to a particular patient. For example, many people with chronic pain do not take medication or have sleep problems, so the formulation will not need to include those. Equally, additional boxes may be added (e.g. the presence of a comorbid condition)—see the paper by Detweiler-Bedell et al. (2008) for a good summary of how a plan for managing patients with multiple comorbidities might work. This sort of model can help both clinician and patient to make sense of the patient's pain problems and identify what might be targeted in treatment to improve things.

Essentially, a case formulation can be considered as a type of hypothesis, or preliminary working model, which we can then test by intervening in specific areas and evaluating the outcome. If necessary, the formulation may be modified as result of these tests, just as we do in scientific experiments. Thus if the patient's assessment reveals high levels of catastrophic beliefs and low levels of pain self-efficacy beliefs, the formulation can represent them in a way that makes the likely effects of these mediating factors clear, and what might be done to modify them. This might be called targeted or tailored treatment (Åsenlöf et al. 2005; Persons 1989; Turkat 1985).

Consistent with the ICD-11 approach, a case formulation can enable the clinician to describe not only the patient's presenting problems, such as persisting pain, distress and interference in daily activities, but also the possible contributions made by biological, psychological and social/environmental factors. In many ways, this can seem more useful to both patient and clinician than a diagnostic term or label, like fibromyalgia, or neuropathic pain, which may have no specific treatment implications without reference to the patient. The treatment implications of this biopsychosocial formulation will be discussed in the next Chapter 12.

Hypothetical case example

A hypothetical example can help to illustrate how a case formulation might be constructed.

A 45-year-old man reports persisting low back pain following a fall at work 12 months ago. Initial radiography did not reveal any abnormalities, though a computed tomography (CT) scan subsequently revealed moderate posterior disc bulging at L4/5, but no apparent compression of neural structures. Neurological examination revealed no neurological abnormality. Heat treatment and manipulation have provided only brief relief of his pain. Simple analgesics and antiinflammatory medication provided little help. His doctor then prescribed low-dose opioids to be taken as needed, but lately he has been taking them on a daily basis without noticeable benefit and he now reports constipation. His doctor is concerned about this. His doctor referred him to a physiotherapist for exercise and advice, but he does not adhere to the exercise plan as he finds they aggravate his pain. But he does find the heat pack on his back comforting when sitting or lying on the couch or in bed.

He describes his pain as almost constantly present and fluctuating in severity. On average, he rates the pain as 6/10 in severity. It is aggravated by most activities and reduced by resting and heat (hot showers and a heat pack). He has been off work since his accident, and he doubts he will be able to return to his old job. His employer was sympathetic initially but now says he has to terminate his job. He does have a workers compensation claim and has been receiving wage replacement income, but the amount is gradually being reduced. The independent insurance doctor told him he could not find anything seriously wrong with him and he should continue with exercises and return to work. He and his wife are having to rely more on her wages to cover their expenses.

Currently, he reports being unable to perform most of his normal house and yard chores as it seems everything he does aggravates his pain. His mood is often depressed, and he reports often feeling useless and frustrated. His score on a depression symptom scale places him in the moderately depressed range for people with chronic pain. Sleep at night is disturbed and the days are marked by lethargy and tiredness. He is comfort eating and has put on over 16 kg in the last year. He reports he and his wife are having more arguments than usual, and he avoids social engagements as they usually involve a lot of sitting. He has gradually lost touch with his old friends, and he has not played golf with them since his fall.

On examination, the patient appears noticeably distressed and walks slowly and spends most of examination session standing and leaning on a chair. He is unable to touch his toes and reports tenderness in his lumbar spine (L3/4). All back movements, rotation, flexion/extension appear reduced and are accompanied by grimaces and reports of increased pain. There is no evidence of muscle wasting and no sensory loss is detected. He reports he can only stand for about 10 minutes before his pain increases and he has to change position. Walking is limited to about 12 minutes and sitting to about 10 minutes. When asked what he thinks is causing his persisting pain he says he is not sure but is concerned something is wrong with his spine and has been missed. He does not feel he can return to work or resume his normal life until his pain is relieved. He was asked to complete self-report questionnaires about his pain, and they indicate he has very low pain self-efficacy (i.e. low confidence in being active while in pain), and he tends to worry a lot about his pain and what it means for his future (his catastrophising score was in the high range for people with pain). Another scale indicated a high level of fear of movement when in pain.

When this diagram (see Fig. 5.2) was shared with the patient, he said he was surprised as he had never looked at his problems like this. He just thought that all he needed was good pain relief and everything would get back to normal. He agreed that the diagram did provide an accurate summary of his problems but he is unsure how he can change anything. This is where his healthcare providers can step in and discuss what might be possible to change and how this could be achieved. This will be explored in the next chapter.

Diagnosis using ICD-11

The aforementioned man's pain is clearly chronic (persisting longer than 3 months) and would meet criteria for the diagnosis of chronic primary low-back pain, which comes under chronic primary musculoskeletal pain.

Chronic primary pain is chronic pain in one or more anatomical regions that is characterised by significant emotional distress (e.g. anxiety, anger/frustration or depressed mood) and functional disability (e.g. interference in daily life activities and reduced participation in social roles). Chronic primary pain is multifactorial, with biological, psychological and social factors contributing to the pain syndrome. The diagnosis is appropriate independently of identified biological or psychological contributors unless a specific diagnosis would better account for the presenting symptoms (Nicholas et al. 2019).

In this case, possible biological contributors might include central sensitisation and increased body weight adding pressure to his spine, but there are not enough to meet criteria for another diagnosis. Several psychological factors are evident, including emotional distress, heightened worry about his pain and fear of movement, avoidance of activities likely to aggravate his pain, poor sleep, as well as very low pain self-efficacy. Social factors in this case might include social isolation, loss of work, financial pressures, insurance company pressure and conflict with his

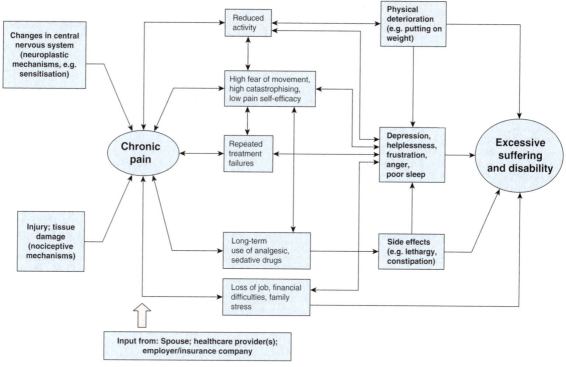

Fig. 5.2 How might a case formulation summarise this man's problems?

wife. These appear likely to be contributing to the man's presentation and problems with his back pain.

His ICD-11 severity code is 233, with pain intensity estimated at 7/10 (code 5 2, moderately severe), pain-related distress at 8/10 (code 5 3, severe) and pain-related disability at 7/10 (code 5 3, severe).

Both the ICD-11 diagnosis and the biopsychosocial case formulation allow us to identify possible targets for intervention tailored to this man's presenting features.

Conclusion

How psychological factors are thought to contribute to the experience and impact of pain will guide all clinical interventions for chronic pain. Ideas about how psychological factors contribute to pain have evolved markedly since the Gate Control Theory was enunciated in 1965. Most recently, the chronic pain diagnoses described in ICD-11 have encouraged clinicians to think about how psychological (as well as biological and environmental) factors might be contributing to the chronic pain and associated distress and disability reported by patients with chronic pain. Importantly, ICD-11 discourages attributing a patient's problems to psychological factors by exclusion. The use of a case formulation approach enables the clinician to consider how any psychological factors identified in their assessment might be contributing to a patient's clinical presentation. In the next chapter, the ways in which a case formulation can be used to guide targeted (or tailored) interventions for chronic pain will be discussed and illustrated.

Review questions	Q

1. How has the Gate Control Theory of pain contributed to pain management?
2. Explain why clinicians should focus their management strategies on mediators rather than modulating factors.

3. Describe how a case formulation approach can guide person-centred, individualised management for patients.

References

American Psychiatric Association DSM-III, 1980. Diagnostic and Statistical Manual of Mental Disorders, 3rd ed. APA, Washington, DC. DSM-III.

American Psychiatric Association DSM-IIIR, 1987. Diagnostic and statistical manual, 3rd rev. ed. APA, Washington, DC.

American Psychiatric Association DSM-IV, 1994. Diagnostic and Statistical Manual of Mental Disorders, 4th ed. APA, Washington, DC.

American Psychiatric Association. DSM-lV-TR, 2000. Diagnostic and statistical manual of mental disorders, 4th ed. APA, Washington, DC.

American Psychiatric Association. DSM-V, 2013. Diagnostic and statistical manual of mental disorders, 5th ed. APA, Washington, DC.

Åsenlöf, P., Denison, E., Lindberg, P., 2005. Individually tailored treatment targeting activity, motor behavior, and cognition reduces pain–related disability, a randomized controlled trial in patients with musculoskeletal pain. J. Pain 6, 588–603.

Blyth, F.M., March, L.M., Nicholas, M.K., Cousins, M.J., 2005. Self-management of chronic pain, a population-based study. Pain 113 (3), 285–292.

Buchbinder, R., Jolley, D., 2004. Population based intervention to change back pain beliefs, three year follow up population survey. Brit. Med. J. 328 (7435), 321.

Chou, R., Shekelle, P., 2010. Will this patient develop persistent disabling low back pain? J. Am. Med. Assoc. 303, 1295–1302.

Cosci, F., Fava, G.A., 2016. The clinical inadequacy of the DSM-5 classification of somatic symptom and related disorders, an alternative trans-diagnostic model. CNS. Spectr. 21, 310–317.

Edwards, R., Dworkin, R.H., Sullivan, M.D., Turk, D.C., Wasan, A.D., 2016. The role of psychosocial processes in the development and maintenance of chronic pain. J. Pain 17 (9 Suppl), T70–T92.

Detweiler-Bedell, J., Friedman, M.A., Leventhal, H., Miller, I.W., Leventhal, E.A., 2008. Integrating co-morbid depression and chronic physical disease management: Identifying and resolving failures in self-regulation. Clinical Psychology Review; 28(8): 1426–1446.

Engel, G., 1977. The need for a new medical model: a challenge for biomedicine. Science 196, 129–136.

Fillingim, R.B., Bruehl, S., Dworkin, R.H., Dworkin, S.F., Loeser, J.D., Turk, D.C., et al., 2014. The ACTTION—American Pain Society Pain Taxonomy (AAPT), an evidence based and multidimensional approach to classifying chronic pain conditions. J. Pain 15, 241–249.

Fishbain, D.A., 1995. DSM-IV, implications and issues for the pain clinician. Am. Pain. Soc. Bull. 5, 6–18.

Frymoyer, J.W., 1988. Back pain and sciatica. N. Engl. J. Med. 318, 291–300.

Guerrero, A.V.S., Maujean, A., Campbell, L., Sterling, M., 2018. A systematic review and meta-analysis of the effectiveness of psychological interventions delivered by physiotherapists on pain, disability and psychological outcomes in musculoskeletal pain conditions. Clin. J. Pain 34, 838–857.

Jackson, T., Wang, Y., Wang, Y., Fan, H., 2014. Self-efficacy and chronic pain outcomes, a meta-analytic review. J. Pain 15, 800–814.

Kori, S.H., Miller, R.P., Todd, D.D., 1990. Kinesiophobia: a new view of chronic pain behaviour. Pain. Manag. 3, 35–43.

Ledingham, A., Cohn, E., Baker, K., Keysor, J., 2020. Exercise adherence, beliefs of adults with knee osteoarthritis over 2 years. Physiother. Theory. Pract. 36 (12), 1363–1378.

Lee, H., Hubscher, M., Moseley, G.L., Kamper, S.J., Traeger, A.C., Mansell, G., et al., 2015. How does pain lead to disability? A systematic review and meta-analysis of mediation studies in people with back and neck pain. Pain 156, 988–997.

Leeuw, M., Goossens, M.E.J.B.,, Linton, S.J., Crombez, G., Boersma, K., Vlaeyen, J.W.S., 2007. The fear-avoidance model of musculoskeletal pain, state of the scientific evidence. J. Behav. Med. 30, 77–94.

Loeser, J.D., 1982. Concepts of pain. In: Stanton-Hicks, M., Boas, R. (Eds.), Chronic Low-Back Pain. Raven Press, New York, pp. 145–148.

Mallen, C.D., Peat, G., Thomas, E., Dunn, K., Croft, P.R., 2007. Prognostic factors for musculoskeletal pain in primary care, a systematic review. Br. J. Gen .Pract. 57, 655–661.

Melzack, R., Wall, P.D., 1965. Pain mechanisms: a new theory. Science 150, 971–979.

Merskey, H., 2000. Beware somatization. Eur. J. Pain 4, 3–4.

Miedema, H.S., Chorus, A.M., Wevers, C.W.J., van der Linden, S., 1998. Chronicity of back problems during working life. Spine 23, 2021–2029.

Mihalko, S.L., Cox, P., Beavers, D.P., Miller, G.D., Nicklas, B.J., Lyles, M., et al., 2019. Effect of intensive diet and exercise on self-efficacy in overweight and obese adults with knee osteoarthritis, The IDEA randomized clinical trial. Transl. Behav. Med. 9, 227–235.

Nicholas, M.K., Asghari, A., Sharpe, L., Brnabic, S., Wood, B.M., Overton, S., et al., 2014. Cognitive exposure versus avoidance in patients with chronic pain, adherence matters. Eur. J. Pain 18 (3), 424–437.

Nicholas, M.K., Blyth, F.M., 2016. Are self-management strategies effective in chronic pain treatment? Pain Manage. 6, 75–88.

Nicholas, M., Vlaeyen, J.W.S., Rief, W., et al., 2019. The IASP classification of chronic pain for ICD-11, chronic primary pain. Pain 160, 28–37.

Persons, J.B., 1989. Cognitive Therapy in Practice: A Case Formulation Approach. Norton & Company, New York, NY.

Pincus, T., McCracken, L., 2013. Psychological factors and treatment opportunities in low back pain. Best. Pract. Res. Clin. Rheumatol. 27, 625–635.

Racine, M., Moulin, D.E., Nielson, W.R., Morley-Forster, P.K., Lynch, M., Clark, A.J., et al., 2016. The reciprocal associations between catastrophizing and pain outcomes in patients being treated for neuropathic pain: a cross-lagged panel analysis study. Pain 157, 1946–1953.

Rief, W., Isaac, M., 2007. Are somatoform disorders "mental disorders"? A contribution to the current debate. Curr. Opin. Psychiatry 20, 143–146.

Schütze, R., Rees, C., Smith, A., Slater, H., Campbell, J.M., O'Sullivan, P., et al., 2018. How can we best reduce pain catastrophizing in adults with chronic noncancer pain? A Systematic Review and Meta-Analysis. J. Pain 19 (3), 233–256.

Sullivan, M.J.L., Adams, H., Martel, M.-O., Scott, W., Wideman, T., 2011. Catastrophizing and perceived injustice, risk factors for the transition to chronicity after whiplash injury. Spine 36 (25S), S244–S249.

Treede, R.D., Rief, W., Barke, A., Aziz, Q., Bennett, M.I., Benoliel, R., et al., 2019. Chronic pain as a symptom and a disease, the IASP classification of chronic pain for the international classification of diseases ICD-11. Pain 160, 19–27.

Troup, J.D.G., Videman, T., 1989. Inactivity and the aetiopathogenesis of musculoskeletal disorders. Clin. Biomech. 4, 173–178.

Turk, D.C., Flor, H., 1999. Chronic pain: a biobehavioral perspective. In: Gatchel, R.J., Turk, D.C. (Eds.), Psychosocial Factors in Pain: Critical Perspectives. Guilford Press, New York, pp. 18–34.

Turk, D.C., Meichenbaum, D., Genes, M., 1983. Pain and Behavioral Medicine: A Cognitive-Behavioral Perspective. Guilford Press, New York, NY.

Turk, D.C., Rudy, T., 1992. Cognitive factors and persistent pain: a glimpse into Pandora's box. Cog. Ther. Res. 16 (2), 99–122.

Turkat, I.D., 1985. In: Behavioral Case Formulation. Plenum Press, New York.

van Hoof, M., Vriezekolk, J.E., Kroeze, R.J., O'Dowd, J.K., van Limbeek, J., Spruit, M., 2021. Targeting self-efficacy more important than dysfunctional behavioral cognitions in patients with longstanding chronic low back pain, a longitudinal study. BMC Musculoskelet. Disord. 22, 824 2021.

Vlaeyen, J.W.S., Linton, S.J., 2002. Fear-avoidance and its consequences in chronic musculoskeletal pain, a state of the art. Pain 85, 317–332.

Vlaeyen, J.W.S., Morley, S.J., 2005. Cognitive behavioral treatments for chronic pain, what works for whom? Clin. J. Pain 21, 1–8.

Von Korff, M., Gruman, J., Schaefer, J., Curry, S., Wagner, E.H., 1997. Collaborative management of chronic illness. Ann. Intern. Med. 127 (12), 1097–1102.

Vos, T., Abajobir, A.A., Abate, K.H., Abbafati, C., Abbas, K.M., Abate, K.H., et al., 2017. Global, regional, and national incidence, prevalence, and years lived with disability for 328 diseases and injuries for 195 countries, 1990-2016, a systematic analysis for the Global Burden of Disease Study 2016. Lancet 390, 1211–1259.

Waddell, G., Bircher, M., Finlayson, D., Main, C.J., 1984. Symptoms and signs: physical disease or illness behaviour? Br. Med. J. 1984;289:739-41.

Woolf, C.J., 2011. Central sensitization, implications for the diagnosis and treatment of pain. Pain 152, S2–15.

Chapter | 6 |

Neuroanatomy of the nociceptive system

Mary P. Galea

LEARNING OBJECTIVES

At the end of this chapter, readers will understand the:
1. Different types of peripheral nociceptors and their associated axons.
2. Organisation of the dorsal horn and the termination patterns of afferent inputs.
3. Pathways involved in transmitting nociceptive information within the nervous system.
4. Areas of the nervous system involved in the perception, integration and response to nociceptive signals.

Overview

This chapter is concerned specifically with the nervous system structures involved in nociception. The historical framework for studying pain has implied that there is a sensory channel for pain in the manner of sensory channels for other sensations (Willis & Coggeshall 1991). It will be clear from the following review that this is not the case, and that pain is a complex, multidimensional phenomenon. Melzack & Casey (1968) suggested that pain needs to be considered in three interacting dimensions: sensory-discriminative, cognitive-evaluative and motivational-affective. The sensory dimension refers to the capacity to analyse the intensity, location, quality and behaviour of pain. The cognitive-evaluative dimension is concerned with the phenomena of anticipation, attention, suggestion and the influence of previous experience and knowledge. Finally, the motivational-affective dimension is the emotional response (fear, anxiety) that controls responses to the pain. Craig (2002) has argued that pain, in conjunction with temperature and itch, is an interoceptive sensation, inherently associated with emotion, and integrated into the homeostatic network that provides a representation of the physiological condition of the body. This view is based on evidence of specific substrates for many features of pain and its modulation.

A study of the anatomical connections of the nociceptive system provides a framework for understanding how all these dimensions of pain are registered and interact within the nervous system. Much of the information comes from studies in animals, including rodents, cats and some in primates. While some features of the nociceptive system are conserved across species, more recent studies have reported differences in humans compared to other species, especially rodents. Appreciating these differences is important for understanding how humans experience pain.

The physiological basis of nociception, particularly the mechanisms of signalling and modulating nociceptive stimuli, will be covered more specifically in the next chapter.

Structure and function of peripheral nociceptors

A receptor is specialised nervous tissue sensitive to a particular change in the environment. A change in the environment provides the stimulus. Normally, a receptor responds preferentially only to one type of stimulus, called the *adequate stimulus*, not in the sense of magnitude, but rather in its specificity to that receptor. Receptors convert the physical energy of the adequate stimulus into electrochemical energy that activates the associated neuron.

Nociceptors are a class of peripheral receptors that respond to tissue-damaging or potentially tissue-damaging stimuli (from Latin *nocere*, to injure). The skin is densely innervated by nociceptors. Nociceptors are also present in other body tissues, including bone, muscle, joint capsules, viscera and blood vessels, as well as the meninges and peripheral nerve sheaths. However, nociceptors have not been found in articular cartilage, synovial membranes, lung parenchyma, visceral pleura, pericardium, brain or spinal cord tissue.

The inference that specialised nociceptors existed was made on the basis of experiments on peripheral nerves in humans using graded electrical stimulation and differential nerve blocks (Adrian 1931; Burgess & Perl 1967; Bessou & Perl 1969). Although derived from neural crest cells like other sensory neurons, nociceptive neurons differ in terms of function, morphology and gene expression. Nociceptive neurons can be subdivided into two types: Aδ neurons and C neurons, which are giving rise to two groups of afferent fibres:

- *small-diameter thinly myelinated fibres (Aδ)* with a conduction velocity of 5 to 30 m/s. Activation is associated with well-localised sensations of sharp, pricking pain.
- *small-diameter, unmyelinated C fibres*, which are ensheathed in bundles by nonmyelinating Schwann cells (Remak Schwann cells, Harty & Monk 2017), conduct slowly (0.5–2 m/s). These fibres transmit diffuse pain sensations that can be dull, poorly localised and persistent (Price & Dubner, 1977).

The terminology A to C is generally used in relation to cutaneous and visceral axons (Erlanger & Gasser 1937). A different terminology (I–IV) has been applied in the case of muscle and joint nerves (Table 6.1).

The structure of nociceptors has been described as unencapsulated or free nerve endings, sensitive to many forms of noxious stimuli (Dubin & Patapoutian 2010). In the skin, the terminals of Aδ fibres remain ensheathed by Schwann cell processes until they penetrate the epidermal basal lamina (Kruger et al. 1981). In the cornea, Aδ fibre nerve endings are thin and elongated, running parallel to the corneal surface, whereas C-fibre endings form clusters of short branches running mostly perpendicular to the surface (MacIver & Tarnelian 1993).

Table 6.1 Classifications of mammalian nerve fibres

Fibre type (Erlanger/ Gasser)	Function	Group (Lloyd)	Function	Average fibre diameter (µm)	Average conduction velocity (m/s)
Aα	Primary muscle spindle afferents, motor fibres to motor neurons	I	Primary muscle spindle afferents	15	95
Aβ	Cutaneous touch and pressure afferents	II	Afferents from tendon organs, afferents from cutaneous mechanoreceptors	8	50
Aγ	Motor fibres to muscle spindles			6	20
Aδ	Cutaneous temperature and pain afferents	III	Afferents from deep pressure receptors in muscle	3	15
B	Sympathetic preganglionic fibres			3	7
C	Cutaneous pain afferents (unmyelinated); sympathetic post-ganglionic fibres	IV	Unmyelinated nerve fibres	0.5	1

Nociceptors in the skin

Nociceptors are complex structures that have heterogeneous properties, responding to multiple stimulus modalities (polymodal). Investigation of responses of specific nociceptors is fraught with difficulty, as a lack of response may indicate a failure to apply a sufficient intensity of stimulation. Moreover, application of the stimulus may induce long-term changes in the response properties of the nociceptor (Meyer et al. 2006).

Aδ nociceptors, although polymodal, can be divided into two main classes on the basis of response to mechanical stimuli, leading to a distinction between mechanically sensitive afferents (MSA) and mechanically insensitive afferents (MIA).

Type I Aδ nociceptors were initially called high-threshold mechanoreceptors (HTM; Burgess & Perl 1967) because they respond with a slowly adapting discharge to strong punctate pressure. These units are densely distributed in hairy and glabrous skin (Campbell et al. 1979). Their receptive fields are distinctive, consisting of a series of sensitive points that may be spread evenly over an area of several square centimetres in proximal areas. In distal areas, such as the glabrous skin of the hands and feet, or on the face, receptive fields are smaller and may comprise only a single point. These units have myelinated axons (Aδ) with a conducting speed of 5 to 25m/s, with a few conducting more quickly in the A–β range (55 m/s). They mediate the 'first' response to pinprick and other intense mechanical stimuli (Basbaum et al. 2009).

Type I Aδ nociceptors were thought to be unresponsive to heat, but have been shown to have very high heat thresholds, usually 53°C or higher (Treede et al. 1998). With maintained heat stimuli, HTM receptors will respond and become sensitised with tissue injury (Basbaum et al. 2009). Meyer et al. (1994) have suggested that the Aδ Type I receptors be termed A-fibre mechano-heat-sensitive receptors (AMHs), as they are responsive to both mechanical and heat stimuli. Heat sensitivity in AMHs is mediated by the vanilloid receptor-like protein 1 (TRPV2) receptors (Caterina et al. 1999).

There is also evidence of A-fibre nociceptors with conduction velocities in the Aβ range, despite the widely held view that large-diameter Aβ afferent fibres transmit signals only from low-threshold mechanoreceptors in the skin. These represent approximately 18% of A-fibre nociceptors in the primate (Treede et al. 1998) and are polymodal, responding to heat stimuli of long duration and moderate pressure mechanical stimuli (Burgess & Perl 1967; Djouhri & Lawson 2004; Treede et al. 1998).

Type II Aδ nociceptors have a lower heat threshold than type I units but very high mechanical thresholds, so they are termed *heat-responsive MIAs*. They may become sensitised to mechanical stimuli after injury. They have been reported in the knee joint (Schaible & Schmidt 1985), viscera (Häbler et al. 1990) and cornea (Tanelian 1991). Some of the cutaneous MIAs may be chemospecific receptors, while others may respond to intense cold or heat stimuli (Meyer et al. 1991). MIAs are not found in glabrous skin. The axons have a mean conduction velocity of 15 m/s and mediate the 'first' acute pain response to noxious heat.

Unmyelinated C fibres are heterogeneous. Most are polymodal, responding to both mechanical and heat stimuli, hence the term C-fibre mechano-heat-sensitive receptor (CMH). Bessou & Perl (1969) have shown that these are the predominant type of C-fibre nociceptor in mammalian skin, comprising about 90% of all afferent C fibres.

The heat-responsive terminals of CMHs lie at varying depths beneath the skin (between 20 and 570 μm) and so their heat threshold is dependent on the temperature at the heat-responsive terminal and not on the rate of temperature increase (Tillman et al. 1995). Mechanical nociceptors with C-axons have a slowly adapting response to mechanical stimuli. They lack the distinctive multipoint receptive fields of the A-fibre units; instead, their fields usually consist of a zone of uniform sensitivity (Iggo 1960; Lynn 1984).

A class of C fibres, called *C-tactile afferents*, have low-threshold mechanoreceptors present only in hairy skin. They have small receptive fields (Wessberg et al. 2003) and respond vigorously to slow and light stroking (Bessou et al. 1971; Vallbo et al. 1999). They mediate pleasant touch (Löken et al. 2009) and have been found to modulate pain (Habig et al. 2017). Some cutaneous C nociceptors can be classified as *pruriceptors*, responding to mechanical, thermal or chemical (e.g. histamine) stimuli and eliciting the sensation of itch (La Motte et al. 2014).

Another way of classifying nociceptors is through identification of neuroanatomical and molecular characteristics (Snider & McMahon 1998). C-fibre neurons can be divided into two groups according to their expression of the plant lectin isolectin IB4A (Stucky 2007). IB4-negative neurons are typically peptidergic, releasing neuropeptides such as substance P and calcitonin gene-related peptide (CGRP), as well as the TrkA neurotrophin receptor. They express the receptor TRPV1 (transient receptor potential vanilloid 1) which makes them sensitive to heat (Immke and Gavva 2006). IB4-positive neurons are nonpeptidergic, expressing the Ret tyrosine kinase receptor for glial-derived neurotrophic factor (GDNF), with ~75% expressing Mrgpr member D (MrgprD) and sensitive to mechanical stimuli (Braz et al. 2014; Dong et al. 2001). Peptidergic neurons are thought to mediate inflammatory pain, while nonpeptidergic neurons are thought to mediate neuropathic pain (Julius & Basbaum 2001). Zylka et al. (2005) have shown that in the mouse, the fibres of these two populations terminate in different layers of the epidermis, but occasionally intertwine.

The chemosensitivity of C-polymodal nociceptors has not been studied as much as their sensitivity to heat and pressure. They can be excited by potassium, histamine, serotonin, bradykinin, capsaicin, mustard oil, acetylcholine and dilute acids, by various means (topical application, intradermal injection, arterial injection) and all in doses that would be painful in humans (see Willis & Coggeshall 1991 for review). Chemicals act on nociceptors by altering the conductance of ion channels in the cell membrane and causing depolarisation (Rang et al. 1991). This may result in sensitisation of the nociceptors, creating an increased responsiveness to stimulation. Further information on peripheral sensitisation will be presented in Chapter 7.

Cold nociceptors have been reported in monkeys (LaMotte & Thalhammer 1982) and in humans (Campero et al. 1996). They respond strongly to prolonged cooling of the skin by ice and weakly to strong pressure, but are not responsive to heat. The threshold for cold pain in humans is about 14°C (Harrison & Davis 1999), but high-threshold cold receptors in the monkey respond only to temperatures below 27°C and are not responsive to mechanical or heat noxious stimuli (LaMotte & Thalhammer 1982). Because of the delay in response between the onset of the stimulus and the report of pain, it has been suggested that cold pain is subserved by deeper receptors than heat pain. The sense of cooling is subserved by primary afferents called cold fibres, which are predominantly Aδ in type. However, cold fibres do not faithfully encode stimuli that induce cold pain (Meyer et al. 2006). Cutaneous Aδ nociceptors have ongoing activity at room temperature. They also respond to temperatures below 0°C and encode stimulus intensity (Simone & Kajander 1997). Cold pain is thought to be mediated by nociceptors located in cutaneous veins (Klement & Arndt 1992).

Skeletal muscle nociceptors

The terminology of Lloyd (1943) is usually used in relation to muscle and joint nerves (Table 6.1). Group III afferent fibres are small-diameter myelinated fibres; group IV fibres are unmyelinated and constitute the majority of muscle nociceptors. Numerous unencapsulated endings can be located in the connective tissue and in the wall of arterioles in skeletal muscle and can be subdivided into mechanical and polymodal types (Stacey 1969). Effective stimuli are high-intensity mechanical forces, as well as endogenous pain-producing substances such as bradykinin, serotonin and potassium ions. Increased levels of adrenaline, as well as hypoxia and impaired metabolism following trauma or unaccustomed exercise, may also activate nociceptors (Kieschke et al. 1988; Mense 1993). Group III afferent fibres are responsive to mechanical stimulation of muscle, including stretch (Mense & Stahnke 1983). Many are activated by exercise and therefore probably function as ergoreceptors. However, a significant proportion of these are nociceptive. Some group III afferents are responsive to the injection of chemicals such as hypertonic sodium chloride (Abrahams et al. 1984).

Approximately 40% of group IV afferents are classified as low-threshold mechanosensitive (LTM) units and respond to gentle muscle stretch or contraction (Hoheisel et al. 2005). These nonnociceptive units control the adjustment of circulation and respiration to the demands of physical exercise (McCloskey & Mitchell 1972). The remaining proportion of group IV afferents are called HTM units (Mense 2009). They are activated with tissue-threatening mechanical stimulation, e.g. when muscle contractions occur during ischaemia (Mense & Meyer 1985). Many are readily activated by pain-producing chemicals (Mense & Meyer 1988) or thermal stimuli (Hertel et al. 1976).

One of the most relevant chemical causes of muscle pain is a drop in tissue pH (an increase in proton concentration), possibly related to tonic contractions leading to ischaemia or accumulation of lactic acid (Mense 2009). The mechanism is related to the large number of acid-sensing ion channels (ASICs) in the membrane of muscle nociceptors (Hoheisel et al. 2004; Sluka et al. 2003). Another cause is a release of adenosine triphosphate (ATP) resulting from damage to muscle cells or an increase in permeability of the muscle cell membrane (Burnstock 2007). Other chemical factors are bradykinin, formed in damaged tissue, and serotonin, prostaglandins and nerve growth factor, which sensitise group IV afferents (see Mense 2009 for review).

Joint nociceptors

Nociceptors in joints are located in the joint capsule and ligaments, bone, periosteum, articular fat pads and around blood vessels, but not in the joint cartilage. They have been studied predominantly in the knee joint. The terminals of group III and group IV sensory nerve endings comprise multiple axonal beads ensheathed by Schwann cell processes, except for some areas of exposed axon membrane containing structural specialisations characteristic of receptive sites. The beads thus represent multiple receptive sites (Heppelmann et al. 1990). Some of these receptors may be nociceptive.

Joint nociceptors can be classified as:
- high-threshold units that discharge only in response to noxious pressure or extreme joint movement (Bessou & Laporte 1961)
- units that respond to strong pressure but not to movement
- units that do not respond to any mechanical stimulus in the normal joint (MIAs or silent nociceptors) (Schaible & Schmidt 1988).

In the normal joint, only the first type is activated, but all joint afferents become sensitised if the joint becomes inflamed (see Chapter 7).

Visceral nociceptors

In somatic tissue such as skin and muscle, there is a clear distinction between mechanorecptive and nociceptive afferents. This is not the case in visceral tissue, for which pain may not be reported even in response to tissue-damaging stimuli. Nociceptors are located in visceral organs, including the heart, gastrointestinal tract and reproductive organs, and in the walls of blood vessels. Pain-producing stimuli in the viscera include inflammation, distension of hollow muscular-walled organs such as the gastrointestinal tract, the urinary tract and the gall bladder, ischaemia in organs such as the heart, and traction in the mesentery. While nociceptive neurons from viscera are considered to be carried mainly in sympathetic afferent nerves, the vagus nerve, which innervates all of the thoracic and abdominal viscera, is important for chemical nociception and the feeling of unpleasantness associated with visceral pain (Bielefeldt & Gebhart 2006).

Recent studies have identified two functionally distinct subpopulations of afferents in human bowel tissue, one in the muscular layer and the other in the serosal layer. The former, but not the latter, are sensitive to tissue stretch. Serosal units have low mechanical sensitivity and are most likely to be nociceptive, given their response to noxious stimuli such as bradykinin and ATP (McGuire et al. 2018). The serosal units travel into the intestine with arterioles and project into the submucosa (Reed & Vanner 2017). Nociceptors in the bowel may be activated by distension and a wide range of mediators originating from the intestinal lumen, including inflammatory mediators such as histamine and bradykinin, neurotrophins such as nerve growth factor, and cytokines such as tumour necrosis factor-α (Reed & Vanner 2017). Microbiota may directly increase nociceptive signalling in the colon in addition to pronociceptive cytokine release from immune cells (Ochoa-Cortes et al. 2010).

Nonneuronal cells

Although signal transduction mechanisms have been considered properties of neurons, nonneuronal cells have been shown to participate in nociception. Immune cells (macrophages and lymphocytes) and glial cells in the peripheral nervous system (Schwann cells and satellite cells) and central nervous system (CNS) (astrocytes and microglia) play a critical role in chronic pain processing (Ji et al. 2016; Milligan & Watkins 2009 for review). Resident immune cells (mast cells, macrophages and neutrophils) are activated in response to injury and sensitise peripheral nociceptors (Ren & Dubner 2010). Intrinsic sensory transduction mechanisms of keratinocytes in the skin can directly elicit firing of nociceptive and tactile sensory afferent fibres (Baumbauer et al. 2015; Pang et al. 2015). A recent study has provided evidence of a previously unrecognised type of specialised glial cell called a nociceptive Schwann cell that projects into the epidermis in direct conjunction with the nociceptive nerve endings, forming a mesh-like network. The nociceptive Schwann cells contribute to the sensation of mechanical pain (Abdo et al. 2019).

Anatomy of referred pain

Pain from stimulation of viscera is frequently localised to the surface of the body, a phenomenon termed *referred pain*. This may be explained by the convergence of nociceptive input for deep and cutaneous tissues onto common somatosensory spinal neurons that also receive afferents from topographically separate body regions (the so-called projection-convergence theory; Ruch 1946). Sensations from the viscera have no separate ascending spinal pathways and are represented within the known somatosensory pathways. The level of the spinal cord to which visceral afferent fibres from the internal organs project depends on their embryonic innervation. Many viscera migrate well away from their embryonic origin during development, and therefore referred pain from the viscera may be perceived at locations remote from the actual site of the stimulus. For example, the heart is derived from endoderm in the neck and upper thorax, so nociceptive afferents from the heart enter the spinal cord through the dorsal roots C3–T5 rather than lower down. Similarly, afferents from the gall bladder enter the spinal cord at T9 rather than at L1, its location later in life. The pain signals carried by these fibres may be referred to the areas of skin via Aδ fibres to the same segment of the spinal cord. Hence, a heart attack causing ischaemia of cardiac muscle can often present as pain in the left shoulder passing into the left arm (the cutaneous segments supplied by C3–T5). In the same way, an inflamed gall bladder can frequently cause pain at the tip of the right scapula, supplied by T9.

Pain may also be referred from tissues other than viscera. This frequently occurs in musculoskeletal conditions and has been explained with reference to patterns of dermatomal, myotomal and sclerotomal territories. However, there is enormous individual variation in these territories, as well as variability in presenting symptoms (Grieve 1994).

Dorsal root ganglion cells

The somata of nociceptive afferents are located in the dorsal root ganglia (DRG) and the equivalent ganglia of cranial nerves V, VII, IX and X. DRG cells are pseudo-unipolar neurons conveying information from the periphery into the spinal cord. These cells can be grouped into two classes based on variations in soma size, diameter of axons, morphology of peripheral terminals and site of central terminations. The division into two size classes has a functional correlate in that, generally, large cells giving rise to large-diameter axons relay low-threshold mechanical and proprioceptive stimuli, and small cells relay nociceptive and thermal stimuli (Lawson 1992). Studies in laboratory animals have shown that small DRG cells stain intensely and contain many organelles and peptides, including substance P (SP), somatostatin, CGRP, vasoactive intestinal peptide (VIP) and galanin (Willis & Coggeshall 1991). However, molecular expression patterns in DRG neurons in humans differ from those in laboratory animals. For example, while many molecules typical of nociceptors (e.g. TRPV1 and CGRP) are expressed in small- and medium-sized neurons in mice, this is not the case in humans, where nociception-related proteins are expressed in neurons of all sizes (Haberberger et al. 2019). Moreover, the separation of nociceptive DRG neurons into peptidergic and nonpeptidergic populations is not so clear-cut in human DRG as the GDNF receptor protein Ret is also present in neurons that express TrkA (Rostock et al. 2018).

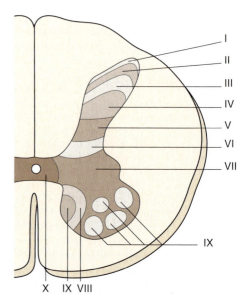

Fig. 6.1 The laminae of the spinal cord based on the description of Rexed (1952, 1954). Laminae I–VI comprise the dorsal horn.

the dorsal root entry zone (DREZ). The bundle of small-diameter fibres contains those involved in nociception, together with fibres involved in temperature and visceral sensation. They divide into short ascending and descending branches that run longitudinally in the dorsolateral fasciculus of Lissauer. Within several segments they leave the tract to synapse with neurons in the dorsal horn.

Primary afferents

As primary afferent fibres in peripheral nerves travel towards the spinal cord, they group to form spinal nerves, each spinal nerve supplying a discrete area of skin (dermatome), and overlapping to a greater or lesser degree the dermatomes of neighbouring spinal nerves. Each spinal nerve splits to form a ventral and dorsal root. The dorsal roots are purely sensory, but a considerable number of small-diameter unmyelinated afferent fibres are located in the ventral root (ventral root afferents; Coggeshall et al. 1974; Light & Metz 1978). These fibres end blindly, terminate in the pia mater or loop back into the dorsal root (Karlsson & Zakrisson 1998).

Sorting of primary afferent fibres occurs in the dorsal roots in primates (Snyder 1977). Large-diameter afferents subserving mechanoreception enter the spinal cord in the medial division of the dorsal root, while small-diameter fibres form a lateral bundle. The fibres enter the cord at

The dorsal horn

The dorsal horn of the spinal cord is the first site for integration and processing of incoming sensory information. The dorsal horn has historically been divided into three broad regions: the marginal zone, the substantia gelatinosa and the nucleus proprius. Rexed (1952, 1954) divided the grey matter of the spinal cord into 10 laminae based on cytoarchitectural criteria, with the dorsal horn encompassing laminae I to V (Fig. 6.1). Further anatomical and physiological studies have since confirmed functional differences in dorsal horn neurons in different laminae, as well as different patterns of projections. In addition, cells, axons and terminals in the different laminae of the dorsal horn have a distinctive chemical profile, which has been shown to change following a lesion (see Willis & Coggeshall 1991 for review).

Primary afferent fibres terminate in different laminae depending on their function (Fig. 6.2):

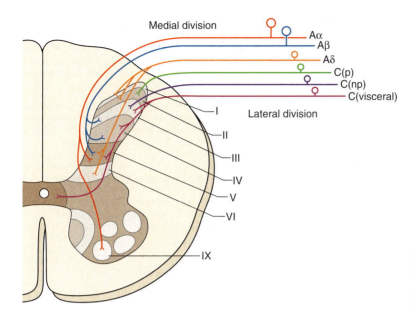

Fig. 6.2 The terminations of afferent fibres in the dorsal horn vary by depth. Large fibres *(Aβ)* enter in the medial division and small fibres *(Aδ and C)* enter in the lateral division of the dorsal root. *C(p)*, peptidergic; *C(np)*, nonpeptidergic.

Lamina I (the marginal zone) contains a high density of projection neurons that process nociceptive information. There are *nociceptive-specific* neurons that are excited solely by nociceptors and *wide dynamic range* neurons (also in lamina V–VI) that respond to both nociceptive and mechanoreceptive input.

Lamina II (the substantia gelatinosa) may be divided into an outer section, lamina IIo, and an inner section, lamina IIi, which has a lower density of neurons (Todd 2010). The most prominent structures in lamina II are complex structures called *glomeruli* through which a primary afferent terminal can make synaptic contact with several peripheral dendrites, axonal terminals and cell bodies (Kerr 1975). Glomeruli are key structures of the dorsal horn because they offer a morphological basis for both presynaptic and postsynaptic modulation of the primary afferent input. They comprise a central primary afferent terminal that makes contact with a group of between four and eight surrounding dendrites and other peripheral axon terminals and are set apart from the surrounding tissue by glial processes (Fig. 6.3). Using morphological criteria, the peripheral terminals appear to have the characteristics of inhibitory synapses and may contain the inhibitory neurotransmitters γ-aminobutyric acid (GABA) or enkephalin. The central terminals have the characteristics of excitatory terminals and may contain CGRP, glutamate, SP, cholecystokinin or serotonin. The glomerulus therefore comprises a complicated arrangement of inhibitory synaptic terminals surrounding an excitatory primary afferent ending.

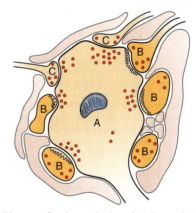

Fig. 6.3 Diagram of a glomerulus based on the work of Kerr (1975). *A*, Central terminal; *B*, dendrites; *C*, dendritic spines from lamina II neurons. *Pink shaded areas* represent glial processes.

The neuropil of *lamina III* resembles that of lamina II, but has slightly larger cells and myelinated axons. *Laminae IV and V* are characterised by neurons of various sizes. Lamina IV has prominent large cells, while lamina V is distinguished by longitudinally oriented myelinated axons. Laminae III, IV and the upper part of lamina V comprise most of the nucleus proprius.

Lamina VI is present only in cervical and lumbosacral enlargements and is a transition zone between the primary afferent-dominated dorsal horn and the ventral horn, with descending input predominating.

A population of neurons responding to noxious mechanical and thermal stimuli has been reported in *lamina X* in the vicinity of the central canal of the spinal cord. In addition to these high-threshold type cells, lamina X also contains neurons that are low threshold and have a wide dynamic range. Many of the cells have convergent input from visceral afferent fibres, and some of these respond only to visceral stimuli (Honda 1985; Honda & Perl 1985).

Somatotopic organisation of dorsal horn

The dorsal horn in the cervical and lumbar enlargements appears to be somatotopically organised with distal regions being represented medially and proximal areas laterally. There is a rostrocaudal representation of the digits, with the first digit being represented most rostrally and the fifth digit most caudally (Brown et al. 1989; Florence et al. 1988; Wilson et al. 1986).

Terminations of afferent fibres in the dorsal horn

The incoming afferent fibres of all types establish a web of connections with dorsal horn neurons, exerting a changing pattern of excitatory and inhibitory inputs that determines the firing of dorsal horn projection neurons and of interneurons that mediate spinal reflex responses (Table 6.2). Normally there is a certain degree of segregation in the termination pattern for different afferent fibre classifications in the dorsal horn, but this may not be the case in pathological situations. Woolf et al. (1992) showed that peripheral nerve injury triggers sprouting of myelinated afferents into lamina II, resulting in the possibility of functional contacts of low-threshold mechanoreceptive afferents with cells that normally have only C-fibre input.

Table 6.2 Terminations of afferent fibres in the dorsal horn

Afferents	Terminal zones in dorsal horn
Large-diameter myelinated fibres	III, IV and V
Small-diameter myelinated fibres (Aδ)	I and V
Unmyelinated fibres (C)	II, III
Visceral projections	II, IV–V and X

Large-diameter myelinated fibres

Collaterals of the large Aβ fibres initially travel ventrally through the dorsal horn but reverse when they reach the deeper laminae and break up to give rise to large flame-shaped arbors as they course dorsally. These terminations are dense in laminae III, IV and V (Fig. 6.2). It has been shown that the distal parts of the arbors of hair-follicle afferents enter the innermost part of lamina II (Brown 1981).

Small-diameter myelinated fibres

Collaterals of Aδ fibres terminate both superficially and deep within the dorsal horn. High-threshold afferents terminate profusely with arborisations in lamina I. Low-threshold hair afferents pass through lamina I to terminate in lamina V (Mense & Prabhakar 1986) and VI (Ralston & Ralston 1982) (Fig. 6.2).

Unmyelinated fibres

Unmyelinated afferents from the skin terminate in the superficial dorsal horn. The peptidergic C-fibre population terminates partly in lamina I but predominantly the outer part of lamina II of the dorsal horn (lamina IIo), while the nonpeptidergic group terminates in the inner part of lamina II, lamina IIi (Zylka et al. 2005). However, there is evidence that these populations overlap in other species (e.g. rat), and in humans, their protein markers intermingle within dorsal root ganglion neurons and in the spinal dorsal horn (Shiers et al. 2021). Lamina IIi has excitatory interneurons expressing the gamma isoform of protein kinase C, which has been implicated in persistent pain post-injury (Malmberg et al. 1997). Sugiura et al. (1989) reported that several branches of C-afferent fibres combined to terminate in a nest-like arrangement extending 400 µm rostrocaudally and 100 µm mediolaterally. In the cervical region, polymodal nociceptor fibre terminations were predominantly in lamina IIi. In the lumbar region, C-polymodal nociceptive fibres bifurcate into an ascending and a shorter descending branch. The rostrocaudal distribution is remarkably long (4600 µm) but the mediolateral extent is restricted (200 µm). Terminations are predominantly in lamina I and IIo, but some branches extend to laminae III and IV (Sugiura et al. 1986) (Fig. 6.2).

Visceral projections

Myelinated axons innervating abdominal and pelvic viscera project to lamina I or deeper laminae V–VI (de Groat et al. 1981; Morgan et al. 1981). Unmyelinated visceral

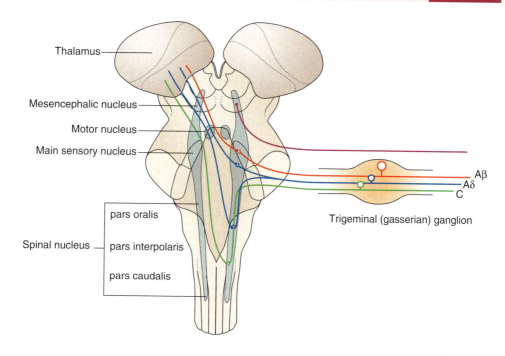

Fig. 6.4 Nuclei of the trigeminal nerve and their afferent connections. The cell bodies of most of the primary sensory neurons are in the trigeminal (Gasserian) ganglion, with the remainder in the mesencephalic nucleus. Small-diameter fibres subserving pain and temperature enter the spinal nucleus and synapse in the pars caudalis. Second-order axons cross the midline to form the trigeminothalamic tract.

afferents terminate in laminae I and II with some extension to lamina III (Gobel et al. 1981; LaMotte 1977). Unlike somatic C fibres which terminate in a reasonably circumscribed region, visceral unmyelinated afferent fibre terminations are more extensive, distributed over several spinal segments rostrocaudally, with ascending and descending branches extending for two to three segments through Lissauer's tract. Terminations are predominantly in laminae I and II but have also been reported in laminae V and X, as well as in contralateral laminae V and X (Sugiura et al. 1989) (Fig. 6.2).

Trigeminal system

Somatic sensation of the head and oral cavity is carried by four cranial nerves: the *trigeminal* (innervates most of the head and oral cavity), the *facial*, the *glossopharyngeal* and the *vagus* nerves (innervate the skin of the external ear, pharynx, nasal cavity and middle ear). The meninges are innervated by the trigeminal and vagus nerves. The trigeminal nerve is the largest cranial nerve, with four nuclei: the motor nucleus, the main sensory nucleus, the spinal nucleus and the mesencephalic nucleus. As is the case with sensory inputs to the rest of the body, tactile

sensation is mediated by large-diameter myelinated fibres, and pain and temperature sensations are mediated by small-diameter myelinated and unmyelinated fibres.

The sensory nuclei of the trigeminal nerve consist of three different parts. From caudal to rostral these are the *nucleus of the spinal tract*, the *main* or *principal sensory nucleus* and the *mesencephalic sensory nucleus* (Fig. 6.4). The fibres of the sensory root enter the pons and course dorsomedially towards the sensory nucleus. About half the fibres divide into ascending or descending branches as they enter the pons; the remainder ascend or descend without division. Many of the latter are very long and descend as the spinal tract of the trigeminal nerve to the caudal end of the medulla where it fuses with the dorsolateral tract of Lissauer in the spinal cord. As the tract descends, collaterals are given off to a long nucleus lying immediately medial to it, the *nucleus of the spinal tract*, which is continuous with the substantia gelatinosa of the dorsal horn. The *spinal nucleus* extends caudally through the whole length of the medulla and into the spinal cord as far as the second cervical segment. In the medulla, the tract and its nucleus are situated beneath the surface, with the upper part producing an elevation called the tuberculum cinereum.

Large-diameter axons of the trigeminal nerve terminate in the *main sensory nucleus*. The majority of neurons in the main sensory nucleus give rise to axons that decussate in the pons and ascend dorsomedial to fibres from the dorsal column nuclei in the medial lemniscus. These ascending fibres (the *trigeminal lemniscus*) synapse in the medial division of the ventral posterior nucleus of the thalamus (VPM). From here, the axons of the thalamic neurons project to the primary somatosensory cortex. This is the principal pathway for tactile perception in the face and is analogous to the dorsal column/medial lemniscal system. The main sensory nucleus of the trigeminal nerve is functionally similar to the dorsal column nuclei.

Pain and temperature are conveyed by smaller-diameter fibres terminating in the spinal part of the nucleus. The spinal trigeminal nucleus can be divided into three morphologically different parts: the *nucleus caudalis*, the *nucleus interpolaris* and the *nucleus oralis*. The nucleus caudalis mediates facial sensation. Like the dorsal horn, it plays an important role in pain and temperature senses, including dental pain, and a lesser role in tactile sensation. The nucleus interpolaris plays a role in mediating sensation from the teeth and the nucleus oralis is thought to be involved with discriminative touch sensation. Structurally and functionally, the nucleus caudalis resembles the dorsal horn on the basis of a number of features: (1) morphology and lamination, (2) laminar distribution of afferent terminals and (3) laminar distribution of projection neurons. The caudal nucleus is sometimes called the *medullary dorsal horn* (Fig. 6.5) because its laminar organisation is similar to the spinal dorsal horn (Dubner & Bennett 1983; Martin 1996).

Lamina I is equivalent to lamina I of the dorsal horn, and the portion of the spinal tract overlying lamina I of the spinal nucleus is the rostral extension of Lissauer's tract. Laminae II is equivalent to the substantia gelatinosa (lamina II), and laminae III and IV, termed the magnocellular nucleus in the trigeminal system, are equivalent to the nucleus proprius (laminae III and IV and the upper part of lamina V) in the dorsal horn. Each of these structures is associated with neurons responding to various types of stimuli. Those in the deep regions respond to both nociceptive and innocuous stimuli (wide dynamic range neurons), while neurons responding specifically to nociceptive or thermal stimuli are located in the substantia gelatinosa. There is an 'onion skin' pattern of representation of parts of the face in the spinal trigeminal nucleus, where regions around the mouth and nose are represented rostrally in the nucleus, while those in more lateral regions of the face are represented more caudally (Brodal 1981).

Sympathetic nervous system

The responses of an organism during pain and stress, which consist of autonomic, neuroendocrine and motor

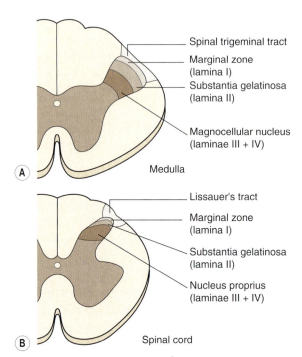

Fig. 6.5 Section through the medulla illustrating the trigeminal dorsal horn in (A). Corresponding areas of the spinal dorsal horn are shown in (B).

responses, are integral components of an adaptive biological system. They are important for the organism to function in a dynamic, challenging and possibly dangerous environment. The typical autonomic responses consist of an activation of various sympathetic pathways to skeletal muscle, skin, heart and viscera, thus leading to an increase of blood flow through skeletal muscle, increased cardiac output, piloerection, sweating and a reduction of blood flow through skin and viscera (Jänig 1995). Under physiological conditions, peripheral sympathetic pathways are distinct with respect to their target organs, and somatosensory pathways are functionally distinct with respect to the peripheral receptors and the corresponding sensations (Jänig 1992). However, following tissue damage this situation may radically change, such that the sympathetic and sensory channels are no longer separated (see Chapter 13).

The *hypothalamus* has a major role in producing responses to emotional changes and needs and is responsible for maintaining homeostasis. Through efferent pathways to autonomic ganglia in the brainstem and spinal cord, the hypothalamus controls sympathetic and parasympathetic functions. The hypothalamus receives inputs from the reticular formation in the brainstem and the amygdala, a collection of nuclei in the temporal lobe that are considered to be part of the limbic system.

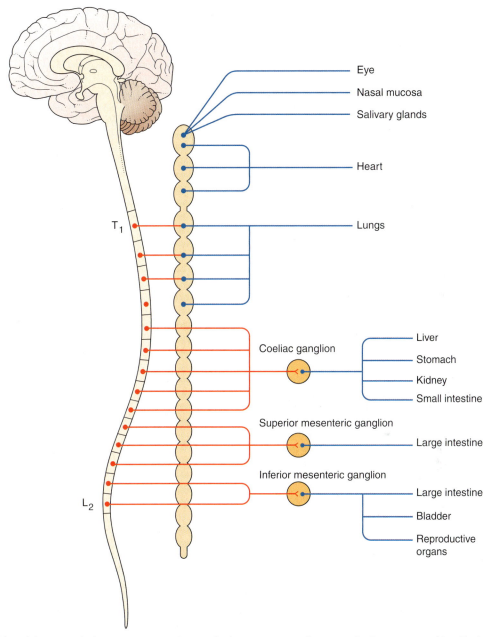

Eye
Nasal mucosa
Salivary glands

Heart

T_1

Lungs

Coeliac ganglion

Liver
Stomach
Kidney
Small intestine

Superior mesenteric ganglion

Large intestine

Inferior mesenteric ganglion

L_2

Large intestine
Bladder
Reproductive organs

Fig. 6.6 Plan of the sympathetic nervous system. Preganglionic neurons are *red*, postganglionic neurons are *blue*. The innervation of blood vessels, sweat glands and piloerector muscles is not shown.

The sympathetic pathways from the hypothalamus descend through the brainstem and spinal cord to synapse in the intermediolateral columns of the spinal cord between T1 and L2. In this area are the cell bodies of the *preganglionic neurons*. The preganglionic axons are myelinated and short (white rami), leaving the CNS via the ventral root and synapsing in the paravertebral *sympathetic chain* (ganglia). The sympathetic chain extends from the base of the skull to the coccyx (Fig. 6.6). The *postganglionic axons* are unmyelinated (grey rami) and rejoin the spinal nerves (Fig. 6.7) accompanying the peripheral nerves to innervate the body wall and blood vessels. Sympathetic

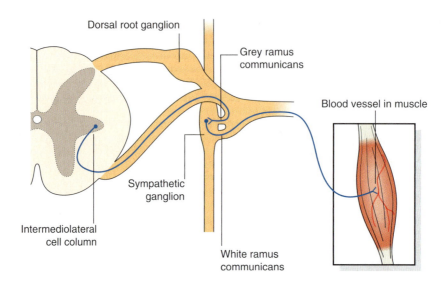

Fig. 6.7 Relationship of sympathetic axons with peripheral nerves.

axons innervating the face and brain arise from the inferior, middle and superior cervical ganglia and follow the carotid and vertebral arteries to their targets.

Spinal cord transmission pathways

Ascending tracts

Somatosensory signals are conveyed along with two major ascending systems in the spinal cord: the anterolateral system and the dorsal column-medial lemniscal system. The latter carries information about tactile sensation and limb proprioception. The anterolateral system relays information predominantly about pain and temperature, but also some tactile information. It comprises three pathways: the spinothalamic tract, the spinoreticular tract and the spinomesencephalic tract (Fig. 6.8).

The spinothalamic tract (STT) originates from neurons along the length of the spinal cord, with a particularly large concentration of STT cells in the uppermost cervical segments, including a large ipsilateral group of neurons in the ventral horn. Below this level, the majority of STT neurons are contralateral to their target. In the primate, STT neurons are located in three main regions: laminae I, IV–VI and VII–X (Apkarian & Hodge, 1989a; Hodge & Apkarian 1990), suggesting anatomically and functionally distinct components based on sites of termination in the thalamus (Craig 2006, 2008; Craig & Zhang 2006). The axons cross the midline in the dorsal and ventral white commissures at a level near the cell body and ascend to the thalamus in the lateral funiculus on the contralateral side. Although

most axons occupy the ventral lateral quadrant of the spinal white matter, some axons, particularly those originating from lamina I cells, ascend to the dorsal lateral quadrant (Apkarian & Hodge 1989b). The STT in the lateral funiculus has a somatotopic organisation. Axons from the most caudal regions of the spinal cord occupy the most dorsolateral position, with axons from progressively more rostral levels joining the tract in more ventromedial positions (Applebaum et al. 1975). In the brainstem, the STT passes dorsolateral to the inferior olivary nucleus in the medulla, then ascends dorsolateral to the medial lemniscus through higher levels of the brainstem to the thalamus. The STT transmits nociceptive and thermal information, as well as touch sensations.

The spinoreticular tract (SRT) in the primate originates from neurons in laminae VII and VIII, as well as the lateral part of lamina V. Some neurons are in lamina X. The majority of neurons giving rise to the SRT are in the uppermost cervical segments, although cells from all levels of the spinal cord are involved (Kevetter et al. 1982). There are two components: a projection to the lateral reticular nucleus (a precerebellar nucleus) and a projection to the pontine and medullary reticular formation, which gives rise to descending pathways to the spinal cord. Most of the projections from the cervical and lumbar enlargements cross the midline near the level of the cell bodies, but some axons originating from cervical segments remain uncrossed. They ascend in the ventral lateral column of the spinal cord with the STT and form a prominent bundle lateral to it in the brainstem. The SRT has no obvious somatotopic organisation and terminates in the following nuclei of the reticular formation: nucleus medullae oblongatae centralis,

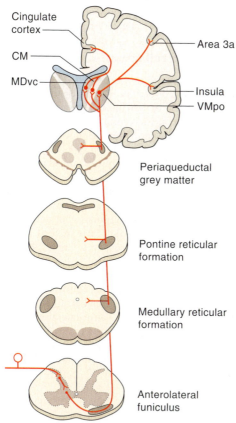

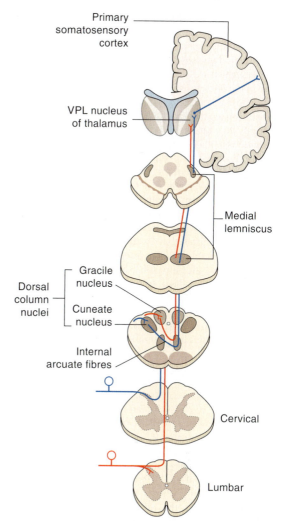

Fig. 6.8 Organisation of the anterolateral system. Primary axons terminate in the dorsal horn. Second-order axons cross the midline and ascend in the anterolateral funiculus in the spinal cord and the spinal lemniscus in the brainstem to terminate in the thalamus. Collaterals of these axons terminate in the reticular formation (spinoreticular axons) and in the periaqueductal grey matter (spinomesencephalic axons) *(shaded)*. Thalamocortical axons from the ventral caudal region of the mediodorsal (MDvc) and centromedian (CM) nuclei then project to the cingulate cortex, while those from the posterior region of the ventral medial (VMpo) nucleus project to area 3a and the insular cortex.

Fig. 6.9 Organisation of the dorsal column-medial lemniscal system. Large-diameter axons enter the spinal cord and ascend in the dorsal columns to the medulla, where they synapse in the dorsal column nuclei (nucleus gracilis and nucleus cuneatus). Second-order axons cross the midline and ascend in the medial lemniscus to terminate in the ventral posterolateral *(VPL)* nucleus of the thalamus. Thalamocortical axons then project to the somatosensory cortex.

lateral reticular nucleus, nucleus reticularis gigantocellularis, nucleus reticularis pontis caudalis and oralis, nucleus paragigantocellularis dorsalis and lateralis, and nucleus subcoeruleus (Mehler et al. 1960).

The *spinomesencephalic tract* (SMT) is a collection of pathways from the spinal cord to several different midbrain nuclei. It originates primarily from neurons in laminae I, V, VII and X (Zhang et al. 1990). The majority of axons cross the midline and ascend with the STT and SRT in the ventral lateral column. The SMT projects to the nucleus cuneiformis, the parabrachial nucleus, the intercollicular nucleus, the deep layers of the superior colliculus, the nucleus of Darkschewitsch, the anterior and posterior pretectal nuclei, the red nucleus, the

Edinger–Westphal nucleus, the interstitial nucleus of Cajal and the periaqueductal grey (PAG) (Yezierski 1988). The SMT is roughly somatotopically organised, with the projection from the cervical enlargement terminating more rostrally than that from the lumbosacral region. The PAG contains neurons that are part of a descending pathway that regulates pain transmission.

Other tracts in the dorsolateral funiculus and the dorsal columns also convey nociceptive information (Fig. 6.9). The *spinocervical tract* (SCT) originates from laminae III and IV at all levels of the cord where neurons respond predominantly to tactile stimuli, but some are activated by noxious stimuli. The axons project ipsilaterally in the dorsolateral funiculus to the lateral cervical nucleus, located just ventrolateral to the dorsal horn in segments C1–C3. The lateral cervical nucleus is quite small in the primate (Mizuno et al. 1967) and may be present in humans, although it is possible that the nucleus may not be distinctly separate from the dorsal horn in some cases (Ha & Morin 1964; Kircher & Ha 1968; Truex et al. 1965). Most of the neurons in the lateral cervical nucleus cross the midline in the ventral white commissure and ascend in the medial lemniscus to midbrain nuclei and to the thalamus.

The *dorsal column-medial lemniscal system* consists of branches of primary afferent fibres conveying tactile and proprioceptive information, as well as the axons of neurons in laminae IV–VI. There are also unmyelinated primary afferent fibres that synapse in the dorsal column nuclei, presumably arising from nociceptors (Patterson et al. 1990). In addition, there is a visceral pain pathway ascending in the dorsal column (Al-Chaer et al. 1998; Hirschberg et al. 1996; Willis et al. 1999). The medially located fasciculus gracilis contains a representation of the lower part of the trunk and lower extremity, whereas the fasciculus cuneatus lateral to it contains a representation of the upper part of the trunk and the upper extremity. This tract projects to the dorsal column nuclei in the medulla, from which axons ascend in the medial lemniscus to the thalamus. The sensory representation in the dorsal column nuclei is somatotopic with caudal parts of the body represented medially in the nucleus gracilis and the rostral regions laterally in the nucleus cuneatus. The trunk representation is in a region between the two nuclei. The distal extremities are represented dorsally and the proximal body ventrally (Johnson et al. 1968).

The ascending pathway from the spinal trigeminal nucleus (especially the caudal and interpolar regions) mediates facial and dental pain. The organisation of this pathway is similar to that of the anterolateral system. This pathway is called the *trigeminothalamic tract* and is predominantly crossed, ascending with the axons of the spinothalamic tract to the thalamus.

Areas of the brain involved in the perception, integration and response to nociception

Brainstem

Lamina I neurons project to three major regions of the brainstem: the catecholamine cell groups, the parabrachial nucleus and the PAG. Neurons from laminae V and VII project mainly to the reticular formation, the lateral reticular nucleus and the tectum, with smaller projections

to the parabrachial nucleus, the ventrolateral medulla and the PAG (Dostrovsky & Craig 2006).

Catecholamine cell groups

The Catecholamine cell groups in the lateral regions of the brainstem secrete dopamine (DA), noradrenaline (norepinephrine (NE)) or adrenaline (epinephrine (E)) are neurotransmitters in the central and peripheral nervous systems as well as hormones in the endocrine system. The neuronal groups containing DA or NE are labelled with the letter A, while those containing E are labelled with the letter C (Hökfelt et al. 1984).

The spinal projections predominantly terminate in the ventrolateral medulla (A1, C1, A5), the nucleus of the solitary tract (A2), the locus coeruleus (A6) and the sub-coerulear and Kölliker-Füse regions in the dorsolateral pons (A7) (Dostrovsky & Craig 2006). These regions are involved in integration of autonomic functions, with the nucleus of the solitary tract (A2) being a relay station for visceral afferents controlling cardiovascular, respiratory and gastrointestinal function (Benna-roch 2020a). Neurons in the ventrolateral medulla (A1) have a projection to the hypothalamus, which triggers the release of adrenocorticotrophic hormone and vasopressin in response to noxious stimulation (Dostrovsky & Craig 2006).

Rostral ventral medulla

Two nuclei that are widely implicated in descending control of nociception are the nucleus raphe magnus and the dorsal raphe nucleus. The nucleus raphe magnus receives inputs from the PAG and the dorsal raphe nucleus and is believed to mediate some of the effects of PAG stimulation. The raphe nuclei and adjacent nuclear groups contain serotonin (5HT) and project via the dorsolateral funiculus of the spinal cord to the superficial laminae of the dorsal horn, where the release of serotonin inhibits wide dynamic range neurons (Lipp 1991). The dorsal raphe nucleus also has ascending projections to the thalamus and hypothalamus, the basal ganglia and the amygdala and has been shown to modulate the activity induced by noxious stimulation of neurons in the thalamus (Wang & Nakai 1994).

The nucleus paragigantocellularis in the ventromedial medulla also receives input from the PAG and gives rise to a large projection to the locus coeruleus, as well as to the nucleus raphe magnus and the spinal cord (Stamford 1995).

Dorsolateral pontine tegmentum

The parabrachial nucleus is a complex of cytoarchitecturally distinct subnuclei surrounding the superior cerebellar peduncles in the dorsolateral pons. It receives projections from the nucleus of the solitary tract containing visceral sensory information, and inputs related to autonomic control, including respiration, fluid balance, blood pressure, cardiovascular function and thermoregulation (Herbert et al. 1990). The lateral parabrachial nucleus receives nociceptive, itch and thermal information from lamina I in the spinal and trigeminal dorsal horn (Craig 1995) as well as the deep dorsal horn, and projects to the PAG (Chiang et al. 2019). Its inputs and reciprocal connections of the parabrachial nucleus with the amygdala, stria terminalis and multiple hypothalamic nuclei indicate a role in homeostasis and the state of the body and contribute to the affective dimension of pain (ibid). Noradrenergic neurons of the pontine tegmentum, mainly from the locus coeruleus (A6), contribute to pain modulation by inhibiting spinothalamic activity in the dorsal horn through binding of noradrenaline on the primary afferent neuron, which directly suppresses the release of SP (Lipp 1991).

Periaqueductal grey matter

The periaqueductal grey matter surrounds the cerebral aqueduct of the midbrain. Anatomically, the PAG can be divided into medial, dorsal, dorsolateral and ventrolateral regions, each region forming longitudinal columns that have a high degree of functional specificity (Bandler et al. 1991; Bandler & Keay 1996; Bandler & Shipley 1994; Henderson et al. 1998). Through these longitudinal columns, the PAG has reciprocal connections with all levels of the nervous system and plays an important role in integrating a large number of functions that are critical to survival through its influence on the nociceptive, autonomic and motor systems (Bandler & Keay 1996; Bandler & Shipley 1994; Behbehani 1995; Bernard & Bandler 1998; Keay & Bandler 1993; Morgan et al. 1998). Functions controlled by the PAG include pain facilitation, analgesia, fear and anxiety, vocalisation, sexual behaviour and cardiovascular control (Behbehani 1995; Bernard & Bandler 1998).

Pain modulation can be demonstrated from electrical stimulation of various regions of the PAG. However, stimulation of the dorsolateral and ventrolateral subregions of the PAG produces different autonomic and motor responses (Lovick 1991; Morgan 1991) based on differing patterns of projections. In addition to the inputs from the spinal cord via the spinomesencephalic tract, the PAG also receives afferents from the parafascicular nucleus of the thalamus, the hypothalamus, the amygdala (Gray & Magnuson 1992), frontal and insular cortex (Hardy & Leichnetz 1981), the reticular formation, locus coeruleus (adrenergic projections) and other catecholaminergic nuclei in the brainstem (Herbert & Saper 1992). The ascending projections from the dorsolateral PAG are to the central lateral and paraventricular thalamic nuclei and

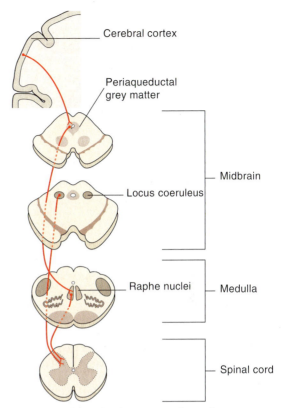

Fig. 6.10 The descending brainstem pathways from periaqueductal grey matter, raphe nucleus and locus coeruleus involved in pain inhibition.

the anterior hypothalamic area (Cameron et al. 1995a). The descending projections are to the locus coeruleus the pericoerulear region and the nucleus paragigantocellularis (Cameron et al. 1995b). The ventrolateral PAG, on the other hand, projects rostrally to the parafascicular and centromedian thalamic nuclei, the lateral hypothalamic area (Cameron et al. 1995a) and the orbital frontal cortex (Coffield et al. 1992). The descending projections are to the pontine reticular formation and the nucleus raphe magnus (Basbaum & Fields 1984; Cameron et al. 1995b). Stimulation of the PAG or the nucleus raphe magnus inhibits spinothalamic tract cells (Fields & Basbaum 1994) (Fig. 6.10). This difference in anatomical connectivity between the dorsolateral and ventrolateral regions of the PAG may provide a basis for their distinct and opposite modulatory influences on pain, autonomic and motor function.

Reticular formation

The reticular formation comprises a number of morphologically and biochemically different groups of

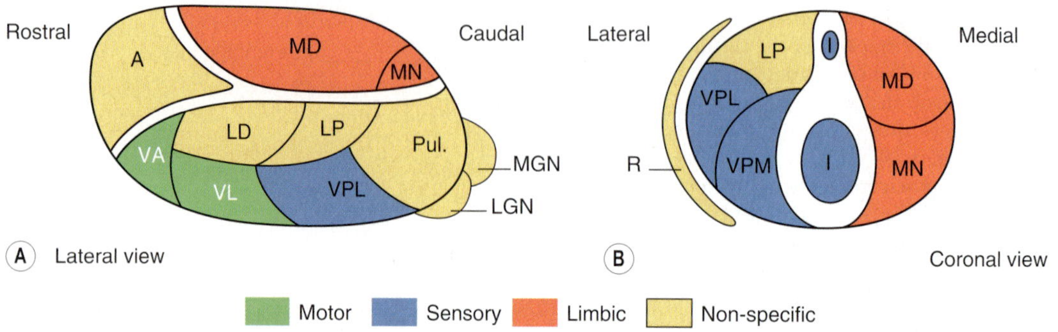

Fig. 6.11 Nuclei of the thalamus in lateral (A) and coronal (B) views. Nuclei associated with limbic functions: *A*, anterior nucleus; *LD*, lateral dorsal nucleus; *MD*, mediodorsal nucleus. Nuclei associated with motor functions: *VA*, ventral anterior nucleus; *VL*, ventral lateral nucleus. Nuclei associated with sensory functions: *LGN*, lateral geniculate nucleus; *MGN*, medial geniculate nucleus; *VPL*, ventral posterolateral nucleus; *VPM*, ventral posteromedial nucleus. Nuclei associated with sensory integration: *LP*, lateral posterior; *Pul*, pulvinar. Nonspecific nuclei: *IL*, intralaminar nuclei; *MN*, midline nuclei.

neurons distributed throughout the medulla, pons and midbrain. There is a projection from the reticular formation to the intralaminar nuclei of the thalamus (Peschanski & Besson 1984), which are known to be involved in the processing of nociceptive information (Kenshalo et al. 1980), as well as a projection to the spinal cord. It is important to note that there are reciprocal connections between the reticular formation and the limbic system. As previously discussed, the nuclei of the reticular formation receive nociceptive inputs through the SRT (Mehler et al. 1960). The reticular formation is involved in several different functions: activation of the brain for behavioural arousal, modulation of segmental stretch reflexes via the reticulospinal tracts, control of breathing and cardiac functions, and modulation of pain.

Thalamus

The thalamus represents the final link in the transmission of impulses to the cerebral cortex, processing almost all sensory and motor information prior to its transfer to cortical areas. The thalamus consists of six groups of nuclei: lateral (ventral and dorsal), medial, anterior, intralaminar, midline and reticular (Fig. 6.11).

- The nuclei of the ventral tier of the lateral group are specific relay nuclei, each receiving specific sensory or motor input and projecting to specific regions of the cerebral cortex. Of this group of nuclei, the *ventral posterolateral (VPL)* and *ventral posteromedial (VPM)* nuclei are concerned with sensation from the body and the face, respectively, while the *ventral anterior (VA)*, *ventral medial (VM)* and *ventral lateral (VL)* nuclei are concerned with motor function. Within the VM, which receives afferents from the basal ganglia (Hendry et al. 1979), is a cytoarchitecturally distinct nucleus in the posterior

region, VMpo, which plays a role in nociception (Craig et al. 1994).
- The nuclei of the dorsal tier of the lateral group and the nuclei of the medial group (*mediodorsal*) are association nuclei, projecting to association cortex (prefrontal association cortex, limbic association cortex, parietal-temporal-occipital association cortex).
- The *anterior nuclei* are specific relay nuclei, with connections to the hypothalamus and the cingulate gyrus.
- The *intralaminar*, *reticular* and *midline nuclei* are nonspecific nuclei, with widespread connections. The intralaminar nuclei receive inputs from the reticular formation in the brainstem.

Termination of spinothalamic afferents in the thalamus

Two subdivisions of the thalamic nuclei receive nociceptive input from spinal projection neurons.

The ventral nuclear group

Spinothalamic afferents from the contralateral side of the spinal cord terminate throughout VPL (Berkley 1980; Boivie 1979; Burton & Craig 1983; Mantyh 1983; Ralston & Ralston 1992). The terminals of spinothalamic axons overlap with those of the medial lemniscus in VPL of monkeys (Mehler et al. 1960) and extend into the ventral posterior inferior nucleus (VPI; Gingold et al. 1991), rostrally into VL (Applebaum et al. 1979; Berkley 1980; Boivie 1979; Burton & Craig 1983; Craig & Burton 1981) and caudally into the posterior nuclei (Ralston & Ralston 1992). There is a somatotopic organisation of spinothalamic terminals in VPL, which appear to be arranged in clusters across the nucleus (Boivie 1979; Mantyh 1983; Mehler et al. 1960). In monkeys and humans, VMpo

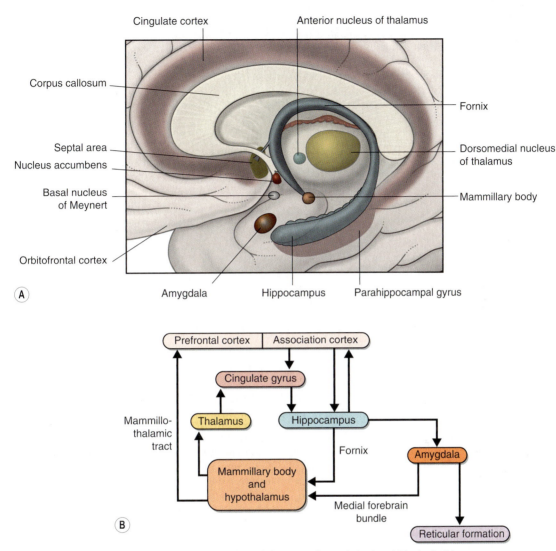

Fig. 6.12 (A) Limbic areas of the brain. (B) Diagram of neural circuits within the limbic system.

receives strong nociceptive and thermoreceptive-specific projections from lamina I (Craig et al. 1994) and projects to insular cortex (Pritchard et al. 1986), and area 3a in the fundus of the central sulcus (Craig 2003). The VMpo is contiguous with the basal region of the ventral medial nucleus (VMb), which receives direct input from the nucleus of the solitary tract (Beckstead 1980), transmitting visceral and gustatory information.

The receptive fields of thalamic neurons responsive to nociceptive stimuli are small and their discharge frequency can be related to the intensity and duration of the stimulus (Kenshalo et al. 1980). These neurons mediate the sensory-discriminative aspects of pain. Neurons in

VPI respond to innocuous mechanical stimuli (Kaas et al. 1984) as well as to nociceptive stimuli (Casey & Morrow 1987). The spinothalamic inputs to the lateral thalamic nuclei, which have direct projections to the primary somatosensory cortex (Gingold et al. 1991), are known as the *neo*-spinothalamic tract. This structure appears to be most prominently developed in primates.

The medial nuclear group

The medial group of thalamic nuclei, particularly the central lateral nucleus (CL), the intralaminar complex and the ventral caudal region of the mediodorsal nucleus (MDvc), receives collaterals of the spinothalamic and trigeminothalamic tracts, as well as inputs from the medullary and pontine reticular formation (Apkarian & Hodge 1989c; Burton & Craig 1983; Craig & Burton 1981; Mantyh 1983), the cerebellum (Asanuma et al. 1983) and the globus pallidus (Nauta & Mehler 1966). Neurons in CL are responsive to the intensity and duration of nociceptive stimuli and have large, often bilateral, receptive fields (Dong et al. 1978). Some spinothalamic tract axons project to both the intralaminar nuclei and VPL, and cells giving rise to these projections have small excitatory receptive fields, with surrounding larger inhibitory areas. Their discharge characteristics indicate that they could mediate discriminative aspects of noxious cutaneous stimulation, such as intensity, duration and localisation. The receptive fields of cells giving rise to projections to the intralaminar nuclei alone have large bilateral receptive fields (Giesler et al. 1981). The diffuse projections of the intralaminar nuclei to many different areas of the cortex have been considered part of a nonspecific arousal system, but it is also possible that their role is concerned with affective states induced by a painful stimulus. These nuclei are characterised by significant numbers of opiate receptors (see Jones 1985 for review). Because these medial projections to the thalamus appeared first in vertebrate evolution, they have been termed the *paleospinothalamic tract*.

Limbic structures

Broca (1878) first described the *limbic lobe* as consisting of the cingulate gyrus, the parahippocampal gyrus as well as the subcallosal gyrus and the hippocampal formation. Papez (1937) suggested that the limbic lobe formed a neural circuit providing the anatomical substrate for emotion. It was MacLean (1955) who recommended the term *limbic system*, which refers to a much more extensive complex of structures including the cingulate cortex, the temporal pole, the anterior portion of the insula, the posterior orbital surface of the frontal lobe and a number of subcortical structures, such as the thalamus, hypothalamus, septal nuclei and the amygdala (Fig. 6.12).

Basal ganglia

Three large subcortical nuclei comprise the basal ganglia: *caudate, putamen* (together called the *corpus striatum*) and the *globus pallidus* (*external and internal components*). There are interconnections with the *subthalamic nucleus* and the *substantia nigra* (comprising the pars reticulata and the pars compacta), which are also considered to be part of the basal ganglia (Fig. 6.13). The basal ganglia have a markedly heterogeneous structure, structurally, neurochemically and functionally. Their role in movement

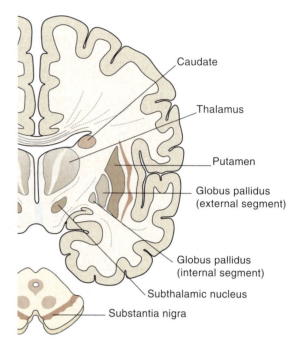

Fig. 6.13 Structures comprising the basal ganglia *(shaded)*.

control is evident from two common motor disorders affecting the basal ganglia, Parkinson's disease and Huntingdon's disease, both of which are caused by deficiencies in specific neurotransmitters.

The striatum receives afferent input from the entire cerebral cortex via the topographically organised corticostriate projection, as well as from other nuclei that comprise the basal ganglia, and projects to the VM, VL, ventral posterior, mediodorsal and centromedian nuclei of the thalamus. Through this circuit, there are projections back to different regions of the cerebral cortex. There are at least four open-loop circuits between the cerebral cortex and basal ganglia: a motor loop concerned with regulation of movement, a cognitive loop concerned with aspects of memory, a limbic loop concerned with emotional aspects of movement and an oculomotor loop concerned with the control of saccadic eye movements (Côté & Crutcher 1991).

Electrophysiological, metabolic and blood-flow studies have demonstrated that neurons in the basal ganglia are responsive to noxious and non-noxious somatosensory information. Nociceptive neurons have been located in the substantia nigra, caudate, putamen and globus pallidus. They have large receptive fields that encode stimulus intensity, while another population of neurons responds selectively to noxious stimuli without coding stimulus intensity (Chudler et al. 1993).

Basal ganglia disease such as Parkinson's disease may be accompanied by changes in pain perception. A recent large study of people with early to moderate Parkinson's disease found that 85% of participants reported pain and 42% reported moderate to severe pain not associated with motor dysfunction (Silverdale et al. 2018). Studies of deep brain stimulation of the subthalamic nucleus show that low-frequency stimulation increases pain thresholds and that abnormal central pain processing occurs in Parkinson's disease (Mostofi et al. 2021). These observations, as well as the anatomical and neurochemical connections of the basal ganglia, have led to the suggestion that they have a role in the sensory-discriminative, affective and cognitive aspects of pain, as well as in the modulation of nociceptive information (Chudler & Dong 1995).

Cerebral cortex

Imaging techniques have shown that in addition to the primary somatosensory cortex (SI) (Bushnell et al. 1999), multiple cortical areas are activated by painful stimuli, including the secondary somatosensory cortex (SII), the anterior cingulate cortex (Talbot et al. 1991), the insula, the prefrontal cortex (Treede et al. 1999) and the supplementary motor area (SMA) (Coghill et al. 1994). Subcortical activity has been observed in the thalamus and cerebellum. There is a distributed cortical system, involving parietal, cingulate and frontal regions, involved in the dynamic coding of pain intensity over time (Porro et al. 1998). These cortical regions also give rise to corticospinal projection (Galea & Darian-Smith 1994) and are also activated during active movement (Colebatch et al. 1991; Deiber et al. 1991; Matelli et al. 1993; Seitz & Roland 1992). Pain-related activation is more widely dispersed across both thalamic and cortical regions than that produced by innocuous vibratory stimuli, which is focused on SI. This distributed cerebral activation reflects the complex nature of pain, involving discriminative, affective, autonomic and motor components (Coghill et al. 1994).

Thalamocortical axons projecting predominantly from the VPL, VPI and CL nuclei relay nociceptive and thermal information to the primary somatosensory area of the cerebral cortex (SI) (Gingold et al. 1991). This area in anthropoid primates is differentiable into three cytoarchitectonic subfields, areas 3a, 3b, 1 and 2 of Brodmann. Each structurally distinct cortical field subserves a specific function, that is, there are functionally different neuron populations in each of these areas, with area 3a in the fundus of the central sulcus receiving proprioceptive inputs from muscle spindles, areas 3b/1 receiving inputs from cutaneous receptors and area 2 receiving input from deep pressure receptors (Kaas et al. 1979). Neurons in areas 3b/1 respond to stimulation of Aδ nociceptors, with

responses tightly coupled to the temporal profile of stimulation, and subserve fast/discriminative first pain (Chudler et al. 1990). The contralateral body surface is represented sequentially in each of these cortical areas. The regions of the body surface with the greatest tactile acuity, the face and the hand, are maximally represented in the cortical projection to the postcentral gyrus. These representational maps are dynamic and they change as a result of experience (Buonomano & Merzenich 1998).

The VPI has connections with SI and the second somatosensory cortex (SII) (Cusick & Gould 1990), but it is not known whether nociceptive inputs to VPI are relayed only to SI or to both SI and SII. SII CL has diffuse cortical projections. Although stimulation of CL gives rise to motor responses (Schlag-Rey & Schlag 1984), spinothalamic projections to CL do not contact thalamocortical neurons projecting to primary motor cortex (Greenan & Strick 1986).

VMpo has projections to the insular cortex and area 3a. Stimulation of the right dorsal posterior insula in awake humans causes localised pain, whereas stimulation of the posterior region of the insular cortex in both hemispheres elicits nonpainful sensations (Ostrowsky et al. 2002). While area 3a has been considered to be a primarily proprioceptive relay to the primary motor cortex, recordings in nonhuman primates have shown that it is highly responsive to cutaneous C-fibre nociceptive stimulation (Whitsel et al. 2019). Area 3a neurons exhibit slow temporal summation during repetitive thermal stimulation of C nociceptors and responses remain elevated for an extended period. Thus area 3a is thought to subserve slow/non-discriminative second pain (Cheng et al. 2015).

The MDvc projects to the anterior cingulate cortex (area 24c). The anterior cingulate cortex receives projections from MDvc and is considered to play a key role in the pain matrix (Tracey & Mantyh 2007). However, Vogt (2009) has proposed a four-region model of the cingulate gyrus, each with unique connections and functional organisation, as each region appears to be involved in different aspects of pain processing. The anterior cingulate cortex (ACC) is involved with pain-related attention, arousal, motor withdrawal. Human imaging studies have shown that this region may be associated with sadness (Ploner et al. 2002). The anterior part of the middle cingulate cortex (MCC) is most consistently involved in response to acute noxious stimulation and with the anterior insula forms a network integrating interoceptive information with emotional salience. The posterior MCC plays a role in reflexive orientation of the body in response to noxious stimuli. The posterior cingulate cortex (PCC) is involved in conscious processing of pain experience (Bennaroch 2020b).

Posterior parietal cortex has connections with the SI cortex and other polymodal association areas, including the limbic system (Cavada & Goldman-Rakic 1989) and is part of a general attentional system. Activation of this region may reflect hypervigilance or super-attentiveness to the sensory information accompanying chronic pain. The role of corticospinal projections from this region on dorsal horn neurons is unknown.

The cingulate cortex is involved in the processing of painful stimuli (Hsieh et al. 1995; Jones et al. 1991; Treede et al. 1999). The cingulate sulcus is a unique region of the limbic system, in that it appears to be involved in affecting and regulating context-relevant motor behaviours (Devinsky et al. 1995). It has been suggested that this region is critical for maintaining a working interaction between the limbic areas and motor areas of the cerebral cortex. Stimulation in the cingulate area (area 24) may also be involved in autonomic responses, such as changes in respiration and cardiovascular function (Hoff et al. 1963; Lofving 1961). Its role might be in linking emotional, motivational and memory-related information generated in limbic areas directly to motor areas (Morecraft & van Hoesen 1998). The ACC contains pain-anticipation-related neurons (Koyama et al. 1998) and therefore has a role in the anticipation of pain that precedes avoidance behaviour.

Neurons in SII and the posterior (granular) insula (Ig) are responsive to a wide range of somatosensory stimuli (Burton & Robinson 1981). The corticospinal projections from these areas terminate in the dorsal horn, but their specific role is unknown. The majority of neurons in SII respond to rapid, transient stimuli such as light touch. 'Complex zones' have been described, which become active during the performance of complex tasks (Burton & Robinson 1981). The posterior insula receives converging information about all five sensory modalities. Its efferent connections include the limbic system through the cingulate gyrus and amygdala (Mesulam & Mufson 1982), as well as the spinal cord (Galea & Darian-Smith 1994); therefore this area might have the function of providing the link between motivational and emotional states with relevant sensory information. Insular cortex is consistently activated by painful stimuli (Coghill et al. 1999; Craig et al. 2000). Noxious heat has been found to activate a region of the anterior insula (Id), which has connections with SI, SII and the cingulate region (area 24) (Mufson & Mesulam 1982) as well as with the amygdala and perirhinal cortex (Friedman et al. 1986). Although stimulation of the anterior insula produces predominantly visceral sensations, it also evokes unusual somatic sensations, movements and sometimes a sense of fear (Penfield & Rasmussen 1955).

Anatomical and imaging data suggest that the sensory-discriminative aspect of pain processing is subserved by a 'lateral' subsystem which includes thalamocortical afferents to SI, SII and posterior insula, whereas the motivational-affective aspect is subserved by a 'medial' subsystem, comprising projections to the anterior cingulate and prefrontal cortices (Albe-Fessard et al. 1985; Kulkarni et al. 2005; Rainville et al. 1997). However, clinically, pain is experienced as a unitary unpleasant bodily experience (Chapman et al. 2001; Talbot et al. 2019).

Corticospinal projections

Corticospinal projections are the only direct link between the sensorimotor cortex and the spinal cord. The origin of corticospinal projections in the primate cortex is more extensive than is commonly recognised. They comprise parallel, somatotopically organised projections to each level of the spinal cord with unique, though overlapping, patterns of termination. In addition to a dense projection from the motor cortex, corticospinal fibres arise from the premotor cortex, the postcentral cortex, especially the posterior parietal areas, the second somatosensory area and the caudal part of the insula. On the medial surface, there are extensive projections to the spinal cord from the SMA and the cortex within the cingulate sulcus (Dum & Strick 1991; Galea & Darian-Smith 1994) (Fig. 6.14).

Each of these cortical regions is distinguished not only by a characteristic cytoarchitecture, but also by a unique set of subcortical connections via the thalamus. The subcortical input to the precentral regions, including SMA and primary motor cortex, is mainly from the cerebellum and basal ganglia, whereas the input to the parietal corticospinal neuron populations is largely somatosensory (Darian-Smith et al. 1990). The ACC and insular cortex have connections with the limbic system (Baleydier & Maugiere 1980; Mesulam & Mufson 1982; Pandya et al. 1981; Vogt & Pandya 1987) and may have particular relevance to avoidance behaviour (Shima et al. 1991). Furthermore, the regions giving rise to corticospinal projections have complex, often reciprocal, cortico-cortical connections (Barbas & Pandya 1987; Cavada & Goldman-Rakic 1989; Preuss & Goldman-Rakic 1991). Both parietal and premotor cortical areas have converging inputs to the motor cortex (Leichnetz 1986; Matelli et al. 1986; Muakkassa & Strick 1979; Petrides & Pandya 1984).

The direct cortical projections to the dorsal horn arise from postcentral cortical areas. However, there are corticospinal projections from other brain areas to other spinal cord laminae-containing spinothalamic neurons. Areas 3b/1 and 2/5 have projections to laminae III–VI, with the greatest concentration medially (Cheema et al. 1984; Coulter & Jones 1977; Ralston & Ralston 1985). Cheema et al. (1984) identified labelling in the superficial laminae of the dorsal horn (laminae I and II) after injections of WGA-HRP into the somatosensory cortex.

The precentral cortical areas have a very wide pattern of termination. Area 4, classical motor cortex, projects

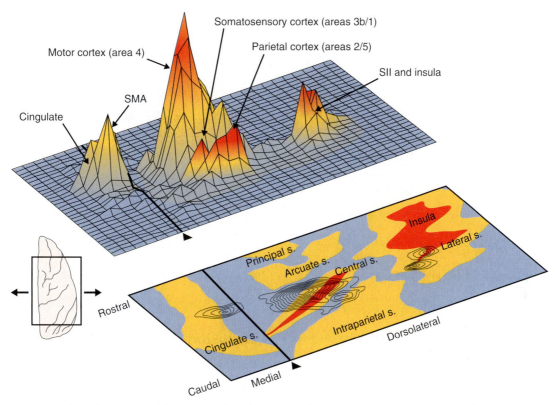

Fig. 6.14 Three-dimensional map and the corresponding contour map of the contralateral corticospinal soma distribution retrogradely labelled by a fluorescent dye injection at the cervical spinal cord. The contour map has been plotted onto the planar projection of the unfolded cortex. Sulci are indicated in yellow and are labelled in the bottom map; area 3a and the insula are shown in red" The heavy *black line* indicated by the *arrowhead* represents the sagittal midline, with the medial surface to the left. The maps show the variation in density of corticospinal projections terminating at mid-cervical levels. The most dense projection is from the primary motor cortex in the dorsal bank of the central sulcus, with smaller projections arising from the medial surface (SMA and rostral cingulate cortex), posterior parietal and insular cortex (including SII). Note the reduction of the corticospinal projection from areas 3a and 3b, compared with that from adjacent areas 4 and 2/5. *SMA*, Supplementary motor area.

predominantly to the intermediate zone (laminae VII and VIII), but the terminals extend into the lateral and medial regions of the ventral horn (lamina IX), as well as extensively, though more sparsely, into the deeper laminae of the dorsal horn (laminae V and VI). The supplementary motor cortex has a similar pattern of termination mainly in the intermediate zone and among the motor neuron pools (Galea & Darian-Smith 1997; Maier et al. 2002). The dorsal caudal cingulate area projects to the dorsolateral portion of the intermediate zone of the spinal cord (where spinothalamic neurons are located), while projections from the ventral caudal cingulate area terminate in the dorsomedial region (in the region of neurons projecting to the dorsal columns). However, there are sparse terminations in the dorsolateral region of the ventral horn and in the dorsal horn (laminae III and IV). These projections appear to be more dense in

the rostral segments of the cervical spinal cord (Dum & Strick 1996) (Fig. 6.15).

Role of corticospinal projections

The corticospinal projections form a parallel, distributed system arising from areas with complex interconnections and converging on different parts of the spinal circuitry. Their role in the modulation of activity in the dorsal horn, particularly in relation to pain, has not been investigated extensively.

Stimulation of SI and SII areas can result in primary afferent depolarisation (PAD) in fibres of the dorsal root (group Ib and II muscle afferents and cutaneous afferents, but not group Ia afferents (Andersen et al. 1964; Carpenter et al. 1963). It appears that sensorimotor cortex stimulation depresses the response of superficial

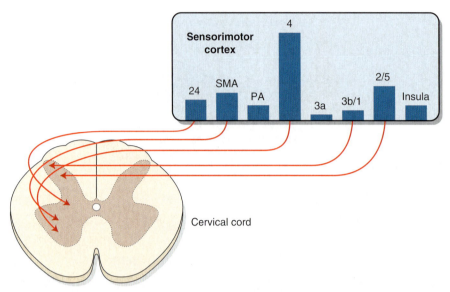

Fig. 6.15 Representation of the known areas of termination of corticospinal projections from different cortical areas. *PA*, postarcuate area; *SMA*, supplementary motor area.

dorsal horn neurons to a subsequent stimulus from the Lissauer tract. This tract is therefore thought to mediate the PAD evoked from multiple neural pathways (Lidierth & Wall 1998). Stimulation of sensorimotor cortex can also elicit both excitatory and inhibitory responses in dorsal horn neurons, particularly in laminae IV and V (Fetz 1968; Lundberg et al. 1962; Wall 1967). These cells receive a wide convergence of cutaneous input, as well as afferent information from muscle and joints. In a study in the monkey by Coulter et al. (1974), stimulation of the pre- or postcentral gyrus produced either a depression of the activity of neurons in the dorsal horn or an excitation followed by depression. Corticospinal projections from motor cortex may be excitatory to spinothalamic neurons, while those from postcentral cortex may inhibit them (Lidierth & Wall 1998; Ralston & Ralston 1985; Yezierski et al. 1983). Corticospinal projections to the superficial laminae (arising predominantly from areas 3b/1) may directly modulate nociceptive-specific neurons (Cheema et al. 1984).

The corticospinal neuron populations can produce indirect effects on the dorsal horn through collaterals to the *dorsal column nuclei*, where the effect is to diminish the postsynaptic responses of the dorsal column nuclei to somatic sensory nerve stimulation (Magni et al. 1959). In addition, there are collaterals to the PAG and the nucleus raphe magnus (Kuypers 1981), which have descending inhibitory connections with the spinal cord. Thus the cerebral cortex, through the corticospinal tract, may exert a modulatory effect on both motor and sensory functions, including pain.

Conclusion

This chapter has provided a review of the nervous system structures involved in nociception and their connections. Nociceptors are involved in signalling painful stimuli. There are several kinds of cutaneous nociceptors that can be activated by one or more kinds of noxious stimuli: mechanical, thermal or chemical. Other nociceptors are found in muscle, joints and viscera. Nociceptive and thermal signals are transmitted along unmyelinated (C) and small-diameter myelinated (Aδ) axons that synapse in the dorsal horn. Second-order neurons arise from different regions of the dorsal horn, cross the midline in the ventral commissure and ascend to the brainstem and thalamus in the anterolateral column. They synapse in a number of brainstem nuclei (including the reticular formation and the PAG) and in several thalamic nuclei (VPL, VPI, VMpo, MD, CL and the intralaminar nuclei). From the thalamus, nociceptive and thermal stimuli are relayed mainly to the SI area of the cerebral cortex. Multiple cortical areas are activated by painful stimuli, including the SII cortex, the ACC, the insula, the prefrontal cortex and the SMA. Pain signals may be modified through descending projections from the brainstem and cerebral cortex. The organisation of these structures suggests that there is a distributed cortical system concerned with the perception of pain. This distributed cerebral activation reflects the complex nature of pain, involving discriminative, affective, autonomic and motor components. An understanding of this complexity can provide insights for the management of pain in the clinical setting.

Review questions

Q

1. What classes of axons convey nociceptive and temperature information?
2. In which ways could nociceptive information be modulated at the level of the dorsal horn?
3. What spinal cord pathways convey nociceptive information to the brain? What are their targets?
4. Which regions of the brain subserve the sensory-discriminative and motivational-affective aspects of pain? How do their connections differ?
5. Name the descending projections to the dorsal horn. What is their role?

References

Abdo, H., Calvo-Enrique, L., Martinez Lopez, J., Song, J., Zhang, M.-D., Usokin, D., et al., 2019. Specialized cutaneous Schwann cells initiate pain sensation. Science 365, 695–699.

Abrahams, V.C., Lynn, B., Richmond, F.J.R., 1984. Organization and sensory properties of small myelinated fibres in the dorsal cervical rami of the cat. J. Physiol. 347, 177–187.

Adrian, E.D., 1931. The messages in sensory nerve fibres and their interpretation. Proc. R. Soc. B 109, 1–18.

Albe-Fessard, D., Berkley, K.J., Kruger, L., Ralston, H.J., Willis, W.D., 1985. Diencephalic mechanisms of pain sensation. Brain Res. Rev. 9, 217–296.

Al-Chaer, E.D., Feng, Y., Willis, W.D., 1998. A role for the dorsal column in nociceptive visceral input into the thalamus of primates. J. Neurophysiol. 79, 3143–3150.

Andersen, P., Eccles, J.C., Sears, T.A., 1964. Cortically evoked depolarization of primary afferent fibers in the spinal cord. J. Neurophysiol. 27, 63–77.

Apkarian, A.V., Hodge, C., 1989a. Primate spinothalamic pathways: I. A quantitative study of the cells of origin of the spinothalamic pathway. J. Comp. Neurol. 288, 447–473.

Apkarian, A.V., Hodge, C., 1989b. Primate spinothalamic pathways: II. The cells of origin of the dorsolateral and ventral spinothalamic pathways. J. Comp. Neurol. 288, 474–492.

Apkarian, A.V., Hodge, C., 1989c. Primate spinothalamic pathways: III. Thalamic terminations of the dorsolateral and ventral spinothalamic pathways. J. Comp. Neurol. 288, 493–511.

Applebaum, A.E., Beall, J.E., Foreman, R.D., Willis, W.D., 1975. Organization and receptive fields of primate spinothalamic tract neurons. J. Neurophysiol. 38, 572–586.

Applebaum, A.E., Leonard, R.B., Kenshalo, D.R., Martin, R.F., Willis, W.D., 1979. Nuclei in which functionally identified spinothalamic tract neurons terminate. J. Comp. Neurol. 188, 575–586.

Asanuma, C., Thach, W.T., Jones, E.G., 1983. Anatomical evidence for segregated focal groupings of efferent cells and their terminal ramifications in the cerebellothalamic pathway of the monkey. Brain Res. Rev. 5, 267–297.

Baleydier, C., Maugiere, F., 1980. The duality of the cingulate gyrus in monkey: neuroanatomical study and functional hypothesis. Brain 103, 525–554.

Bandler, R., Keay, K.A., 1996. Columnar organization in the midbrain periaqueductal gray and the integration of emotional expression. Prog. Brain. Res. 107, 285–300.

Bandler, R., Shipley, M.T., 1994. Columnar organization in the midbrain periaqueductal gray: modules for emotional expression? [published erratum appears in Trends Neurosci 1994 Nov 17(11):445]. Trends. Neurosci. 17, 379–389.

Bandler, R., Carrive, P., Zhang, S.P., 1991. Integration of somatic and autonomic reactions within the midbrain periaqueductal gray: viscerotopic, somatotopic and functional organization. Prog. Brain. Res. 87, 269–305.

Barbas, H., Pandya, D.N., 1987. Architecture and frontal cortical connections of the premotor cortex (area 6) in the rhesus monkey. J. Comp. Neurol. 256, 211–228.

Basbaum, A.I., Fields, H.L., 1984. Endogenous pain control systems: brainstem spinal pathways and endorphin circuitry. Annu. Rev. Neurosci. 7, 309–338.

Basbaum, A.I., Bautista, D.M., Scherrer, G., Julius, D., 2009. Cellular and molecular mechanisms of pain. Cell 139 (2), 267–284.

Baumbauer, K.M., DeBerry, J.J., Adelman, P.C., Miller, R.H., Hacisuka, J., Lee, K.H., et al., 2015. Keratinocytes can modulate and directly initiate nociceptive responses. Elife 4, e09674.

Beckstead, R.M., 1980. The nucleus of the solitary tract in the monkey: projections to the thalamus and brain stem nuclei. J. Comp. Neurol. 190, 259–282.

Behbehani, M.M., 1995. Functional characteristics of the midbrain periaqueductal gray. Prog. Neurobiol. 46, 575–605.

Bennaroch, E.E., 2020a. Physiology and pathophysiology of the autonomic nervous system. Con. Autonom. Dis. 26, 12–24.

Bennaroch, E.E., 2020b. What is the role of the cingulate cortex in pain? Neurology 95, 729–732.

Berkley, K., 1980. Spatial relationships between the terminations of somatic and motor pathways in the rostral brainstem of cats and monkeys. I. Ascending somatic sensory inputs to lateral diencephalon. J. Comp. Neurol. 193, 283–317.

Bernard, J.F., Bandler, R., 1998. Parallel circuits for emotional coping behaviour: new pieces in the puzzle. J. Comp. Neurol. 401, 429–436.

Bessou, P., Laporte, Y., 1961. Étude des recepteurs musculaires innervés par les fibres afferentes du groupe III (fibres myelinisées fines), chez le chat. Arch. Ital. Biol. 99, 293–321.

Bessou, P., Perl, E.R., 1969. Response of cutaneous sensory units with unmyelinated fibres to noxious stimuli. J. Neurophysiol. 32, 1025–1043.

Bessou, P., Burgess, P.R., Perl, E.R., Taylor, C.B., 1971. Dynamic properties of mechanoreceptors with unmyelinated (C) fibers. J. Neurophysiol. 34, 116–131.

Bielefeldt, K., Gebhart, G.F., 2006. Visceral pain: basic mechanisms. In: McMahon, S.B., Koltzenburg, M. (Eds.), Wall and Melzack's Textbook of Pain, fifth ed. Elsevier, Philadelphia, pp. 721–736.

Boivie, J., 1979. An anatomical reinvestigation of the termination of the spinothalamic tract in the monkey. J. Comp. Neurol. 186, 343–370.

Braz, J., Solorzano, C., Wang, X., et al., 2014. Transmittmg pain and itch messages: a contemporary view of the spinal cord circuits that generate Gate Control. Neuron 82, 522–536.

Broca, P., 1878. Anatomie comparée de circonvolutions cérébrales. Le grand lobe limbique et la scissure limbique dans le série des mammifères. Rev. Anthropol. 1, 385–498.

Brodal, A., 1981. Neurological Anatomy in Relation to Clinical Medicine. Oxford University Press, New York.

Brown, P.B., Brushart, T.M., Ritz, L.A., 1989. Somatotopy of digital nerve projections to the dorsal horn in the monkey. Somatosens. Mot. Res. 6, 309–317.

Brown, A.G., 1981. Organization in the Spinal Cord. Springer, Berlin.

Buonomano, D.V., Merzenich, M.M., 1998. Cortical plasticity: from maps to synapses. Annu. Rev. Neurosci. 21, 149–186.

Burgess, P.R., Perl, E.R., 1967. Myelinated afferent fibres responding specifically to noxious stimulation of the skin. J. Physiol. (Lond.) 190, 541–562.

Burnstock, G., 2007. Physiology and pathophysiology of purogenic neurotransmission. Physiol. Rev. 87, 659–797.

Burton, H., Craig, A.D., 1983. Spinothalamic projections in cat, raccoon and monkey: a study based on anterograde transport of horseradish peroxidase. In: Macchi, G., Rustioni, A., Spreafico, R. (Eds.), Somatosensory Integration in the Thalamus. Elsevier, Amsterdam, pp. 17–41.

Burton, H., Robinson, C.J., 1981. Organization of the SII parietal cortex. Multiple somatic sensory representations within and near the second somatic sensory area of the cynomolgus monkeys. In: Woolsey, C.N. (Ed.), Cortical Sensory Organization. Multiple Sensory Areas, vol. 1. Humana Press, New Jersey, pp. 67–119.

Bushnell, M.C., Duncan, G.H., Hofbauer, R.K., Ha, B., Chen, J.-I., Carrier, B., 1999. Pain perception: is there a role for primary somatosensory cortex? Proc. Nat. Acad. Sci. USA 96, 7705–7709.

Cameron, A.A., Khan, I.A., Westlund, K.N., Cliffer, K.D., Willis, W.D., 1995a. The efferent projections of the periaqueductal gray in the rat: a Phaseolus vulgaris-leucoagglutinin study. I. Ascending projections. J. Comp. Neurol. 351, 568–584.

Cameron, A.A., Khan, I.A., Westlund, K.N., Willis, W.D., 1995b. The efferent projections of the periaqueductal gray in the rat: a Phaseolus vulgaris-leucoagglutinin study. II. Descending projections. J. Comp. Neurol. 351, 585–601.

Campbell, J.N., Meyer, R.A., LaMotte, R.H., 1979. Sensitization of myelinated nociceptive afferents that innervate monkey hand. J. Neurophysiol. 42, 1669–1679.

Campero, M., Serra, J., Ochoa, J.L., 1996. C-polymodal nociceptors activated by noxious low temperature in human skin. J. Physiol. 497, 565–572.

Carpenter, D., Lundberg, A., Norrsell, U., 1963. Primary afferent depolarization evoked from the sensorimotor cortex. Acta. Physiol. Scand. 59, 126–142.

Casey, K.L., Morrow, T.J., 1987. Nociceptive neurons in the ventral posterior thalamus of the awake squirrel monkey: observations in identification, modulation and drug effects. In: Besson, J.-M., Guilbaud, D., Peschanksi, M. (Eds.), Thalamus and Pain. Elsevier, Amsterdam, pp. 211–226.

Caterina, M.J., Rosen, T.A., Tominaga, M., Brake, A.J., Julius, D., 1999. A capsaicin-receptor homologue with a high threshold for noxious heat. Nature 398, 436–441.

Cavada, C., Goldman-Rakic, P.S., 1989. Posterior parietal cortex in rhesus monkey: II. Evidence for segregated corticocortical networks linking sensory and limbic areas with the frontal lobe. J. Comp. Neurol. 287, 422–445.

Chapman, C.R., Nakamura, Y., Donaldson, G.W., Bradshaw, D.H., Flores, L., Chapman, C.N., 2001. Sensory and affective dimensions of phasic pain are indistinguishable in the self-report and psychophysiology of normal laboratory subjects. J. Pain 2, 279–294.

Cheema, S.S., Rustioni, A., Whitsel, B.L., 1984. Light and electron microscopic evidence for a direct corticospinal projection to superficial laminae of the dorsal horn in cats and monkeys. J. Comp. Neurol. 225, 276–290.

Cheng, J.C., Erpelding, N., Kucyi, A., DeSouza, D.D., Davis, K.D., 2015. Individual differences in temporal summation of pain reflects pronociceptive and antinociceptive brain structure and function. J. Neurosci. 35, 9689–9700.

Chiang, M.C., Bowen, A., Schier, L.A., Tupone, D., Uddin, O., Heinricher, M.M., 2019. Parabrachial complex: a hub for pain and aversion. J. Neurosci. 39, 8225–8230.

Chudler, E.H., Dong, W.K., 1995. The role of the basal ganglia in nociception and pain. Pain 60, 3–38.

Chudler, E.H., Anton, F., Dubner, R., Kenshalo, D.R., 1990. Responses of nociceptive SI neurons in monkeys and pain sensation in humans elicited by noxious thermal stimulation: effect of interstimulus interval. J. Neurophysiol. 63, 559–569.

Chudler, E.H., Sugiyama, K., Dong, W.K., 1993. Nociceptive responses of neurons in the neostriatum and globus pallidus of the rat. J. Neurophysiol. 69, 1890–1903.

Coffield, J.A., Bowen, K.K., Miletic, V., 1992. Retrograde tracing of projections between the nucleus submedius, the ventrolateral orbital cortex, and the midbrain in the rat. J. Comp. Neurol. 321, 488–499.

Coggeshall, R.E., Coulter, J.D., Willis, W.D., 1974. Unmyelinated axons in the ventral roots of the cat lumbosacral enlargement. J. Comp. Neurol. 153, 39–58.

Coghill, R.C., Talbot, J.D., Evans, A.C., et al., 1994. Distributed processing of pain and vibration by the human brain. J. Neurosci. 14, 4095–4108.

Coghill, R.C., Sang, C.N., Maisog, J.M., Iadarola, M.J., 1999. Pain intensity processing within the human brain: a bilateral distributed mechanism. J. Neurophysiol. 82, 1934–1943.

Colebatch, J.G., Deiber, M.-P., Passingham, R.E., Friston, K.J., Frackowiak, R.S.J., 1991. Regional cerebral blood flow during voluntary arm and hand movements in human subjects. J. Neurophysiol. 65, 1392–1401.

Côté, L., Crutcher, M.D., 1991. The basal ganglia. In: Kandel, E.R., Schwartz, J.H., Jessell, T.M. (Eds.), Principles of Neural Science, third ed. Elsevier, New York, pp. 647–659.

Coulter, J.D., Jones, E.G., 1977. Differential distribution of corticospinal projections from individual cytoarchitectonic fields in the monkey. Brain. Res. 129, 335–340.

Coulter, J.D., Maunz, R.A., Willis, W.D., 1974. Effects of stimulation of sensorimotor cortex on primate spinothalamic neurons. Brain. Res. 65, 351–356.

Craig, A.D., Burton, H., 1981. Spinal and medullary lamina I projection to nucleus submedius in medial thalamus: a possible pain center. J. Neurophysiol. 45, 443–466.

Craig, A.D., Zhang, E.-T., 2006. Retrograde analyses of spinothalamic projections in the macaque monkey: input to posterolateral thalamus. J. Comp. Neurol. 499, 953–964.

Craig, A.D., Bushnell, M.C., Zhang, E.-T., Blomqvist, A., 1994. A thalamic nucleus specific for pain and temperature sensation. Nature 372, 770–773.

Craig, A.D., Chen, K., Bandy, D., Reiman, E.M., 2000. Thermosensory activation of insular cortex. Nat. Neurosci. 3, 184–190.

Craig, A.D., 1995. Distribution of brainstem projections from spinal lamina I neurons in the cat and monkey. J. Comp. Neurol. 361, 225–248.

Craig, A.D., 2002. How do you feel? Interception: the sense of the physiological condition of the body. Nat. Rev. Neurosci. 3, 655–666.

Craig, A.D., 2003. Pain mechanisms: labeled lines versus convergence in central processing. Annu. Rev. Neurosci. 26, 1–30.

Craig, A.D., 2006. Retrograde analyses of spinothalamic projections in the macaque monkey: input to ventral posterior nuclei. J. Comp. Neurol. 499, 965–978.

Craig, A.D., 2008. Retrograde analyses of spinothalamic projections in the macaque monkey: input to ventral lateral nucleus. J. Comp. Neurol. 508, 315–328.

Cusick, C.G., Gould, H.J., 1990. Connections between area 3b of the somatosensory cortex and subdivisions of the ventroposterior nuclear complex and the anterior pulvinar in squirrel monkeys. J. Comp. Neurol. 292, 83–102.

Darian-Smith, C., Darian-Smith, I., Cheema, S.S., 1990. Thalamic projections to sensorimotor cortex in the macaque monkey: use of multiple retrograde tracers. J. Comp. Neurol. 299, 17–46.

de Groat, W.C., Nadelhaft, I., Milne, R., Booth, A.M., Morgan, C., Thor, K., 1981. Organisation of the sacral parasympathetic reflex pathways to the urinary bladder and large intestine. J. Auton. Nerv. Syst. 3 (2–4), 135–160.

Deiber, M.-P., Passingham, R.E., Colebatch, J.G., Friston, K.J., Nixon, P.D., Frackowiak, R.S.J., 1991. Cortical areas and the selection of movement: a study with positron emission tomography. Exp. Brain. Res. 84, 393–402.

Devinsky, O., Morrell, M.J., Vogt, B.A., 1995. Contributions of anterior cingulate cortex to behaviour. Brain 118, 279–306.

Djouhri, L., Lawson, S.N., 2004. Aβ-fiber nociceptive primary afferent neurons: a review of incidence and properties in relation to other afferent A-fiber neurons in mammals. Brain. Res. Rev. 46, 131–145.

Dong, W.K., Ryu, H., Wagman, I.H., 1978. Nociceptive responses in medial thalamus and their relationship to spinothalamic pathways. J. Neurophysiol. 41, 1592–1613.

Dong, X., Han, S.-K., Zylka, M.J., et al., 2001. A diverse family of GPCRs expressed in specific subsets of nociceptive sensory neurons. Cell 106, 619–632.

Dostrovsky, J.O., Craig, A.D., 2006. Ascending projection systems. In: McMahon, S.B., Koltzenburg, M. (Eds.), Wall and Melzack's Textbook of Pain, fifth ed. Elsevier, Philadelphia, pp. 187–203.

Dubin, A.E., Patapoutian, A., 2010. Nocicpetors: the sensors of the pain pathway. J. Clin. Investig. 120, 3760–3772.

Dubner, R., Bennett, G.J., 1983. Spinal and trigeminal mechanisms of nociception. Ann. Rev. Neurosci. 6, 381–418.

Dum, R.P., Strick, P.L., 1991. The origin of corticospinal projections from the premotor areas in the frontal lobe. J. Neurosci. 11, 667–689.

Dum, R.P., Strick, P.L., 1996. Spinal cord terminations of the medial wall motor areas in macaque monkeys. J. Neurosc. 16, 6513–6525.

Erlanger, J., Gasser, H.S., 1937. Electrical Signs of Nervous Activity. University of Pennsylvania Press, Philadelphia.

Fetz, E.E., 1968. Pyramidal tract effects on interneurons in the cat lumbar dorsal horn. J. Neurophysiol. 31, 69–80.

Fields, H.L., Basbaum, A.I., 1994. Central nervous system mechanisms of pain modulation. In: Wall, P.D., Melzack, R. (Eds.), Textbook of Pain. Churchill Livingstone, Edinburgh, pp. 243–257.

Florence, S.L., Wall, J.T., Kaas, J.H., 1988. The somatotopic pattern of afferent projections from the digits to the spinal cord and cuneate nucleus in macaque monkeys. Brain. Res. 452, 388–392.

Friedman, D.P., Murray, E.A., O'Neill, J.B., Mishkin, M., 1986. Cortical connections of the somatosensory fields of the lateral sulcus of macaques: evidence of a corticolimbic pathway for touch. J. Comp. Neurol. 252, 323–347.

Galea, M.P., Darian-Smith, I., 1994. Multiple corticospinal neuron populations in the macaque monkey are specified by their unique cortical origins, spinal terminations and connections. Cerebr. Cortex. 4, 166–194.

Galea, M.P., Darian-Smith, I., 1997. Corticospinal projection patterns following unilateral cervical spinal cord section in the newborn and juvenile macaque monkey. J. Comp. Neurol. 381, 282–306.

Giesler, G.J., Spiel, H.R., Willis, W.D., 1981. Organization of spinothalamic tract axons within the rat spinal cord. J. Comp. Neurol. 195, 243–252.

Gingold, S.I., Greenspan, J.D., Apkarian, A.V., 1991. Anatomic evidence of nociceptive inputs to primary somatosensory cortex: relationship between spinothalamic terminals and thalamocortical cells in squirrel monkeys. J. Comp. Neurol. 308, 467–490.

Gobel, S., Falls, W.M., Humphrey, E., 1981. Morphology and synaptic connections of ultrafine primary axons in lamina I of the spinal dorsal horn: candidates for the terminal axonal arbors of primary neurones in unmyelinated (C) axons. J. Neurosci. 1, 1163–1179.

Gray, T.S., Magnuson, D.J., 1992. Peptide immunoreactive neurons in the amygdala and the bed nucleus of the stria terminalis project to the midbrain central gray in the rat. Peptides 13, 451–460.

Greenan, T.J., Strick, P.L., 1986. Do thalamic regions which project to rostral primate motor cortex receive spinothalamic input? Brain. Res. 362, 384–388.

Grieve, G.P., 1994. Referred pain and other clinical features. In: Boyling, J.D., Palastanga, N. (Eds.), Grieve's Modern Manual Therapy, The Vertebral Column, second ed. Churchill Livingstone, London.

Ha, H., Morin, F., 1964. Comparative anatomical observations of the cervical nucleus, *N. cervicalis lateralis*, of some primates. Anat. Rec. 148, 374–375.

Haberberger, R.V., Barry, C., Dominegz, N., et al., 2019. Human dorsal root ganglia. Front. Cell Neurosci. 13, 271.

Habig, K., Schänzer, A., Schirner, W., Lautenschläger, G., Dassinger, B., Olausson, H., et al., 2017. Low threshold unmyelinated mechanoafferents can modulate pain. BMC. Neurol. 17, 184.

Häbler, H.-J., Jänig, W., Koltzenburg, M., 1990. Activation of unmyelinated fibres by mechanical stimuli and inflammation of the urinary bladder in the cat. J. Physiol. (Lond.) 425, 545–562.

Hardy, S.G.P., Leichnetz, G.R., 1981. Cortical projections to the periaqueductal gray in the monkey: a retrograde and orthograde horseradish peroxidase study. Neurosci. Lett. 22, 97–101.

Harrison, J.L.K., Davis, K.D., 1999. Cold-evoked pain varies with skin type and cooling rate: a psychophysical study in humans. Pain 83, 123–135.

Harty, B.L., Monk, K.R., 2017. Unwrapping the unappreciated: recent progress in Remak Schwann cell biology. Curr. Opin. Neurobiol. 47, 131–137.

Henderson, L.A., Keay, K.A., Bandler, R., 1998. The ventrolateral periaqueductal gray projects to caudal brainstem depressor regions: a functional-anatomical and physiological study. Neuroscience 82, 201–221.

Hendry, S.H.C., Jones, E.G., Graham, J., 1979. Thalamic relay nuclei for cerebellar and certain related fiber systems in the cat. J. Comp. Neurol. 185, 679–714.

Heppelmann, B., Messlinger, K., Neiss, W.F., Schmidt, R.F., 1990. Ultrastructural three-dimensional reconstruction of group III and group IV sensory nerve endings ('free nerve endings') in the knee joint of the cat: evidence for multiple receptive sites. J. Comp. Neurol. 292, 103–116.

Herbert, H., Saper, C.R., 1992. Organization of medullary adrenergic and noradrenergic projections to the periaqueductal gray matter in the rat. J. Comp. Neurol. 314, 34–52.

Herbert, H., Moga, M.M., Saper, C.B., 1990. Connections of the parabrachial nucleus with the nucleus of the solitary tract and the medullary reticular formation in the rat. J. Comp. Neurol. 293, 540–580.

Hertel, H.C., Howaldt, B., Mense, S., 1976. Responses of group IV and group III muscle afferents to thermal stimuli. Brain. Res. 113, 201–205.

Hirschberg, R.M., Al-Chaer, E.D., Lawand, N.B., Westlund, K.N., Willis, W.D., 1996. Is there a pathway in the posterior funiculus that signals visceral pain? Pain 67, 291–305.

Hodge, C.J., Apkarian, A.V., 1990. The spinothalamic tract. Crit. Rev. Neurobiol. 5, 363–397.

Hoff, E.C., Kell, J.F., Carroll, M.N., 1963. Effects of cortical stimulation and lesions on cardiovascular function. Physiol. Rev. 43, 68–114.

Hoheisel, U., Reinöhl, J., Unger, T., Mense, S., 2004. Acidic pH and capsaicin activate mechanosensitive group IV muscle receptors in the rat. Pain 110, 149–157.

Hoheisel, U., Unger, T., Mense, S., 2005. Excitatory and modulatory effects of inflammatory cytokines and neurotrophins on mechanosensitive group IV muscle afferents in the rat. Pain 114, 168–176.

Hökfelt, T., Martensson, O., Björklund, A., Kleinau, S., Goldstein, M., 1984. Distribution maps of tyrosine-hydroxylaseimmunoreactive neurons in the rat brain. In: Björklund, A., Hökfelt, T. (Eds.), Handbook of Chemical Neuroanatomy Part 1, vol. 2. Elsevier, Amsterdam, pp. 277–379.

Honda, C.N., Perl, E.R., 1985. Functional and morphological features of neurons in the midline region of the caudal spinal cord in the cat. Brain. Res. 340, 285–295.

Honda, C.N., 1985. Visceral and somatic afferent convergence onto neurons near the central canal in the sacral spinal cord of the cat. J. Neurophysiol. 53, 1059–1078.

Hsieh, J.-C., Belfrage, M., Stone-Elander, S., Hansson, P., Ingvar, M., 1995. Central representation of chronic ongoing neuropathic pain studied by positron emission tomography. Pain 63, 225–236.

Iggo, A., 1960. Cutaneous mechanoreceptors with C fibres. J. Physiol. (Lond.) 152, 337–353.

Immke, D.C., Gavva, N.R., 2006. The TRPV1 receptor and nociception. Semin. Cell. Dev. Biol. 17, 582–591.

Jänig, W., 1992. Pain and the sympathetic nervous system: pathophysiological mechanisms. In: Bannister, R., Mathias, C. (Eds.), Autonomic Failure. Oxford University Press, Oxford, pp. 231–251.

Jänig, W., 1995. The sympathetic nervous system in pain. Eur. J. Anaesthesiol. 12 (Suppl. 10), 53–60.

Ji, R.-R., Chamessian, A., Zhang, Y.-Q., 2016. Pain regulation by non-neuronal cells and inflammation. Science 354, 572–577.

Johnson, J.I., Welker, W.I., Pubols, B.H., 1968. Somatotopic organization of raccoon dorsal column nuclei. J. Comp. Neurol. 132, 1–44.

Jones, A.K.P., Brown, W.D., Friston, K.J., Qi, L.Y., Frackowiack, R.S.J., 1991. Cortical and subcortical localization of response to pain in man using positron emission tomography. Proc. R. Soc. Ser. B 244, 39–44.

Jones, E.G., 1985. The Thalamus. Plenum Press, New York.

Julius, D., Basbaum, A.I., 2001. Molecular mechanisms of nociception. Nature 413, 203–210.

Kaas, J.H., Nelson, R.J., Sur, M., Lin, C.-S., Merzenich, M.M., 1979. Multiple representations of the body within the primary somatosensory cortex of primates. Science 204, 521–523.

Kaas, J.H., Nelson, R.J., Sur, M., Dykes, R.W., Merzenich, M.M., 1984. The somatotopic organization of the ventroposterior thalamus of the squirrel monkey, *Saimiri sciureus*. J. Comp. Neurol. 226, 111–140.

Karlsson, M., Zakrisson, M., 1998. Relation between putative afferent axons and the glia limitancs in rat motor roots. J. Peripher. Nerv. Syst. 3, 47–53.

Keay, K.A., Bandler, R., 1993. Deep and superficial noxious stimulation increases Fos-like immunoreactivity in different regions of the midbrain periaqueductal gray of the rat. Neurosci. Lett. 154, 23–26.

Kenshalo, D.R., Giesler, G.J., Leonard, R.B., Willis, W.D., 1980. Responses of neurons in primate ventral posterior lateral nucleus to noxious stimuli. J. Neurophysiol. 43, 1594–1614.

Kerr, F.W.L., 1975. Neuroanatomical substrates of nociception in the spinal cord. Pain 1, 325–356.

Kevetter, G.A., Haber, L.H., Yezierski, R.P., Chung, J.M., Martin, R.F., Willis, W.D., 1982. Cells of origin of the spinoreticular tract in the monkey. J. Comp. Neurol. 207, 61–74.

Kieschke, J., Mense, S., Prabhakar, N.R., 1988. Influence of adrenaline and hypoxia on rat muscle receptors in vitro. In: Hamann, W., Iggo, A. (Eds.), Progress in Brain Research. Elsevier, Amsterdam, pp. 91–97.

Kircher, C., Ha, H., 1968. The nucleus cervicalis lateralis in primates including the human. Anat. Rec. 160, 376.

Klement, W., Arndt, J.O., 1992. The role of nociceptors of cutaneous veins in the mediation of cold pain in man. J. Physiol. 449, 73–83.

Koyama, T., Tanaka, Y.Z., Mikami, A., 1998. Nociceptive neurons in macaque anterior cingulate activate during anticipation of pain. Neuroreport 9, 2663–2667.

Kruger, L., Perl, E.R., Sedivec, M.J., 1981. Fine structure of myelinated mechanical nociceptor endings in cat hairy skin. J. Comp. Neurol. 198, 137–154.

Kulkarni, B., Bentley, D.E., Elliott, R., Youell, P., Watson, A., Derbyshire, S.W.G., et al., 2005. Attention to pain localization and unpleasantness discriminates the functions of the medial and lateral pain systems. Eur. J. Neurosci. 21, 3133–3142.

Kuypers, H.G.J.M., 1981. Anatomy of the descending pathways. In: Brooks, V.B., Brookhart, J.M., Mountcastle, V.B. (Eds.), Handbook of Physiology Section 1: The Nervous System, Volume II, Motor Control, Part 1. American Physiological Society, Bethesda, pp. 597–666.

La Motte, R.H., Dong, X., Ringkamp, M., 2014. Sensory neurons and circuits mediating itch. Nat. Rev. Neurosci. 15, 19–31.

LaMotte, R.H., Thalhammer, J.G., 1982. Response properties of high-threshold cutaneous cold receptors in the primate. Brain. Res. 244, 279–287.

LaMotte, C., 1977. Distribution of the tract of Lissauer and dorsal horn fibres in the primate spinal cord. J. Comp. Neurol. 172, 529–562.

Lawson, S.N., 1992. Morphological and biochemical cell types of sensory neurons. In: Scott, S.A. (Ed.), Sensory Neurons: Diversity, Development and Plasticity. Oxford University Press, Oxford, pp. 27–59.

Leichnetz, G.R., 1986. Afferent and efferent connections of the dorsolateral precentral gyrus (area 4, hand/arm region) in the macaque monkey, with comparisons to area 8. J. Comp. Neurol. 254, 260–292.

Lidierth, M., Wall, P.D., 1998. Dorsal horn cells connected to the Lissauer tract and their relation to the dorsal root potential in the rat. J. Neurophysiol. 80, 667–679.

Light, A.R., Metz, C.B., 1978. The morphology of the spinal cord efferent and afferent neurons contributing to the ventral roots of the cat. J. Comp. Neurol. 179, 501–516.

Lipp, J., 1991. Possible mechanisms of morphine analgesia. Clin. Neuropharmacol. 14, 131–147.

Lloyd, D.P.C., 1943. Neuron patterns controlling transmission of ipsilateral hindlimb reflexes in cat. J. Neurophysiol. 6, 293–315.

Lofving, B., 1961. Cardiovascular adjustments induced from the rostral cingulate gyrus. Acta. Physiol. Scand. 53, 1–82.

Löken, L.S., Wessberg, J., Morrison, I., McGlone, F., Olausson, H., 2009. Coding of pleasant touch by unmyelinated afferents in humans. Nat. Neurosci. 12 (5), 547–548.

Lovick, T.A., 1991. Interactions between descending pathways from the dorsal and ventrolateral periaqueductal gray matter in the rat. In: Depaulis, A., Bandler, R. (Eds.), The Midbrain Periaqueductal Gray Matter. Plenum Press, New York, pp. 101–120.

Lundberg, A., Norrsell, U., Voorhoeve, P., 1962. Pyramidal effects on lumbosacral interneurons activated by somatic afferents. Acta. Physiol. Scand. 56, 220–229.

Lynn, B., 1984. The detection of injury and tissue damage. In: Wall, P.D., Melzack, R. (Eds.), Textbook of Pain. Churchill Livingstone, Edinburgh, pp. 19–33.

MacIver, M.B., Tanelian, D.L., 1993. Structural and functional specialization of Aδ and C fiber free nerve endings innervating rabbit corneal epithelium. J. Neurosci. 13, 4511–4524.

MacLean, P.D., 1955. The limbic system ('visceral brain') and emotional behaviour. Arch. Neurol. Psychiatr. 73, 130–134.

Magni, F., Melzack, R., Moruzzi, G., Smith, C.J., 1959. Direct pyramidal influences on the dorsal column nuclei. Arch. Ital. Biol. 97, 357–377.

Maier, M.A., Armand, J., Kirkwood, P.A., Yang, H.-W., Davis, J.N., Lemon, R.N., 2002. Differences in the corticospinal projections from primary motor cortex and supplementary motor area to macaque upper limb motoneurons: an anatomical and electrophysiological study. Cerebr. Cortex 12, 281–296.

Malmberg, A.B., Chen, C., Tonegawa, S., Basbaum, A.I., 1997. Preserved acute pain and reduced neuropathic pain in mice lacking PKC gamma. Science 278, 279–283.

Mantyh, P.W., 1983. The spinothalamic tract in the primate: a reexamination using wheatgerm agglutinin conjugated to horseradish peroxidase. Neuroscience 9, 847–862.

Martin, J.H., 1996. Neuroanatomy. Text and Atlas, second ed. Appleton & Lange, Stamford, CT.

Matelli, M., Camarda, R., Glickstein, M., Rizzolatti, G., 1986. Afferent and efferent projections of the inferior area 6 in the macaque monkey. J. Comp. Neurol. 251, 281–298.

Matelli, M., Rizzolatti, G., Bettinardi, V., et al., 1993. Activation of precentral and mesial motor areas during the execution of elementary proximal and distal arm movements: a PET study. Neuroreport 4, 1295–1298.

McCloskey, D.I., Mitchell, J.H., 1972. Reflex cardiovascular and respiratory responses originating in exercising muscle. J. Physiol. 234, 173–186.

McGuire, C., Boundouki, G., Hockley, J.F.R., Reed, D., Cibert-Goton, V., Peiris, M., et al., 2018. Ex vivo study of human visceral nociceptors. Gut 67, 86–96.

Mehler, W.R., Feferman, M.E., Nauta, W.J.H., 1960. Ascending axon degeneration following anterolateral cordotomy. An experimental study in the monkey. Brain 83, 718–751.

Melzack, R., Casey, K.L., 1968. Sensory, motivational, and central control determinants of pain. A new conceptual model. In: Kenshalo, R. (Ed.), The Skin Senses. Thomas, Springfield, IL, pp. 423–443.

Mense, S., Meyer, H., 1985. Different types of slowly conducting afferent units in cat skeletal muscle and tendon. J. Physiol. 363, 403–417.

Mense, S., Meyer, H., 1988. Bradykinin-induced modulation of the response behaviour of different types of feline group III and IV muscle receptors. J. Physiol. 398, 49–63.

Mense, S., Prabhakar, N.R., 1986. Spinal terminations of nociceptive afferent fibres from deep tissues in the cat. Neurosci. Lett. 66, 169–174.

Mense, S., Stahnke, M., 1983. Responses in muscle afferent fibres of slow conduction velocity to contractions and ischaemia in the cat. J. Physiol. 342, 383–397.

Mense, S., 1993. Nociception from skeletal muscle in relation to clinical muscle pain. Pain 54, 241–289.

Mense, S., 2009. Algesic agents exciting muscle nociceptors. Exp. Brain. Res. 196, 89–100.

Mesulam, M.-M., Mufson, E.J., 1982. Insula in the Old World monkey: efferent cortical output and comments on function. J. Comp. Neurol. 212, 38–52.

Meyer, R.A., Davis, K.D., Cohen, R.H., Treede, R.-D., Campbell, J.N., 1991. Mechanically insensitive afferents (MIAs) in cutaneous nerves of monkey. Brain. Res. 561, 252–261.

Meyer, R.A., Campbell, J.N., Raja, S.N., 1994. Peripheral neural mechanisms of nociception. In: Wall, P.D., Melzack, R. (Eds.), Textbook of Pain. Churchill Livingstone, Edinburgh, pp. 13–44.

Meyer, R.A., Ringkamp, M., Campbell, J.N., Raja, S.N., 2006. Peripheral mechanisms of cutaneous nociception. In: McMahon, S.B., Koltzenburg, M. (Eds.), Wall and Melzack's Textbook of Pain, fifth ed. Elsevier, Philadelphia, pp. 3–34.

Milligan, E.S., Watkins, L.R., 2009. Pathological and protective roles of glia in chronic pain. Nat. Rev. Neurosci. 10 (1), 23–36.

Mizuno, N., Nakano, K., Imaizumi, M., Okamoto, M., 1967. The lateral cervical nucleus of the Japanese monkey (*Macaca fuscata*). J. Comp. Neurol. 129, 375–384.

Morecraft, R.J., van Hoesen, G.W., 1998. Convergence of limbic input to the cingulate motor cortex in the rhesus monkey. Brain. Res. Bull. 45, 209–232.

Morgan, C., Nadelhaft, I., de Groat, W.C., 1981. The distribution of visceral primary afferents from the pelvic nerve to Lissauer's tract and spinal gray matter and its relationship to the sacral parasympathetic nucleus. J. Comp. Neurol. 201 (3), 415–440.

Morgan, M.M., Whitney, P.K., Gold, M.S., 1998. Immobility and flight associated with antinociception produced by activation of the ventral and lateral/dorsal regions of the rat periaqueductal gray. Brain. Res. 804, 159–166.

Morgan, M.M., 1991. Differences in antinociception evoked from dorsal and ventral regions of the caudal periaqueductal gray matter. In: Depaulis, A., Bandler, R. (Eds.), The Midbrain Periaqueductal Gray Matter. Plenum Press, New York, pp. 139–150.

Mostofi, A., Morgante, F., Edwards, M.J., Brown, P., Pereira, E.A.C., 2021. Pain in Parkinson's disease and the role of the subthalamic nucleus. Brain 44 (5), 1342–1350.

Muakkassa, K.F., Strick, P.L., 1979. Frontal lobe inputs to primate motor cortex: evidence for four somatotopically organized 'premotor' areas. Brain. Res. 177, 176–182.

Mufson, E.J., Mesulam, M.-M., 1982. Insula of the Old World monkey. II Afferent cortical input and comments on the claustrum. J. Comp. Neurol. 212, 23–37.

Nauta, W.J.H., Mehler, W.R., 1966. Projections of the lentiform nucleus in the monkey. Brain. Res. 1, 3–42.

Ochoa-Cortes, F., Ramos-Lomas, T., Miranda-Morales, M., Ian Spreadbury, Ibeakanma, C., Barajas-Lopez, C., et al., 2010. Bacterial cell products signal to mouse colonic nociceptive dorsal root ganglia neurons. Am. J. Physiol. Gastrointest. Liver Physiol. 299, G723–G732.

Ostrowsky, K., Magnin, M., Ryvlin, P., Isnard, J., Guenot, M., Maugière, 2002. Representation of pain and somatic sensation in the human insula: a study of responses to direct electrical cortical stimulation. Cereb. Cortex. 12 (4), 376–385.

Pandya, D.N., Van Hoesen, G.W., Mesulam, M.M., 1981. Efferent connections of the cingulate gyrus in the rhesus monkey. Exp. Brain. Res. 42, 319–330.

Pang, Z., Sakamoto, T., Tiwan, V., Kim, Y.-S., Yang, F., Dong, X., et al., 2015. Selective keratinocyte stimulation is sufficient to evoke nociception in mice. Pain 156, 656–665.

Papez, J.W., 1937. A proposed mechanism of emotion. Arch. Neurol. Psychiatr. 38, 725–743.

Patterson, J.T., Coggeshall, R.E., Lee, W.T., Chung, K., 1990. Long ascending unmyelinated primary afferent axons in the rat dorsal column: immunohistochemical localizations. Neurosci. Lett. 108, 6–10.

Penfield, W., Rasmussen, T., 1955. The Cerebral Cortex of Man. Macmillan, New York.

Peschanski, M., Besson, J.M., 1984. A spino-reticulo-thalamic pathway in the rat: an anatomical study with reference to pain transmission. Neuroscience 12, 165–178.

Petrides, M., Pandya, D.N., 1984. Projections to the frontal cortex from the posterior parietal region in the rhesus monkey. J. Comp. Neurol. 228, 105–116.

Ploner, M., Gross, J., Timmermann, L., Schnitzler, A., 2002. Cortical representation of first and second pain sensations in humans. Proc. Nat. Acad. Sci. USA 99, 12444–12448.

Porro, C.A., Cettolo, V., Francescato, M.P., Baraldi, P., 1998. Temporal and intensity coding of pain in human cortex. J. Neurophysiol. 80, 3312–3320.

Preuss, T.M., Goldman-Rakic, P.S., 1991. Ipsilateral cortical connections of granular frontal cortex in the strepsirrhine primate Galago, with comparative comments on anthropoid primates. J. Comp. Neurol. 310, 507–549.

Price, D.D., Dubner, R., 1977. Mechanisms of first and second pain in the peripheral and central nervous system. J. Invest. Dermatol. 69, 167–171.

Pritchard, T.C., Hamilton, R.B., Morse, J.R., Norgren, R., 1986. Projections of thalamic, gustatory and lingual areas in the monkey, macaca fascicularis. J. Comp. Neurol. 244, 213–228.

Rainville, P., Duncan, G.H., Price, D.D., Carrier, B., Bushnell, M.C., 1997. Pain affect encoded in human anterior cingulate but not somatosensory cortex. Science 277, 968–971.

Ralston, H.J., Ralston, D.D., 1982. The distribution of dorsal root axons to laminae IV, V, and VI of the macaque spinal cord: a qualitative electron microscopic study. J. Comp. Neurol. 212, 435–448.

Ralston, D.D., Ralston, H.J., 1985. The terminations of corticospinal tract axons in the macaque monkey. J. Comp. Neurol. 242, 325–337.

Ralston, H.J., Ralston, D.D., 1992. The primate dorsal spinothalamic tract: evidence for a specific termination in the posterior nuclei (Po/SG) of the thalamus. Pain 48, 107–118.

Rang, H.P., Bevan, S., Dray, A., 1991. Chemical activation of nociceptive peripheral neurons. Br. Med. Bull. 47, 534–548.

Reed, D.E., Vanner, S.J., 2017. Emerging studies of human visceral nociceptors. Am. J. Physiol. Gastrointest. Liver Physiol. 312, G201–G207.

Ren, K.R., Dubner, R., 2010. Interactions between the immune and nervous systems in pain. Nat. Med. 16, 1267–1276.

Rexed, B., 1952. The cytoarchitectonic organization of the spinal cord in the cat. J. Comp. Neurol. 96, 415–495.

Rexed, B., 1954. A cytoarchitectonic atlas of the spinal cord in the cat. J. Comp. Neurol. 100, 297–379.

Rostock, C., Schrenk-Siemens, K., Pohle, J., et al., 2018. Human vs mouse nociceptors – similarities and differences. Neuroscience 387, 13–27.

Ruch, T.C., 1946. Visceral sensation and referred pain. In: Fulton, J.F. (Ed.), Howell's Textbook of Physiology, fifteenth ed. Saunders, Philadelphia, pp. 385–401.

Schaible, H.G., Schmidt, R.F., 1985. Effects of an experimental arthritis on the sensory properties of fine articular afferent units. J. Neurophysiol. 54, 1109–1122.

Schaible, H.G., Schmidt, R.F., 1988. Time course of mechanosensitivity changes in articular afferents during a developing experimental arthritis. J. Neurophysiol. 60, 2180–2195.

Schlag-Rey, M., Schlag, J., 1984. Visuomotor functions of central thalamus in monkey. I. Unit activity related to spontaneous eye movements. J. Neurophysiol. 51, 1149–1174.

Seitz, R.J., Roland, P.E., 1992. Learning of sequential and finger movements in man: a combined kinematic and positron emission tomography (PET) study. Eur. J. Neurosci. 4, 154–165.

Shiers, S.I., Sankaranarayanan, I., Jeevakumar, V., et al., 2021. Convergence of peptidergic and non-peptidergic protein markers in the human dorsal root ganglion and spinal dorsal horn. J. Comp. Neurol. 529, 2771–2778.

Shima, K., Aya, K., Mushiake, H., Inase, M., Aizawa, H., Tanji, J., 1991. Two movement-related foci in the primate cingulate cortex observed in signal-triggered and self-paced forelimb movements. J. Neurophysiol. 65, 188–202.

Silverdale, M.A., Kobylecki, C., Kass-Illiyya, et al., 2018. A detailed clinical study of 1957 participants with early/moderate Parkinson's disease. Park. Relat. Disord. 56, 27–32.

Simone, D.A., Kajander, K.C., 1997. Responses of A-fiber nociceptors to noxious cold. J. Neurophysiol. 77, 2049–2060.

Sluka, K.A., Price, M.P., Breese, N.M., Stucky, C.L., Wemmie, J.A., Welsh, M.J., 2003. Chronic hyperalgesia induced by repeated acid injections in muscle is abolished by the loss of the ASIC3, but not ASIC1. Pain 106, 229–239.

Snider, W.D., McMahon, S.B., 1998. Tackling pain at the source: new ideas about nociceptors. Neuron 20, 629–632.

Snyder, R., 1977. The organization of the dorsal root entry zone in cats and monkeys. J. Comp. Neurol. 174, 47–70.

Stacey, M.J., 1969. Free nerve endings in skeletal muscle of the cat. J. Anat. 105, 231–254.

Stamford, J.A., 1995. Descending control of pain. Br. J. Anaesth. 75, 217–227.

Stucky, C.L., 2007. IB4-positive neurons, role in inflammatory pain. In: Schmidt, R.F., Willis, W.D. (Eds.), Encyclopedia of Pain. Springer Berlin, Heidelberg.

Sugiura, Y., Lee, C.L., Perl, E.R., 1986. Central projections of identified unmyelinated (C) fibers innervating mammalian skin. Science 234, 358–361.

Sugiura, Y., Terui, N., Hosoya, Y., 1989. Difference in distribution of central terminals between visceral and somatic unmyelinated (C) primary afferent fibers. J. Neurophysiol. 62, 834–840.

Talbot, J.D., Marrett, S., Evans, A.C., Meyer, E., Bushnell, M.C., Duncan, G.H., 1991. Multiple representations of pain in human cerebral cortex. Science 251, 1355–1358.

Talbot, K., Madden, V.J., Jones, S.L., Moseley, G.L., 2019. The sensory and affective components of pain: are they differentially modifiable dimensions or inseparable aspects of a unitary experience: a systematic review. Br. J. Anaesth. 123, e263–e271.

Tanelian, D.I., 1991. Cholinergic activation of a population of corneal afferent nerves. Exp. Brain. Res. 86, 414–420.

Tillman, D.B., Treede, R.-D., Meyer, R.A., Campbell, J.N., 1995. Response of C fibre nociceptors in the anaesthetized monkey to heat stimuli: estimates of receptor depth and threshold. J. Physiol. 485, 753–765.

Todd, A.J., 2010. Neuronal circuitry for pain processing in the dorsal horn. Nat. Rev. Neurosci. 11, 823–836.

Tracey, I., Mantyh, P.W., 2007. The cerebral signature for pain perception and its modulation. Neuron 55, 377–391.

Treede, R.-D., Meyer, R.A., Campbell, J.N., 1998. Myelinated mechanically insensitive afferents from monkey hairy skin: heat-response properties. J. Neurophysiol. 80, 1082–1093.

Treede, R.-D., Kenshalo, D.R., Gracely, R.H., Jones, A.K.P., 1999. The cortical representation of pain. Pain 79, 105–111.

Truex, R.C., Taylor, M.J., Smythe, M.Q., Gildenberg, P.L., 1965. The lateral cervical nucleus of cat, dog and man. J. Comp. Neurol. 139, 93–104.

Vallbo, A.B., Olausson, H., Wessberg, J., 1999. Unmyelinated afferents constitute a second system coding tactile stimuli of the human hairy skin. J. Neurophysiol. 81, 2753–2763.

Vogt, B.A., Pandya, D.N., 1987. Cingulate cortex of the rhesus monkey: II Cortical afferents. J. Comp. Neurol. 262, 271–289.

Vogt, B.A., 2009. Pain and emotion interactions in subregions of the cingulate gyrus. Nat. Rev. Neurosci. 6, 533–544.

Wall, P.D., 1967. The laminar organization of dorsal horn and effects of descending impulses. J. Physiol. 188, 403–423.

Wang, Q.-P., Nakai, Y., 1994. The dorsal raphe: an important nucleus in pain modulation. Brain. Res. Bull. 34, 575–585.

Wessberg, J., Olausson, H., Fernstrom, K.W., Vallbo, A.B., 2003. Receptive field properties of unmyelinated tactile afferents in the human skin. J. Neurophysiol. 89, 1567–1575.

Whitsel, B.L., Vierck, C.J., Waters, R.S., Tommerdahl, M., Favorov, O.V., 2019. Contributions of nociresponsive area 3a to normal and abnormal somatosensory perception. J. Pain 20, 405–419.

Willis, W.D., Coggeshall, R.E., 1991. Sensory Mechanisms of the Spinal Cord, second ed. Plenum, New York.

Willis, W.D., Al-Chaer, E.D., Quast, M.J., Westlund, K.N., 1999. A visceral pathway in the dorsal column of the spinal cord. Proc. Nat. Acad. Sci. USA 96, 7675–7679.

Wilson, P., Meyers, D.E., Snow, P.J., 1986. The detailed somatotopic organization of the dorsal horn in the lumbosacral enlargement of the cat spinal cord. J. Neurophysiol. 55, 604–617.

Woolf, C.J., Shortland, P., Coggeshall, R.E., 1992. Peripheral nerve injury triggers central sprouting of myelinated afferents. Nature 355, 75–78.

Yezierski, R.P., Gerhart, K.D., Schrock, R.J., Willis, W.D., 1983. A further examination of effects of cortical stimulation on primate spinothalamic tract cells. J. Neurophysiol. 49, 424–441.

Yezierski, R.P., 1988. Spinomesencephalic tract: projections from the lumbosacral spinal cord of the rat, cat, and monkey. J. Comp. Neurol. 267, 131–146.

Zhang, D., Carlton, S.M., Sorkin, L.S., Willis, W.D., 1990. Collaterals of primate spinothalamic tract neurons to the periaqueductal gray. J. Comp. Neurol. 296, 277–290.

Zylka, M.J., Rice, F.L., Anderson, D.J., 2005. Topographically distinct epidermal nociceptive circuits revealed by axonal tracers targeted to *Mrgprd*. Neuron 45, 17–25.

Chapter 7

Neurophysiology of pain

Hubert van Griensven and Teodora Trendafilova

LEARNING OBJECTIVES

At the end of this chapter, readers will understand the:
1. Neurophysiology underlying somatic and visceral pain.
2. Mechanisms of sensitisation in the peripheral and central nervous system.
3. Control of nociceptive processing by the brain.

Introduction

Chapter 6 dealt with the neuroanatomical substrate of nociception and pain, i.e. the structures that make the perception and modulation of pain possible. This chapter focuses on the neurophysiology of pain or function. Structure and function are closely related, for example the makeup and location of nociceptors determines their functional properties. Familiarisation with aspects of Chapter 6, specifically nociceptors and nociceptive neurones, dorsal horn and brain, is therefore recommended.

The sensory nervous system provides us with an awareness of the internal and external environment of our bodies. The detection of influences that create actual or potential tissue damage is referred to as *nociception*, defined as the neural process of encoding noxious stimuli (IASP 2021) or the translation of these noxious influences into neural signals. Nociception is a protective mechanism that helps us to avoid harmful influences or withdraw from them. If we are injured, nociception promotes behaviours that aid recovery, such as protecting the affected area of the body, adapting activities and communicating to others that we are not well.

Tissue damage generates pain through the stimulation of nociceptors, but pain is not purely the consequence of nociception. For example, nociceptive pain can be enhanced or suppressed through modulation in the central nervous system (CNS). Conversely, nociceptive fibres can be stimulated (electrically, for example) without creating pain. It is therefore incorrect to speak of pain receptors, pain fibres and pain pathways.

Pain is defined as *an unpleasant sensory and emotional experience associated with, or resembling that associated with, actual or potential tissue damage* (IASP 2021). This makes it clear that pain is an experience rather than a physiological mechanism, and that this experience does not necessarily involve nociception. That said, pain is likely to *feel like* an indication of tissue damage. This presents challenges to clinicians: if a patient reports pain, is this pain experience an accurate reflection of a tissue pathology? The answer to this question requires an understanding of the neurophysiological mechanisms that may create, maintain, enhance or reduce the experience of pain. This understanding is also essential when it comes to providing a patient with a realistic explanation for their pain.

This chapter starts by introducing aspects of pain physiology and explaining the characteristics and mechanisms of nociception. This helps clinicians to judge whether a patient's pain is likely to be nociceptive and therefore suggestive of tissue pathology. Next, the way nociceptive signals are processed in the CNS, specifically the spinal cord, is discussed. Nociception can be altered considerably in the spinal cord, through suppression or amplification of nociceptive signals. Insight into these processes is important for understanding how pain perception may differ from what is going on with the tissues. The final part of the chapter explains modulation of nociception by the brain.

A note of caution: much of the information in this chapter is based on laboratory findings. It is plausible that it applies to the clinical situation, because it closely resembles what we observe in and hear from patients. However, preclinical or laboratory research often investigates the response to a stimulus, while persistent pain is often spontaneous. Extrapolation of reductionist research findings to the complexity of human existence must be done with a sense of epistemic humility: understanding is always limited and subject to change. This extrapolation is likely to benefit from a field called *translational pain research*, which aims to bridge the gap between scientific research and clinical practice (Mao 2012; Mouraux et al. 2021).

Mechanisms of nociception

Innervation and sensory responses differ between tissue types and organs. Cutaneous sensation has been studied most and is the type of sensation that humans are most aware of. It is often used as a model for sensory research and will be used as a general introduction into sensory neurophysiology and nociception. Differences with deeper tissues including viscera will be noted.

Note: *nociceptive pain* is a term used only when the somatosensory nervous system is intact and functioning normally. Pain associated with damage or disease of the somatosensory nervous system itself is classed as *neuropathic pain* and is the subject of Chapter 13.

Nociceptive neurons of the unmyelinated type C or the thin myelinated type Aδ have different response characteristics and are associated with certain aspects of the pain experience. Aδ neurones respond quickly and have a short adaptation time. Pain associated with Aδ stimulation is sharp and localised. Because of these characteristics, Aδ information is classed as *discriminative*. On the other hand, stimulation of C fibres leads to a slow onset and a slow decay of action potentials. C-fibre pain is likely to be diffuse, i.e. difficult to localise with precision.

Nociceptors are receptors at the peripheral terminal of a nociceptive neurone. They have a high stimulation threshold, i.e. they respond only to stimuli outside the normal and healthy range unless sensitised (next section). Unlike mechanoreceptors with their highly specialised structures, most nociceptors consist of free nerve endings. Some are sensitive selectively to nociceptive mechanical, thermal or chemical stimuli (Basbaum 2021). *Polymodal nociceptors* respond to two or more of these types of stimuli (ibid). So-called *sleeping* or *silent nociceptors* do not respond to noxious stimuli until they are exposed to tissue inflammation (Perl 2007).

First and second pain

Lewis established that a brief noxious stimulation produces an initial flash of pain, followed by a longer-lasting and often more intense pain (Lewis 1942). He referred to the two sensations as *first pain* and *second pain*. The difference was most pronounced when the stimulus was delivered to the hands or feet but diminished closer to the trunk (ibid). This was explained by the different conduction times: the higher diameter and myelin sheath offer Aδ fibres a faster conduction speed compared with C fibres (Price & Dubner 1977). Due to these differences between C and Aδ fibres, acute tissue trauma may initially be felt as sharp and localised pain, followed by a wave of deep and longer-lasting pain (van Cranenburgh 2000). Second pain is often thought of as an aspect of persistent pain (Eckert et al. 2017).

The difference in sensation between the two systems can be demonstrated quite simply through nerve compression, for instance by crossing one's legs (Price 1999). Aβ fibres, which are most reliant on circulation, stop functioning first so the limb 'falls asleep'. As soon as this happens (i.e. when sensitivity to light touch disappears), a sharp pinch will mainly activate Aδ fibres. It will feel a little strange but immediate and sharp. This corresponds with *first pain*. If compression persists, the Aδ neurones also become blocked, the skin becomes very numb but the same pinch will still activate C fibres. The sensation is delayed, feels dull and outlasts the pinch. This corresponds with *second pain*.

Nociceptors contain populations of *receptor channels*, ion channels with binding sites for certain ligands (specific ions or molecules). Examples include acid-sensing ion channels (ASICs) activated by ischaemia and other acidity, and a range of transient receptor potential channels (TRPs) responsive to stimuli such as extreme temperatures and capsaicin (chili pepper extract). Response characteristics of a nociceptor are thus determined by its receptor channel population. When receptor channels are activated, they allow specific ions to flow across the cell membrane of the neuron, leading to depolarisation and generation of action potentials. This process of encoding stimuli into patterns of action potentials in neurons is called *transduction*.

Peripheral sensitisation

Peripheral sensitisation is the increased responsiveness and reduced threshold of nociceptive neurons in the periphery to the stimulation of their receptive fields (IASP 2021). An example is a fresh bruise, which may not be felt spontaneously but which can be acutely sensitive to gentle pressure (mechanical allodynia). It will also respond more strongly to painful stimuli (primary hyperalgesia, as opposed to secondary hyperalgesia due to changes in the CNS).

Peripheral sensitisation is typically the result of tissue damage and inflammation, associated with the release of a host of ions and molecules referred to as *ligands*. Some ligands bind to *metabotropic receptors*, which do not open ion channels but alter responsiveness of the neuron internally (Siegelbaum et al. 2021). When activated, these receptors create internal processes (second messenger chemicals) that affect the ion channels, making them more likely to open (Fig. 7.1). Activation of metabotropic receptors underpins the development of persistent pain. For a review of peripheral sensitisation, please see Dawes et al. (2013). At least two types of metabotropic receptors are involved. Prostaglandins, bradykinin, adrenaline and ATP bind to *G-protein receptors*. Cytokines such as tumour necrosis factor-alpha (TNF-α) and interleukins (IL) bind to tyrosine kinases (TrK). TrK also has binding sites for neurotrophic factors such as nerve growth factor (NGF), which tissues release in small quantities under normal circumstances. Activation of TrK by neurotrophic factors generates chemical signals inside the neuron, which are transported along the axon to the cell body. This influences gene transcription in the nucleus, and therefore the makeup of the neuron. NGF levels are increased during inflammation, altering expression of brain-derived neurotrophic factor (BDNF) and contributing to sensitisation of nociceptive neurones (Basbaum 2021).

Neurogenic inflammation

Although nociceptive neurones are afferents or sensory neurones, they play an active role in the regulation of tissue inflammation through the release of neuropeptides. These neuropeptides, specifically substance P (SP) and calcitonin gene-related peptide (CGRP), are produced in the cell body, transported through the axons and stored in the neurone's peripheral terminals. They may be released when nociceptive fibres are activated and have a local proinflammatory and vasodilatory effect (Basbaum 2021). This can be observed as an area of redness and oedema (flare). This 'fuelling' of local inflammatory processes is known as *neurogenic inflammation*. It does not take place if the peripheral nerve is blocked proximally (LaMotte et al. 1991). Neuropeptides also sensitise nociceptors through release of histamine from mast cells, creating allodynia and hyperalgesia to mechanical stimuli and heat in the flare area (Raja et al. 1984). This affects sensitivity to stroking and sharpness, but not blunt pressure (Meyer et al. 2006).

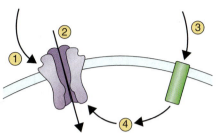

Fig. 7.1 Ligands and receptors. Some ligands bind with receptors on ion channels *(1)*, opening them and allowing specific ions to pass the neuronal membrane *(2)*. Ligands may also bind with *metabotropic receptors (3)*, which do not open ion channels but activate internal processes *(4)*, releasing second messenger chemicals that sensitise the ion channels internally. (Based on Siegelbaum, S., Clapham, D., Marder, E., 2021. Modulation of synaptic transmission and neuronal excitability: second messengers. In: Kandel, E., Koester, J., Mack, S., Siegelbaum, S. (Eds.), Principles of Neural Science. Mc Graw Hill, New York, pp. 301–323.)

Deep somatic nociception

In joints, nociceptors from Aδ and C fibres respond only to extreme mechanical stimuli such as end of range overpressures, but also tissue damage (Schaible 2013). They will also develop peripheral sensitisation and become mechanosensitive in response to inflammation and arthritic conditions (ibid). Periosteum is innervated by high- and low-threshold mechanoreceptors, which can also be sensitised by inflammatory mediators (Nencini & Ivanusic 2016). Responses from neurones in bone marrow have been investigated less, but mechanical sensitisation in response to increased intraosseal pressure has been found (ibid).

Group III and IV muscle afferents have a high stimulation threshold, although some group IV receptors contribute to mechanical stimuli in the normal range, possibly to function as *ergoceptors* which play a role in local homeostatic regulation (Mense 2013). Tissue damage and inflammation produce peripheral sensitisation of nociceptors in muscles, producing mechanical allodynia (ibid). Muscle nociceptors also respond to muscle activity under ischaemic conditions.

Visceral nociception

Innervation and pain perception are different for viscera and are not consistent across organs—please refer to Bielefeld & Gebhart (2013) and Mayer & Gebhart (1994) for reviews. The types of stimuli which provoke pain can be quite different from those causing somatic pain. For example, distention of the bowel and other hollow organs can be painful, while cutting the bowel does not cause any pain whatsoever (Bielefeld & Gebhart 2013; Ness & Gebhart 1990). Visceral activity is generally not perceived consciously, but nociceptive stimulation can generate diffuse

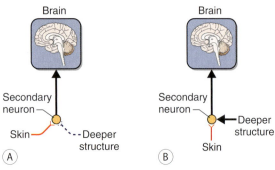

Fig. 7.2 The two main theoretical models of referred pain. (A) The convergence-projection model suggests that areas of skin and deeper tissues such as joints or viscera have an equal influence on the secondary neurone in the dorsal horn. (B) The convergence-facilitation model suggests that nociceptive stimulation from deeper structures creates pain by facilitating cutaneous input into secondary neurones in the dorsal horn.

pain that is difficult to localise (Mayer & Raybould 1990). The pain refers to more superficial structures (see later) and can therefore be mistaken for somatic pain. This is one of the mechanisms of so-called masqueraders, i.e. pain suggestive of a musculoskeletal problem is in fact the consequence of internal pathologies. Visceral pain can be associated with hyperalgesia in superficial somatic tissues (see, e.g. Sarkar et al. 2000), but also in other viscera (Giamberardino et al. 2010). Referred pain and hyperalgesia across viscera and to different tissues are thought to be mediated through shared segmental innervation (Brumovsky & Gebhart 2010).

Referred pain

Referred pain is pain felt at a distance from and in tissues distinct from the origin of nociceptive stimulation. It is a normal feature of the nervous system and must therefore be distinguished from peripheral or central neuropathic pain (see Chapter 13). Referred pain is thought to be a consequence of the convergence of sensory input in the dorsal horn. Referred pain is not a subjective phenomenon and can be associated with measurable hyperalgesia (Coutinho et al. 2000; Sarkar et al. 2000).

Pain referral can be said to be from deep to superficial structures (Arendt-Nielsen et al. 2000), e.g. visceral pain or deep musculoskeletal pain tends to be felt in musculoskeletal and cutaneous tissues. This may be at least in part related to the observation that the number of somatic afferents in the dorsal root far outweighs the number of visceral afferents (Proacci & Maresca 1993). Referred pain also tends to be from proximal structures to the periphery, e.g. from hip to thigh and knee, or from spinal ligaments to a limb.

Two theories offer the most plausible explanation for referred pain (Fig. 7.2) (Arendt-Nielsen et al. 2000;

McMahon 1997). The *convergence-projection theory* suggests that afferents from deep tissues share second-order neurones with more superficial tissues. Examples of deep structures may be viscera, spinal ligaments or joint capsules. Due to the shared secondary pathways, the brain has no way of distinguishing between nociceptive input from a deep structure and a superficial somatic structure innervated by the same spinal segment. It is likely to interpret the pain as coming from the more superficial structures, presumably because this is where most sensation normally comes from and because superficial somatic innervation is more refined. The *convergence-facilitation theory* poses that nociceptive input from deeper tissues is not perceived directly but sensitises secondary neurones. The theory suggests that sensory input from superficial structures arriving at the same secondary neurones will thus be facilitated, so that innocuous sensations from those structures may now be perceived as painful.

Nociceptive processing in the dorsal horn

Projection neurones—the role of the spinal cord in pain signalling

The neurones projecting from the peripheral nervous system (first-order neurones) into the spinal cord synapse onto second-order neurones. These can be either interneurones or projections neurones. The latter carries the signal from

Projection neurones

Lamina I projection neurones send signals into the brainstem, to areas such as the rostral ventromedial medulla (RVM), which in turn sends descending signals back to the spinal cord, creating a feedback loop. In addition, superficial projection neurones signal to higher brain centres in the thalamus, the periaqueductal grey (PAG) and the parabrachial area (PB) (Dickenson et al. 1997; Todd 2002). The projection neurones in deeper laminae form a large part of the spinothalamic tract and send information predominantly to the thalamus. The signals from the thalamus are then transmitted to the cortical centres of pain which include the insular, anterior cingulate and prefrontal cortices (Tracey & Mantyh, 2007). The major ascending tract for pain and temperature, where the axons of superficial and deep projection neurones join together and ascend to the brainstem and thalamus, is known as the spinothalamic or anterolateral tract system (ALT). Other tracts ascending from the dorsal horn include the spinocervical to the sensory cortex and the postsynaptic dorsal column pathway to the medulla. Much less is known about these two tracts (Abraira & Ginty 2013; Brown 1983).

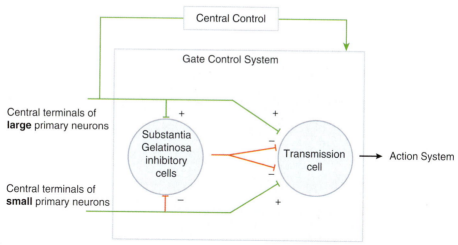

Fig. 7.3 The gate control theory of pain. Large and small primary neurones project to the dorsal horn where they both excite transmission cells and thus engage the action system. However, large fibres activate inhibitory cells of the substantia gelatinosa, while small fibres inhibit them. Therefore the gate will be opened depending on the balance between large and small cell input into the spinal cord. (From Melzack, R., Wall, P.D., 1996. Pain mechanisms: a new theory. A gate control system modulates sensory input from the skin before it evokes pain perception and response. Pain Forum 5 (1), 3 -11, Figure 4)

the dorsal horn to the brain and is found mainly in lamina I and deeper laminae III–VI (see Chapter 6).

In the dorsal root ganglia and periphery, sensory encoding is largely modality-specific, i.e. certain populations of neurones are largely responsible for specific sensations including nociception. However, at the level of the CNS, this is more complex and there are neurones which respond to a variety of stimuli (i.e. wide-dynamic range neurones (WDR)) (Moayedi & Davis 2013). Yet pain and touch, for example, are perceived separately. This integration and deciphering of nociceptive signalling in the CNS has prompted the generation of several theories of pain.

Synaptic circuits—function depending on neuronal interplay

One of the main theories about the integration of information in the spinal cord is the gate control theory (Fig. 7.3) (Melzack & Wall 1965). It suggests that both large and small primary afferents transmit signals to the brain, but also interact with neurones in substantia gelatinosa (SG) which serve as a 'gate'. These gate neurones are excited by large and inhibited by small peripheral afferents. Gate neurones inhibit transmission to the brain, so their excitation (by large fibres) leads to stronger inhibition, while nociceptive input from small fibres leads to weaker inhibition and opening of the gate. This theory also applies to pathological pain states, where reduced spinal cord inhibition opens the gate and allows innocuous signals to be interpreted as pain. This phenomenon is known as *tactile allodynia*.

There have been other models attempting to explain nociceptive coding in the spinal cord (Koch et al. 2018; Ma 2010; Prescott et al. 2014). The *labelled line theory* suggests that information about each sensory modality is carried by a dedicated line of neurones, from the periphery to the CNS. However, this fails to account for neurones in the spinal cord responding to multiple modalities, as well as their ability to adapt to neuronal stimulation by functional and structural changes (neuronal plasticity). The *intensity theory* proposes that nociception is the result of a series of subthreshold stimulations which, under certain summation conditions, can be experienced as pain. It was first postulated by Erb (1874), who suggested that every sensation was capable of producing pain if it reached sufficient intensity (Dallenbach 1939). Although more sophisticated, this theory still does not include neuronal plasticity, as at the time the nervous system was considered 'hard-wired' and fixed (Moayedi & Davis 2013).

The *pattern theory* suggests that each sensory modality produces a specific firing pattern, which serves as a code that is deciphered by the spinal cord. Finally, the *combinatorial theory* posits that pain perception depends on the combination of active peripheral fibres and the intensity of their activity. Both theories propose levels of plasticity within the local circuits.

The number of pain theories reflects the difficulties in the field to understand the neural code of pain perception: how is it possible that a large amount of sensory information seemingly converges in the spinal cord but is still perceived very precisely as touch, temperature, itch or pain? This is an important question in pathological states, where pain may be generated in response to

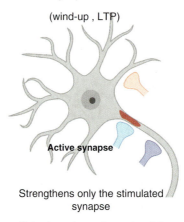

Homosynaptic mechanisms

(wind-up , LTP)

Heterosynaptic mechanisms

Active synapse

Active synapse

Strengthens only the stimulated synapse

(linked to primary hyperalgesia)

Spreads to nonstimulated synapses

(linked to secondary hyperalgesia and tactile allodynia)

Central sensitisation is likely to include both homo- and heterosynaptic processes

Fig. 7.4 Homosynaptic and heterosynaptic mechanisms in central sensitisation. Homosynaptic mechanisms involve activity-dependent potentiation of a single synapse, caused by continuous signalling through that same synapse *(left panel)*. Heterosynaptic potentiation develops when one set of synapses (conditioning input) are sensitised and this leads to stimulation of other, nonactivated groups of synapses *(right panel)*. *LTP,* Long-term potentiation. (Adapted from Latremoliere, A., Woolf, C.J., 2009. Central sensitization: a generator of pain hypersensitivity by central neural plasticity. J. Pain. 10 (9), 895-926.)

the wrong stimuli or without any obvious stimulation (Prescott et al. 2014). Therefore understanding microcircuits involved in nociception, using more sophisticated experiments and computer modelling, is of great importance in deciphering the neural code of pain perception, especially in pathological conditions (Prescott et al. 2014). This will allow us to evaluate the existing pain theories and postulate new ones.

Activity-dependent plasticity and nociplastic pain

A reason that the neural code is difficult to decipher is that spinal cord neurones exhibit activity-dependent changes in structure and function, i.e. neuronal plasticity. These changes become clinically significant in states of nerve damage or inflammation, which can then lead to nociplastic pain (see Nociplastic pain box). The mechanism underlying the development of this pain will be discussed here.

Repeated nociceptive stimulation can cause an increased output of second-order neurones in the dorsal horn. One associated phenomenon is *wind-up* (Mendell & Wall 1965). Wind-up is *homosynaptic*, i.e. it affects only the synapse between the primary and secondary neurones involved. It disappears within seconds after the stimulation is terminated (Fig. 7.4). Clinically, it is thought to manifest as *temporal summation*, i.e. a repeated stimulus is experienced as increasingly intense (Eide 2000).

Nociplastic pain

Patients may display a heightened responsiveness to sensory input, despite a lack of evidence of a nociceptive or neuropathic cause. This may be due to altered activity in the sensory CNS and is called *nociplastic pain* (IASP 2021). It may manifest as *allodynia* (pain in response to signals which are normally not painful, such as light touch), hyperalgesia (enhanced response to painful stimuli) and spreading pain and sensitivity (Woolf 2011). Nociplastic changes may occur throughout the sensory CNS. A specific mechanism is *central sensitisation* (CS, see later), the increased responsiveness of nociceptive neurones in the dorsal horn. CS can only be established by measuring input and output of neurones in vitro, so it is more appropriate to use the term *nociplastic pain* in clinic (van Griensven et al. 2020).

Temporal summation has been explored in various pain disorders. For example, a significant proportion of patients with neuropathic pain have been found to have facilitated temporal summation (Felsby et al. 1996; Maier et al. 2010). In patients with spinal cord injury, wind-up-like pain may be more prevalent in painful than non-painful de-innervated skin areas (Eide et al. 1996). Facilitated wind-up pain has also been found in postherpetic neuralgia (Eide et al. 1994), chronic postsurgical pain (Pud et al. 1998), fibromyalgia (Staud 2013) and irritable bowel syndrome (Rössel et al. 1999). For further detail, see Arendt-Nielsen et al. (2018), Herrero et al. (2000) and Woolf (2011).

Strong or persistent stimulation may spread the heightened sensitivity to adjacent synapses in the same secondary neurone (heterosynaptic), ultimately affecting the full cell and creating longer-lasting changes (see Fig. 7.4). This *central sensitisation* (CS), defined as *the increased responsiveness of nociceptive neurones in the central nervous system to their normal or subthreshold afferent input* (IASP 2021), means that secondary nociceptive neurones respond more strongly to peripheral nociceptive input and may also develop a new sensitivity to nonnoxious input. CS is strongly associated with the development of chronic pain (Latremoliere & Woolf 2009). Unlike wind-up, CS may last for minutes, hours or even longer (ibid). In the absence of further nociceptive stimuli, it is expected to fade away—see later. Reducing sources of nociception, therefore, may be relevant even in patients displaying nociplastic pain (see The importance of the periphery in maintaining CS Box).

In summary, CS includes both homosynaptic and heterosynaptic mechanisms. It may be a result of injury to the peripheral tissues, inflammation, nerve damage or wind-up-inducing repetitive stimulation (Cervero et al. 1984; Cook et al. 1987; Hylden et al. 1989; Li et al. 1999; Woolf & Thompson 1991). Most of these injuries produce heterosynaptic plasticity, i.e. the activation of synapses that were not originally stimulated. This is thought to underlie clinical manifestations of CS such as allodynia or secondary hyperalgesia (Latremoliere & Woolf 2009).

The importance of the periphery in maintaining CS

This has long been the subject of debate. Neurophysiological evidence suggests that once induced, some peripheral input is required to maintain CS. Indeed, skin anaesthesia reduces pain behaviour in preclinical models of CS (e.g. formalin or capsaicin injection) (Dickenson & Sullivan 1987; McCall et al. 1996; Taylor et al. 1995). Another preclinical study suggested that low levels of intermittent firing in dorsal root ganglia neurones may contribute to sustained pain behaviour in CS (Chisholm et al. 2018). In a study of patients with persistent CRPS, local anaesthetic blocks abolished allodynia and spontaneous pain, with symptoms returning after waning of anaesthesia (Gracely et al. 1992).

The importance of peripheral input is becoming increasingly clear, even in patient populations where CS has been thought to be independent of peripheral changes. For instance, there is strong evidence that small fibres degenerate (Grayston et al. 2019) and surviving silent nociceptors become hyperexcitable and fire spontaneously (Serra et al. 2014) in patients with fibromyalgia, thus potentially contributing to the maintenance of CS. Removal of a peripheral driver, for instance through joint replacement, may reverse even structural changes in the brain (Gwilym et al. 2010). Although CS may be independent of an (obvious) peripheral driver (Baron et al. 2013), evidence suggests that peripheral drivers are likely required to maintain CS in patients. It is therefore important to carefully assess and manage peripheral sources of pain where possible, even in patients with long-standing and nociplastic pain.

Dorsal horn neurones—an integrated network

The spinal cord is a dynamic circuit of many neurones which constantly interact. CS is the result of converging mechanisms which continuously interact through feedback loops across different neuronal circuits. Therefore heightened sensitivity in the spinal cord likely represents the attempt of this integrated network to establish a dynamic equilibrium in a state of continuous stimulation. This explains why any activity-dependent changes, once established, affect a large network of cells and not only single neurones. Although the next section focuses on single neurone changes, neurones belong to a network and pain perception depends on microcircuits within the spinal cord.

Basic biology of CS
Synaptic transmission

Neuronal communication is achieved through synaptic transmission. Electrical impulses (action potentials) are propagated along nociceptive neurones to their central terminals in the dorsal horn of the spinal cord. When the action potentials reach the synapse with the secondary neurone, they trigger the release of chemical messengers, known as neurotransmitters, into the synaptic gap. These neurotransmitters bind to receptors, located in the postsynaptic membrane of the secondary neurone, triggering the generation of action potentials in the respective second neurone. The main excitatory neurotransmitter, glutamate, binds to AMPA and NMDA receptors.

Phases and maintenance of CS

The initial stages of CS are associated with functional plasticity where the conditioning stimulus leads to the voltage-dependent activation of NMDA receptors. Under normal conditions, glutamate activates both AMPA and NMDA receptors, but NMDA receptors remain blocked by a magnesium (Mg^{2+}) ion. Persistent nociceptive input may lower the membrane potential enough to remove the Mg^{2+} block, generating a major influx of Ca^{2+} and initiation of CS (Mayer et al. 1984). This is complemented by AMPA receptors, voltage-gated Ca^{2+} channels and intracellular stores. Other neurotransmitters and receptors are also implicated. One example is substance P which binds to neurokinin 1 (NK1) G-protein-coupled receptors, expressed by most projection neurones (Khasabov et al. 2002; Mantyh et al. 1997; Willis 2002). The binding of substance P to this receptor produces long-lasting depolarisation which allows for the summation of incoming action potentials, contributing to wind-up and CS (Dougherty & Willis 1991; Henry 1976; Xu et al. 1992). CGRP and BDNF have similar functions when released by small-diameter primary neurones (Heppenstall & Lewin 2001; Kerr et al. 1999; Thompson et al. 1999; Zhou & Rush 1996).

Calcium as a second messenger

The increases in intracellular Ca^{2+} lead to a cascade of events which maintain and define the heightened sensitivity. This includes activation of kinases which change NMDA and AMPA receptors both functionally (by increasing their activity) and anatomically (by laying down more receptors in the membrane). This ultimately leads to increased activity (Carvalho et al. 2000; Chen & Roche 2007; Galan et al. 2004; Lau & Zukin 2007). An example of structural changes in the synapse is the increase in a type of AMPA receptor subunit called GluR1. GluR1-containing receptors allow much more Ca^{2+} influx in comparison to the GluR2-containing ones which are expressed under normal conditions. This leads to an increase in synaptic transmission (synaptic strength) (Banke et al. 2000; Battaglia 2016; Esteban et al. 2003; Galan et al. 2004). These initial changes usually lead to a short-lasting sensitisation, but prolonged accumulation of intracellular Ca^{2+} can cause more sustained synaptic facilitation. This second phase of CS involves a number of further modifications (Hu et al. 2003; Ji et al. 1999; Lever et al. 2003; Simonetti et al. 2013). A growing body of evidence also shows *structural* changes during prolonged CS, including increased dendritic and synaptic density (Kuner 2017; Lu et al. 2015; Simonetti et al. 2013; Tan et al. 2012).

Glial role in central sensitisation

The development of CS is affected not only by neurones. Glial cells, including oligodendrocytes, microglia and astrocytes also play a crucial role. Microglia have a surveillance function. Cell-threatening changes in the environment, such as invading pathogens, toxic chemicals or neuronal injury, can lead to microglial activation (Dheen et al. 2007). Astrocytes constitute 40% to 50% of all glial cells (Watkins et al. 2007). They wrap and modulate neuronal synapses and have been shown to support neurones by providing neurotransmitter precursors. Like microglia,

astrocytes also become activated in response to threatening environmental changes, but they also respond to signals from activated microglia (Bradesi 2010). Finally, oligodendrocytes are important in axonal myelination.

Current evidence suggests that both microglia and astrocytes can become activated in response to injury and inflammation (such as CFA or formalin administration) (Cao & Zhang 2008). Once activated, glial cells release proinflammatory cytokines, chemokines, prostaglandins and nerve growth factors, which can sensitise neurones. There are many pathways that have been explored in the context of glia and CS. For example, release of the cytokine TNF by microglia leads to glutamate release from C-fibre terminals in the dorsal horn, causing enhanced neurotransmission and potentiation of pathological pain (Ji et al. 2018). Other cytokines such as IL-1β produced by both microglia and astrocytes can affect CS presynaptically (increased glutamate release) and postsynaptically (increased function of NMDA receptors) (Cao & Zhang 2008; Guo et al. 2007; Ji et al. 2018; Kawasaki et al. 2008). For other signalling pathways implicated in the role of glial function in CS see Bradesi (2010) and Ji et al. (2018).

Information about clinical therapies linked to glial cell modulation is sparse. In many cases, positive responses seen in mice do not translate into successful treatment in humans. For example, the antibiotic minocycline is a glial cell modulator and has been shown to be beneficial in neuropathic pain and opioid tolerance in rodents (Hutchinson et al. 2008; Popiolek-Barczyk et al. 2014), but was recently found to have low efficacy in humans (Arout et al. 2019). Therefore much more data are needed to fully understand the potential of glial cells as a therapeutic target in pain management.

CS in clinical care

Despite our understanding, CS still represents a major clinical challenge. Historically, heightened central sensitivity, especially when occurring without clear pathology, was considered psychosomatic (Woolf 2011). Today, although CS is a well-studied neurobiological phenomenon, there are still challenges arising from the variety of possible central adaptations, as well as diagnostic and therapeutic difficulties. It is important to make a distinction between CS and psychological conditions such as depression and anxiety (van Griensven et al. 2020). The two can influence each other but, as described in this chapter, CS has its own physiological causes and mechanisms.

Interestingly, a recent comprehensive review of the neuroimaging literature in five central sensitivity syndromes (fibromyalgia, chronic fatigue syndrome, irritable bowel syndrome, temporomandibular joint disorder and vulvodynia syndrome) shows that evoked sensory stimulation is associated with augmentation to painful and nonpainful stimulation in different brain regions, although the heterogeneity between and within these syndromes makes the identification of a clear CS signature challenging (Walitt et al. 2016). Neuroimaging techniques in the spinal cord are more complex. Nonetheless, spinal cord functional magnetic resonance imaging (fMRI) studies in healthy subjects has shown increased spinal cord grey matter activation after capsaicin sensitisation, in comparison to nonsensitised, innocuous or noxious heat application (Rempe et al. 2015). Moreover, capsaicin sensitisation led to activation of more segments, both ipsi- and contralateral to the site of stimulation (ibid). A similar fMRI study compared control subjects with fibromyalgia patients, showing enhanced dorsal horn activity and aftersensations in the fibromyalgia group (Bosma et al. 2016). These advances in neuroimaging point to a possible future biomarker for CS, which would be a significant step towards the diagnosis and treatment of this phenomenon.

In clinic, ongoing, spontaneous and widespread pain as well as severe, long-lasting pain following usually innocuous stimuli, can raise the suspicion of a central contribution to a patient condition (van Griensven et al. 2020). The diagnosis of CS currently relies on measurement of input and output of a neural system, which is not possible in vivo. It is therefore prudent to refer to nociplastic pain rather than CS. However, surrogate biomarkers for CS may be established using quantitative sensory testing for cold/heat and mechanical hyperalgesia in areas which are secondary (ipsilateral but innervated by a different segmental level)

or even tertiary (contralateral) to the primary site (Zhu et al. 2019). Other methods include dynamic mechanical hyperalgesia (painful sensation in response to light touch), temporal summation (exacerbated pain ratings during and after a series of repeated stimulation), spatial summation (heightened pain sensation when using, for example, an increasing area of simultaneous pinprick stimulation) and conditioned pain modulation (see later and van Griensven et al. (2020).

Descending inhibition and facilitation

Modulation of nociceptive processing is influenced by sensory input and local regulation in the dorsal horn. In addition, the brain can exert a powerful influence through inhibitory and facilitatory pathways descending to the spinal cord (Fig. 7.5).

LeBars et al. (1979a, 1979b) discovered that painful stimulation was able to inhibit nociceptive transmission by lumbar neurones receiving both Aβ and C fibres (i.e. WDR cells). They found that this effect was observed only when the brain and spinal cord were intact and concluded that the effect had to be mediated by supraspinal processes. Because the inhibition could be brought on by painful stimulation even in areas innervated by other spinal segments, they called it *diffuse noxious inhibitory control (DNIC)*. It is now known that DNIC is in part mediated by

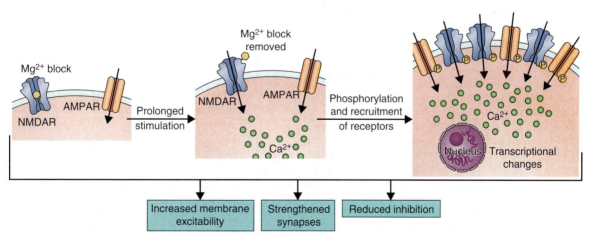

Fig. 7.5 The main neurobiological changes implicated in central sensitisation at spinal cord level. (A) Glutamate opens ion channels with α-amino-3-hydroxy-5-methyl-4-isoxazolepropionic acid receptors *(AMPAR)* and N-methyl-D-aspartate receptors *(NMDAR)*, but NMDAR remains closed by a magnesium block (Mg^{2+}). (B) Prolonged stimulation leads to removal of the Mg^{2+} block and an influx of calcium (Ca^{2+}). (C) The increased concentration of intracellular Ca^{2+} leads to enhanced recruitment and responsiveness of receptors (synaptic strength). Biochemical signals influence DNA transcription in the nucleus of the neurone, creating structural changes that reinforce sensitisation.

neurones in the caudal medulla (*subnucleus reticularis dorsalis* (*SRD*)), the activity of which increases according to the intensity of nociceptive stimulation received (Villanueva 2009). SRD neurones regulate activity in the thalamus (an important relay centre for nociceptive information), the deep dorsal horn (laminae V–VII, see Chapter 6) and several other regions (ibid). There is evidence to suggest that the DNIC does not work well in patients with damage to caudal medulla (De Broucker et al. 1990).

The DNIC-SRD network regulates nociceptive signals as they enter the spinal cord, and as they are processed in the brain stem. It is likely that it forms the physiological basis of the clinical observation that one pain can inhibit another (*counter-irritation*) (Yarnitsky 2015). It is possible to apply TENS or acupuncture in this way, for example (see Chapter 16). In research, the effectiveness of DNIC is assessed by testing whether a noxious test stimulus is moderated by a separate noxious conditioning stimulus, applied either simultaneously or sequentially (Nir & Yarnitsky 2015; Ramaswamy & Wodehouse 2021). This is referred to as *conditioned pain modulation* (CPM). A number of studies have demonstrated reduced efficiency of CPM in patients with chronic pain conditions, suggesting poor pain modulation in these groups (Ossipov & Porreca 2014).

Another network that has been shown to be important for the modulation of nociceptive processing involves the *PAG* and the *RVM*. Nociceptive stimulation can activate the PAG, which in turn stimulates the RVM. The RVM also receives input from higher centres involved in cognition and emotions, which is likely to account for the influence of psychological factors on nociceptive processing in the dorsal horn (Heinricher 2015). RVM neurones descend to the dorsal horn, where their release of serotonin (5-HT) inhibits firing of neurones in laminae I, II and V (Heinricher & Fields 2013). A similar descending pathway from the *locus coeruleus* (LC) exerts its inhibitory influence on the dorsal horn by releasing noradrenaline (NA, also known as norepinephrine) (ibid). Both descending pathways work largely through volume transmission rather than synaptic communication (Todd 2010). The PAG-RVM network has been shown to also be activated in life-threatening situations (Heinricher & Fields 2013), producing what is known as stress-induced analgesia (Butler & Finn 2009). This is likely to account for experiences of survivors of life-threatening accidents and attacks, who may not become aware of pain from injuries until they are out of immediate danger. The network is also involved in offset analgesia, the observation that a small reduction in nociceptive stimulation has a greater than expected analgesic effect when combined with the expectation of pain relief (Ligato et al. 2017). Offset analgesia suggests that expectation of pain relief may generate actual pain relief through stimulation of the PAG, so assessment of patient expectation and early pain relief may be important therapeutic strategies (Fields 2018).

Although the discussion above focuses on central inhibition of pain, the influence of the SRD and the RVM on the dorsal horn can also be facilitatory (Villanueva & Fields 2004). The RVM contains descending neurones which inhibit nociceptive transmission (*off cells*), but also *on cells* which are implicated in facilitation. It has been implicated in the development of hypersensitivity (allodynia and hyperalgesia) in inflammation and neuropathy (Gardell et al. 2003). Acute inflammation and nerve injury may shift regulation towards facilitation (Heinricher & Fields 2013; Porreca et al. 2002), but inhibitory systems become active once inflammation and nociceptive input reduce (Dubner & Ren 2004). In humans, the factors influencing nociceptive facilitation and inhibition are likely to be complex and context-specific.

Conclusion

This chapter has highlighted the role functional and structural changes in the nervous system can play in the origin and maintenance of persistent pain. An understanding of the mechanisms underlying these changes enables the clinician to assess, treat and manage their pain patient more holistically and effectively. Establishing and addressing a pathology and tissue diagnosis remains as important as ever, but it should be complemented by an assessment of the pain mechanisms involved.

Neural circuitry in the dorsal horn is important for the regulation of nociceptive processing and therefore pain perception. This circuitry is influenced considerably by neural pathways descending from the brain. Another aspect of brain function relevant for pain is cortical representation, which is covered in Chapter 13 together with its implications for therapy.

Review questions   Q

1. What is the difference between nociception and pain?
2. What pain characteristics would suggest that a nociceptive pain is mediated by Aδ fibres, or by C fibres?
3. What are the mechanisms responsible for primary and secondary hyperalgesia?
4. What is referred pain? How is it different from neuropathic pain?
5. Describe a physiological mechanism which explains how distraction can suppress nociceptive input.
6. What are the main theories describing the integration of information at the level of the spinal cord?
7. What is CS?

References

Abraira, V.E., Ginty, D.D., 2013. The sensory neurons of touch. Neuron. 79 (4), 618–639.

Arendt-Nielsen, L., Laursen, R., Drewes, A., 2000. Referred pain as an indicator for neural plasticity. In: Sandkühler, J., Bromm, B., Gebhart, G. (Eds.), Nervous System Plasticity and Chronic Pain. Elsevier, Amsterdam, pp. 344–356.

Arendt-Nielsen, L., Morlion, B., Perrot, S., Dahan, A., Dickenson, A., Kress, H.G., et al., 2018. Assessment and manifestation of central sensitisation across different chronic pain conditions. Eur. J. Pain 22 (2), 216–241.

Arout, C.A., Waters, A.J., MacLean, R.R., Compton, P., Sofuoglu, M., 2019. Minocycline does not affect experimental pain or addiction-related outcomes in opioid maintained patients. Psychopharmacology 236 (10), 2857–2866.

Banke, T.G., Bowie, D., Lee, H., Huganir, R.L., Schousboe, A., Traynelis, S.F., 2000. Control of GluR1 AMPA receptor function by cAMP-dependent protein kinase. J. Neurosci. 20 (1), 89–102.

Baron, R., Hans, G., Dickenson, A.H., 2013. Peripheral input and its importance for central sensitization: central sensitization. Ann. Neurol. 74 (5), 630–636.

Basbaum, A., 2021. Pain. In: Kandel, E., Koester, J., Mack, S., Siegelbaum, S. (Eds.), Principles of Neural Science, sixth ed. McGraw Hill, New York, p. 470. 407.

Battaglia, A.A., 2016. An Introduction to Pain and its Relation to Nervous System Disorders. 2016. Wiley Blackwell, Oxford, p. 440.

Bielefeld, K., Gebhart, G., 2013. Visceral pain: basic mechanisms. In: McMahon, S., Koltzenburg, M., Tracey, I., Turk, D. (Eds.), Wall & Melzack's Textbook of Pain. Saunders, Philadelphia, pp. 703–717.

Bosma, R.L., Mojarad, E.A., Leung, L., Pukall, C., Staud, R., Stroman, P.W., 2016. FMRI of spinal and supra-spinal correlates of temporal pain summation in fibromyalgia patients. Hum. Brain. Mapp. 37 (4), 1349–1360.

Bradesi, S., 2010. Role of spinal cord glia in the central processing of peripheral pain perception. Neuro. Gastroenterol. Motil. 22 (5), 499–511.

Brown, A.G., 1983. Neuronal organization in the dorsal horn of the spinal cord. Acta. Morphol. Hung. 31 (1–3), 87–99.

Brumovsky, P., Gebhart, G., 2010. Visceral organ cross-sensitization – an integrated perspective. Auton. Neurosci. 153 (1–2), 106.

Butler, R., Finn, D., 2009. Stress-induced analgesia. Prog. Neurobiol. 88 (3), 184–202.

Cao, H., Zhang, Y.-Q., 2008. Spinal glial activation contributes to pathological pain states. Neurosci. Biobehav. Rev. 32 (5), 972–983.

Carvalho, A.L., Duarte, C.B., Carvalho, A.P., 2000. Regulation of AMPA receptors by phosphorylation. Neurochem. Res. 25 (9–10), 1245–1255.

Cervero, F., Shouenborg, J., Sjölund, B.H., Waddell, P.J., 1984. Cutaneous inputs to dorsal horn neurones in adult rats treated at birth with capsaicin. Brain Res. 301 (1), 47–57.

Chen, B.S., Roche, K.W., 2007. Regulation of NMDA receptors by phosphorylation. Neuropharmacology 53 (3), 362–368.

Chisholm, K.I., Khovanov, N., Lopes, D.M., La Russa, F., McMahon, S.B., 2018. Large scale in vivo recording of sensory neuron activity with GCaMP6. Eneuro. 5 (1).

Cook, A.J., Woolf, C.J., Wall, P.D., McMahon, S.B., 1987. Dynamic receptive field plasticity in rat spinal cord dorsal horn following C-primary afferent input. Nature 325 (6100), 151–153.

Coutinho, S., Su, X., Sengupta, J., Gebhart, G., 2000. Role of sensitized pelvic nerve afferents from the inflamed rat colon in the maintenance of visceral hyperalgesia. In: Sandkühler, J., Bromm, B., Gebhart, G. (Eds.), Nervous System Plasticity and Chronic Pain. Elsevier, Amsterdam, pp. 375–387.

Dallenbach, K.M., 1939. Pain: history and present status. Am. J. Psychol. 52 (3), 331.

Dawes, J., Andersson, D., Bennett, D., Bevan, S., McMahon, S., 2013. Inflammatory mediators and modulators of pain. In: McMahon, S., Koltzenburg, M., Tracey, I., Turk, D. (Eds.), Wall & Melzack's Textbook of Pain. Saunders, Philadelphia, pp. 48–67.

De Broucker, T., Cesaro, P., Willer, J., Le Bars, D., 1990. Diffuse noxious inhibitory controls in man. Involvement of the spinoreticular tract. Brain 113 (1223), 1234.

Dheen, S.T., Kaur, C., Ling, E.-A., 2007. Microglial activation and its implications in the brain diseases. Curr. Med. Chem. 14 (11), 1189–1197.

Dickenson, A.H., Sullivan, A.F., 1987. Evidence for a role of the NMDA receptor in the frequency dependent potentiation of deep rat dorsal horn nociceptive neurones following C fibre stimulation. Neuropharmacology 26 (8), 1235–1238.

Dickenson, A.H., Chapman, V., Green, G.M., 1997. The pharmacology of excitatory and inhibitory amino acid-mediated events in the transmission and modulation of pain in the spinal cord. Gen. Pharmacol. 28 (5), 633–638.

Dougherty, P.M., Willis, W.D., 1991. Enhancement of spinothalamic neuron responses to chemical and mechanical stimuli following combined micro-iontophoretic application of N-methyl-D-aspartic acid and substance P. Pain 47 (1), 85–93.

Dubner, R., Ren, K., 2004. Brainstem modulation of pain. In: Villanueva, L., Dickenson, A., Ollat, H. (Eds.), The Pain System in Normal and Pathological States: A Primer for Clinicians. IASP Press, Seattle, pp. 107–120.

Eckert, N., Vierck, C., Simon, C., Cruz-Almeida, Y., Fillingim, R., Riley 3rd, J., 2017. Testing assumptions in human pain models: psychophysical differences between first and second pain. J. Pain. 18 (3), 266–273.

Eide, P.K., 2000. Wind-up and the NMDA receptor complex from a clinical perspective. Eur. J. Pain. 4 (1), 5–15.

Eide, P.K., Jørum, E., Stubhaug, A., Bremnes, J., Breivik, H., 1994. Relief of post-herpetic neuralgia with the Symbol receptor antagonist ketamine: a double-blind, cross-over comparison with morphine and placebo. Pain 58 (3), 347–354.

Eide, P.K., Jorum, E., Stenehjem, A.E., 1996. Somatosensory findings in patients with spinal cord injury and central dysaesthesia pain. J. Neurol. Neurosurg. Psychiatr. 60 (4), 411–415.

Esteban, J.A., Shi, S.H., Wilson, C., Nuriya, M., Huganir, R.L., Malinow, R., 2003. PKA phosphorylation of AMPA receptor subunits controls synaptic trafficking underlying plasticity. Nat. Neurosci. 6 (2), 136–143.

Felsby, S., Nielsen, J., Arendt-Nielsen, L., Jensen, T.S., 1996. NMDA receptor blockade in chronic neuropathic pain: a comparison of ketamine and magnesium chloride. Pain 64 (2), 283–291.

Fields, H., 2018. How expectations influence pain. Pain 159 (9), S3–S10.

Galan, A., Laird, J.M.A., Cervero, F., 2004. In vivo recruitment by painful stimuli of AMPA receptor subunits to the plasma membrane of spinal cord neurons. Pain 112 (3), 315–323.

Gardell, L., Vanderah, T., Gardell, S., Wang, R., Ossipov, M., Lai, J., et al., 2003. Enhanced evoked excitatory transmitter release in experimental neuropathy requires descending facilitation. J. Neurosci. 23 (23), 8370–8379.

Giamberardino, M., Constantini, R., Affaitati, G., Fabrizio, A., Lapenna, D., Tafuri, E., et al., 2010. Viscero-visceral hyperalgesia: characterization in different clinical models. Pain 151, 307–322.

Gracely, R.H., Lynch, S.A., Bennett, G.J., 1992. Painful neuropathy: altered central processing maintained dynamically by peripheral input. Pain 51 (2), 175–194.

Grayston, R., Czanner, G., Elhadd, K., Goebel, A., Frank, B., Üçeyler, N., et al., 2019. A systematic review and meta-analysis of the prevalence of small fiber pathology in fibromyalgia: implications for a new paradigm in fibromyalgia etiopathogenesis. Semin. Arthritis. Rheum. 48 (5), 933–940.

Guo, W., Wang, H., Watanabe, M., Shimizu, K., Zou, S., LaGraize, S.C., et al., 2007. Glial-cytokine-neuronal interactions underlying the mechanisms of persistent pain. J. Neurosci. 27 (22), 6006–6018.

Gwilym, S.E., Filippini, N., Douaud, G., Carr, A.J., Tracey, I., 2010. Thalamic atrophy associated with painful osteoarthritis of the hip is reversible after arthroplasty: a longitudinal voxel-based morphometric study. Arthritis. Rheum. 62 (10), 2930–2940.

Heinricher, M., 2015. Descending control mechanisms and persistent pain after surgery. In: Wilder-Smith, O., Arendt-Nielsen, L., Yarnitsky, D., Vissers, K. (Eds.), Postoperative Pain. Science and Clinical Practice. Wolters Kluwer, Philadelphia, pp. 59–68.

Heinricher, M., Fields, H., 2013. Central nervous system mechanisms of pain modulation. In: McMahon, S., Koltzenburg, M., Tracey, I., Turk, D. (Eds.), Wall & Melzack's Textbook of Pain. Saunders, Philadelphia, pp. 129–142.

Henry, J.L., 1976. Effects of substance P on functionally identified units in cat spinal cord. Brain Res. 114 (3), 439–451.

Heppenstall, P.A., Lewin, G.R., 2001. BDNF but not NT-4 is required for normal flexion reflex plasticity and function. Proc. Natl. Acad. Sci. U. S. A. 98 (14), 8107–8112.

Herrero, J.F., Laird, J.M.A., Lopez-Garcia, J.A., 2000. Wind-up of spinal cord neurones and pain sensation: much ado about something? Prog. Neurobiol. 61 (2), 169–203.

Hu, H.J., Glauner, K.S., Gereau, R.W., 2003. ERK integrates PKA and PKC signaling in superficial dorsal horn neurons. I. Modulation of A-type K+ currents. J. Neurophysiol. 90 (3), 1671–1679.

Hutchinson, M.R., Northcutt, A.L., Chao, L.W., Kearney, J.J., Zhang, Y., Berkelhammer, D.L., et al., 2008. Minocycline suppresses morphine-induced respiratory depression, suppresses morphine-induced reward, and enhances systemic morphine-induced analgesia. Brain Behav. Immun. 22 (8), 1248–1256.

Hylden, J.L.K., Nahin, R.L., Traub, R.J., Dubner, R., 1989. Expansion of receptive fields of spinal lamina I projection neurons in rats with unilateral adjuvant-induced inflammation: the contribution of dorsal horn mechanisms. Pain 37 (2), 229–243.

IASP, 2021. Terminology. Available from: https://www.iasp-pain.org/Education/Content.aspx?ItemNumber=1698.

Ji, R.R., Baba, H., Brenner, G.J., Woolf, C.J., 1999. Nociceptive-specific activation of ERK in spinal neurons contributes to pain hypersensitivity. Nat. Neurosci. 2 (12), 1114–1119.

Ji, R.-R., Nackley, A., Huh, Y., Terrando, N., Maixner, W., 2018. Neuroinflammation and central sensitization in chronic and widespread pain. Anesthesiology 129 (2), 343–366.

Kawasaki, Y., Zhang, L., Cheng, J.-K., Ji, R.-R., 2008. Cytokine mechanisms of central sensitization: distinct and overlapping role of interleukin-1beta, interleukin-6, and tumor necrosis factor-alpha in regulating synaptic and neuronal activity in the superficial spinal cord. J. Neurosci. 28 (20), 5189–5194.

Kerr, B.J., Bradbury, E.J., Bennett, D.L., Trivedi, P.M., Dassan, P., French, J., et al., 1999. Brain-derived neurotrophic factor modulates nociceptive sensory inputs and NMDA-evoked responses in the rat spinal cord. J. Neurosci. 19 (12), 5138–5148.

Khasabov, S.G., Rogers, S.D., Ghilardi, J.R., Peters, C.M., Mantyh, P.W., Simone, D.A., 2002. Spinal neurons that possess the substance P receptor are required for the development of central sensitization. J. Neurosci. 22 (20), 9086–9098.

Koch, S.C., Acton, D., Goulding, M., 2018. Spinal circuits for touch, pain, and itch. Annu. Rev. Physiol. 80, 189–217.

Kuner R, Flor H. Structural plasticity and reorganisation in chronic pain. Nat Rev Neurosci. 2016 15;18(1):20–30. https://doi:10.1038/nrn.2016.162. Erratum in: Nat Rev Neurosci. 2017 Feb;18(2):158. Erratum in: Nat Rev Neurosci. 2017 Jan 20;18(2):113. PMID: 27974843.

LaMotte, R., Shain, C., Simone, D., Tsai, E., 1991. Neurogenic hyperalgesia: psychophysical studies of underlying mechanisms. J. Neurophysiol. 66 (1), 190–211.

Latremoliere, A., Woolf, C.J., 2009. Central sensitization: a generator of pain hypersensitivity by central neural plasticity. J. Pain. 10 (9), 895–926.

Lau, C.G., Zukin, R.S., 2007. NMDA receptor trafficking in synaptic plasticity and neuropsychiatric disorders. Nat. Rev. Neurosci. 8 (6), 413–426.

LeBars, D., Dickenson, A., Besson, J.-M., 1979a. Diffuse noxious inhibitory controls (DNIC). 1. Effects on dorsal horn convergent neurones in the rat. Pain 6, 283–304.

LeBars, D., Dickenson, A., Besson, J.-M., 1979b. Diffuse noxious inhibitory controls (DNIC). 2. Lack of effect on non-convergent neurones, supraspinal involvement and theoretical implications. Pain 6, 305–327.

Lever, I.J., Pezet, S., McMahon, S.B., Malcangio, M., 2003. The signaling components of sensory fiber transmission involved in the activation of ERK MAP kinase in the mouse dorsal horn. Mol. Cell. Neurosci. 24 (2), 259–270.

Lewis, T., 1942. Pain. Macmillan, New York.

Li, J., Simone, D.A., Larson, A.A., 1999. Windup leads to characteristics of central sensitization. Pain 79 (1), 75–82.

Ligato, D., Peterson, K., Mørch, C., Arendt-Nielsen, L., 2017. Offset analgesia: the role of peripheral and central mechanisms. Eur. J. Pain. 22 (1), 142–149.

Lu, J.N., Luo, C., Bali, K.K., Xie, R.G., Mains, R.E., Eipper, B.A., et al., 2015. A role for Kalirin-7 in nociceptive sensitization via activity-dependent modulation of spinal synapses. Nat. Commun. 6, 6820.

Ma, Q., 2010. Labeled lines meet and talk: population coding of somatic sensations. J. Clin. Invest. 120 (11), 3773–3778.

Maier, C., Baron, R., Tölle, T.R., Binder, A., Birbaumer, N., Birklein, F., et al., 2010. Quantitative sensory testing in the German Research Network on Neuropathic Pain (DFNS): somatosensory abnormalities in 1236 patients with different neuropathic pain syndromes. Pain 150 (3), 439–450.

Mantyh, P.W., Rogers, S.D., Honore, P., Allen, B.J., Ghilardi, J.R., Li, J., et al., 1997. Inhibition of hyperalgesia by ablation of lamina I spinal neurons expressing the substance P receptor. Science 278 (5336), 275–279.

Mao, J., 2012. Current challenges in translational pain research. Trends. Pharmacol. Sci. 33 (11), 568–573.

Mayer, E., Gebhart, G., 1994. Basic and clinical aspects of visceral hyperalgesia. Gastroenterology 107, 271–293.

Mayer, E., Raybould, H., 1990. Role of visceral afferent mechanisms in functional bowel disorders. Gastroenterology 99, 1688–1704.

Mayer, M.L., Westbrook, G.L., Guthrie, P.B., 1984. Voltage-dependent block by Mg^{2+} of NMDA responses in spinal-cord neurons. Nature 309 (5965), 261–263.

McCall, W.D., Tanner, K.D., Levine, J.D., 1996. Formalin induces biphasic activity in C-fibers in the rat. Neurosci. Lett. 208 (1), 45–48.

McMahon, S., 1997. Are there fundamental differences in the peripheral mechanisms of visceral and somatic pain? Behav. Brain. Sci. 20, 381–391.

Melzack, R., Wall, P.D., 1965. Pain mechanisms: a new theory. Science 150, 971–979.

Melzack, R., Wall, P.D., 1996. Pain mechanisms: a new theory. A gate control system modulates sensory input from the skin before it evokes pain perception and response. Pain Forum 5 (1), 3–11.

Mendell, L.M., Wall, P.D., 1965. Responses of single dorsal cord cells to peripheral cutaneous unmyelinated fibres. Nature 206 (4979), 97–99.

Mense, S., 2013. Basic mechanisms of muscle pain. In: McMahon, S., Koltzenburg, M., Tracey, I., Turk, D. (Eds.), Wall & Melzack's Textbook of Pain. Saunders, Philadelphia, pp. 620–628.

Meyer, R., Ringkamp, M., Campbell, J., Raja, S., 2006. Peripheral mechanisms of cutaneous nociception. In: McMahon, S., Koltzenburg, M. (Eds.), Wall and Melzack's Textbook of Pain, 5 ed. Churchill Livingstone, Edinburgh, pp. 3–34.

Moayedi, M., Davis, K.D., 2013. Theories of pain: from specificity to gate control. J. Neurophysiol. 109 (1), 5–12.

Mouraux, A., Bannister, K., Becker, S., Finn, D., Pickering, G., Pogatzki-Zahn, E., et al., 2021. Challenges and opportunities in translational pain research –An opinion paper of the working group on translational pain research of the European pain federation (EFIC). Eur. J. Pain. 00, 1–26.

Nencini, S., Ivanusic, J., 2016. The physiology of bone pain. How much do we really know? Front. Physiol. 7 (157).

Ness, T., Gebhart, G., 1990. Visceral pain: a review of experimental studies. Pain 41, 167–234.

Nir, R., Yarnitsky, D., 2015. Conditioned pain modulation. Curr. Opin. Support. Palliat. Care. 9 (2), 131–137.

Ossipov, M., Porreca, F., 2014. Central mechanisms of pain. In: Raja, S., Sommer, C. (Eds.), Pain 2014. Refresher Courses. IASP Press, Washington DC, pp. 13–22.

Perl, E., 2007. Ideas about pain, a historical view. Nat. Rev. 8, 71–80.

Popiolek-Barczyk, K., Rojewska, E., Jurga, A.M., Makuch, W., Zador, F., Borsodi, A., et al., 2014. Minocycline enhances the effectiveness of nociceptin/orphanin FQ during neuropathic pain. BioMed Res. Int. 2014, 762930.

Porreca, F., Ossipov, M., Gebhart, G., 2002. Chronic pain and medullary descending facilitation. Trends. Neurosci 25 (6), 319–325.

Prescott, S.A., Ma, Q., De Koninck, Y., 2014. Normal and abnormal coding of somatosensory stimuli causing pain. Nat. Neurosci. 17 (2), 183–191.

Price, D., 1999. Psychological Mechanisms of Pain and Analgesia. IASP Press, Seattle.

Price, D., Dubner, R., 1977. Mechanisms of first and second pain in the peripheral and central nervous systems. J. Invest. Dermatol. 69, 167–171.

Proacci, P., Maresca, M., 1993. The historical development of the concepts of hyperalgesia and referred pain. In: Vecchiet, L., Albe-Fessard, D., Lindblom, U., Giamberardino, M. (Eds.), New Trends in Referred Pain and Hyperalgesia. Elsevier, Amsterdam, pp. 275–285.

Pud, D., Eisenberg, E., Spitzer, A., Adler, R., Fried, G., Yarnitsky, D., 1998. The NMDA receptor antagonist amantadine reduces surgical neuropathic pain in cancer patients: a double blind, randomized, placebo controlled trial. Pain 75 (2), 349–354.

Raja, S., Campbell, J., Meyer, R., 1984. Evidence for different mechanisms of primary and secondary hyperalgesia following heat injury to the glabrous skin. Brain 107, 1179–1188.

Ramaswamy, S., Wodehouse, T., 2021. Conditioned pain modulation—a comprehensive review. Clin. Neurophysiol. 51, 197–208.

Rempe, T., Wolff, S., Riedel, C., Baron, R., Stroman, P.W., Jansen, O., et al., 2015. Spinal and supraspinal processing of thermal stimuli: an fMRI study. J. Magn. Reson. Imag. 41 (4), 1046–1055.

Rössel, P., Drewes, A.M., Peterse, P., 1999. Pain produced by electric stimulation of the rectum in patients with irritable bowel syndrome: further evidence of visceral hyperalgesia. Scand. J. Gastroenterol. 34 (10), 1001–1006.

Sarkar, S., Aziz, Q., Woolf, C., Hobson, A., Thompson, D., 2000. Contribution of central sensitisation to the development of non-cardiac chest pain. Lancet 356, 1154–1159.

Schaible, H., 2013. Joint pain: basic mechanisms. In: McMahon, S., Koltzenburg, M., Tracey, I., Turk, D. (Eds.), Wall & Melzack's Textbook of Pain. Saunders, Philadelphia, pp. 609–619.

Serra, J., Collado, A., Solà, R., Antonelli, F., Torres, X., Salgueiro, M., et al., 2014. Hyperexcitable C nociceptors in fibromyalgia: C nociceptors in fibromyalgia. Ann. Neurol. 75 (2), 196–208.

Siegelbaum, S., Clapham, D., Marder, E., 2021. Modulation of synaptic transmission and neuronal excitability: second messengers. In: Kandel, E., Koester, J., Mack, S., Siegelbaum, S. (Eds.), Principles of Neural Science. Mc Graw Hill, New York, pp. 301–323.

Simonetti, M., Hagenston, A.M., Vardeh, D., Freitag, H.E., Mauceri, D., Lu, J.N., et al., 2013. Nuclear calcium signaling in spinal neurons drives a genomic program required for persistent inflammatory pain. Neuron. 77 (1), 43–57.

Staud, R., 2013. The important role of CNS facilitation and inhibition for chronic pain. 8 (6), 639–646.

Tan, A.M., Samad, O.A., Fischer, T.Z., Zhao, P., Persson, A.K., Waxman, S.G., 2012. Maladaptive dendritic spine remodeling contributes to diabetic neuropathic pain. J. Neurosci. 32 (20), 6795–6807.

Taylor, B.K., Peterson, M.A., Basbaum, A.I., 1995. Persistent cardiovascular and behavioral nociceptive responses to subcutaneous formalin require peripheral nerve input. J. Neurosci. 15 (11), 7575–7584.

Thompson, S.W., Bennett, D.L., Kerr, B.J., Bradbury, E.J., McMahon, S.B., 1999. Brain-derived neurotrophic factor is an endogenous modulator of nociceptive responses in the spinal cord. Proc. Natl. Acad. Sci. U. S. A. 96 (14), 7714–7718.

Todd, A.J., 2002. Anatomy of primary afferents and projection neurones in the rat spinal dorsal horn with particular emphasis on substance P and the neurokinin 1 receptor. Exp. Physiol. 87 (2), 245–249.

Todd, A., 2010. Neuronal circuitry for pain processing in the dorsal horn. Nat. Rev. 11, 823–836.

Tracey, I., Mantyh, P.W., 2007. The cerebral signature for pain perception and its modulation. Neuron 55 (3), 377–391.

van Cranenburgh, B., 2000. Pijn: Vanuit Een Neurowetenschappelijk Perspectief. Elsevier Gezondheidszorg, Maarssen.

van Griensven, H., Schmid, A., Trendafilova, T., Low, M., 2020. Central sensitization in musculoskeletal pain: lost in translation? J. Orthop. Sports. Phys. Ther. 50 (11), 592–596.

Villanueva, L., 2009. Diffuse noxious inhibitory control (DNIC) as a tool for exploring dysfunction of endogenous pain modulatory systems. Pain 143 (3), 161–162.

Villanueva, L., Fields, H., 2004. Endogenous central mechanisms of pain modulation. In: Villanueva, L., Dickenson, A., Ollat, H. (Eds.), The Pain System in Normal and Pathological States: A Primer for Clinicians. IASP Press, Seattle, pp. 223–243.

Walitt, B., Ceko, M., Gracely, J.L., Gracely, R.H., 2016. Neuroimaging of central sensitivity syndromes: key insights from the scientific literature. Curr. Rheumatol. Rev. 12 (1), 55–87.

Watkins, L.R., Hutchinson, M.R., Ledeboer, A., Wieseler-Frank, J., Milligan, E.D., Maier, S.F., 2007. Norman Cousins Lecture. Glia as the 'bad guys': implications for improving clinical pain control and the clinical utility of opioids. Brain Behav. Immun. 21 (2), 131–146.

Willis, W.D., 2002. Long-term potentiation in spinothalamic neurons. Brain Res. Rev. 40 (1–3), 202–214.

Woolf, C.J., 2011. Central sensitization: implications for the diagnosis and treatment of pain. Pain 152 (3), S2–S15.

Woolf, C.J., Thompson, S.W.N., 1991. The induction and maintenance of central sensitization is dependent on N-methyl-d-aspartic acid receptor activation; implications for the treatment of post-injury pain hypersensitivity states. Pain 44 (3), 293–299.

Xu, X.J., Dalsgaard, C.J., Wiesenfeld-Hallin, Z., 1992. Spinal substance P and N-methyl-D-aspartate receptors are coactivated in the induction of central sensitization of the nociceptive flexor reflex. Neuroscience 51 (3), 641–648.

Yarnitsky, D., 2015. Role of endogenous pain modulation in chronic pain mechanisms and treatment. Pain 156, S24–S31.

Zhou, X.F., Rush, R.A., 1996. Endogenous brain-derived neurotrophic factor is anterogradely transported in primary sensory neurons. Neuroscience 74 (4), 945–953.

Zhu, G.C., Böttger, K., Slater, H., Cook, C., Farrell, S.F., Hailey, L., et al., 2019. Concurrent validity of a low-cost and time-efficient clinical sensory test battery to evaluate somatosensory dysfunction. Eur. J. Pain 23 (10), 1826–1838.

Section | 2 |

Assessment and management of pain

Chapter 8

Assessing pain

Jenny Strong and Hubert van Griensven

LEARNING OBJECTIVES

At the end of this chapter, readers will be able to:
1. Understand the place of self-report measures, observational measures and physiological measures in understanding an individual's pain experience.
2. Be aware of developments in pain measurement.
3. Describe commonly used pain assessment frameworks and dimensions.
4. Describe pain measurement tools for different dimensions of pain.
5. Be aware of common-sense considerations in assessment tool selection.

Overview

'Pain assessment and measurement remain imperfectly solved problems for clinicians and researchers. It remains a clinical art to combine patients reports, behavioural observations, and physiological measurements with the history, physical exam, laboratory information, and overall clinical context in guiding clinical judgements and therapeutic interventions'. These words of Berde & McGrath (2009) on pain measurement remain apposite today.

Earlier chapters discussed the multifaceted and all-encompassing experience of pain and the burden upon individuals, families and society. To reflect this, the person who lives with pain should be central in the pain assessment process. Healthcare professionals must gain a comprehensive understanding of the intensity, experiences and impact of their patient's pain. It is not enough to ask, 'How intense is your pain on a 0–10 scale?' Each healthcare professional must carefully assess the multidimensional aspects of the patient's pain and use this to design personalised treatment and management plans and to determine progress.

Unfortunately, several meta-analyses of chronic pain clinical trials have observed that the heterogeneity of pain outcome measures is a major obstacle to meaningful comparison of treatments (e.g. Hayden et al. 2005). There have been calls for the use of agreed outcome measures across trials to enable meta-analyses of clinical trials (e.g. Dworkin et al. 2005; Turk et al. 2008). Fortunately, a number of recent developments through international consensus enable clinicians and researchers to undertake the necessary and sufficient assessment of a person's pain. Beginning this century, international consensus meetings have synthesised comprehensive yet parsimonious sets of tools for best practice clinic and research. There is general consensus across these outcome measure sets, including Initiative on Methods, Measurement, and Pain Assessment in Clinical Trials (IMMPACT) from Canada and the United States, electronic Persistent Pain Outcome Collaboration (ePPOC) from Australia and New Zealand, and the British Pain Society in the United Kingdom.

This chapter will provide the pain therapist with knowledge about types of pain measures and when their use may be indicated, based on prominent international pain assessment and measurement guidelines. It starts with a brief consideration of the development of our pain assessment toolkit. Next it adds a dimension that we consider to be at the epicentre of pain assessment: the patient's goals. Principles of pain assessment will then be outlined, before providing two case studies for insight into the clinical reasoning that underpins pain evaluation.

Recent history of pain measurement

The search for the best way of measuring and understanding a person's pain is not new. Beecher (1959), based on his observations of soldiers injured during battle and civilians with similar injuries, declared that pain is 'in very large part determined by other factors [than the size of the wound or injury]'. Around that time, Prof Ronald Melzack, described as 'the father of pain management' (McAllister 2019), turned his attention to improving understanding the nature of and measurement of pain. He recognised that assessing a patient's pain intensity alone was inadequate. With the assistance of his colleague Torgerson, he went on to quantify pain descriptors he had gathered from many patients and developed the McGill Pain Questionnaire (MPQ).

In 1988, Williams (1988) developed a core set of reliable and valid pain measures. This set included physical, functional, behavioural/cognitive and emotional measures, as well as measures for economic and sociocultural factors. In the 1990s, various authors provided their views on the necessary dimensions for pain assessment. For example, Deyo et al. (1998) discussed the need for reduced heterogeneity of chronic pain outcome measures. They proposed a standard set of outcome measures for low back pain clinical trials, which included a six-item patient outcome set that asked about bothersomeness of pain and interference with normal work over the preceding week, days with reduced activities or inability to work over the preceding 4 weeks, satisfaction if the symptoms remained and satisfaction with medical care. They further recommended that if clinicians had enough time, they could also use either the Roland Morris Questionnaire or the Oswestry Disability Questionnaire, and either the EuroQol or the SF-12. Strong et al. (2002) proposed that therapists consider the patient's description of their pain, their responses to that pain, and the impact of that pain on the patient's life as core aspects of pain measurement.

The following decade saw groups of clinicians and scientists coming together to agree on measurement frameworks. In North America, the IMMPACT developed a set of agreed core outcome domains and essential or preferred measures to be used for each domain in clinical trials (Dworkin et al. 2005; Turk et al. 2003). The aim was to determine the effectiveness of interventions and improve chronic pain management.

With the IMMPACT recommendations published in 2005, one might have expected to see greater adherence to the use of the recommended measurement tools. However, in 2011, Segerdahl provocatively titled her commentary in the journal *Pain* 'Pain outcome variables – a never ending story' (Segerdahl 2011). There remains outcome measure heterogeneity in chronic pain clinical trials (Morley et al. 2013), such as a new core outcome set for clinical trials with patients with nonspecific low back pain (e.g. Chiarotto et al. 2018a), or the International Classification of Functioning, Disability and Health's Low Back Pain Core Set (Bagraith et al. 2018; Cieza et al. 2004).

In 2011, the Australian and New Zealand College of Anaesthetists Faculty of Pain Medicine and the Australian Pain Society spearheaded an initiative to progress pain outcome measurement following the rollout of the National Pain Strategy (Tardif et al. 2015). The resultant ePPOC was implemented in 2013. The uptake of ePPOC has been impressive, with over 50 adult and paediatric pain treatment facilities across Australia and New Zealand now routinely using ePPOC or the Paeds ePPOC Collaboration (Nicholas et al. 2019).

More recently, a working group of experts from the British Pain Society and the Faculty of Pain Medicine of the Royal College of Anaesthetists developed a set of outcome measures to enhance patient care and aid in benchmarking pain services (British Pain Society & Faculty of Pain Medicine 2019).

Key considerations for therapists when choosing pain measurement tools must be the reliability, validity, sensitivity and clinical utility of the tool. Reliability refers to the extent to which an outcome measure is consistent, for instance across time and raters. Validity refers to the extent to which it measures what it claims to be measuring. Sensitivity refers to the ability of a measurement tool to detect change over time or differences between different groups. These terms are not to be confused with the concepts of the sensitivity and specificity of a *clinical* test, which refers to the ability of a test to correctly identify the presence of a disease and to correctly identify when a patient does not have the disease (Swift et al. 2020). Clinical utility refers to the suitability of the measurement tool to be used in routine practice. While geographical location may dictate the outcome measures to be used, there will also be context specific and theoretical reasons for some measurement tool selection. For example, the cognitive abilities of the patient, their developmental level and their familiarity with the language should be taken into account. The chapters on communication (Chapter 3), pain in childhood (Chapter 19), pain in the elderly (Chapter 20) and pain amongst indigenous populations (Chapter 22) provide more specific guidance in this regard. This current chapter describes commonly used measurement tools.

Types of pain measures

This section discusses the three different categories of pain measurement. The reflective exercise in Box 8.1 is a useful way to consider which category of pain measurement might be most suitable. The reader is encouraged to do the exercise and to consider the potential benefits and limitations of each type of pain measurement for someone with a migraine.

Self-report

As suggested in the Reflective Exercise, there are three types of pain measures: self-report, observational and physiological measures. In self-report, the patient provides information about their pain. Self-report measures often involve rating pain and function on a metric scale. A therapist might ask the patient to rate their highest, lowest, current and average levels of pain. Pain diaries are another example. They help measure the impact of the pain on the patient's life. Pain diaries can be relatively structured so that the necessary information can be recorded at regular intervals. They may include ratings of pain intensity, rest and activity, medication consumption and current mood. With the growth of technology, apps on mobile devices are being frequently used to facilitate the completion of pain self-report (Zhao et al. 2019).

Self-report is considered the gold standard of pain measurement because it is consistent with the definition of pain as a subjective experience (Melzack & Katz 2002). However, this subjective nature also poses a dilemma: the patient's perception and report of their pain are likely to be influenced by other factors. To illustrate, the pain rating that the reader provided on a 0- to 10-pain intensity scale in Box 8.1 may be influenced by the patient's desire for analgesia or a desire to meet the clinician's wishes. Moreover, the patient's perceived level of pain is likely to be influenced by the suffering caused by that pain (Price 1999). For example, a new low-intensity pain may be a cause of great distress in someone with a history of cancer. de Williams et al. (2000) found that many patients could not separate their pain intensity from their distress when completing a pain rating scale.

There has been controversy about the validity of self-report data. For example, the level of pain reported by chronic pain patients may not be related to self-report of physical disability (Patrick & D'Eon 1996). The dilemma here is that clinicians intuitively expect that the extent of disability should be proportionately related to the severity of the pain. When they are not, clinicians are inclined to assume that the patient's self-report of pain intensity is exaggerated. This may be so, but physical performance, perceived level of physical performance and pain intensity reports are different constructs, all of which provide valid clinical information about a patient with chronic pain. Validity of self-report is enhanced by recent comprehensive normative data for many pain measurement tools, so healthcare professionals are urged to compare their patient's report against these available data (e.g. Nicholas et al. 2008, 2019). Finally, self-report measures rely on the person's ability to communicate their pain. It is therefore not always possible for infants, young children, people with a disability that impairs communication or people from different cultures and countries (see Chapters 19, 20 and 22).

Observational measures

Observational measures rely on an observer, typically the clinician or someone well known to the patient. The measure usually relates to the patient's behaviour or activity performance. Observational measures can be useful to complement the self-report given by the patient. They allow assessment of progress and provide patients with information about functional gains. The latter is important for patients who are focused on pain and may not notice functional gains. Observational measures are also useful to identify areas of concern, particularly about the patient's functional performance and ergonomic factors related to work.

There is no behaviour that is an indicator of pain alone, so observation must be correlated with self-report. For example, clutching the abdomen may be due to pain, but it might also be due to nausea or psychological distress. To know what a behaviour signifies, one needs to ask the person. The advantage of collaborative reporting between patient and observer was noted in a study by Ahlers et al. (2008), wherein ICU nurses were found to underestimate critically ill patients' level of pain in comparison to the patients' self-assessment. It is important to remember that observational measures cannot provide purely objective pain measurement. Rather, these measures reflect the therapist's objective *and* subjective measurement of the patient's pain. The housemate's observational measurement of your migraine in Box 8.1 may be affected by her inexperience with migraines and the observation that you are lying down and appear to be relaxing. Case study 8.1 shows an example where observational measurement is needed.

Observation is an essential part of the health professional's toolkit. For example, when a health professional is providing a care item for a patient with minimal language, observation of body language is crucial to avoid pain.

Physiological measures

Pain can cause biological changes in heart rate, respiration, sweating, muscle tension and other changes associated with a stress response (Turk & Okifuji 1999). These biological changes can be used as an indirect measure of acute pain. That said, biological response to acute pain may stabilise over time, e.g. breathing or heart rate may show a change at the sudden onset of pain, but these changes are likely to return to normal even if the pain persists (Melzack & Katz 2002). Physiological measures may be useful in situations where observational measures are difficult. For example, the Critical-Care Pain Observation Tool (C-CPOT) has been developed and tested for use with critically ill adults who cannot communicate verbally (Gélinas et al. 2009).

Another type of physiological measure is quantitative sensory testing (QST), which aims to identify neurophysiological mechanisms underlying a patient's pain (Chapter 7). For a comprehensive testing protocol, see Rolke et al. (2006).

Contemporary consensus pain outcome measurement frameworks

This section provides a review of the pain outcome measurement frameworks introduced earlier in the chapter, IMMPACT (Dworkin et al. 2005; Turk et al. 2008), ePPOC (Australian Health Services Research Institute 2020; Tardif et al. 2015) and the British Outcome Measures (British Pain Society & Faculty of Pain Medicine 2019).

Table 8.1 shows the recommended assessment domains from the frameworks. The frameworks recommend consideration of the nature of pain, its impact and how it interferes with a person's functioning. They also consider emotional functioning associated with the pain. IMMPACT and ePPOC include the patient's rating of change over the course of treatment. Only the British

Outcome Measures specify the measurement of quality of life, while IMMPACT records symptoms and adverse events reported over the treatment (crucial for clinical trials) and patient disposition (e.g. adherence). Finally, ePPOC records health service use and medication use.

The sections that follow discuss tools that may be used to measure each assessment domain. Measures which describe pain are usually based on self-report, typically in the form of questionnaires, pain rating scales and pain drawings. Pain can be described in terms of its intensity, its quality (e.g. burning, aching, dull, sharp, etc.), its frequency and its location. A patient's description of their pain serves several purposes. A baseline description of the pain allows for assessment of change. Ideally, pain should be assessed before, during and after treatment.

Pain intensity

A patient's self-report of their pain intensity has been described as 'the most valid measure of the experience' (Melzack & Katz 2002). Self-report of pain intensity is reliable and valid (Jamison 1996). Clinicians should ask their patient to gauge the intensity or severity of their pain. As mentioned earlier in this chapter, the patient may be asked to give a number to describe their worst pain, least pain, current pain and average pain. Fig. 8.1 illustrates a few ways to measure pain intensity.

Numerical Rating Scale (NRS)

All assessment frameworks recommend the use of a numerical 0- to 10-pain intensity scale, where 0 = no pain and 10 = worst possible pain. A score of less than or equal to 4 is considered mild pain, 4 to 6 moderate and greater than 6 severe (Chien et al. 2017).

Various studies have supported the psychometric properties of the NRS in adult patients (Childs et al. 2005; Jensen et al. 1986, 1989; Strong et al. 1991), and children and adolescents (Castarlenas et al. 2017). For example, Ferraz et al. (1990) reported high test–retest reliability (r = 0.95 and 0.96) in patients with arthritis. The construct validity of the NRS was supported with correlations of 0.79 with a visual analogue scale, and 0.85 with a 0 to 100 scale in patients with chronic back pain, and a loading of 0.89 on a single factor using exploratory factor analysis (Strong et al. 1991). The NRS was found to be sensitive to age and gender differences in patients with back pain, with older men reporting less intense pain than younger men or women (Strong 1992).

The NRS has good clinical utility: it is quick, easy to use and gives a score that can be interpreted. It is useful for healthcare professionals to appreciate if the pain intensity of their patient is mild, moderate or severe.

Nicholas et al. (2019) reported that the average pain intensity score on an NRS for 13,343 patients admitted

CASE STUDY 8.1

Mr Ron Longley (a pseudonym) was a 92-year-old man who lived in the dementia care unit at a residential care facility. He had been residing in the facility for the past 10 months. He was married, and his wife attended every morning to sit with him, but as she was herself frail, she was unable to provide much physical care for Ron. Ron needed assistance to get out of bed, and while he initially had the ability to walk with assistance, he now refused to walk. He preferred to sit in the chair in his room all day. He stopped attending to his self-cares, which upset his wife, who told staff that Ron had been very particular with his grooming and appearance and hygiene. By this stage, Ron was nonverbal.

The facility care staff found it increasingly difficult to get Ron out of bed, into the shower chair for his ablutions, and into his bedside chair. When he was helped into standing position, he would groan as in agony, and flail his arms to get the staff away from him. He would then slump back in his chair and rock from side to side. This was very difficult for the care staff and also distressing for Ron's wife, who explained how he had been the gentlest of people all his life.

The residential care facility asked the general practitioner to review Ron, to help with his ongoing management and care. The general practitioner felt that Ron was in pain and suggested an opioid patch to help alleviate his pain. However, Ron's wife, though frail, had worked as a hospital social worker, and she did not think that opioids should be the first line of action to help relieve her husband's distress. Her son had given her the Australian Pain Society's Pain in Residential Aged Care Facilities: Management Strategies (Goucke 2019), and she had carefully read the document. She therefore met with the general practitioner and requested the residential care facility obtain a review from both a physiotherapist and an occupational therapist.

This referral has come to you. How will you approach this pain assessment review, and what measurements will you use to shape your recommendations to support Ron's care?

Clearly, given Ron's nonverbal state, self-report measures will be inappropriate. You decide to meet with the patient and his wife, and chat with her about what she has been observing every day she has been up visiting her husband. You then liaise with the care staff and arrange to observe the next day during the morning self-care rituals. You have downloaded a copy of the Abbey Pain Scale (Abbey et al. 2004) to guide your observations. This scale looks at vocalisations made by the patient, his facial expressions, change in his body language, behavioural changes, physiological changes and physical changes.

The next morning, you arrive early to be able to observe Ron's behaviour when the staff get him out of bed and into the shower chair for his daily ablutions and showering. At first, Ron seems calm, but the instant his feet make contact with the floor, his expression changes and he whimpers. When the staff assist him into standing so they can transfer him into the shower chair he groans and tries to push the care staff away. With difficulty, he is transferred into the shower chair and wheeled into the en-suite bathroom. He calms while toileting, but once in the shower cubicle, the shower water is turned on, and he starts to groan and frail his arms. You check the water temperature and are assured that it is lukewarm water, not too hot and not too cold.

After his shower, Ron is settled into his chair by the window of his unit. He dozes and seems calm. When his wife arrives, you ask her permission to look more closely at Ron's feet.

Why would you be wanting to examine Ron's feet?

HINT: What are the signs and symptoms of complex regional pain syndrome (CRPS) (see Chapter 13)? This is an exercise we encourage you to complete before you return to this case study.

Please write down the important signs and symptoms of CRPS. Given that Ron is nonverbal, what should you focus on? Clearly, you need to be alert to the *signs* of complex regional pain syndrome, as Ron is unable to tell you about *symptoms* he is experiencing. You have made several observations during the morning's personal care regime. You also speak with his wife about her observations.

Case formulation

You suspect that Ron is suffering pain due to CRPS. You have observed his agitation and distress when he is moved into weight-bearing, and his agitation when the shower water streams onto his lower limbs.

What are the best management strategies for managing the pain of CRPS, especially in a patient who is living with dementia? Please refer to Chapter 14 where neuropathic pain is discussed.

to Australasian Pain Clinics was 6.4 (SD = 1.8). These patients were reporting a severe level of pain at the start of their pain management treatment.

Visual Analogue Scales (VAS)

VAS are scales that consist of a 100-mm line with anchors stating 'No pain' at one end and 'Worst possible pain' or similar at the other. The line may be of horizontal or vertical orientation. A horizontal VAS may be preferred (Strong 1992), although elderly patients may find the VAS confusing (Gagliese & Melzack 1997). The patient is asked to mark the line at a point corresponding to the severity of their pain. The score is the number of millimetres from the 'No pain' anchor, i.e. a figure between 0 and 100, measured with a ruler.

TABLE 8.1 Domains of the pain measurement frameworks

IMMPACT	ePPOC	Outcome measures	Pain textbook
Pain intensity, pain location, pain description and pain qualities	Pain severity, pain location and frequency	Pain quantity (pain intensity)	Pain description—pain intensity, pain quality, and pain location
Physical functioning	Pain interference	Pain interference	Impact of pain
Emotional functioning	Emotional distress	Emotional distress and functioning	Patient responses to pain
Patient rating of global improvement and treatment satisfaction	Patient rating of change	Quality of life	
Symptoms and adverse events	Health service usage		
Patient disposition	Medication usage		

Test–retest reliability has been reported as good, with correlation coefficients of 0.94 and 0.71 (Ferraz et al. 1990). However, reliability of the VAS may be affected if the length of the line is not 100 mm, which can occur when the scale is photocopied, or if measurement is not accurate. A study by Peters et al. (2007) comparing psychometric properties of different pain rating scales indicated that most mistakes were made on the VAS. The construct validity of the VAS has been shown to be good, with a factor loading of 0.87 on a single pain intensity factor, and a correlation of 0.79 with the NRS (Strong et al. 1991). The VAS has been shown to have scale ratio properties, i.e. a 50% reduction in perceived pain correlates well with a similar reduction in VAS rating (Price 1999). The sensitivity of the VAS has been supported (British Pain Society 2019).

Visual tools

Variations of the VAS have been developed over time, such as the PAULA the PAIN-METER (PAULA) (Machata et al. 2009). This visual tool features five faces with different expressions. The patient uses a slider to place their feelings within this emotional range. PAULA was developed to accommodate patients struggling with perceptual-cognitive impairment following general anaesthesia. One side of the scale facing away from the patient depicts a VAS scale, enabling the clinician to assign a numerical score. Reliability of PAULA compares favourably with the VAS (Machata et al. 2009).

Pain quality

Pain quality measures may hint at mechanisms underlying the patient's pain (Jensen et al. 2013). The Brief Pain Inventory, which is recommended in IMMPACT, ePPOC, the British Pain Measures and the Brief Pain Inventory - Long Form includes a list of 15 pain descriptors that include adjectives like burning, nagging, aching, and miserable. Patients are asked which descriptors describe their pain (Cleeland & Ryan 1994).

A well-known and widely used pain quality assessment is the McGill Pain Questionnaire (MPQ) (Melzack 1975; Melzack & Torgerson 1971). The MPQ has been translated into many languages, including Japanese (Hasegawa et al. 2001), French (Boureau et al. 1992), Norwegian (Strand & Ljunggreg 1997) and German (Stein & Mendl 1988). It contains a list of 78 pain descriptors, organised into 20 categories relating to the sensory (categories 1–10), affective (categories 11–15) and evaluative (category 16) dimensions of a person's pain. A miscellaneous class (categories 17–20) is included. Patients are asked to select one descriptor from each of the 20 categories. Quantitative scores derived from the MPQ are number of words chosen, pain rating index total, as well as the sensory index, affective index and evaluative index. Reliability and validity of the MPQ are well established (Melzack & Katz 1994).

Melzack (1987) developed the short-form MPQ (SF-MPQ) for clinical and research situations where time is limited. It consists of 15 descriptors (such as throbbing, heavy and sickening) which patients are asked to rate on a four-point scale where 0 = none, 1 = mild, 2 = moderate and 3 = severe. Dworkin and his colleagues (2009) developed a revised version, the SF-MPQ-2, which expanded on the descriptor items and modified the intensity scale to a 0 to 10 scale. It provides four factors: continuous pain, intermittent pain, neuropathic pain and affective pain (Dworkin et al. 2009). A recent systematic review supported the internal consistency of the

Visual analogue scale (horizontal)

No pain ——————————————————| Pain as bad
as it could be

Numeric rating scale

Please indicate on the line below the number between
0 and 100 that best describes your pain.
A zero (0) would mean 'no pain' and a one hundred (100)
would mean 'pain as bad as it could be'.

Please write only one number. ——

Box scale

If a zero means 'no pain', and a ten (10) means 'pain as bad as it
could be', on this scale of 0-10, what is your level of pain?
Put an 'X' through that number.

0	1	2	3	4	5	6	7	8	9	10

Verbal rating scale

( ) No pain
( ) Some pain
( ) Considerable pain
( ) Pain which could not be more severe

Behavioural rating scale

( ) No pain
( ) Pain present, but can easily be ignored
( ) Pain present, cannot be ignored, but does not interfere with everyday activities
( ) Pain present, cannot be ignored, interferes with concentration
( ) Pain present, cannot be ignored, interferes with all tasks except taking care of
basic needs such as toileting and eating
( ) Pain present, cannot be ignored, rest or bedrest required

Fig. 8.1 Pain intensity measures.

SF-MPQ-2, with α ranging from 0.88 to 0.96, partial support for test–retest reliability, but conflicting findings on the factor structure (Jumbo et al. 2021). The SF-MPQ-2 was found in one of the reviewed studies to be responsive to change (Jumbo et al. 2021).

While some researchers have utilised the MPQ in a quantitative way (e.g. Lowe et al. 1991), its primary value for clinicians is its ability to identify subjective features of a person's pain experience and to detect subtle clinical changes. Jerome et al. (1988) suggested that attention be given to the specific words chosen by patients on the MPQ rather than concentrating on the total scores obtained. From these words chosen, the therapist can obtain an idea of features of a person's pain. Certain types of pain are associated with distinctive words associated with them (Melzack & Katz 2002), e.g. shooting and burning for a patient with phantom limb pain. On the other hand, descriptors chosen by a patient may be unexpected and invite further exploration.

Pain location

A pain drawing consists of outline drawings of the human body, front and back, on which the patient indicates where the pain is by shading the painful area (Margolis et al. 1986) or by indicating the type of symptom (e.g. pins and needles, ache, burning pain) using symbols (Ransford et al. 1976). IMMPACT and ePPOC recommend measurement of the pain location. The pain drawing provides a simple way to gain a graphic representation of patient's pain. Scoring systems have been developed to use with the pain drawing. Margolis et al. (1986, 1988) derived total body pain scores based on the total area shaded as painful.

The pain drawing can assist in clinical reasoning because it provides useful information about the location and distribution of the patient's pain. Seroussi (2015) suggested that practitioners may suspect a chronic pain syndrome by scanning their pain drawings. Pain drawings that do not follow typical anatomical patterns may alert us to the patient having complex problems.

An alternative method to gain an understanding of the location of a patient's pain is offered by ePPOC, which lists 21 body sites and asks the patient to indicate where they feel pain (e.g. face/jaw/temple or calf-left/right). This system does provide an easily quantifiable body location. However, a patient endorsing that they have pain in their left calf does not give as much information to the clinician as their pain drawing where, for example, the whole of the left calf is shaded in.

Pain frequency

ePOCC asks the patient if their pain is always present, often present, occasionally present, rarely present. The MPQ and the Brief Pain Inventory (see later) also enquire about the pattern of the pain that the patient experiences.

To conclude this brief overview of **pain description**, the use of self-report measures of pain intensity, pain quality and pain location is recommended. Such an evaluation helps the clinician to better understand the patient's pain. It allows the patient to feel they have fully communicated the way their pain feels to them and to feel understood (also see Chapter 3). A thorough evaluation can be invaluable in the establishment of the therapeutic relationship.

Pain interference

One of the greatest burdens for the person with persistent pain may be a loss of former roles and in many cases a loss of identity (e.g. Daker-White et al. 2014; van Griensven 2016). For health professionals to enable their patients to achieve their best level of function, it is important to measure the impact of the pain. Tools for the measurement of this dimension include:

1. The Brief Pain Inventory (BPI) (Cleeland & Ryan 1994);
2. The Multidimensional Pain Inventory (MPI) (Kerns et al. 1985);
3. The Oswestry Back Pain Questionnaire (OLBPQ) (Fairbank et al. 1980);
4. The Pain Disability Index (PDI) (Tait et al. 1990);
5. The Roland Morris Questionnaire (RMQ) (Roland & Morris 1983); and
6. The Overactivity in Persistent Pain Assessment (OPPA) (Andrews et al. 2021).

The Brief Pain Inventory (BPI)

The BPI is a simple yet comprehensive self-report measure that obtains information on pain location, pain intensity, pain medications, pain relief and the interference the pain has caused in the individual's life (Cleeland & Ryan 1994; Dworkin et al. 2005). The Pain Interference Scale of the BPI consists of seven items that are rated on a 0 to 10 scale, where 0 = no interference and 10 = maximal interference. A total pain interference score is calculated by summing the scores on these seven items and taking the average. While the BPI was originally developed for use with patients with cancer pain, it is now widely used with patients with chronic, noncancer pain (Tan et al. 2004). It has been translated into many languages. The reliability and validity of the BPI have been supported by a number of studies (Cleeland & Ryan 1994; Nicholas et al. 2019; Radbruch et al. 1999). Keller and colleagues (2004) reported good reliability, with an internal consistency alpha coefficient of 0.94 for patients with arthritis and 0.93 for patients with low back pain. The construct validity was supported, with factor loadings for the seven interference factor items ranging from 0.59 to 0.91, and a correlation of 0.81 with the Roland Disability Questionnaire (Keller et al. 2004). The BPI was found to be sensitive to differences in disability levels and to change over time (Keller et al. 2004). In a recent systematic review, test–retest reliability for the BPI was found, with an intraclass correlation coefficient (ICC) of 0.83, as was internal consistency, with Cronbach's α coefficients ranging from 0.82 to 0.96 (Jumbo et al. 2021). Support was also found for the factor structure and sensitivity (Jumbo et al. 2021).

The mean pain interference score of 12,611 patients attending an Australasian pain facility was 6.4 (1.8).

The Multidimensional Pain Inventory (MPI)

The MPI is a 54-item self-report questionnaire that examines the impact of the pain on a person's life, the response of a significant other to that person's pain and the impact the pain has on an individual's ability to complete instrumental activities of daily living (Kerns et al. 1985). Items are scored on a 0 to 6 scale, where 0 = no, never and 6 = yes, very much. It is quick to administer. There are 12 subscales (pain interference, support, pain severity, life control, affective distress, negative responses by significant other, solicitous responses by significant other, distracting responses by significant other, interference with household chores, outdoor work, activities away from home, and social activities. (Kerns et al. 1985). These are grouped into three categories: measuring pain features, pain responses by significant others and general activities. Patients can be assigned to one of three distinctive groups: Adaptive Coper, Interpersonally Distressed or Dysfunctional (Turk & Rudy 1988). The MPI provides a broader impression of the patient's pain and associated aspects, e.g. how supportive their spouse is and how limited activity is. The MPI has been translated into many languages other than English, including Swedish (Bergstrom et al. 1998) and Turkish (Cetin et al. 2016).

Kerns et al. (1985) reported Cronbach's α coefficients of between 0.70 and 0.90 and test–retest reliability coefficients between 0.62 and 0.91, thus supporting the reliability of the tool. Its validity was supported by correlations with other measures including marital satisfaction and pain severity (Kerns et al. 1985). Wittink and colleagues (2004) reported good Cronbach's α values, ranging from 0.69 to 0.92 and good sensitivity for change for the pain severity, interference and outdoor work domains of the MPI. It has been described as 'an easily accessible, reliable and valid self-report questionnaire' (McKillop & Nielson 2011). The three MPI clusters were found to be associated with expected scores on the alternate measures including the Oswestry Disability Index (ODI) and the Beck Depression Inventory and to have good clinical utility (Choi et al. 2013).

The Oswestry Low Back Pain Disability Questionnaire (ODQ)

The ODQ (Fairbank et al. 1980) is one of the most frequently used self-report tools to measure the physical limitations experienced due to low back pain. It has also been adapted for use with patients with neck pain and general back pain (Fairbank & Pynsent 2000). It consists of 10 questions about the patient's limitations in sitting, standing, walking, lifting, having sex, socialising, sleeping, personal care and travelling. One item assesses pain intensity. Items are scored on a 0 to 5 scale, where 0 = no difficulty and 5 = maximal difficulty. A score out of 50 is obtained and converted to a percentage (Fairbank et al. 1980).

The ODQ has good reliability, with Cronbach's α coefficients ranging from 0.71 to 0.90 (Fairbank et al. 2000). Wittink et al. (2004) reported a Cronbach's α coefficient of 0.86. The ODI correlated at –0.79 with the Back Pain

Functional Scale and at 0.81 with the PDI, supporting its validity (Koc et al. 2018; Soer et al. 2015). It is sensitive to change, with an ICC of 0.83 (Gronblad et al. 1993). These features, combined with its brevity, make it a useable assessment of lifestyle effects for patients with low back pain. It has been described as the 'gold standard' measurement tool for measuring pain interference in patients with low back pain (British Pain Society 2019) and has been translated into several languages other than English, including Polish (Miekisiak et al. 2013).

The Pain Disability Index (PDI)

The PDI (Tait et al. 1987, 1990) is a self-report measure that asks patients to rate how much the pain interferes with seven areas of functioning. It measures voluntary activities (work, social) and obligatory activities (self-care). Each item is scored on an 11-point scale where 0 = no interference and 10 = total interference. A total score is calculated by summing the scores for each item, with a possible total score between 0 and 70. The PDI is a reliable tool, with a high internal consistency, with Cronbach's α values of 0.86 (Tait et al. 1990) and 0.87 (Strong et al. 1994). Factor loadings ranged from 0.56 to 0.91 in the Tait et al.'s study (1990), to 0.51 to 0.78 in the Strong's study (1992). In terms of validity, higher scores (signifying greater disability) on the PDI were significantly associated with greater depression, less feelings of control over the pain and a greater desire for support (Strong 1992). Gronblad et al. (1993) found a correlation of 0.81 between the PDI and the ODI, supporting the construct validity of the PDI. Good test–retest reliability (when tested over a 1-week interval) was good, with an ICC of 0.91 (Gronblad et al. 1994).

The PDI can be used with all types of pain and is quick to administer. The PDI has been translated into several languages other than English, including Dutch (Soer et al. 2015). Reference values for the PDI have been provided, drawn from 6997 patients from Canada and the Netherlands (Soer et al. 2015). The average baseline PDI score for these patients was 37.7 (SD = 14.2).

The Roland Morris Disability Questionnaire (RMDQ)

The RMDQ is a 24-item self-report questionnaire for use with patients with back pain (Roland & Morris 1983). Each item is a sentence that describes a different movement or function about physical activity, rest, psychosocial aspects, household management, eating and the frequency of the pain (Koc et al. 2018). Patients are asked to endorse items that apply to them. A total score out of 24 is obtained, where 0 = no disability and 24 = total disability (Roland & Fairbank 2000). The British Pain Society (2019) reports the RMDQ to have good internal consistency, with a Cronbach's α values between 0.83 and 0.95, and good test–retest reliability, with ICCs between 0.83 and 0.93. Koc et al. (2018) found a correlation between the RMDQ and the Back Pain Functional Scale of r = −0.693.

The Overactivity in Persistent Pain Assessment (OPPA)

The OPPA is a new seven-item multifaceted self-report tool that assesses average pain intensity, overactivity and subsequent pain, frequency with which the patient aggravates their pain by doing too much, the pain levels after such aggravation, recovery times and behaviours the patient engages in after such occasions of overactivity (Andrews et al. 2021). A Cronbach's α value of 0.78 supports acceptable internal consistency of the measure, and good test–retest reliability with an ICC of 0.83 (Andrews et al. 2021). The validity of the OPPA was supported by good construct validity, with significant Spearman's correlations between the OPPA and Pain and Activities Relations Questionnaire (McCracken & Samuel 2007) and the Depression Anxiety Stress Scales 21 (Lovibond & Lovibond 1995), and good structural validity, with a factor analysis supporting one factor, labelled overactivity severity (Andrews et al. 2021). See Fig. 8.2 for the OPPA.

Observed tests

The impact of pain on a person's functioning can also be assessed by measuring the patient's ability to perform actual tasks that are the same as or related to everyday life tasks. These tasks may be compound measures of pain, breathing, leg strength and other factors. Abdel-Moty et al. (1996) observed that both patients with chronic low back pain and healthy volunteers, when asked to self-predict their ability to stair-climb and squat and then do these activities, showed significant underreporting of their physical abilities. They recommended the use of both self-report and actual functional performance. Harding et al. (1994) developed a battery of measures for assessing the physical functioning of patients with chronic pain. The 5-minute walking test, 1-minute standing-up test, 1-minute stair-climbing test and endurance for holding the arms horizontal test were found to be reliable, valid and useful (Harding et al. 1994). The length, duration or number of repetitions of these tests can be tailored to the local setting and patient population, as long as they are applied in a standardised manner.

A compound measure of distance and speed is the shuttle walking test, in which a 10-metre distance needs to be walked in gradually shortening times (Singh et al. 1992). The functional reach measure provides an indication of pain, upper body function, balance and breathing (Duncan et al. 1990).

To summarise, several tools for measuring pain interference and a patient's physical functioning are available. The selection will likely be determined by the local setting and patient demographics, in addition to the patients' cognitive abilities and their ability to understand the language spoken.

Measurement of emotional distress and emotional functioning

A person's response to pain is very personal, based on physiology, personality, previous life experiences, family and culture. How someone responds to and is distressed by the pain is often demonstrated by behavioural and psychological reactions or changes, so therapists need to understand features (Flaherty 1996). There is a raft of tools, including the Beck Depression Inventory (BDI) (Beck et al. 1961), the Depression Anxiety Stress Scales (DASS-21) (Lovibond & Lovibond 1995), the Pain Self-Efficacy Questionnaire (PSEQ) (Nicholas 1994) and the Pain Catastrophising Scale (PCS) (Sullivan et al. 1995). It must be remembered, however, that interpretation of results on such measures needs to be carefully considered, as scale items with a somatic focus may be directly impacted by the patient's pain condition. For example, if a patient reports that they are not sleeping and are exhausted every day, this may be due to the pain rather than their mood state.

Beck Depression Inventory (BDI)

The BDI (Beck et al. 1961) is a widely used, self-report measure which can be used to evaluate the level of depression experienced by patients with chronic pain. It consists of 21 items, that are scored on a 0 to 3 scale, where 0 = normal mood and 3 = most depressed mood. A total score out of 63 is therefore obtained, with higher scores indicating higher levels of depression (Beck et al. 1961). It has been considered reliable for both clinical and research use, although many of the psychometric studies have been conducted on the revised BDI-II (British Pain Society 2019). Its use, however, is restricted, and so it is not useful for occupational and physical therapists, although therapists need to understand its value and the information it provides about patients. A score of 18 or higher suggests the patient is depressed (Kerns & Haythornthwaite 1988), so the therapist should be extra vigilant and should communicate with the psychiatrist or psychologist of the treating team, or the general practitioner.

Depression, Anxiety and Stress Scales (DASS)

The original DASS was a 42-item questionnaire (Lovibond & Lovibond 1995). Each item is scored on a four-point

Likert scale (0 = did not apply to me at all to 3 = applied to me very much or most of the time) in the past 7 days. The Cronbach's α coefficients for the subscales are good, with 0.91 for depression, 0.84 for anxiety and 0.90 for stress (Lovibond & Lovibond 1995). The Anxiety scale was highly correlated with the Beck Anxiety Inventory (*r* = 0.81), while the Depression scale was correlated at 0.74 with the BDI (Crawford & Henry 2003), thus supporting the construct validity, although, as Crawford & Henry (2003) observed, much of the development and psychometric work was conducted with a university student sample. The psychometrics of the DASS were then examined using a large community sample of adults in the United Kingdom (Crawford & Henry 2003). Good Cronbach's α values were found for the scales (0.947, 0.897 and 0.933, respectively), while adequate discriminant and convergent validity was found, with correlation coefficients ranging from 0.62 to 0.78 with other scales including the Hospital Anxiety and Depression Scale (Zigmond & Snaith 1983). A three-factor model was also supported by confirmatory factor analysis (Crawford & Henry 2003).

More recently, the DASS has been shortened to a 21-item version, the DASS-21 (Henry & Crawford 2005). Internal consistency of experimental groups for each of the subscales is reported to be good, with α scores of 0.88 for Depression, 0.82 for Anxiety and 0.90 for Stress.

Overactivity in persistent pain assessment (OPPA)

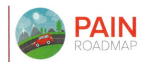

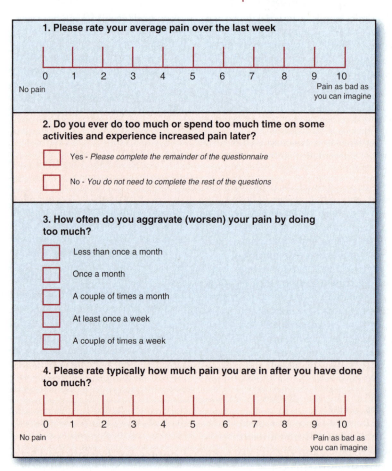

1. Please rate your average pain over the last week

0 1 2 3 4 5 6 7 8 9 10
No pain   Pain as bad as you can imagine

2. Do you ever do too much or spend too much time on some activities and experience increased pain later?

☐ Yes - *Please complete the remainder of the questionnaire*

☐ No - *You do not need to complete the rest of the questions*

3. How often do you aggravate (worsen) your pain by doing too much?

☐ Less than once a month

☐ Once a month

☐ A couple of times a month

☐ At least once a week

☐ A couple of times a week

4. Please rate typically how much pain you are in after you have done too much?

0 1 2 3 4 5 6 7 8 9 10
No pain   Pain as bad as you can imagine

Fig. 8.2 The overactivity in persistent pain assessment (OPPA). (Reprinted with kind permission of Dr. Nicole Andrews, Research Fellow, RECOVER Injury Research Centre, The University of Queensland)

5. What are you normally like after you have done too much?

☐ I find it is a bit more difficult to complete my everyday activities but I am able to push through and do them the same way I normally do

☐ I find it is a lot harder to complete my everyday activities and I need to change the way I do some activities

☐ I can't do all my daily activities but I can do some easy activities or easier parts of the activities

☐ I find it difficult to even do easy activities and need to rest either in an arm chair or in bed

☐ I find it extremely difficult to move and need assistance with basic activities such as going to the toilet and showering

6. How long does it normally take you to recover after you have done too much?

☐ An hour or less

☐ A couple of hours

☐ A day

☐ Two days

☐ Three or more days

7. Please indicate if you ever do any of the following after you have done too much?

☐ Take more of my prescribed pain medication

☐ Use other drugs to cope with my pain including alcohol

☐ Present to the emergency department

Scoring

Frequency	/5
Severity of pain exacerbation	/5
Impact on occupational performance	/5
Recovery time	/5
Maladaptive coping	/5
Total	**/25**

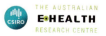

Fig. 8.2, cont'd

Pain Self-Efficacy Questionnaire (PSEQ)

A self-efficacy expectation, combined with an outcome expectation (i.e. the belief that a particular behaviour will result in a certain outcome) may influence a person's avoidance of, or participation in, an activity (Bandura 1977). Self-efficacy beliefs may explain in part the variability between a patient's skill level and their performance outside the treatment setting (Strong 1995). For example, while a patient may have the physical capacity to stand, sit, bend their knees and carry objects while walking, they might not believe they are capable of completing cooking activities. The most frequently used measure of pain self-efficacy is the PSEQ (Nicholas 1994).

The PSEQ is a 10-item Likert questionnaire, designed specifically for chronic pain, where patients are asked to rate their confidence in performing activities despite pain. The scale used is 0 = not at all confident to 6 = completely confident. Total scores range from 0 to 60, with larger scores signalling stronger self-efficacy. It is a valid and reliable tool (Nicholas 1994, 2008). The PSEQ is shown in Fig. 8.3.

Chiarotto et al. (2018b) used confirmatory factor analysis on PSEQ data from 161 patients with neck pain and found one underlying factor that explained 74.4% of the variance, along with significant negative correlations with the PCS (r = −0.538) and the Tampa Scale of Kinesiophobia (TSK) (r = −0.38), providing support for the structural validity and construct validity of the PSEQ.

The average PSEQ scores for the large Australasian patient data set on admission to a pain treatment facility was 20.7 (SD = 13.3), indicating low self-efficacy (Nicholas et al. 2019).

Pain Catastrophising Scale (PCS)

The PCS consists of 13 statements where patients are asked to indicate on a 0 to 4 scale how much this refers to them (Sullivan et al. 1995). The scale anchors are 0 = not at all to 4 = all the time. It has three subscales: rumination (four items), magnification (three items) and helplessness (six items). A total score out of 52 can be calculated, as well as the subscale scores out of 16, 12 and 24, respectively. The greater the score, the greater the catastrophising. While early reports supported the psychometric properties of the PCS, including its internal consistency (Sullivan et al. 1995), more recent studies have questioned the three subscales. For example, de Pielech et al. (2014) found no support for a three-factor structure, using exploratory factor analysis on the PCS-Child version, and the PCS-Parent version, and suggested that the total PCS score be used. Similarly, Akbari et al.'s (2020) study with patients with chronic pain and their partners, while finding Cronbach's α coefficients

of 0.86 for the total score, 0.71 for the rumination subscale, 0.66 for the magnification subscale and 0.78 for the helplessness subscale, supported a two-factor solution rather than a three-factor solution. Finally, patients may find the term *catastrophising* negative and stigmatising. A new measure, developed together with patients and combining catastrophising and self-efficacy, is called the Concerns About Pain Scale (Amtmann et al. 2018). Scores correspond well with the PCS (Amtmann et al. 2020).

The average total PCS scores from the Australasian database on admission for pain management was 29.8 (SD = 13.9) (Nicholas et al. 2019).

Alternative pain impact tools are being developed regularly, and clinicians are advised to keep up to date with emerging literature. They should be guided by pain assessment frameworks developed through consensus meetings, while being attentive to the specific context of their patient population.

Global rating of change (GRC)

GRC scales require the patient to rate how much their condition has changed, either positively or negatively, over a period of time (Kamper et al. 2009). This can be used to either map the clinical condition over time or decide if the treatment being administered is helping the individual. A change of more than 1.35 points on an 11-point GRC may be clinically important (Kamper et al. 2009).

Various authors suggest GRC scales with different scale ranges. For example, the ePPOC uses an overall rating of change on a 0 to 3 scale, where 0 = unchanged and 3 = much better, and a rating of change in physical abilities on a seven-point scale from −3 = very much worse and 3 = very much better (ePPOC clinical reference manual, 2020). Kamper et al. (2009) suggest the use of an 11-point scale, where −5 = very much worse, 0 = unchanged and 5 = completely recovered. The question to be asked in a GRC scale is something like 'With respect to your … [back pain], how would you describe yourself now as compared to before the … [pain education program] commenced' (Kamper et al. 2009). GRC scales have been reported to have excellent test–retest reliability (ICC = 0.90) (Costa et al. 2008) and good construct validity, with significant positive correlations to change scores on the ODI (r = 0.78) and the RMQ (0.50) (Fritz & Irrgang 2001; Stewart et al. 2007).

Quality of life measurement

EuroQoL-5D is a health outcome measure which contains six items (see https://euroqol.org/eq-5d-instruments/). The latest version is the EQ-5D-5L (2021). This simple-to-use self-report tool taps a person's mobility, their ability to look after themselves, do regular activities, the presence of pain or discomfort and feelings of sadness or worry. A

Name: _____   Date: _____

Please rate how **confident** you are that you can do the following things **at present** despite the pain. To indicate your answer circle one of the numbers on the scale under each item, where 0 = not at all confident and 6 = completely confident.
For example:

Not at all confident   0   1   2   (3)   4   5   6   Completely confident

Remember, this questionnaire is not asking whether or not you have been doing these things, but rather how confident you can do them at present, **despite the pain.**

1. I can enjoy things, despite the pain

    Not at all confident   0   1   2   3   4   5   6   Completely confident

2. I can do most of the household chores (e.g. tidying up, washing dishes, etc.) despite the pain.

    Not at all confident   0   1   2   3   4   5   6   Completely confident

3. I can socialize with my friends or family members as often as I used to do, despite the pain.

    Not at all confident   0   1   2   3   4   5   6   Completely confident

4. I can cope with my pain in most situations.

    Not at all confident   0   1   2   3   4   5   6   Completely confident

5. I can do some form of work, despite the pain.
    (Work includes housework, paid and unpaid work.)

    Not at all confident   0   1   2   3   4   5   6   Completely confident

6. I can still do many of the things I enjoy doing, such as hobbies or leisure activity, despite the pain.

    Not at all confident   0   1   2   3   4   5   6   Completely confident

7. I can cope with my pain without medication.

    Not at all confident   0   1   2   3   4   5   6   Completely confident

8. I can still accomplish most of my goals in life, despite the pain.

    Not at all confident   0   1   2   3   4   5   6   Completely confident

9. I can live a normal lifestyle, despite the pain.

    Not at all confident   0   1   2   3   4   5   6   Completely confident

10. I can gradually become more active, despite the pain.

    Not at all confident   0   1   2   3   4   5   6   Completely confident

Fig. 8.3 The pain self-efficacy questionnaire. (Reprinted with kind permission of Professor Michael Nicholas, Director, Pin Education and Pain Management Programs The University of Sydney Pain Management Research Institute Faculty of Medicine and Health.)

sixth item is a global evaluation of the state of the person's health on a 0 to 100 scale, where 0 = worst health and 100 = best health.

Measurement of goals

One important dimension not mentioned in the pain measurement frameworks discussed thus far in this chapter is how to best determine the goals of the individual patient. Oft times, a patient's immediate and only identified goal when they come into the treatment setting is to just take away the pain. Health professionals need to help their patients to identify additional goals they would like to achieve in their lives and work with them to develop strategies to attain them. Goals might be as varied as taking grandchildren to the park for a picnic, returning to a full-time job or being able to look after the garden and plant vegetables.

One well-validated and reliable tool that focuses on goal setting is the Canadian Occupational Performance Measure (COPM) (Law et al. 1990). The COPM uses a semistructured interview, in which the patient is encouraged to identify their performance levels and satisfaction with five areas they identify as goals, across the spectrum of self-care, productivity and leisure activities (Law et al. 1990). The COPM has been translated into several languages other than English, including Danish (Larsen et al. 2021) and Turkish (Torpil et al. 2021). Test–retest reliability has been reported as good, with ICCs between 0.75 and 0.99 (Law et al. 1990; Torpil et al. 2021).

A study examining the construct validity of the COPM Performance Scale found nonsignificant correlations with the PDI of –0.26 and the RAND-36 health survey (–0.01 to 0.250) (Nieuwenhuizen et al. 2014), but this study had a small sample size of 57, introducing potential of a type II error. A recent study (2021) supported the clinical utility of the COPM, while COPM was found to be responsive to change (Raquel et al. 2021).

Case study 8.2 illustrates the range of information that can be available to the clinician prior to their first interaction with the patient, when that patient has provided pre-intervention data on an outcome measurement system like ePPOC.

CASE STUDY 8.2

Mrs Amanda Nguyen (a pseudonym) was a 54-year-old woman who presented to the pain clinic with excruciating pain in her lower back, with the pain radiating down the back of her left leg to her calf.

Mrs Nguyen lived with Fred, her partner of 28 years. Fred was a successful businessman, running their own furniture importation business. They had one son, Leo, who was aged 24. Two years ago, Leo had finished his university degree and moved to another city to take up work. Amanda had helped in the family business with book-keeping and stock inventory responsibilities since Leo had started school. However, for the past 18 months, Amanda's pain had escalated, to the point where she was unable to assist in the workplace. She now stayed at home, tried to rest and seemed to have lost interest in her former activities.

She reported that the pain had come on gradually, with no obvious attributing cause, about 18 months ago. She had been referred to the pain clinic by her general practitioner (GP) 9 months ago. The pain clinic had a long wait list. Her GP had initially prescribed rest and simple analgesics. When these did not alleviate her pain, the GP ordered X-rays, which revealed nothing 'sinister', just some minor degenerative changes to be expected in a 54-year-old person. The GP had referred her to physiotherapy, but Amanda said it had aggravated her pain when she last went to see a physiotherapist, and she refused to go back. Her GP then suggested a referral to a psychologist and an occupational therapist as part of the Australian Department of Health Chronic Disease Management—GP Services package. Amanda was not interested in this option. As she said to her GP, she needed to see a pain specialist who could 'fix her'.

On presentation to the pain clinic, Amanda appeared uncomfortable and quite teary. In the waiting room, she exhibited several pain behaviours, including grimacing and verbal utterances when she moved position in her seat. In the interview room, Amanda explained that the pain started like a pulling and aching pain, and then it got worse with constant aching and shooting and burning pain down the back of her leg. Amanda said the pain was always present during the day and the night, but sometimes it was worse. She found it hard to get to sleep and always woke early, long before the birds started chirping to herald in the dawn.

She was taking Targin 5 mg/2.5 mg twice a day and 50 mg Panadol 4 hourly. She said the medications made no difference to her pain, but she did not want to stop taking the medications in case things 'got even worse'.

Amanda described her pain as being 11 out of 10, it was 'that bad'. She said the pain had ruined everything in her life. She said she felt overwhelmed with the pain and could not do things she used to do, like working in the family business and going to her monthly book club meetings. She couldn't concentrate to read the book, let alone drive

CASE STUDY 8.2—Cont'd

to the meeting and sit for a few hours. She reported that she was not sleeping well, mostly snatching only 3 hours of sleep each night. She said she would wake up irritable and exhausted and was despondent.

She said that Fred was getting angry with her, telling her that she needed to do more to help around the home, even if she wasn't well enough to do her work in the office. While she understood that her inability to do the office work had put added financial pressure on the business and on Fred, she said she felt he was abandoning her. She said since Leo had moved interstate, she had no one to support her.

If you were the intake therapist when Amanda attended her first outpatient appointment, what assessments would you use with Amanda to obtain a clearer picture of her pain problem and of her experience and goals?

As Amanda lives in Australia, she was asked to complete the ePPOC prior to her attendance at the pain clinic.

You therefore start by going to the ePOCC portal to review Amanda's preadmission results. You find the following scores:

Brief Pain Inventory Interference Scale—average score: 7.4—severe
Depression and Anxiety Scale—Depression: 26—severe
Depression and Anxiety Scale—Anxiety: 21—severe
Depression and Anxiety Scale—Stress: 25—moderate
Pain Self-Efficacy Questionnaire: 18—severe
Pain Catastrophising Scale: 41—severe

You realise that Amanda is in a high level of distress. You know that Amanda will be seen next by the pain physician, so you will alert her to your concerns about the patient's level of distress. You then devote the first part of your intake appointment encouraging Amanda to tell her story. You want to gain her trust before you launch into your discipline-specific assessment battery. You also plan to carefully observe Amanda's verbal and nonverbal behaviours during your interview session. Please refer to the chapters on communication (Chapter 3), psychological interventions (Chapter 12) and self-management (Chapter 10).

Conclusion

Health professionals need to be considerate and thorough in the assessment and measurement of a patient's pain, which are the cornerstones of good pain management. The selection of appropriate pain measurement tools can be guided by the relevant national pain consensus frameworks, as relevant to the individual patient. However, therapists must not be constrained by such frameworks and choose measures which are appropriate to their patients. The therapist needs to remember that there is some time to establish a collaborative relationship by getting to know the person and their individual situation, to allow for the patient to expand on formal assessment items and to elaborate on their responses, to actively listen to the patient, and to understand the implications of the pain on the patient's life.

Therapists should choose measures which have acceptable validity and reliability and are manageable in the clinical setting. Therapists need to be attentive to their patients, listen to their words, observe their behaviours and abilities, and integrate the information into their clinical decision making. Careful and thorough assessment of a patient's pain is both an art and a science. It provides the foundation for successful pain management.

Resources for health professionals

British Pain Society https://www.britishpainsociety.org/
ePPOC https://www.uow.edu.au/ahsri/eppoc/
Euroquol—EQ5D https://euroqol.org/eq-5d-instruments/how-can-eq-5d-be-used/
IMMPACT http://www.immpact.org/
NSW Government Agency for Clinical Innovation https://aci.health.nsw.gov.au/networks/pain-management/resources
Pain Australia https://www.painaustralia.org.au/

Review questions

1. What dimensions of the patient's pain problem should be measured by the health professional?
2. Name one measurement tool of pain quality and describe how this data can be helpful for clinicians.
3. Identify three reasons why therapists need to obtain self-report data on a patient's pain.
4. What is a reliable measure of a patient's pain intensity?
5. How might you measure the functional implications of a patient's pain, and the impact it has on an individual's life?

References

Abbey, J., deBellis, A., Piller, N., Esterman, A., Giles, L., Parker, D., et al., 2004. The Abbey Pain Scale: a 1-minute numerical indicator for people with end-stage dementia. Int. J. Palliat. Nurs. 10, 6–13.

Abdel-Moty, A.R., Maguire, G.W., Kaplan, S.H., Johnson, P., 1996. Stated versus observed performance levels in patients with chronic low back pain. Occup. Ther. Health Care 10 (1), 3–23.

Ahlers, S.J.G.M., van Gulik, L., van der Veen, A.M., van Dongen, H.P.A., Bruins, P., Belitser, S.V., et al., 2008. Comparison of different pain scoring systems in critically ill patients in a general ICU. Crit. Care 12, R15.

Akbari, F., Dehghani, M., Mohammadi, S., 2020. Factor structure and invariance of the pain catastrophising scale in patients with chronic pain and their spouses. Psychol. 66, 50–56.

Amtmann, D., Liljenquist, K., Bamer, A., Bocell, F., Jensen, M., Wilson, R., et al., 2018. Measuring pain catastrophizing and pain-related self-efficacy: expert panels, focus groups, and cognitive interviews. Patient 11, 107–117.

Amtmann, D., Bamer, A., Liljenquist, K., Cowan, P., Salem, R., Turk, D., et al., 2020. The Concerns about Pain (CAP) Scale: a patient-reported outcome measure of pain catastrophizing. J. Pain 21, 1198–1211.

Andrews, N.J., Chien, C.-W., Ireland, D., Varnfield, M., 2021. Overactivity assessment in chronic pain: the development and psychometric evaluation of a multi-faceted self-report assessment. Eur. J. Pain 25, 225–242. https://doi.org/10.1002/ejp.1664.

Australian Health Services Research Institute, 2020. ePPOC Clinical Reference Manual Australian Version 2 Dataset. University of Woolloongong. https://documents.uow.edu.au/content/groups/public/@web/@chsd/documents/doc/uow263481.pdf.

Bagraith, K.S., Strong, J., Meredith, P.J., McPhail, S.M., 2018. What do clinicians consider when assessing chronic low back pain? A content analysis of multidisciplinary pain centre team assessments of functioning, disability, and health. Pain 159, 2128–2136. https://doi.org/10.1097/j.pain.0000000000001285.

Bandura, A., 1977. Self-efficacy: toward a unifying theory of behavioral change. Psychol. Rev. 84, 191–215. https://doi-org.ezproxy.library.uq.edu.au/10.1037/0033-295X.84.2.191.

Beck, A.T., Ward, C.H., Mendelson, M., et al., 1961. An inventory for measuring depression. Arch. Gen. Psychiatr. 4, 561–571. https://doi.org/10.1001/archpsyc.1961.02710120031004.

Beecher, H.K., 1959. Measurement of Subjective Responses. Oxford University Press, New York.

Bergstrom, G., Jensen, B.I., Bodin, L., Linton, J.S., Nygren, L.A., Carlsson, G.S., 1998. Reliability and factor structure of the multidisciplinary pain inventory – Swedish language version (MPI-S). Pain 75, 101–110.

Berde, C., McGrath, P., 2009. Pain measurement and Beecher's challenge: 50 years later. Anesthesiology 111, 473–474.

Boureau, F., Luu, M., Doubrere, J.F., 1992. Comparative study of the validity of four French McGill Pain Questionnaire (MPQ) versions. Pain 50, 59–65. https://doi.org/10.1097/AJP.0000000000000406.

British Pain Society & Faculty of Pain Medicine (January 2019). Outcome Measure. https://www.britishpainsociety.org/static/uploads/resources/files/Outcome_Measures_January_2019.pdf.

Castarlenas, E., Jensen, M., von Baeyer, C., Miro, J., 2017. Psychometric properties of the Numerical Rating Scale to assess self-reported pain intensity in children and adolescents: a systematic review. Clin. J. Pain 33, 376–383.

Cetin, A.A., Bektas, H., Ozdogan, M., 2016. The west haven yale multidimensional pain inventory: reliability and validity of the Turkish version in individuals with cancer. Eur. J. Oncol. 20, 1–9. https://doi.org/10.1016/j.ejon.2015.2015.03.007.

Chiarotto, A., Boers, M., Deyo, R.A., Buchbinder, R., Corbin, T.P., Costa, L.O.P., et al., 2018a. Core outcome measurement instruments for clinical trials in non-specific low back pain. Pain 159, 481–495. https://doi.org/10.1097/j.pain.0000000000001117.

Chiarotto, A., Falla, D., Polli, A., Monticone, M., 2018b. Validity and responsiveness of the Pain Self-Efficacy Questionnaire in patients with neck pain disorders. J. Orthopaed. Sport. Phy. Med. 48 (3), 204–216. https://www.jospt.org/doi/10.2519/jospt.2018.7605.

Chien, C.-W., Bagraith, K.S., Khan, A., Deen, M., Syu, J.-J., Strong, J., 2017. Establishment of cutpoints to categorize the severity of chronic pain using composite ratings with Rasch analysis. Eur. J. Pain 21, 82–91. https://doi.org/10.1002/ejp.906.

Choi, Y.H., Mayer, T.G., Williams, M., Gatchel, R.J., 2013. The clinical utility of the Multidimensional Pain Inventory (MPI) in characterizing chronic disabling occupational musculoskeletal disorders. J. Occup. Rehabil. 23, 239–247. https://doi.org/10.1007/s10926-012-9393-x.

Cieza, A., Ewert, T., Ustun, B., Chatterji, S., Kostanjsek, N., Stucki, G., 2004. Development of ICF core sets for patients with chronic conditions. J. Rehabil. Med. 44 (Suppl. l), 9–11. https://doi.org/10.1080/16501960410015353.

Cleeland, R.C., Ryan, K., 1994. Pain assessment: global use of the brief pain inventory. Annal. Acad. Med. 23, 129–138.

Childs, J.D., Piva, S.R., Fritz, J.M., 2005. Responsiveness of the Numeric Rating Scale in patients with low back pain. Spine 30, 1331–1334.

Costa, L.O.P., Maher, C.G., Latimer, J., Ferreira, P.H., Ferreira, M.L., Pozi, G.C., et al., 2008. Clinimetric testing of three self-report outcome measures for low back pain patients in Brazil: which one is best? Spine 33, 2459–2463. https://doi.org/10.1097/BSR.0b013e3181849dbe.

Crawford, J.R., Henry, J.D., 2003. The Depression Anxiety Stress Scales (DASS): normative data and latent structure in a large non-clinical sample. Br. J. Clin. Psychol. 42, 111–131. https://doi.org/10.1348/014466503321903544.

Daker-White, G., Donovan, J., Campbell, R., 2014. Redefined by illness: meta-ethnography of qualitative studies on the experience of rheumatoid arthritis. Disabil. Rehabil. 36, 1061–1071. https://doi.org/10.3109/09638288.2013.829531.

de Pielech, M., Ryan, M., Logan, D., Kaczynski, K., White, M.T., Simons, L.E., 2014. Pain catastrophizing in children with chronic pain and their parents: proposed clinical reference points and re-examination of the PCS measure. Pain 155, 2360–2367. https://doi.org/10.1016/j.pain.2014.08.035.

De Williams, A.C., Davies, H.T.O., Chadury, Y., 2000. Simple pain rating scales hide complex idiosyncratic meanings. Pain 85, 457–463. https://doi.org/10.1016/s0304-3959(99)00299-7.

Deyo, R.A., Battie, M., Beurskens, A.J., Bombardier, C., Croft, P., Koes, B., et al., 1998. Outcome measures for low back pain research: a proposal for standardized use. Spine 23 (18), 2003–2013.

Duncan, P., Weiner, D., Chandler, J., Studenski, S., 1990. Functional reach: a new clinical measure of balance. J. Gerontol. 45, 192–197.

Dworkin, R., Turk, D., Farrar, J., Haythornthwaite, J.A., Jensen, M.P., Katz, N.P., et al., 2005. Core outcomes for chronic pain clinical trials: IMMPACT recommendations. Pain 113, 9–19. https://doi.org/10.1016/j.pain.2004.09.012.

Dworkin, R.H., Turk, D.C., Revick, D.A., Harding, G., Coyne, K.S., Peirce-Sander, S., et al., 2009. Development and initial validation of an expanded and revised version of the Short-form McGill Pain Questionnaire (SF-MPQ-2). Pain 144, 35–42. https://doi.org/10.1016/j.pain.2009.02.007.

Ferraz, M.B., Quaresma, M.R., Aquino, L.R., Atra, E., Tugwell, P., Goldsmith, C.H., 1990. Reliability of pain scales in the assessment of literate and illiterate patients with rheumatoid arthritis. J. Rheumat 17, 1022–1024.

Fairbank, J.C., Pynsent, P.B., 2000. The Oswestry disability Index. Spine 25, 2940–2953.

Fairbank, J.C.T., Couper, J., Davies, J.B., et al., 1980. The Oswestry low back disability questionnaire. Physiotherapy 66, 271–273.

Flaherty, S.A., 1996. Pain measurement tools for clinical practice and research. J. Am. Assoc. Nurse. Anesth. 64, 133–140.

Fritz, J.M., Irrgang, J.J., 2001. A comparison of a modified Oswestry low back pain disability questionnaire and the Quebec back pain disability scale. Phys. Ther. 81, 776–788. https://doi.org/10.1093/ptj/81.2.776.

Gagliese, L., Melzack, R., 1997. Chronic pain in elderly people. Pain 70, 3–14. https://doi.org/10.1016/s0304-3959(96)03266-6.

Gélinas, C., Fillion, L., Puntillo, K.A., 2009. Item selection and content validity of the Critical-Care Pain Observation Tool for non-verbal adults. J. Adv. Nurs. 65, 203–216. https://doi.org/10.1111/j.1365-2648.2008.04847.x.

Goucke, C.R. (Ed.), 2019. Pain in Residential Aged Care Facilities: Management Strategies, second ed. Australian Pain Society, Sydney.

Gronblad, M., Hupli, M., Wennerstrand, P., Jarvinen, E., Lukinmaa, A., Kouri, J.-P., et al., 1993. Intel-correlation and test-retest reliability of the Pain Disability Index (PDI) and the Oswestry Disability Questionnaire (ODQ) and their correlation with pain intensity in low back pain patients. Clin. J. Pain 9 (3), 189–195.

Gronblad, M., Jarvinen, E., Hurri, H., Hupli, M., Karaharju, E., 1994. Relationship of the Pain Disability Index (PDI) and the Oswestry Disability Questionnaire (ODQ) with three dynamic physical tests in a group of patients with chronic low-back and leg pain. Clin. J. Pain 10 (3), 197–203.

Harding, V.R., de Williams, A.C., Richardson, P.H., Nicholas, M.K., Jackson, J.L., Richardson, I.H., et al., 1994. The development of a battery of measures for assessing physical functioning of chronic pain patients. Pain 58, 367–375. https://doi.org/10.1016/0304-3959(94)90131-7.

Hasegawa, M., Hattori, S., Mishima, M., Matsaumoto, I., Kimura, T., Baba, Y., et al., 2001. The MPQ Japanese version, reconsidered: confirming the theoretical structure. Pain. Res. Manag. 6, 173–180. https://doi.org/10.1155/2001/718236.

Hayden, J.S.A., van Tulder, M.V., Malmivaara, A.V., Koes, B.W., 2005. Meta-analysis: exercise therapy for nonspecific low back pain. Ann. Intern. Med. 142, 765–775. https://doi.org/10.7326/0003-4819-142-9-200505030-00013.

Henry, J.D., Crawford, J.R., 2005. The short-form version of the Depression Anxiety Stress Scales (DASS-21); construct validity and normative data in a large, non-clinical sample. Br. J. Clin. Psychol. 44, 227–239. https://doi.org/10.1348/014466505X29657.

Jamison, R.N., 1996. Psychological factors in chronic pain: assessment and treatment issues. J. Back. Musculoskelet. Rehabil. 7, 79–95.

Jensen, M.P., Karoly, P., Braver, S., 1986. The measurement of clinical pain intensity: a comparison of six methods. Pain 27, 117–126. https://doi.org/10.1016/0304-3959(86)90228-9.

Jensen, M., Karoly, P., O'Riordan, E., Bland, F., Burns, R., 1989. The subjective experience of acute pain. An assessment of the utility of 10 indices. Clin. J. Pain 5 (2), 153–160.

Jensen, M.P., Johnson, L.E., Gertz, K.J., Galer, B.L., Gammaitoni, A.R., 2013. The words patients use to describe chronic pain: implications for measuring pain quality. Pain 154, 2722–2728. https://doi.org/10.1016/j.pain.2013.08.003.

Jerome, A., Holroyd, K.A., Theofanous, A.G., Pingel, J.D., Lake, A.E., Saper, J.R., 1988. Cluster headache pain vs other vascular headache pain: differences revealed with two approaches to the McGill Pain Questionnaire. Pain 34, 35–42. https://doi.org/10.1016/0304-3959(88)90179-0.

Jumbo, S.U., MacDermid, J.C., Kalu, M.E., Packham, T.L., Athwal, G.S., Faber, K.J., 2021. Measurement properties of the brief Pain Inventory- Short Form (BPI-SF), and the revised short McGill Pain Questionnaire Version-2 (SF-MPQ-2) in pain-related musculoskeletal conditions. A systematic review. Clin. J. Pain 37, 454–474. https://doi.org/10.1097/AJP.0000000000000933.

Kamper, S.J., Maher, C.G., Mackay, G., 2009. Global Rating of Change Scales: a review of strengths and weaknesses and considerations for design. J. Man. Manip. Ther. 17, 163–170. https://doi.org/10.1179/jmt.2009.17.3.163.

Keller, S., Bann, C., Dodd, S., Schein, J., Mendoza, T., Cleeland, C.S., 2004. Validity of the Brief Pain Inventory for use in documenting the outcomes of patients with noncancer pain. Clin. J. Pain 20 (5), 309–318.

Kerns, R.D., Haythornthwaite, J., 1988. Depression among chronic pain patients: cognitive-behavioral analysis and effect on rehabilitation outcome. J. Consult. Clin. Psychol. 56 (6), 870–876. https://doi.org/10.1037/0022-006X.56.6.870.

Kerns, R.D., Turk, D.C., Rudy, T.E., 1985. The West Haven-Yale Multidimensional Pain Inventory (WHYMPI). Pain 23, 145–156. https://doi.org/10.1016/0304-3959(85)90004-1.

Koc, M., Bayer, B., Bayer, K., 2018. A comparison of back pain functional scale with roland morris disability questionnaire, oswestry disability index, and short-form 36-health survey. Spine 43, 877–882. https://doi.org/10.1097/BRS.0000000000002431.

Larsen, E.A., Winge, C.J., Christensen, J.R., 2021. Clinical utility of the Danish version of the Canadian occupational performance measure. Scand. J. Occup. Ther. 28, 239–250. https://doi.org/10.1080/11038128.2019.1634130.

Law, M., Baptiste, S., McColl, M., Opzoomer, A., Polatajko, H., Pollock, N., 1990. The Canadian Occupational Therapy Performance Measure: an outcome measure for occupational therapy. Can. J. Occup. Ther. 57, 82–87. https://doi.org/10.1177/000841749005700201.

Lovibond, S.H., Lovibond, P.F., 1995. Manual for the Depression Anxiety Stress Scales. Psychology Foundation, Sydney.

Lowe, N.K., Walker, S.N., MacCallum, R.C., 1991. Confirming the theoretical structure of the McGill Pain Questionnaire in acute clinical pain. Pain 46, 57–62. https://doi.org/10.1016/0304-3959(91)90033-T.

Machata, A.M., Kabon, B., Willschke, H., et al., 2009. A new instrument for pain assessment in the immediate post-operative period. Anaesthesia 64, 392–398. https://doi.org/10.1111/j.1365-2044.2008.05798.x.

Margolis, R.B., Tait, R.C., Krause, S.J., 1986. A rating system for use with patient pain drawings. Pain 24, 57–65. https://doi.org/10.1016/0304-3959(86)90026-6.

Margolis, R.B., Chibnall, J.T., Tait, R.C., 1988. Test–retest reliability of the pain drawing instrument. Pain 33, 49–51. https://doi.org/10.1016/0304-3959(88)90202-3.

McAllister, M.J., 2019. The Passing of Ron Melzack, PhD. "The Father of Pain Management". Institute for Chronic Pain. https://www.instituteforchronicpain.org/blog/item/218-the-passing-of-ron-malzack-phd.

McKillop, J.M., Nielson, W.R., 2011. Improving the usefulness of the Multidimensional pain inventory. Pain Res. Manag. 16, 239–244. https://doi.org/10.1155/2011/873424.

McCreacken, L.M., Samuel, V.M., 2007. The role of avoidance, pacing, and other activity patterns in chronic pain. Pain 130, 119–125.

McCracken, L.M. & Samuel, V.M. (2007). The role of avoidance, pacing, and other activity patterns in chronic pain. Pain, 130 (1-2), 119–125.

Miekisiak, G., Kollataj, M., Dobrogowski, J., Kloc, W., Libionka, W., Banach, M., et al., 2013. Validation and cross-cultural adaptation of the Polish version of the Oswestry Disability Index. Spine 34, E237–E243.

Melzack, R., 1975. The McGill Pain Questionnaire: major properties and scoring methods. Pain 1, 277–299. https://doi.org/10.1016/0304-3959(75)90044-5.

Melzack, R., 1987. The short-form McGill pain questionnaire. Pain 30 (2), 191–197. https://doi.org/10.1016/0304-3959(87)91074-8.

Melzack, R., Katz, J., 1994. Pain measurement in persons in pain. In: Wall, P.D., Melzack, R. (Eds.), Textbook of Pain, third ed. Churchill Livingstone, New York, pp. 337–351.

Melzack, R., Katz, J., 2002. The problem of pain; measurement in clinical settings. In: Burchiel, K.J. (Ed.), Surgical Management of Pain. Thieme Medical Publishers, New York, pp. 78–96.

Melzack, R., Torgerson, W.S., 1971. On the language of pain. Anesthesiology 34 (1), 50–59.

Morley, S., Williams, A., Eccleston, C., 2013. Examining the evidence about psychological treatments for chronic pain: time for a paradigm shift? Pain 154, 1929–1931. https://doi.org/10.1016/j.pain.2013.05.049.

Nicholas, M., 1994. Pain Self-Efficacy Questionnaire (PSEQ): Preliminary Report. Unpublished Paper. University of Sydney Pain Management and Research Centre, St Leonards.

Nicholas, M.K., Asghari, A., Blyth, F.M., 2008. What do the numbers mean? Normative data in chronic pain measures. Pain 134, 158–173. https://doi.org/10.1016/j.pain.2007.04.007.

Nicholas, M.K., Costa, D.S.J., Blanchard, M., Tardif, H., Asghari, A., Blyth, F., 2019. Normative data for common pain measures in chronic pain clinic populations: closing a gap for clinicians and researchers. Pain 160, 1156–1165. https://doi.org/10.1097/j.pain.0000000000001496.

Nieuwenhuizen, M.G., deGroot, S., Janssen, T.W.J., van der Maas, L.C.C., Becjerman, H., 2014. Canadian occupational performance measure performance scale: validity and responsiveness in chronic pain. JRRD (J. Rehabil. Res. Dev.) 51, 727–746. https://doi.org/10.16821/JRRD.2012.12.0221.

Patrick, L., D'Eon, J., 1996. Social support and functional status in chronic pain patients. Can. J. Rehabil. 9, 195–201.

Peters, M.L., Patijn, J., Lamé, I., 2007. Pain assessment in younger and older pain patients: psychometric properties and patient preference of five commonly used measures of pain intensity. Pain. Med. 8, 601–610. https://doi-org.ezproxy.library.uq.edu.au/10.1111/j.1526-4637.2007.00311.x.

Price, D., 1999. The dimensions of pain experience. In: Price, D. (Ed.), Psychological Mechanisms of Pain and Analgesia. IASP Press, Seattle.

Radbruch, L., Loick, G., Kiencke, P., Lindena, G., Sabatowski, R., Grond, S., et al., 1999. Validation of the German version of the brief pain inventory. J. Pain. Symptom. Manag. 18, 180–187. https://doi.org/10.1016/s0885-3924(99)00064-0.

Ransford, A., Cairns, D., Mooney, V., 1976. The pain drawing as an aid to the psychologic evaluation of patients with low-back pain. Spine 1 (2), 127–134.

Raquel, C.-T., Villafane, J.H., Medina-Porqueres, I., Garcia-Orza, S., Valdes, K., 2021. Convergent validity and responsiveness of the COPM for the evaluation of therapeutic outcomes for patients with carpometacarpal osteoarthritis. J. Hand. Ther. 34, 1439–1445. https://doi.org/10.1016/j.ht.2020.03.011.

Roland, M., Fairbank, J., 2000. The roland-morris disability questionnaire and the oswestry disability questionnaire. Spine 25, 3115–3124.

Roland, M., Morris, R., 1983. A study of the natural history of back pain: part I: development of a reliable and sensitive measure of disability in low-back pain. Spine 8 (2), 141–144.

Rolke, R., Magerl, W., Campbell, K., Schalber, C., Caspari, S., Birklein, F., et al., 2006. Quantitative sensory testing: a comprehensive protocol for clinical trials. Eur. J. Pain 10, 77–88.

Segerdahl, M., 2011. Commentary pain outcome variables – a never ending story? Pain 152, 961–962. https://doi.org/10.1016/j.pain.2011.03.008.

Seroussi, R., 2015. Chronic pain assessment. Phys. Med. Rehabil. Clin. 26, 185–199. https://doi.org/10.1016/j.pmr.2014.12.009.

Singh, S., Morgan, M., Scott, S., Walters, D., Hardman, A., 1992. Development of a shuttle walking test of disability in patients with chronic airways obstruction. Thorax 47, 1019–1024.

Stein, C., Mendl, G., 1988. The German counterpart to McGill pain questionnaire. Pain vol, 251–255. https://doi.org/10.1016/0304-3959(88)90074-7.

Stewart, M., Maher, C., Refshauge, K., Bogduk, N., Nicholas, M., 2007. Responsiveness of pain and disability measures for chronic whiplash. Spine 32, 580–585. https://doi.org/10.1097/01.brs.0000256380.71056.6d.

Strand, L.I., Ljunggren, A.E., 1997. Different approximations of the McGill Pain Questionnaire in the Norwegian language: a discussion of content validity. J. Adv. Nurs. 26, 772–779. https://doi-org.ezproxy.library.uq.edu.au/10.1046/j.1365-2648.1997.00383.x.

Strong, J., 1992. Chronic low back pain: towards an integrated psychosocial assessment model. Doctoral dissertation, The University of Queensland, The University of Queensland Research Repository. http.

Strong, J., 1995. Self-efficacy and the patient with chronic pain. In: Schacklock, M. (Ed.), Moving in on Pain. Butterworth-Heinemann, Melbourne.

Strong, J., Ashton, R., Chant, D., 1991. Pain intensity measurement in chronic low back pain. Clin. J. Pain 7 (3), 209–218.

Strong, J., Ashton, R., Stewart, A., 1994. Chronic low back pain: toward an integrated psychosocial assessment model. J. Consult. Clin. Psychol. 62, 1058–1063. https://doi.org/10.1037/0022-006X.62.5.1064.

Strong, J., Sturgess, J., Unruh, A.M., Vicenzino, B., 2002. Pain assessment and measurement. In: Strong, J., Unruh, A.M., Wright, A., Baxter, G.D.P. (Eds.), A Textbook for Therapists. Churchill Livingstone, Edinburgh, pp. 123–147.

Soer, R., Koke, A.J.A., Speijer, B.L.G.N., Vroomen, P.C.A.K., Smeets, R.J.E.M., Coppes, M.H., et al., 2015. Reference values of the Pain Disability Index in patients with painful musculoskeletal spinal disorders. Spine 40, E545–E551.

Sullivan, M.J.L., Bishop, S.R., Pivik, J., 1995. The pain catastrophizing scale: development and validation. Psychol. Assess. 7, 524–532. https://doi.org/10.1037/1040-3590.7.4.524.

Swift, A., Heale, R., Twycross, A., 2020. What are sensitivity and specificity? Evid. Base. Nurs. 23, 2–4. https://doi.org/10.1136/ebnurs-2019-103225.

Tait, R.C., Pollard, A., Margolis, R.B., Duckro, P.N., Krause, S.J., 1987. The Pain Disability Index: psychometric and validity data. Arch. Phys. Med. Rehabil. 68, 438–441.

Tait, R.C., Chibnall, J.T., Krause, S., 1990. The pain disability Index: psychometric properties. Pain 40 (2), 171–182. https://doi.org/10.1016/0304-3959(90)90068-O.

Tan, G., Jensen, M.P., Thornby, J.I., Shanti, B.F., 2004. Validation of the brief Pain Inventory for chronic non-malignant pain. J. Pain 5, 133–137. https://doi.org/10.1016/j.pain.2003.12.005.

Tardif, H., Blanchard, M., Fenwick, N., Blissett, C., Eager, K., 2015. Electronic Persistent Pain Outcomes Collaboration National Report, 2014. Australian Health Services Institute Research Institute, Wollongong. https://doi.org/10.1093/pm/pnw201.

Torpil, B., Caglar, G.E., Bumin, G., Pkcetin, 2021. Validity and reliability of the Canadian Occupational Performance Measure (COPM-TR) for people with multiple sclerosis. Occup. Ther. Health. Care 35, 306–317. https://doi.org/10.1080/07380577.2021.1933673.

Turk, D.C., Okifuji, A., 1999. Assessment of patients' reporting of pain: an integrated perspective. Lancet 353 (9166), 1784–1788. https://doi.org/10.1016/s01406736(99)10309-4.

Turk, D.C., Rudy, T.E., 1988. Toward an empirically derived taxonomy of chronic pain patients: integration of psychological assessment data. J. Consult. Clin. Psychol. 56, 233–238. https://doi.org/10.1037/0022-006X.56.2.233.

Turk, D.C., Dworkin, R.H., Allen, R.R., Bellamy, N., Brandenburg, N., Carr, D.B., et al., 2003. Core outcome domains for chronic pain clinical trials: IMMPACT recommendations. Pain 106, 337–345. https://doi.org/10.1016/j.pain.2003.08.001.

Turk, D., Dworkin, R., Revicki, D., Harding, G., Burke, L.B., Cella, D., et al., 2008. Identifying important outcome domains for chronic pain clinical trials: an IMMPACT survey of people with pain. Pain 137 (2), 276–285. https://doi.org/10.1016/j.pain.2007.09.002.

Van Griensven, H., 2016. Patients' experiences of living with persistent back pain. Int. J. Osteopath. Med. 19, 44–49.

Williams, R.C., 1988. Towards a set of reliable and valid measures for chronic pain assessment and outcome research. Pain 35, 239–251. https://doi.org/10.1016/0304-3959(88)90133-9.

Wittink, H., Turk, D.C., Carr, D.B., Sukiennik, A., Rogers, W., 2004. Comparison of the redundancy, reliability, and responsiveness to change among SF-36, oswestry disability index and multidimensional pain inventory. Clin. J. Pain 20, 133–142.

Zhao, P., Lancey, R., Varghese, E., 2019. Mobile applications for pain management: an app analysis for clinical use. BMC Med. Inf. Decis. Making 19, 106. https://doi.org/10.1186/s12911-019-0827-7.

Zigmond, A.S., Snaith, R.P., 1983. The hospital anxiety and depression scale. Acta. Psychiatrica. Scandinavia 67, 361–370. https://doi.org/10.1111/j.1600-0447.1983.tb09716.x.

Chapter 9

Pain education for patients

Joletta Belton and Joost van Wijchen

Learning objectives

At the end of this chapter, readers will be able to:
1. Recognise the challenges of pain education.
2. Summarise current pain education research.
3. Describe various frames of reference that can be used in relation to pain education.
4. Understand the concept of co-creation of pain education.
5. Compare current ways of delivering pain education to the concept that effective pain education is a dialogue and mutual learning and teaching process.
6. Apply conversational pain education approaches with patients in practice.

Introduction

Pain education for patients has grown in interest and practice in recent years. It seems intuitive that patient education is important. Patients seek care to understand their pain and what can be done about it. But what do we mean by *pain education for patients* and are we doing it well? Can we do it better?

This chapter explores these questions, starting with current trends and research about patient education about pain.

Next, it explores challenges of pain education and what might be missing. Then it suggests how these challenges may be addressed, including a vision for education that is more collaborative and is focused on transformative learning. The chapter finishes with the clinical encounter and discusses strategies to better help patients make sense of their pain and know what to do about it. Throughout the chapter new ways of looking at patient education are brought in, with ideas from philosophy, critical pedagogy, patient engagement and narrative medicine. There are a number of *Reflective Practice* exercises throughout to enable clinicians to engage with the ideas presented. The authors hope this chapter sparks the reader's curiosity and creativity when it comes to teaching and learning and that it will help improve their experience of pain education in the clinical encounter.

This chapter is the start of a conversation about pain education for patients, not a definitive conclusion. The ways in which we teach, educate, learn and apply what we know are always evolving, for patients and clinicians alike.

Current pain education for patients

Pain education may first have started with back schools, where patients were provided information about biomechanics, posture and anatomy as part of a programme that encouraged self-management (Parreira et al. 2017). Back schools began in 1969 (Straube et al. 2016), but despite their longevity, recent systematic reviews and meta-analyses have concluded there is no solid evidence in favour of them (Parreira et al. 2017; Straube et al. 2016). In recent years, there has been a shift away from biomedical and biomechanical explanations for pain, which can inadvertently lead patients to believe their bodies are fragile, vulnerable and in need of protection (Darlow et al. 2013). There has been a shift towards frameworks that involve teaching patients about pain biology. This type of education has many names, including pain neuroscience education, pain neurophysiology education and therapeutic neuroscience education. For ease, we will refer to all of these as *pain science education*. The most well-known approaches to teaching patients about pain science are *Explain Pain* (Butler & Moseley 2015), and *Therapeutic Neuroscience Education: Teaching Patients about Pain* (Louw & Puentedura 2013). These books are based on the premise that pain biology is readily understood by patients and the public and that understanding pain biology can change the experience of pain (Moseley & Butler 2015a).

Current reviews of pain science education for patients

Recent systematic reviews and meta-analyses of pain science education for patients have come to varying conclusions. In general, the evidence is of low-to-moderate quality and trends towards small benefits in the short, medium and long term. Most recent reviews agree that pain science education should not be used as a standalone treatment (Bülow et al. 2021; Marris et al. 2021; Tegner et al. 2018; Wood & Hendrick 2019). A recent review and meta-analysis by Marris et al. (2021; 14 studies, 1024 participants) supports the idea that pain education combined with other treatments delivers more clinically and patient-relevant outcomes (Moseley & Butler, 2015a). When people receive pain education—including pain science education, back school, cognitive behavioural therapy, or training in self-management or coping skills—alongside other physical therapy interventions, they improve significantly more than control groups.

In one of the most favourable reviews, Tegner et al. (2018; 7 studies, 313 participants) found moderate-quality evidence for clinically relevant pain relief just after intervention and at 3-month follow-up when pain science education was used as an intervention in patients with chronic low back pain. The effect on disability just after the intervention and at around 3-month follow-up was also positive, but with lower quality of evidence and smaller effect sizes (Tegner et al. 2018). Reviews by Wood & Hendrik (2019; 8 studies, 615 participants) and Watson et al. (2019; 12 studies, 755 participants) showed lower quality of evidence and smaller effect sizes favouring pain science education for both pain relief and disability in the short and medium terms. Watson et al. (2019) concluded that pain science education does not produce clinically relevant effects on pain or disability ratings. A review by Bülow et al. (2021; 18 studies, 1559 participants) found low-quality evidence in support of pain science education on measures of pain intensity in the short and longer terms (around 1 year after the intervention) and on disability ratings and psychological distress immediately after the intervention.

Patient experiences of pain science education

Pain science education is proposed to provide benefits through pain reconceptualisation (Watson et al. 2019). Reconceptualisation does not happen for all patients, though, and has been described as 'partial and patchy' (King et al. 2016). The relevance of pain science education varied widely across participants, with perceived reconceptualisation of pain ranging from zero to full reconceptualisation (ibid). When reconceptualisation occurred it correlated with increased knowledge and understanding of pain biology, as well as meaningful improvements in pain, function and well-being (ibid). Pain ratings have even been found to improve for some people up to a year after a pain science education intervention, suggesting that positive impacts can be sustainable (Bülow et al. 2021).

When pain reconceptualisation occurs, patients most value learning that even when pain is present, they are safe and not necessarily injured or damaged; that thoughts and emotions can influence pain; and that pain can change over time (Leake et al. 2021). The concepts from *Explain Pain* rated as most important by patients were that pain is a heightened protective response that is changeable (ibid). These findings suggest that pain science education can help some patients see their pain as less threatening and provide hope that their pain experience can change.

Some patients experience no benefit from pain science education at all (King et al. 2016). Other patients cannot see how it applies to their pain, even when the information made sense and was interesting (King et al. 2016 2018). This echoes the frustrations found in other studies, where patients have expressed that while explanations may be insightful, they can also be 'frustratingly impractical' (Keen et al. 2021). They have asked for practical information about pain, which they can apply in their lives day-to-day (Kennedy et al. 2017).

Summary of current trends and research

Research on pain education consistently finds positive outcomes with small effect sizes, similar to those found in other treatments for pain. However, it is not clear what content or methods make patient education successful, or for whom (Coster & Norman 2009). Positive outcomes are thought to be a result of patient education's effect on knowledge, skills and health behaviours (Simonsmeier et al. 2021), and there appears to be no difference between different types of education (Marris et al. 2021). Moreover, patient education is generally low-cost and low-harm and is able to change multiple parameters of a person's health condition, from physiological to psychological, including reducing medication and healthcare use and improving pain and function (Simonsmeier et al. 2021).

For many people with pain, understanding their pain differently has been lifechanging. As Drew Leder (2016) wrote: 'In my own case … the pain came to feel less sinister, severe, and overpowering. Knowing that "there is something I can do" made all the difference.' This is powerful and is a sentiment shared by many people living with pain, including one of the authors of this chapter (Belton 2019). But there is more to do. Even with the most favourable interpretations of current evidence, the number needed to treat (NNT) for pain science education is about four (Moseley & Butler 2017). This is better than most treatments for pain, including medications, yet it still means three out of four people do not receive a clinically significant benefit of at least 50% reduction of pain after 1 year (Box 9.1).

Challenges

Pain information has become more accurate with advances in pain science, but merely providing more or more accurate information is not as helpful as we may hope (Wittink & Oosterhaven 2018). Pain education is beneficial for many patients, but the development of solutions that help more people requires different questions to be asked. For example:

Why might patients find pain education interesting, but not useful?

Before addressing this question, it is beneficial to unpick the 'education' in pain education. How can education be conceptualised and operationalised?

What is education?

Patient education has been described as a planned and systematic approach to providing patients with information about their health, diagnoses and/or treatment based on their individual needs and circumstances (Simonsmeier et al. 2021). This is a common way of viewing education, but there is some unease with this definition. Perhaps unintentionally, it has created roles where the

clinician is the provider of information and the patient the passive recipient (Matthews 2014; see also Chapter 3). This unidirectional provision of information has been referred to as a *banking model of education*, in which the teacher deposits knowledge in the patient who is assumed to retrieve it later (Freire 1972). Providing patients with evidence-based information or explanations about their pain is thought to improve their understanding and empower them to make necessary changes (Matthews 2014). Although these explanations are well-intentioned (Launer 2018), this transmission of knowledge does not often lead to meaningful change (Matthews 2014). This can be frustrating for clinicians and patients alike.

To overcome some challenges that traditional patient education has faced, it may be helpful to approach education in the clinical environment as collaborative, relational and multidirectional. Rather than a one-way flow of information, education may be seen as an exchange where patients and clinicians learn from and with one another. This is aligned with what patients prefer in the clinical encounter (Haverfield et al. 2018). In this exchange, patients are active participants, sharing their unique knowledge and expertise of themselves, their lives and their pain with their clinician. The clinician learns not only about the patient's symptoms and medical history, but also about the impact of pain on their life; their needs, values, and goals; and their hopes and fears. In essence, the clinician learns the patient's story. This provides the clinician with a better understanding of what might be most useful to discuss with the patient regarding pain, the patient's diagnosis and possible treatments or strategies.

To summarise, pain education should not be something clinicians do to or give to a passive patient. Education is co-constructive learning and a way of becoming more capable. In this way, pain education becomes a dynamic, collaborative, transformative process that fosters learning and change. Through conversation and learning from and with one another, patient and clinician come to a shared understanding of what is happening and decide—together—what to do about it (Low 2020). By bringing together the patient's story and the clinician's relevant training, expertise and knowledge of current research, a narrative about pain can be cocreated that is more accurate and therapeutic, and makes both biological and biographical sense (Brody 1994; Launer 2018; Low 2020). In this narrative-based approach, pain education emphasises learning that bridges the gap between receiving or knowing information (and perhaps finding it interesting but not relevant), and applying that knowledge in ways that enable the person with pain to become more capable and live more fully (Robeyns 2005). This helps the patient move from having knowledge to being capable and able to act on that knowledge (Fraser & Greenhalgh 2001) (Box 9.2).

BOX 9.2 **Reflective practice—conceptualising education**

As education is a concept, we would like to invite you to explore your conceptualisations of pain education. What does pain education mean for you? In the light of being a clinician? In the light of being a citizen? Connected to education are the concepts of learning and teaching. Again, broad terms which are conceptualised in various ways. How would you conceptualise those? Would those differ in various contexts? Would they change when the context of the clinical encounter moves to the patient's daily life?

BOX 9.3 **Reflective practice—frames of reference P**

As pain education and conceptualisations don't happen in a vacuum but are seen within a frame of reference, we would like to invite you to explore the frames of reference you use in contexts and cases of individual patients. Are there similarities and differences?

Complexity of pain

One of the greatest challenges facing pain educators is the complexity of the pain experience itself. Pain is incredibly hard to define (Cohen et al. 2018), let alone explain. While pain education has improved tremendously over the years, the 'bio' aspect of the biopsychosocial framework is still heavily emphasised (Mescouto et al. 2020). It has merely shifted from biomedical, biomechanical and pathoanatomical explanations of pain to biological or neurophysiological explanations (Mescouto et al. 2020; Stilwell & Harman 2019). New explanations tend to be brain- or neurocentric, e.g. pain is seen as a protective output of the brain (Moseley & Butler 2017; Stilwell & Harman 2019) and the brain effectively creates pain (Moseley & Butler 2015b).

These explanations often fail to capture the lived experience of pain and its impacts. This can lead to pushback from patients, who can interpret these explanations as suggestions that pain is 'all in their head' (Stilwell & Harman 2019). Alternatively, patients may find the information impractical and not relevant to their pain or their lives (Keen et al. 2021; Kennedy et al. 2017; King et al. 2016, 2018). Therefore the view of pain education and what it means in the clinical encounter needs to be expanded. There is a great base, founded on pain science and the clinical expertise of health professionals. What might be missing are the more subjective and intersubjective aspects of the pain experience, which are just as legitimate, real and important as the science (Cohen et al. 2018). Through conversation and narrative-based approaches, we can view pain education as a dynamic, collaborative process between clinician and patient (Launer 2018; Low 2020). Education thus becomes a transformative endeavour for the unique person, in their particular situation, with all the inherent complexities therein (Donaldson 2019).

This is important because pain affects, and is affected by, many factors in people's lives. Its most distressing aspects are often not the associated sensations and symptoms, but rather how the pain experience reverberates to every corner the patient's life (Smith & Osborne 2007). Pain is often less a threat to our tissues and more a threat to our sense of self, our relationships, our ability to think and express ourselves, and our way of being in and relating to the world (Biro 2010; Bunzli et al. 2016; Smith & Osborne 2007). There is often a sense of incoherence (Thompson 2016), chaos (Frank 2013) and being torn apart from oneself and one's world (Toye et al. 2021). People with pain also experience and fear stigma, judgement, disbelief and delegitimisation (Froud et al. 2014), all of which can contribute to 'the painfulness of pain' (Leder 2016). However, these aspects of the pain experience are often not addressed or even acknowledged (Froud et al. 2014). In many ways, pain care has merely shifted from identifying and fixing a pathology to identifying and fixing unhelpful beliefs or behaviours (Mescouto et al. 2020).

For this reason, this chapter presents a collaborative and relational approach to pain education. When patients and clinicians learn from and with one another, pain education becomes a collaborative effort where the content is relevant to the patient's unique pain experience and circumstances and allows them to act on what they've learned. To provide pain education that is more helpful for more people, we can consider the use of other frames of reference, such as a capability approach (Robeyns 2005) or a framework of salutogenesis (Eriksson 2017). This would shift care to a focus on capability and health promotion, rather than deficits and disease (Box 9.3).

Solutions

Frameworks for understanding pain and health

Most approaches to understanding and explaining pain are still individualistic and are often bio- or neurocentric (Mescouto et al. 2020). Yet we are inseparable from the people and world around us (Coninx & Stilwell 2021) including systems, policies, culture, and the prevailing beliefs and ideas of the day (Nicholls et al. 2016; also see Chapter 4). To address this, different frameworks have been proposed to move beyond the way the biopsychosocial model is currently implemented.

It is important to recognise that health professionals use frames of reference in their practice, either explicitly or implicitly. These frames of reference include many elements, from education and training to clinical guidelines to expertise gained through experience. When making decisions in the clinical encounter, frames of reference act as lenses through which thought and action occur, which have been referred to as *mindlines* (Gabbay & le May 2010, 2016). Mindlines guide clinical reasoning and action, yet they are flexible and adapt as new information, or new lenses, become available. This section introduces a few different lenses or frames of reference that may help improve pain education in practice.

An *enactive approach to pain* combines biology and phenomenology and views pain as an emergent process that occurs when bodily integrity is threatened (Stilwell & Harman 2019). This is consistent with the current definition of pain and pain science explanations, but suggests that pain emerges from a whole person (not just the brain or the periphery) who is inseparable from the world around them (Stilwell & Harman 2019). It places more emphasis on sense-making and how pain changes the ways we understand ourselves and navigate our environment (Stilwell et al. 2020).

Similarly, *connectivity* recognises humans as connected, intersubjective and codependent beings (Nicholls et al. 2016). We are not just connected with other people, but also with sociopolitical systems and structures, technology, the environment, culture and the prevailing thoughts and ideas of our professional and social circles (see Chapter 4). Acknowledging these connections and our common humanity may lead to a different approach in healthcare, where clinician and patient are seen as intra-active—a part of the same system—rather than interactive—two separate systems interacting. This approach is less stigmatising, judgemental and paternalistic and moves from facilitating independence to enabling fruitful connections (Nicholls et al. 2016). This requires learning what these fruitful and varied connections may look like, and how they may best be facilitated, from people living with pain. We need more collaborative, cooperative and community-based approaches to redefining health and healthcare.

In this sense, *critical pedagogy* might be very helpful. Critical pedagogy sees education as a collaborative process in which the learner also teaches, and the teacher also learns. It is not about providing knowledge, but rather about co-constructing contextual knowledge (Dawkins-Moultin et al. 2016). Critical pedagogy includes three main elements: continuous dialogue and reflection, identifying and naming the problem of the learner, and learning and working together in order to find solutions to the problem (Dawkins-Moultin et al. 2016; Matthews 2014). This avoids the pitfalls of the banking model of education, as there are no predetermined problems, solutions or outcomes (Matthews 2014). Instead, education becomes a dynamic exchange, a process of learning that emancipates the learner and allows them to become freer and more capable in the world (Robeyns 2005).

Table 9.1 summarises frameworks mentioned in this chapter.

TABLE 9.1 Different frames for considering pain education

Salutogenesis	Focusing on what creates health and (re)establishes a sense of coherence, where our experiences make sense and are manageable and meaningful
Capability approach	Moving beyond providing information or transmitting knowledge (which may establish competency) to helping patients be able to adapt to current circumstances, generate new knowledge and become more capable
Connectivity	A recognition that people are codependent beings who are connected to the people, structures, systems, culture, environment, and ideas around us and looking for ways to make fruitful connections
Enactivism	Viewing pain as emergent from the whole person who is situated in and inseparable from the world around them, which they have to navigate differently when they experience pain
Narrative-based approach	Listening closely to people's stories to better understand them and their pain, acknowledging and validating their experiences, and working together to cocreate new narratives about those experiences that may be more therapeutic and foster healing
Critical pedagogy	Approaching education as a collaborative and flexible endeavour that fosters transformation through continual reflection and dialogue, identifying and naming problems together, and cocreating solutions
Mindlines	How you bring all you know together in the clinical environment

Cocreating pain education

How can pain education for patients incorporate first-person, lived experience, and intersubjective ways of understanding pain with what we know of pain science? One way is through qualitative research that provides context and understanding of what works for patients when it comes to pain education (Simonsmeier et al. 2021). It may be even more important to understand why and how they think pain education works. Involving patient partners in the research and the development of educational methods, programmes and resources for health professionals is also a recommended place to start (Bombard et al. 2018; Brand et al. 2021). The inclusion of lived experience perspectives provides a potential to dramatically change how healthcare professionals think about pain and the way they discuss pain with patients. This can also be done through storytelling, narratives, poetry, photography and art (Brand et al. 2021; Padfield & Zakrzewska 2021). Doing so can help humanise patients and provide insight into the profound loss, struggle and suffering that can accompany pain (Toye et al. 2015).

In addition to research and codeveloping education for healthcare professionals, lived experience perspectives can also be incorporated into the development and delivery of pain education for patients. This may make pain education more accessible, relevant and useful for people living with pain (Karazivan et al. 2015). Involving people with pain enables them to share how to put knowledge into practice and apply the information in day-to-day life. Education that includes application of learning is more effective (and engaging) than just transferring information via lectures or educational materials (Simonsmeier et al. 2021). This is aligned with patients' desire to learn practical ways of managing or living with their pain (Kennedy et al. 2017). Pain education should improve and help patients' lives and not be an additional burden.

Peer mentors or coaches can also be providers of pain education and support in clinical and healthcare environments. Peer support has been around for a long time in other areas of health, particularly mental and behavioural health, and has significant benefits (Shalaby & Agyapong 2020). Learning from and with peers can lead to a powerful, relieving sense of no longer being alone (Toye et al. 2021). It can offer hope and a window to possibility. Trained peer facilitators can lend understanding and support, as well as practical ways of integrating pain education into daily life in ways that health professionals may not be able to (McKeon et al. 2021; Shalaby & Agyapong 2020). Not only do the patients benefit from this, their peer facilitators often find a sense of purpose and meaning in the experience as well (McKeon et al. 2021; Toye et al. 2021) (Box 9.4).

Improving pain education in the clinical encounter

As suggested, asking different questions may lead to improvements in pain education for patients. Pain education can be beneficial for patients, reducing the threatening and sinister nature of pain and opening the door to new possibilities. We can ask:

> *How we can we make the experience of pain less threatening, and living a full life more possible, for more people living with pain?*

Patients seek the expertise, knowledge and guidance of clinicians to help make sense of their pain and find a way forward. In this search for answers, they may reject explanations that are too different from their beliefs, goals or understanding (Darlow et al. 2013), or those that are too vague or simplistic (Stilwell et al. 2020). Coconstruction of knowledge and education minimises this risk.

In order to best help a patient make sense of *their* pain, we need to know more about them and their pain experience. What is their experience like? What does the pain mean to them? What do they think is happening? What are their expectations? What are their needs? What are their values and goals? What have they stopped doing because of pain? Why? What worries them most? What matters most to them?

By learning more about the person with pain, clinicians can better understand their experience and go beyond explanations of pain biology. It can include an exploration of the person's story, and how the clinician's knowledge and training can best be incorporated to develop a new understanding of pain. This is not to say that pain biology has no place in pain education; rather, it is highlighting where it may be situated to achieve better outcomes. In this way, education includes helping patients share their experience of pain and give voice to it. It facilitates working together, through dialogue and reflection, to find solutions that work best for that person within their personal contexts and environments. The following sections bring these ideas from critical pedagogy together with a narrative-based approach to facilitate learning and transformation in the clinical encounter.

Intersubjectivity

Pain is invisible. The only way we know of another's pain is if they tell or show us that they are in pain. By its very nature, then, pain is intersubjective (Charon 2021). Entering into a dialogue moves from the division of the subjective experience of the person in pain and the objective knowledge and expertise of the clinician, towards an intersubjective knowledge and way of knowing. In this intersubjective space, which has been called *the third space* (Cohen et al. 2018) or *safe container* (Miciak et al. 2018), the person's story becomes something that can be explored alongside other forms of evidence (Morris 2013). In this space, everyone's perspective matters and enters into a dynamic interaction, like a dance (Cohen et al. 2018). In this third space or safe container, a therapeutic relationship can be established, with a sense of the presence of the other (Miciak et al. 2018). This sense of presence and being fully present are what create true intersubjectivity (Charon 2021). First, we have to find ourselves, next we find each other and finally we exchange perspectives.

Receiving stories (listening)

Before a patient can develop a new understanding of their pain and new stories about their experiences, their current story must be heard (Braeuninger-Weimer et al. 2019; Frank 2013; Toye et al. 2021). During the assessment, there is a distinct 'need to know' on behalf of the clinician, as well as a 'need to be known' on behalf of the patient (Brody 1994). How does this knowing develop? It usually starts with the patient's story—often referred to as taking a history or, preferably, receiving a story. When a patient shares their story and it is well heard by a trusted, attentive clinician, they gain a critical distance from the tale being told and can begin to see their story differently (Frank 2013). They can learn a lot about their own pain and what may be done about it, simply through being able to express themselves (Charon 2021; Frank 2013; see Chapter 3). Watson et al.'s review (2019) found that patients really valued being able to tell their own story. It enhanced their ability, and perhaps willingness, to reconceptualise their pain. If, on the other hand, the person's story is not heard or is dismissed, the opportunity for recovery may be lost (Charon 2021).

Acknowledgement, validation

A common theme among people living with pain is a sense of being invalidated, so validation of both pain and the person in pain is a critical step towards healing (Toye et al. 2021). Many patients experience a sense of relief, of a burden being lifted, when they are given the opportunity to put words to their experience (Stewart & Ryan 2020). There is even greater benefit when those stories are acknowledged (Bunzli et al. 2016) and believed (Braeuninger-Weimer et al. 2019; Haverfield et al. 2018). Charon calls this witnessing our pain (2021). Patients want to be listened to and heard without being judged or stigmatised, and believed without their reports being dismissed or trivialised, which is common in the absence of objective findings (Haverfield et al. 2018; Kim et al. 2021). Being heard without judgement or doubt helps to establish trust and openness (Haverfield et al. 2018), frees up the capacity to take on new information, such as pain education (Braeuninger-Weimer et al. 2019), and instils confidence in making decisions with a healthcare provider regarding the treatment plan (Kim et al. 2021). When clinicians recognise their patient's pain and suffering and show their desire to join the patient to addressing these, they open a door to care (Charon 2021).

Conversations inviting change

Pain education in the clinical environment can be seen as a back and forth, a conversation, that allows for the cocreation of new, more therapeutic narratives that make biological *and* biographical sense for the person in pain. Through this exchange and permission to tell their story, patients can gain critical distance from the story they are telling and begin to see things in a different light (Frank 2013). Arthur Frank said that we don't just tell stories about ourselves and our experiences, we also create ourselves in the telling (2013). In this process, they may repeat some of the same stories because they have yet to make sense of things and are still working through it (ibid). This IS learning. The patient may be able to begin to connect their own dots, question what doesn't make sense, name challenges, see possibility where before they only saw barriers and begin to come to a new account of their reality (Dawkins-Moultin et al. 2016; Launer 2018). Every story has a potential to change in the next retelling (Launer 2018). Clinicians have a crucial role to play in what new stories are being told.

One approach to achieving this is through *conversations inviting change* (Launer 2018). This approach emphasises curiosity, exploration and flexibility, rather than jumping in with explanations of pain, which may not be relevant to the person at that time. It is important to know first how the patient is currently making sense of things, and what they would like to know (ibid). Launer stresses the importance of going in with an intentional stance of not knowing and not making assumptions, while being curious about both the person in pain and the conversation itself. Following the patient's story and language, the clinician can ask relevant questions that may make space for the patient to change their own story. 'Good questioning is often (although not always) a better way of creating openness and possibility' (ibid). These questions are important to patients, as they demonstrate the clinician is listening and paying close attention to their story (Haverfield et al. 2018).

The questions and the ensuing conversation also allow the clinician to share information that the patient finds useful and enable an exploration of possible treatment plans (Haverfield et al. 2018). Importantly, the purpose of asking relevant questions is not to persuade someone to think a certain way or to fix their story for them (Launer 2018). One cannot force a new narrative onto a person, as in the banking model of education, which leads to frustrations for both patient and clinician. One can, however, invite change and work with patients to cocreate new narratives that tell a better account of their reality. The aim is to help patients think about their story and their pain in new ways that make sense for them and their particular contexts, values, goals and lives (Launer 2018).

When met with resistance to changing a particular narrative, rather than forcing a chosen narrative, the clinician can meet the resistance with curiosity. If the conversation seems stuck or stilted, creative ways of facilitating conversation may be considered, such as using stories or metaphors (Loftus 2011; Stewart & Ryan 2020; see Chapter 3), videos (Toye et al. 2015), photographs or art (Padfield & Zakrzewska 2021).

Patient-led goal setting

Conversations about a person's individual pain experience and what can be done affords the opportunity for patient-led goal setting. Goals are often set for patients by healthcare professionals, which may not align with or be relevant to what they want for themselves (Gardner et al. 2019). Through conversation and dialogue, what matters most to the person in pain can be known and incorporated into the treatment plan and patient goals. Structured, patient-led goal setting combined with pain science education has been shown to produce clinically meaningful improvements in pain and disability ratings, quality of life scores and greater self-efficacy (ibid). These changes are maintained in the medium and long terms (2- and 12-month follow-ups, respectively) (ibid).

Co-construction of narratives and goals

The biographical and social disruption that occurs as a result of pain often leads to a search for meaning and a

TABLE 9.2 Pain education in practice

Listening (receiving stories)

Acknowledgement and validation

Conversations that invite change

Patient-led goal setting

Co-construction of new narratives

BOX 9.5 **Reflective practice—understanding the patient to understand their pain**

Does the idea of educating through dialogue, reflection and conversation resonate with you? What about working together to identify and name the challenges the patient is facing? How might that help determine what resources and information might be helpful when devising solutions? What are the challenges to such an approach? In what ways might this improve your experience of providing education in the clinical encounter?

need to make sense of what is happening (Frank 2013). This may be where pain education that has a focus on collaborative, transformative learning can have its greatest effect. The meanings of pain can change over time, which in turn can change our pain experience (Belton 2019). For some, these changes may include regaining a sense of coherence (Eriksson 2017; Thompson 2016); reconnecting with their self, others and the world around them (Toye et al. 2021); or finding new purpose in helping others who are also living with pain (McKeon et al. 2021). Frank (2013) calls this a *quest narrative*, where we are able to reinterpret our past, find purpose and new meaning in the present and regain a sense of a viable future. Facilitating this change is a fundamental part of pain education.

Taken together, inviting change in an intersubjective space and allowing patients to lead goal setting can serve the educational purpose of co-constructing a new narrative about pain that makes sense and can be acted upon (Eriksson 2017). These cocreated narratives can be aligned with pain science and particular diagnoses, while also being relevant to and making sense for the individual and their life story (Bunzli et al. 2016). There is a shift from educating about pain science to incorporating pain science and clinical expertise into the interpretations, meanings, beliefs and story of the person living with pain who has sought their guidance. New narratives can help people with pain to see the world and their place in it differently, helping them uncover possibilities they did not see before, enabling them to become more capable and engage with life more fully (Robeyns 2005) (Table 9.2) (Box 9.5).

Conclusion

Pain education—or making sense of pain together?

Learning more about what pain is, and perhaps more importantly what it isn't, helps people to understand their pain in new ways and change the meaning of their experiences. This has to be done in a way that makes biological or scientific sense and also biographical sense. Merely replacing the patient's narrative with a clinical, biomedical or pain science narrative, as can happen in a banking model of education, is often not helpful and can understandably be met with resistance. It can be seen as another form of 'fixing', only shifted from bodies to minds and from joints and discs to beliefs, thoughts and stories. Pain education for patients should be about making sense of pain in ways that are meaningful to the individual. This is predicated on the healthcare professional's own knowledge and comfort with the complexities of chronic pain and their communication skills (see Chapters 2 and 3). The topics throughout this book are not separate concepts, they are integrally connected.

This chapter has not outlined what to teach about pain or how to teach it. That was intentional and we hope it has become clear why. Pain education will be different for each individual (patients *and* clinicians), and also for each group, context, culture and therapeutic environment. Pain

BOX 9.6 **Reflective practice—picking one thing to do differently**

A lot of concepts and ideas about education and learning have been shared in this chapter, some of which may be new. What is one thing you can try in your next clinical encounter?

education in the clinical environment is a collaboration where the clinician learns from and with the person living with pain, while the person living with pain learns from and with the clinician. Together, patient and clinician can cocreate a new story and new meanings and create a therapeutic plan that makes sense for that particular individual.

Pain education is evolving. Where traditionally most educational interventions or initiatives have been led by researchers and clinicians, there is now a move towards cocreation and codevelopment of research, education and learning. The more multiple ways of knowing pain can be brought together—including scientific research; clinical training, expertise, and experience; and the expertise, insights, and knowledge of people living with pain—the better we can understand, teach and treat pain. Bringing those ways of knowing to light will reveal more frames to view the complex problem of pain. Hopefully education will continue to be disrupted, challenged and changed, not just for patients, but for health professionals too (Box 9.6).

References

Belton, J., 2019. Exploring the meanings of pain: my pain story. In: van Rysewyk, S. (Ed.), Meanings of Pain: Volume 2: Common Types of Pain and Language. Springer, Cham, pp. 1–15.

Biro, D., 2010. Listening to Pain: Finding Words, Compassion, and Relief. W.W. Norton & Company, New York.

Bombard, Y., Baker, G.R., Orlando, E., Fancott, C., Bhatia, P., Casalino, S., et al., 2018. Engaging patients to improve quality of care: a systematic review. Implement Sci. 13 (1), 98.

Brand, G., Sheers, C., Wise, S., Seubert, L., Clifford, R., Griffiths, P., et al., 2021. A research approach for co-designing education with healthcare consumers. Med. Educ. 55 (5), 574–581.

Braeuninger-Weimer, K., Anjarwalla, N., Pincus, T., 2019. Discharged and dismissed: a qualitative study with back pain patients discharged without treatment from orthopaedic consultations. Eur. J. Pain 23 (8), 1464–1474. https://doi.org/10.1002/ejp.1412.

Brody, H., 1994. My story is broken; Can you help me fix it?": medical ethics and the joint construction of narrative. Lit. Med. 13 (1), 79–92. https://doi.org/10.1353/lm.2011.0169.

Bülow, K., Lindberg, K., Vaegter, H.B., Juhl, C.B., 2021. Effectiveness of pain neurophysiology education on musculoskeletal pain: a systematic review and meta-analysis.

Pain Med. 22 (4), 891–904. https://doi.org/10.1093/pm/pnaa484.

Bunzli, S., Smith, A., Schütze, R., O'Sullivan, P., 2016. The lived experience of pain-related fear in people with chronic low back pain. In: van Rysewyk, S. (Ed.), Meanings of Pain. Springer, Cham.

Butler, D., Moseley, L., 2015. Explain Pain, second ed. NOI Group Publications.

Charon, R., 2021. How to listen for the talk of pain. In: Padfield, D., Zakrzewska (Eds.), Encountering Pain: Hearing, Seeing, Speaking. UCL Press, London, UK.

Cohen, M., Quintner, J., van Rysewyk, S., 2018. Reconsidering the international association for the study of pain definition of pain. Pain Rep. 3 (2), e634. https://doi.org/10.1097/PR9.0000000000000634.

Coninx, S., Stilwell, P., 2021. Pain and the field of affordances: an enactive approach to acute and chronic pain. Synthese 199 (3–4), 7835–7863.

Coster, S., Norman, I., 2009. Cochrane reviews of educational and self-management interventions to guide nursing practice: a review. Int. J. Nurs. Stud. 46 (4), 508–528. https://doi.org/10.1016/j.ijnurstu.2008.09.009.

Darlow, B., Dowell, A., Baxter, G.D., Mathieson, F., Perry, M., Dean, S., 2013. The enduring impact of what clinicians say to people with low back pain. Ann. Fam. Med. 11 (6), 527–534. https://doi.org/10.1370/afm.1518.

Dawkins-Moultin, L., McDonald, A., McKyer, L., 2016. Integrating the principles of socioecology and critical pedagogy for health promotion health literacy interventions. J. Health Commun. 21 (Suppl. 2), 30–35. https://doi.org/10.1080/10810730.2016.1196273.

Donaldson, J.P., 2019. Travelling in Troy with an Instructional Designer. Hybrid Pedagogy https://hybridpedagogy.org/travelling-in-troy/.

Eriksson, M., 2017. The sense of coherence in the salutogenic model of health. In: Mittelmark, M.B., Sagy, S., Eriksson, M., BauerJürgen, G.F., Pelikan, M., Lindström, B., Espnes, G.A. (Eds.), The Handbook of Salutogenesis. Springer, Cham.

Frank, A., 2013. The Wounded Storyteller: Body, Illness, and Ethics, second ed. The University of Chicago Press Chicago, IL.

Fraser, S.W., Greenhalgh, T., 2001. Coping with complexity: educating for capability. BMJ (Clinical Research Ed) 323 (7316), 799–803. https://doi.org/10.1136/bmj.323.7316.799.

Freire, P., 1972. Pedagogy of the Oppressed. Herder and Herder, New York.

Froud, R., Patterson, S., Eldridge, S., Seale, C., Pincus, T., Rajendran, D., et al., 2014. A systematic review and meta-synthesis of the impact of low back pain on people's lives. BMC Muscoskel. Disord. 15 (50). https://doi.org/10.1186/1471-2474-15-50.

Gabbay, J., le May, A., 2010. Practice-Based Evidence for Healthcare: Clinical Mindlines. Routledge, Abingdon, OX.

Gabbay, J., le May, A., 2016. Mindlines: making sense of evidence in practice. Br. J. Gen. Pract.: J. Roy. Coll. Gen. Pract. 66 (649), 402–403. https://doi.org/10.3399/bjgp16X686221.

Gardner, T., Refshauge, K., McAuley, J., Hübscher, M., Goodall, S., Smith, L., 2019. Combined education and patient-led goal setting intervention reduced chronic low back pain disability and intensity at 12 months: a randomised controlled trial. Br. J. Sports Med. 53 (22), 1424–1431. https://doi.org/10.1136/bjsports-2018-100080.

Haverfield, M.C., Giannitrapani, K., Timko, C., Lorenz, K., 2018. Patient-centered pain management communication from the patient perspective. J. Gen. Intern. Med. 33 (8), 1374–1380. https://doi.org/10.1007/s11606-018-4490-y.

Karazivan, P., Dumez, V., Flora, L., Pomey, M.-P., Del Grande, C., Ghadiri, D.P., et al., 2015. The patient-as-partner approach in health care. Acad. Med. 90 (4), 437–441. https://doi.org/10.1097/ACM.0000000000000603.

Keen, S., Lomeli-Rodriguez, M., Williams, A., 2021. Exploring how people with chronic pain understand their pain: a qualitative study. Scand. J. Pain 21 (4), 743–753.

Kennedy, D., Wainwright, A., Pereira, L., Robarts, S., Dickson, P., Christian, J., et al., 2017. A qualitative study of patient education needs for hip and knee replacement. BMC Muscoskel. Disord. 18 (1), 413. https://doi.org/10.1186/s12891-017-1769-9.

Kim, K., Rendon, I., Starkweather, A., 2021. Patient and provider perspectives on patient-centered chronic pain management. Pain Manag. Nurs. 22 (4), 470–477. https://doi.org/10.1016/j.pmn.2021.02.003.

King, R., Robinson, V., Elliott-Button, H.L., Watson, J.A., Ryan, C.G., Martin, D.J., 2018. Pain reconceptualisation after pain neurophysiology education in adults with chronic low back pain: a qualitative study. Pain Res. Manag. 3745651. https://doi.org/10.1155/2018/3745651. 2018.

King, R., Robinson, V., Ryan, C.G., Martin, D.J., 2016. An exploration of the extent and nature of reconceptualisation of pain following pain neurophysiology education: a qualitative study of experiences of people with chronic musculoskeletal pain. Patient Educ. Counsel 99 (8), 1389–1393. https://doi.org/10.1016/j.pec.2016.03.008.

Launer, J., 2018. Narrative-Based Practice in Health and Social Care: Conversations Inviting Change, second ed. Routledge, Abingdon, OX.

Leake, H.B., Moseley, G.L., Stanton, T.R., O'Hagan, E.T., Heathcote, L.C., 2021. What do patients value learning about pain? A mixed-methods survey on the relevance of target concepts after pain science education. Pain 162 (10), 2558–2568.

Leder, D., 2016. The experiential paradoxes of pain. J. Med. Philos. 41 (5), 444–460. https://doi.org/10.1093/jmp/jhw020.

Loftus, S., 2011. Pain and its metaphors: a dialogical approach. J. Med. Humanit. 32 (3), 213–230. https://doi.org/10.1007/s10912-011-9139-3.

Louw, A., Puentedura, E., 2013. Therapeutic Neuroscience Education: Teaching Patients about Pain. International Pain & Spine Institute Minneapolis, MN.

Low, M., 2020. Above and beyond statistical evidence. Why stories matter for clinical decisions and shared decision making. In: Anjum, R., Copeland, S., Rocca, E. (Eds.), Rethinking Causality, Complexity and Evidence for the Unique Patient. Springer, Cham.

Marris, D., Theophanous, K., Cabezon, P., Dunlap, Z., Donaldson, M., 2021. The impact of combining pain education strategies with physical therapy interventions for patients with chronic pain: a systematic review and meta-analysis of randomized controlled trials. Physiother. Theory Pract. 37 (4), 461–472. https://doi.org/10.1080/09593985.2019.1633714.

Matthews, C., 2014. Critical pedagogy in health education. Health. Educ. J 73 (5), 600–609. https://doi.org/10.1177/0017896913510511.

McKeon, G., Mastrogiovanni, C., Chapman, J., Stanton, R., Matthews, E., Steel, Z., et al., 2021. The experiences of peer-facilitators delivering a physical activity intervention for emergency service workers and their families. Ment. Health Phys. Act. 21, 100414. https://doi.org/10.1016/j.mhpa.2021.100414.

Mescouto, K., Olson, R.E., Hodges, P.W., Setchell, J., 2020. A critical review of the biopsychosocial model of low back pain care: time for a new approach? Disabil. Rehabil. 1–15.

Miciak, M., Mayan, M., Brown, C., Joyce, A.S., Gross, D.P., 2018. The necessary conditions of engagement for the therapeutic relationship in physiotherapy: an interpretive description study. Arch. Physiother. 8, 3. https://doi.org/10.1186/s40945-018-0044-1.

Morris, D.B., 2013. Narrative and pain: towards an integrative model. In: Moore, R.J. (Ed.), Handbook of Pain and Palliative Care. Springer New York, NY. https://doi.org/10.1007/978-1-4419-1651-8_38.

Moseley, G.L., Butler, D.S., 2017. Explain Pain Supercharged: The Clinican's Manual. Noigroup Publications, Adelaide.

Moseley, G.L., Butler, D.S., 2015a. Fifteen years of explaining pain: the past, present, and future. J. Pain 16 (9), 807–813.

Moseley, G.L., Butler, D.S., 2015b. The Explain Pain Handbook: Protectometer. Noigroup Publications.

Nicholls, D.A., Atkinson, K., Bjorbækmo, W.S., Gibson, B.E., Latchem, J., Olesen, J., et al., 2016. Connectivity: an emerging concept for physiotherapy practice. Physiother. Theory Pract.

32 (3), 159–170. https://doi.org/10.3109/09593985.2015.11 37665.

Padfield, D., Zakrzewska, J.M., 2021. Encountering Pain: Hearing, Seeing, Speaking. UCL Press, Chicago, IL.

Parreira, P., Heymans, M.W., van Tulder, M.W., Esmail, R., Koes, B.W., Poquet, N., et al., 2017. Back Schools for chronic non-specific low back pain. Cochrane Database Syst. Rev. 8 (8), CD011674. https://doi.org/10.1002/14651858.CD011674.pub2.

Robeyns, I., 2005. The capability approach: a theoretical survey. J. Hum. Dev. 6 (1), 93–117. https://doi.org/10.1080/146498805200034266.

Simonsmeier, B.A., Flaig, M., Simacek, T., Schneider, M., 2021. What sixty years of research says about the effectiveness of patient education on health: a second order meta-analysis. Health Psychol. Rev. 1–25.

Shalaby, R., Agyapong, V., 2020. Peer support in mental health: literature review. JMIR Ment. Health. 7 (6), e15572. https://doi.org/10.2196/15572.

Smith, J.A., Osborn, M., 2007. Pain as an assault on the self: an interpretative phenomenological analysis of the psychological impact of chronic benign low back pain. Psychol. Health 22 (5), 517–534. https://doi.org/10.1080/14768320600941756.

Stewart, M., Ryan, S.-J., 2020. Do metaphors have therapeutic value for people in pain? A systematic review. Pain Rehabilitation: Journal of the Physiotherapy Pain Association 48, 10–23.

Stilwell, P., Harman, K., 2019. An enactive approach to pain: beyond the biopsychosocial model. Phenomenol. Cognitive Sci. 18, 637–665. https://doi.org/10.1007/s11097-019-09624-7.

Stilwell, P., Stilwell, C., Sabo, B., Harman, K., 2020. Painful Metaphors: Enactivism and Art in Qualitative Research. Advance online publication. https://doi.org/10.1136/medhum-2020-011874. Medical Humanities, medhum-2020-011874.

Straube, S., Harden, M., Schröder, H., Arendacka, B., Fan, X., Moore, R.A., et al., 2016. Back schools for the treatment of chronic low back pain: possibility of benefit but no convincing evidence after 47 years of research-systematic review and meta-analysis. Pain 157 (10), 2160–2172. https://doi.org/10.1097/j.pain.0000000000000640.

Tegner, H., Frederiksen, P., Esbensen, B.A., Juhl, C., 2018. Neurophysiological pain education for patients with chronic low back pain: a systematic review and meta-analysis. Clin. J. Pain 34 (8), 778–786. https://doi.org/10.1097/AJP.0000000000000594.

Thompson, B.L., 2016. Making sense: regaining self-coherence. In: van Rysewyk, S. (Ed.), Meanings of Pain. Springer, Cham. https://doi.org/10.1007/978-3-319-49022-9_19.

Toye, F., Belton, J., Hannink, E., Seers, K., Barker, K., 2021. A healing journey with chronic pain: a meta-ethnography synthesizing 195 qualitative studies. Pain Med. 22 (6), 1333–1344. https://doi.org/10.1093/pm/pnaa373.

Toye, F., Jenkins, S., Seers, K., Barker, K., 2015. Exploring the value of qualitative research films in clinical education. BMC Med. Educ. 15, 214. https://doi.org/10.1186/s12909-015-0491-2.

Watson, J.A., Ryan, C.G., Cooper, L., Ellington, D., Whittle, R., Lavender, M., et al., 2019. Pain neuroscience education for adults with chronic musculoskeletal pain: a mixed-methods systematic review and meta-analysis. J. Pain 20 (10), 1140.e1–1140.e22. https://doi.org/10.1016/j.jpain.2019.02.011.

Wittink, H., Oosterhaven, J., 2018. Patient education and health literacy. Musculoskelet. Sci. Pract. 38, 120–127. https://doi.org/10.1016/j.msksp.2018.06.004.

Wood, L., Hendrick, P.A., 2019. A systematic review and meta-analysis of pain neuroscience education for chronic low back pain: short-and long-term outcomes of pain and disability. Eur. J. Pain 23 (2), 234–249. https://doi.org/10.1002/ejp.1314.

Chapter 10

Participating in life roles through self-management

Nicole E. Andrews

LEARNING OBJECTIVES

At the end of this chapter, readers will understand the:
1. Importance of an individual's life roles.
2. Assessment tools and approaches for establishing important life roles and barriers to role participation.
3. Benefits of activity modulation as an intervention for chronic pain.
4. Practical application of activity modulation to increase role participation.

Overview

I am an occupational therapist, a researcher, a mother, a friend, an artist, a survivor. These are some of my life roles. Life roles are sets of connected behaviours, obligations and norms as conceptualised by a society (Pawar 2017). They hold specific meaning for the person performing them and to those around them. Established through choice and need, life roles are normally intertwined with a person's identity and self-worth (Scott et al. 2017b).

Some life roles persist while others change over time, as people go through planned and unplanned life transitions. Chronic pain can have a substantial impact on one's ability to participate in desired and meaningful life roles

(Hadi et al. 2019). Treatment often focuses on assisting individuals to rediscover past roles or develop new roles. This chapter focuses specifically on activity modulation as a self-management strategy for increasing one's capacity to participate in desired life roles.

Establishing treatment direction and options

Successfully engaging in life roles demands certain routines of skilled action (Kielhofner & Burke 1980) and lends itself to a client-centred participation-focused assessment (Scott et al. 2017a). Key aspects of this approach are considered below.

Establishing important life roles

Semistructured interviewing can be valuable for establishing important life roles throughout one's lifespan. The clinician encourages individuals to share their life story. Focus is placed on the activity or occupational choices across the lifespan, critical life events and the impact of life events on occupational choices. The Occupational Performance History Interview (OPHI-II) (Kielhofner et al. 2001) provides a semistructured interview proforma to gather this information. Feedback from both individuals and health professionals have suggested that the OPHI-II interview is helpful for building rapport, generating insights into an individual's life experiences, treatment planning and goal setting (Apte et al. 2005).

An additional tool is the Role Checklist Version 3: Satisfaction and Performance (Scott et al. 2017b). This short 10-item screening tool assesses current role participation, satisfaction with role performance, reasons for nonparticipation and desired future role engagement. Over 90% of occupational therapists and occupational therapy students find the Role Checklist Version 3 useful for treatment planning (Scott et al. 2019).

Examining current routine and role performance

Once important life roles are established, it is helpful to gain a more thorough understanding of current role performance and routine. Semistructured interviews can be used to establish what activities are performed, when, in what context, with whom and how often. Typical daily and weekly routines can be identified through this process, and discrepancies between desired and current role participation start to become apparent.

When assessing routine within the pain field, it is important to consider whether individuals pace their daily activities or engage in overactivity behaviour, as this can significantly interfere with typical routines. Overactivity in the context of chronic pain refers to engagement in high levels of physical activity or prolonged sedentary task engagement that significantly exacerbates pain intensity, resulting in a period of reduced functional capacity (Andrews et al. 2015b; Philips 1988). Individuals often describe being unable to do even basic activities, such as showering, while pain is significantly exacerbated (Andrews et al. 2015c). These periods of incapacity can last up to a few days, making it difficult to participate in life roles such as being a worker or grandparent (Andrews et al. 2015c). Activity pacing can counter this by breaking up and scheduling activities to prevent activity-related pain exacerbations (Andrews & Deen 2016; Nielson et al. 2013). Individuals who pace activity effectively are likely to have more stable pain levels and a consistent routine. The Overactivity in Persistent Pain Assessment (OPPA) is a short assessment tool that can be used to determine overactivity severity and its impact on one's routine (Andrews et al. 2021).

Establishing specific functional difficulties and barriers to participation

This final assessment component focuses on collecting and interpreting information to more specifically identify problems and barriers related to activity participation. Activities that the individual can't do, has difficulties doing, avoids doing or which severely exacerbate pain intensity should be identified in the following areas: (1) self-care; (2) household chores and house maintenance; (3) work, study and volunteering; and (4) leisure and social. The physical, sensory-motor, cognitive and psychosocial dimensions of tasks and activities should be considered when determining possible reasons for the problems experienced.

Specific attention should be given to activity avoidance which, in the context of chronic pain, is commonly described as a reduction in physical or other daily activities as a means to avoid pain escalation (Lethem et al. 1983; Philips 1988). Avoiding activity means having the capacity (physical and mental) to engage in that activity but choosing not to (Andrews et al. 2015a). Activity avoidance has received much empirical attention in the pain field through the fear-avoidance model (Lethem et al. 1983; Vlaeyen & Linton 2000). According to this model, catastrophic interpretations of pain can lead to a fear of pain and avoidance of activity. However, catastrophising thoughts and fear of pain are not the only reasons why individuals with pain avoid activities. Other common reasons for avoidance include feeling judged by others, positive reinforcement by family and health professionals, and apathy (Pincus et al. 2006).

Once specific issues and barriers are identified, treatment targets and plans can be formulated. The rest of this chapter focuses on activity modulation as a self-management treatment strategy to address barriers to participation in roles identified as important to the individual.

Activity modulation as a self-management treatment for persistent pain

Activity modulation refers to the regulation of activity level and/or rate in the service of an adaptive goal or goals (Andrews & Deen 2016; Nielson et al. 2013). Activity modulation encompasses three components: (1) activity adaption, (2) (re)commencing or increasing activity and (3) ceasing or decreasing activity. Possible treatment directions based on barriers and problems identified during assessment are displayed in Fig. 10.1 and specific treatment strategies are discussed later.

Activity adaptation

Simply put, activity adaption requires changing the tools, equipment, method or technique used to perform an activity to make it easier to complete. Adaptations are not designed to change the outcome or purpose of an activity but to alter the way it is performed to make it more aligned with the individual's functional capacity and abilities. Activity adaption should be considered in the following scenarios: (1) when an individual cannot do an activity or needs assistance to complete an activity, (2) when an individual describes difficulties completing an activity or (3) when an individual reports that an activity severely aggravates their pain. Three ways to adapt activities are discussed here.

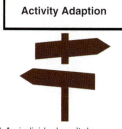

Activity Adaption

1) An individual can't do an activity/ normally requires assistance
OR
2) An individual describes difficulties completing an activity
OR
3) An individual reports that an activity causes severe pain exacerbations

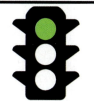

(Re) commencing and increasing activities

An individual has identify that an activity is something that they either want to do or need to do

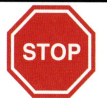

Decreasing and ceasing activities

1) An individual reports feeling overwhelmed or overloaded
OR
2) An individual reports having no time for valued or important activities
OR
3) An activity is severely aggravating pain and is not deemed essential/ important

Fig. 10.1 Treatment targets for identified barriers to role participation.

Activity pacing

Activity pacing is the most commonly used activity adaption technique in the pain field. While the definition of activity pacing varies, it generally refers to strategies used to divide one's daily activities into smaller, more manageable portions, and scheduling activity portions throughout the day in a way that should not exacerbate pain (Birkholtz et al. 2004; Jamieson-Lega et al. 2013; Nielson et al. 2013). Activity pacing is one of the most highly endorsed pain management strategies among health professionals (Brown 2002; Torrance et al. 2011). Outcome studies evaluating the effectiveness of pacing as an intervention are sparse, but research suggests that it can decrease fatigue interference and help establish more consistent activity levels across the week for role participation (Guy et al. 2019).

Examples of activity pacing strategies are:
- **Taking regular short breaks** while completing a task can enable individuals to complete activities and socialise without aggravating pain. For example, a lady who wishes to play bowls with friends can sit down and rest in between bowls, to ensure that she is not standing for prolonged periods of time (which normally aggravates her pain).
- **Alternating postures while doing an activity** can enable individuals to participate in activities for longer than if they maintain the same posture/body position throughout. Common examples are alternating between standing and sitting while working at a computer, preparing meals or doing artwork. Individuals with hand pain aggravated by using a computer mouse can also alter their hand position by regularly switching between an ergonomic mouse and touchpad.
- **Alternating between hard and easy tasks** can keep pain levels at a manageable level, allowing individuals to be more productive throughout the day. For example, a husband who has difficulties vacuuming could vacuum one room, sit down and fold clothes, vacuum another room and then make his wife a cup of coffee.

Scheduling activities using dairies/schedulers or using timers as a reminder to change postures/activities can help individuals to use activity pacing strategies effectively.

Assistive technology

Assistive technology (AT) includes any item, piece of equipment or product used to increase, maintain or improve the functional capabilities of people with disabilities (WHO 2014). They can be acquired commercially from community pharmacies, rehabilitation equipment suppliers, department stores or digital retailers. Examples include:
- **Aids for daily living** such as long handle reachers, modified cutlery, dressing and showering aids, electric cleaning products and ergonomic cooking utensils
- **Seating and positioning** such as adapted seating, lumbar support cushions, coccyx cut-out cushions and sit-to-stand desks
- **Mobility aids** such as electric or manual wheelchairs, walkers and crutches
- **Car or vehicle modifications** such as spinner knobs, reversing cameras and blind-spot detectors
- **Recreational aids** to enable participation in social, leisure and community activities such as long-handled gardening tools, raised garden beds, adaptive controls for video games, bowling arms, adaptive fishing rods and seating systems for boats

- **Sleep solutions** such as mattress overlays, weighted blankets, water-based pillows and sound machines
- **Computer access aids** such as modified or alternative keyboards, ergonomic mice and voice-to-text software
- **Home or workplace modifications** include structural adaptations such as ramps, bathroom changes and automatic door openers
- **Electronic environmental control systems** that control appliances like the telephone, TV, blinds, air conditioning and light switches.

AT is identified by the United Nations Convention on the Rights of Persons with Disabilities (UNCRPD) as a human rights obligation of both states and international donors. The 157 countries that have ratified the UNCRPD must ensure the availability of high-quality, affordable AT products (Khasnabis et al. 2015). In addition, AT is recommended for pain associated with arthritis in several international guidelines (Bannuru et al. 2019; Fernandes et al. 2013; Forestier et al. 2009).

Therapists should, however, exercise caution when prescribing or recommending AT solutions for people with pain. If used incorrectly, AT can contribute to activity avoidance, which may worsen physical deconditioning and increase pain over time. Products that significantly restrict movement, such as mobility aids, splints and braces, should be considered high risk. AT should only be prescribed after a comprehensive functional assessment has been undertaken that takes into consideration psychosocial factors. The aim for prescription should always be to increase activity participation and allow the individual to do more overall. Education should be provided to ensure that AT is used appropriately.

Other forms of activity adaption

Other forms of activity adaption include changing the technique or posture/positioning used to complete a task. Examples of technique changes include one-handed dressing techniques, sliding objects instead of lifting and storing frequently used kitchen items within easy reach. Posture or positioning changes may involve using ergonomic principles to set up a workstation, changing the position of a car seat or sitting to do gardening.

Recommencing and increasing activities

Helping individuals to do more of the things they need or want to do should be a core component of any treatment program for pain management. While sometimes it is easier to start a treatment program by helping individuals to adapt to the activities they are having difficulties with, helping individuals to do more overall should always be the enduring treatment goal. Some general principles and strategies to help individuals either recommence or gradually increase activities are presented later.

Recommencing activities

Health professionals should work with individuals to develop a plan that decreases stress, anxiety and fear about activity engagement. This often involves setting realistic baselines or starting points and using adaptation strategies to ensure that recommencing activities doesn't cause severe pain exacerbations. There are three ways to adapt activities when establishing a baseline level:

- **Downscaling or only doing a portion of the activity** such as going for a 500-m walk instead of a 1-km walk, starting to garden using a small garden bed, or focusing on one room in the house when recommencing cleaning
- **Engaging in similar but easier activities in a particular interest area** such as coaching instead of playing a sport, crocheting instead of knitting, or powerboating instead of sailing
- **Using assistive technology** such as gardening using a raised garden bed or using an electric turbo cleaning brush to clean the bath.

Gradually increasing activity

Graded activity

Graded activity for the management of chronic pain was first described in a seminal work by Fordyce (1976). Based on operant conditioning principles, graded activity uses predetermined quotas to increase activity levels and positively reinforce healthy behaviour. Activity levels should be increased gradually to avoid severe pain aggravations and negative responses to activity engagement. Activities can be increased by either difficulty level, speed, time or outputs (e.g. half a basket of laundry or two knitted beanies). If severe pain aggravation occurs because the increase was too large, individuals should return to the last quotum and try to increase the activity more gradually. Available evidence suggests that graded activity in the short term and intermediate term is more effective at reducing pain severity and disability than no intervention or minimal intervention (López-de-Uralde-Villanueva et al. 2016; Macedo et al. 2010).

Graded exposure

Graded exposure is used as a treatment strategy for individuals who avoid activities predominately due to fear. Graded exposure encourages a confrontation response by exposing individuals to specific situations of which they are fearful during rehabilitation. Health professionals assist individuals to create a hierarchy of feared activities and expose them to the least feared activity first. After exposure, the health professional helps individuals to appraise the consequences of the exposure and addresses irrational and counterproductive beliefs. Once negative associations with the activity engagement are extinguished, activities higher in the hierarchy are undertaken using the same method. Current evidence suggests that graded exposure is as effective as graded activity for reducing pain severity and disability, but more effective at decreasing pain catastrophising than graded activity in the short term (López-de-Uralde-Villanueva et al. 2016; Macedo et al. 2010).

Weaning assistive technology
High-risk AT such as mobility aids, splints and braces should be weaned if they are no longer useful or indicated, to increase movement and activity levels over time. This process can be gradual. For example, a splint could initially be removed while the individual participates in prescribed exercises or certain activities. This may be progressed to a certain number of hours per day without the splint until eventually the individual is confident they can do all activities without the splint. Similar to graded exposure, health professionals may consider creating a hierarchy of scenarios in order to assist with graduated weaning.

Increasing motivation and the role of family and loved ones

Family members can unintentionally reinforce avoidance behaviour. Wanting to care for a loved one by taking over all painful activities can decrease autonomy and self-efficacy. When family members worry about activities that cause pain, this often compounds these fears within the person in pain. Wherever possible, health professionals should include family and loved ones in treatment planning or encourage individuals with pain to share educational resources with their loved ones.

Health professionals should also work with individuals to develop a plan to increase accountability and motivation. Strategies that could be utilised include (1) setting graded activity goals with friends or family members, (2) setting timeframes for when a task or activity is completed by, (3) keeping track of progress and (4) celebrating small wins.

Decreasing and ceasing activities

While it may seem counterproductive, there are certain instances where individuals may benefit from decreasing or ceasing certain activities in order to increase engagement in valued life roles. Decreasing or ceasing activities should be considered if (1) an individual reports feeling overwhelmed

or overloaded, (2) an individual reports having no time for valued or important activities or (3) an activity that is severely aggravating pain is deemed not important. Specific treatment strategies are discussed later.

Values clarification

Value clarification exercises can be used to help individuals identify activities within life roles which are most important and which should be given more time and attention. An example is a mother who spends much time and effort trying to keep the house clean and tidy. She prioritises these activities because of perceived societal or family expectations. This perception may, however, be inaccurate, and the mother's actions may not align with her values of being present and available to spend quality time with her family.

Delegation

Delegation involves assigning activities and tasks to another person. This technique is commonly used to establish family chore schedules, giving the individual with pain the capacity to focus on more important tasks and goals. Delegation can also help individuals to recommence activities by delegating a portion of the activity to a family member. For instance, an individual with pain may hang out half of the laundry with a family member hanging the other half. They may then build up this activity over time.

Community-based support

Community-based assistance with cleaning, shopping, gardening and home maintenance can allow individuals to focus on other roles such as work, parenting or volunteering. Health professionals should provide education and establish clear therapy goals when referring to these services.

Prioritisation lists

Prioritisation lists can help individuals when they are feeling overwhelmed or overloaded. An example is displayed in Table 10.1. Health professionals should assist individuals to determine the priority of activities by weighing up activity deadlines, consequences of noncompletion and activities that may be delegated.

TABLE 10.1 Prioritisation list template

Activity	When do I need to complete this activity?	What will happen if this doesn't get done?	Can I delegate this activity?	Priority ranking

Conclusion

This chapter has provided an overview of core assessment and treatment strategies to enable individuals to increase their participation in desired life roles. The primary aim of the therapeutic approach is to enable individuals to be able to do more of the things they need to or want to do. While altering physical capacity, pain perception or psychological functioning is not the primary target, improvements in these outcomes can be observed when focusing on increasing participation in desired life roles. The approach can therefore be used as a stand-alone intervention or in combination with other approaches described in this textbook.

Review questions   Q

1. What is a life role?
2. What information should be considered when establishing problems and barriers related to role participation?
3. What are the three components of activity modulation?
4. Name three activity pacing strategies.
5. What is the difference between graded activity and graded exposure?
6. In what contexts is decreasing or ceasing activities indicated?

References

Andrews, N., Deen, M., 2016. Defining activity pacing: is it time to jump off the merry-go-round? J. Pain 17 (12), 1359–1362.

Andrews, N.E., Chien, C.W., Ireland, D., Varnfield, M., 2021. Overactivity assessment in chronic pain: the development and psychometric evaluation of a multifaceted self-report assessment. Eur. J. Pain 25 (1), 225–242.

Andrews, N.E., Strong, J., Meredith, P.J., 2015a. Avoidance or incapacitation: a discussion on definition and validity of objective measures of avoidance, persistence, and overactivity. Clin. J. Pain 31 (7), 670–672.

Andrews, N.E., Strong, J., Meredith, P.J., 2015b. Overactivity in chronic pain: is it a valid construct? Pain 156 (10), 1991–2000. https://doi.org/10.1097/j.pain.0000000000000259.

Andrews, N.E., Strong, J., Meredith, P.J., Gordon, K., Bagraith, K.S., 2015c. "It's very hard to change yourself": an exploration of overactivity in people with chronic pain using interpretative phenomenological analysis. Pain 156 (7), 1215–1231. https://doi.org/10.1097/j.pain.0000000000000161.

Apte, A., Kielhofner, G., Paul-Ward, A., Braveman, B., 2005. Therapists' and clients' perceptions of the occupational performance history interview. Occup. Ther. Health. Care 19 (1-2), 173–192. https://doi.org/10.1080/J003v19n01_13.

Bannuru, R.R., Osani, M.C., Vaysbrot, E.E., Arden, N.K., Bennell, K., Bierma-Zeinstra, S.M.A., et al., 2019. OARSI guidelines for the non-surgical management of knee, hip, and polyarticular osteoarthritis. Osteoarthritis. Cartilage 27 (11), 1578–1589. https://doi.org/10.1016/j.joca.2019.06.011.

Birkholtz, M., Aylwin, L., Harman, R.M., 2004. Activity pacing in chronic pain management: one aim, but which method? Part one: introduction and literature review. Br. J. Occup. Ther. 67 (10), 447–452.

Brown, C.A., 2002. Occupational therapists' beliefs regarding treatment options for people with chronic pain. Br. J. Occup. Ther. 65 (9), 398–404.

Fernandes, L., Hagen, K.B., Bijlsma, J.W., Andreassen, O., Christensen, P., Conaghan, P.G., et al., 2013. EULAR recommendations for the non-pharmacological core management of hip and knee osteoarthritis. Ann. Rheum. Dis. 72 (7), 1125–1135. https://doi.org/10.1136/annrheumdis-2012-202745.

Fordyce, W.E., 1976. Behavioral methods for chronic pain and illness. CV Mosby Co, St Louis.

Forestier, R., André-Vert, J., Guillez, P., Coudeyre, E., Lefevre-Colau, M.M., Combe, B., et al., 2009. Non-drug treatment (excluding surgery) in rheumatoid arthritis: clinical practice guidelines. Joint. Bone. Spine 76 (6), 691–698. https://doi.org/10.1016/j.jbspin.2009.01.017.

Guy, L., McKinstry, C., Bruce, C., 2019. Effectiveness of pacing as a learned strategy for people with chronic pain: a systematic review. Am. J. Occup. Ther. 73 (3), 7303205060p7303205061-7303205060p7303205010. https://doi.org/10.5014/ajot.2019.028555.

Hadi, M.A., McHugh, G.A., Closs, S.J., 2019. Impact of chronic pain on patients' quality of life: a comparative mixed-methods study. J. Patient Exp. 6 (2), 133–141. https://doi.org/10.1177/2374373518786013.

Jamieson-Lega, K., Berry, R., Brown, C.A., 2013. Pacing: a concept analysis of the chronic pain intervention. Pain Res. Manag. 18 (4), 207–213. https://doi.org/10.1155/2013/686179.

Khasnabis, C., Mirza, Z., MacLachlan, M., 2015. Opening the GATE to inclusion for people with disabilities. Lancet 386 (10010), 2229–2230. https://doi.org/10.1016/s0140-6736(15)01093-4.

Kielhofner, G., Burke, J.P., 1980. A model of human occupation, part 1. Conceptual framework and content. Am. J. Occup. Ther. 34 (9), 572–581. https://doi.org/10.5014/ajot.34.9.572.

Kielhofner, G., Mallinson, T., Forsyth, K., Lai, J.S., 2001. Psychometric properties of the second version of the Occupational Performance History Interview (OPHI-II). Am. J. Occup. Ther. 55 (3), 260–267. https://doi.org/10.5014/ajot.55.3.260.

Lethem, J., Slade, P.D., Troup, J.D., Bentley, G., 1983. Outline of a fear-avoidance model of exaggerated pain perception--I. Behav. Res. Ther. 21 (4), 401–408. https://doi.org/10.1016/0005-7967(83)90009-8.

López-de-Uralde-Villanueva, I., Muñoz-García, D., Gil-Martínez, A., Pardo-Montero, J., Muñoz-Plata, R., et al., 2016. A systematic review and meta-analysis on the effectiveness of graded activity and graded exposure for chronic nonspecific low back pain Pain Med. 17 (1), 172–188. https://doi.org/10.1111/pme.12882.

Macedo, L.G., Smeets, R.J., Maher, C.G., Latimer, J., McAuley, J.H., 2010. Graded activity and graded exposure for persistent nonspecific low back pain: a systematic review. Phys. Ther. 90 (6), 860–879. https://doi.org/10.2522/ptj.20090303.

Nielson, W.R., Jensen, M.P., Karsdorp, P.A., Vlaeyen, J.W., 2013. Activity pacing in chronic pain: concepts, evidence, and future directions. Clin. J. Pain 29 (5), 461–468. https://doi.org/10.1097/AJP.0b013e3182608561.

Pawar, P., 2017. Model of Human Occupation (MOHO). Available from: https://occupationaltherapyot.com/model-of-human-occupation-moho-frame-of-reference/.

Philips, C., 1988. The psychological management of chronic pain. Springer, New York.

Pincus, T., Vogel, S., Burton, A.K., Santos, R., Field, A.P., 2006. Fear avoidance and prognosis in back pain: a systematic review and synthesis of current evidence. Arthritis. Rheum. 54 (12), 3999–4010. https://doi.org/10.1002/art.22273.

Scott, P.J., Cacich, D., Fulk, M., Michel, K., Whiffen, K., 2017a. Establishing concurrent validity of the Role Checklist Version 2 with the OCAIRS in measurement of participation: a pilot study. Occup. Ther. Int. 2017, 6493472. https://doi.org/10.1155/2017/6493472.

Scott, P.J., McKinney, K., Perron, J., Ruff, E., Smiley, J., 2017b. Measurement of participation: the Role Checklist Version 3: satisfaction and performance. In: Huri, M. (Ed.), Occupational Therapy -Occupation Focused Holistic Practice in Rehabilitation. IntechOpen, London.

Scott, P.J., McKinney, K.G., Perron, J.M., Ruff, E.G., Smiley, J.L., 2019. The revised Role Checklist: improved utility, feasibility, and reliability. OTJR Occup. Particip. Health 39 (1), 56–63. https://doi.org/10.1177/1539449218780618.

Torrance, N., Smith, B.H., Elliott, A.M., Campbell, S.E., Chambers, W.A., Hannaford, P.C., et al., 2011. Potential pain management programmes in primary care. A UK-wide questionnaire and Delphi survey of experts. Fam. Pract. 28 (1), 41–48.

Vlaeyen, J.W.S., Linton, S.J., 2000. Fear-avoidance and its consequences in chronic musculoskeletal pain: a state of the art. Pain 85 (3), 317–332. https://doi.org/10.1016/s0304-3959(99)00242-0.

World Health Organization, 2014. WHO global disability action plan 2014-2021: better health for all people with disability. World Health Organization, Geneva.

Chapter | 11 |

Exercise therapy

Lewis Rawson, Nadine E. Foster, and Melanie A. Holden

LEARNING OBJECTIVES

At the end of this chapter, readers will be able to:
1. Understand principles of exercise prescription.
2. Understand the prevalence and impact of three common musculoskeletal pain problems.
3. Discuss research evidence for exercise as an intervention for persistent musculoskeletal pain.
4. Understand characteristics of successful exercise programmes for patients with pain.

Introduction

Chronic or persistent musculoskeletal (MSK) pain is a major health problem. Modern pain management approaches focus on preventing unnecessary disability and minimising morbidity, following biopsychosocial principles (Jordan et al. 2010). Exercise is a core treatment option within these approaches, reflected in the guidelines from the UK National Institute for Health and Clinical Excellence guidance for chronic pain (NICE 2021a). It includes general exercise, specific body-region exercises for strengthening, flexibility, control and balance, continuing normal physical activities and increasing overall physical activity levels. This chapter discusses the role of exercise in the management of persistent pain, with specific attention to low back pain (LBP), knee pain and hand pain. It considers the particular importance of exercise adherence and its importance for longer-term outcomes for people with persistent pain, before concluding with implications for clinical practice and research.

Definitions and principles

Physical activity is any bodily movement produced by the skeletal muscles that results in energy expenditure (www.cdc.gov/nccdphp/dnpa/physical/terms). Within this, exercise is planned, structured and repetitive movement to maintain or improve physical fitness (e.g. cardiovascular fitness, muscle strength, endurance and flexibility) and psychological wellbeing (ACSM 2021). Therapeutic exercise is the systematic implementation of planned physical movements, postures or activities to remediate or prevent impairments, enhance function, fitness and wellbeing (APTA 2001). The focus of this chapter is on therapeutic exercise for persistent MSK pain, with reference to beneficial general physical activity and lifestyle changes.

A therapeutic exercise programme for someone with persistent MSK pain may have several goals, such as pain reduction, improvement of function, increased muscle strength, endurance or motor control, improved range of movement or flexibility or improved coordination and balance. A collaborative approach is recommended, and goals should be agreed upon with the patient (see Chapter 3). Exercise recommendations should be informed by relevant clinical findings, but also by how the problem is affecting the individual, their general health (including other comorbidities and other MSK pain), previous exercise experience and attitude towards exercise. A number of design variables for the exercise programme must be considered (Fig. 11.1), including the type of exercise prescribed, the volume of exercise (e.g. number of repetitions and sets of a strength exercise, or walking distance),

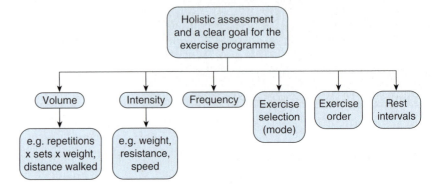

Fig. 11.1 Exercise programme design variables.

exercise intensity (e.g. weight for a resistance exercise or walking speed), frequency (the number of times the programme is completed per week) and duration.

The design variables should be based on physiological principles (see McArdle et al. 1996); Glynn & Fiddler 2009; Hurley & Bearne 2009). They can be summarised as follows:

- Specificity. Any exercise will train a system for the particular task being carried out, e.g. strength training effects will be specific to the muscle groups used, as well as the range and speed of the exercise. Exercises must therefore be chosen appropriately.
- Overload. To achieve a training effect, a system must be exercised at a level beyond which it is normally accustomed to. Achieving the appropriate overload for an individual requires a careful choice of variables, e.g. frequency, intensity, duration and mode of exercise. In patients with persistent pain, this may produce symptoms and psychological resistance, so a tailored behavioural approach may be more appropriate (Åsenlöf et al. 2009).
- Adaptation. The system being exercised will gradually adapt to the overload or training stimulus, for as long as the training stimulus continues to be increased. A limit may be reached where the tissue or system can no longer adapt further.
- Individuality. Different individuals will respond to a given exercise training stimulus in different ways and have exercise preferences based on many factors. Exercise programmes should meet the individual's preferences, capabilities and needs.
- Reversibility. The beneficial effects of exercise begin to be lost as soon as regular training stops, in a similar timeframe as it takes to train the system.

As mentioned, psychological factors must be considered when prescribing exercise for pain patients, because effort and determination are required to realise its benefits. These factors include motivation, self-efficacy to exercise or confidence in the ability to exercise, and personal or internal control (Bandura 1977; Friedrich et al. 2005; McAuley 1992; Marcus et al. 1992). Patient education and coaching alongside the therapeutic exercise programme is therefore

important, to increase understanding of the (pain) problem, challenge unhelpful beliefs and enhance motivation and confidence. These aspects can be enhanced by taking into consideration personal preferences (e.g. for individual or group-based exercise), potential benefits of peer support and social interaction, exercise tailored to the needs of the individual, agreeing specific and meaningful personal short- and long-term goals, and the role of supervision, review and positive reinforcement (Åsenlöf et al. 2009).

Within a biopsychosocial model, goals of an exercise programme should include achievement of specific functional tasks. The required combination of strength, endurance, control, range of movement and balance should be reflected in the choice of exercise, to optimise the chance of carry-over into activities of daily living. It is important to exercise regularly, i.e. at least 2 to 3 times per week, so usually a home exercise programme is required, tailored to the individual and adapted for their home environment and lifestyle. New exercises are started slowly, increased gradually and performed moderately.

The following three sections consider exercise for the most common types of persistent MSK pain.

Example 1: Exercise for persistent nonspecific LBP

The problem

LBP is a very common condition, with a lifetime prevalence as high as 84% (Walker 2000). In the United Kingdom, LBP is the fourth most common reason for consulting a general practitioner and the most common MSK reason. An estimated 6%–9% of people registered with a GP in the United Kingdom consult for LBP every year (Croft et al. 1998; Dunn & Croft 2005), equating to approximately five million people per year (Maniadakis & Gray 2000). Many people also seek care for LBP from MSK therapists such as physiotherapists and osteopaths. LBP is responsible for large personal, societal and financial burdens as many patients with LBP develop persistent pain with a relapsing and recurrent pattern to their symptoms, with implications for their ability to work and take part in social activities. The proportion of patients who continue to experience back pain 12 months after onset is reported to be in the region of 42%–75% (Hestbaek et al. 2003).

It is recognised that only a small proportion of persistent back pain can be attributed to a specific underlying disease or pathology. For patients presenting in primary care with LBP, approximately 1% have serious spinal pathology such as a systemic inflammatory condition or cancer, and around a further 5% have nerve root pain/radicular pain (Waddell 2004). These patients often require a specific diagnosis. Management frequently involves onward referral to secondary care clinicians such as rheumatologists and orthopaedic surgeons. However, most patients have no such pathology as mentioned, so they are often categorised as having *nonspecific LBP*. The evidence presented below focuses on exercise for adults with persistent nonspecific LBP.

Clinical guidelines

Clinical guidelines for the management of LBP have been developed in several countries. The quality of clinical guidelines for the management of LBP has been improving (Bouwmeester et al. 2009). Although some inconsistencies may remain (O'Connell et al. 2017), exercise is recommended in all guidelines for persistent LBP (Dagenais et al. 2010). The most recent UK publication is NICE (2021b) guidance for LBP and sciatica in over 16s. It recommends advising all patients presenting with persistent nonspecific LBP to exercise, be physically active and to carry on with normal activities as much as possible. In addition, exercise is recommended as the core treatment for back pain, should self-management not prove successful. Exercise programmes may include biomechanical, aerobic, mind–body or a combination of approaches (NICE 2021b).

Exercise for persistent nonspecific LBP: the evidence

Exercise therapies are the most widely used type of non-invasive interventions for the management of LBP, with a large body of evidence supporting its use. Systematic reviews of randomised controlled trials (RCTs) of exercise interventions consistently report exercise as achieving equivalent or better outcomes for patients than comparison interventions.

A systematic review by Hayden et al. (2005a) included 43 RCTs (3907 individuals) and investigated the effectiveness of exercise in people with persistent nonspecific LBP. It found strong evidence (consistent findings in multiple high-quality trials) that exercise therapy is as effective as other conservative interventions, although evidence that exercise therapy is superior to other interventions was conflicting, i.e. there were inconsistent findings in multiple trials. The meta-analyses showed pooled mean improvements in pain of 10.2 points (95% confidence interval (CI): 1.31–19.09) compared to no treatment, and 5.93 points (95% CI: 2.21–9.65) compared to other conservative interventions. Pooled mean improvements in function were 3.00 points (95% CI: 0.53–6.48) compared to no treatment, and 2.37 points (95% CI: 0.74–4.0) compared to other conservative interventions. The exercise interventions that showed better outcomes than comparison interventions were generally based in healthcare rather than general population settings, were designed and delivered individually, and commonly included strengthening and trunk stability exercises.

A later systematic review included only higher-quality studies of exercise therapy (Hettinga et al. 2007). The results suggested that the inclusion of smaller RCTs in systematic reviews leads to overestimation of effectiveness. The higher-quality studies supported the use of exercise, particularly strengthening exercises, aerobic exercises, general exercises, hydrotherapy and McKenzie exercises for individuals with persistent pain. Further support that exercise is beneficial for LBP is provided by the systematic review by Macedo et al. (2009), which also suggested that no one type of exercise appears superior. Motor control exercise for LBP was superior to minimal intervention, with mean differences in pain scores at short term, medium term and long term of −14.3 (95% CI: −20.4 to −8.1), −13.6 (95% CI: −22.4 to −4.1) and −14.4 (95% CI: −23.1 to −5.7), respectively. Improvements in function were seen but at long-term follow-up only, with a difference to the comparison groups of −10.8 (95% CI: −18.7 to −2.8). However, motor control exercise was not more effective than other forms of exercise for LBP.

A further comprehensive review of RCTs for persistent nonspecific LBP included 37 RCTs (3957 individuals) (van Middelkoop et al. 2010). Compared to usual care, exercise therapy improved posttreatment pain intensity and disability, and long-term function. The review concluded that evidence from RCTs demonstrates that exercise is effective for persistent LBP, that the effects tend to be small. In line with previous reviews, it concluded that there was no evidence that one particular type of exercise is clearly more effective than others and that it was unclear which patients benefit most from which type of exercise. Of 11 studies that compared different exercise interventions, only two studies found statistically significant differences in pain and disability outcomes: aerobic exercise was found to be better than a flexion exercise regime in one low-quality study and motor control exercise was shown to be slightly better than general exercises in one high-quality study. Pooling of data was not undertaken due to the heterogeneity of the interventions in the studies.

A Cochrane systematic review of 249 RCTs of exercise for chronic low back pain (CLBP) in adults reported that exercise therapy is more beneficial than usual care, no care or placebo comparisons (Hayden et al. 2021a, b). This included therapist-prescribed, group and aerobic exercise programmes. Exercise resulted in clinically important improvements in pain (95% CI: –12.6 to –5.6) and function (95% CI: –8.3 to –5.3), but these did not meet the minimal clinically important thresholds due to the risk of bias.

In addition to specific exercise regimes, graded activity and graded exposure have been shown to be superior to minimal intervention in both the short and medium terms on improving pain (pooled mean change at short term: –6.2 (95% CI: –9.4 to –3.0), medium term: –5.5 (95% CI: –9.9 to –1.0)) and disability (pooled mean change at short term: –6.5 (95% CI: –10.1 to –3.0), medium term –3.9 (95% CI: –7.4 to –0.4)) in individuals with persistent nonspecific LBP (Macedo et al. 2010). However, graded activity and exposure were not better compared to other forms of exercise.

Effect of exercise on work disability

A systematic review has shown that intensive exercise interventions that include aerobic capacity, muscle strength, endurance and coordination training which have some relation to the work environment can reduce the number of sick days in employed individuals with persistent LBP (Schonstein et al. 2003). It must be noted that the interventions included in this review also incorporated cognitive behavioural approaches. More recently, a systematic review and meta-analysis of 23 RCTs showed a statistically significant effect of exercise on work disability in the long term (odds ratio 0.66; 95% CI: 0.48–0.92) but not in the short or medium term, compared to usual care or other exercise interventions (Oesch et al. 2010). As before, there was no evidence of the superiority of any particular type of exercise. In addition, a small effect on sickness absence was found in pooled results (mean difference of –0.18 (95% CI: –0.37 to 0.0)) of five studies of physical conditioning in workers with persistent nonspecific LBP, although conflicting results were found when compared to other exercise interventions (Schaafsma et al. 2010). Hayden et al. (2021a, b) found that only 14% of studies that met inclusion criteria for a recent Cochrane review included outcomes regarding work status, so no conclusions could be drawn in this regard.

Factors improving outcomes with exercise

Exercise therapy incorporates a wide range of heterogeneous interventions which can vary in terms of duration, frequency, setting, dosage and level or absence of supervision. A Bayesian meta-regression of 43 trials examined the characteristics of exercise interventions providing the best outcomes were examined (Hayden et al. 2005b). It concluded that exercise interventions were more effective when individually designed rather than standardised, when exercise programmes were supervised and when carried out over longer time periods. A separate examination of the impact of a variety of study characteristics on the small but significant improvements of pain and disability seen in included trials showed that only exercise dosage was significantly associated with effect sizes (Ferreira et al. 2010).

Hayden et al. (2021b), in a meta-analysis of 217 RCTs, reviewed the efficacy of different forms of exercise for CLBP. They reported that although Pilates, McKenzie and functional restoration programmes may be the most beneficial forms of exercise, all forms of exercise therapy, with the exception of stretching alone, resulted in clinical improvement. The study recommended consideration of a form of exercise that the patient enjoys, with the goal of improving adherence.

Safety of exercise in persistent NSLBP

Exercise in persistent nonspecific LBP is safe. No safety concerns have been raised in the large number of RCTs, although adverse events are rarely reported. Hayden et al. (2021a, b) reported that the rate of adverse events, which included muscular soreness and increased back pain symptoms, was 0.02 to 0.6 per person.

Summary

In summary, therapeutic exercise is the most commonly used conservative intervention for the management of individuals with persistent nonspecific LBP. The variable quality of RCTs presents challenges to interpreting the evidence with many published studies having moderate to high risk of bias. Exercise therapy is effective for managing individuals with persistent nonspecific LBP, but which individuals benefit most from which exercise is still uncertain. In addition, adherence to exercise regimes is poor, so strategies to improve adherence should be considered. This issue is considered later in this chapter.

Example 2: Exercise for knee pain in older adults

The problem

Knee pain is a common MSK complaint caused by acute injuries such as meniscal tears and ligament ruptures, as well as chronic conditions such as osteoarthritis. An estimated 25% of adults aged 40 years and over suffer with

CASE STUDY 11.1

Low back pain

A patient with persistent LBP attends an initial appointment with you. His history and clinical examination findings are presented here.

A 48-year-old warehouse worker has a 6-month history of LBP with some radiation to the left buttock and thigh. He finds difficulty with prolonged flexion activities but also gets increasing discomfort if he walks for longer than 20 minutes. He has minimal sleep disturbance when the pain is severe. The pain started after a few busy days at work, 'picking and packing'. Since then the pain has varied greatly in intensity and location. When the pain has been severe, the patient has taken 1 to 4 days off work. He has found that 'taking it easy' helps to settle the pain. His lifestyle outside work is sedentary and he has no active hobbies other than occasional gardening. His general health is fair although he is on medication for hypertension and high cholesterol.

Today he describes his pain as 4 out of 10 in the lower back and 2 out of 10 in the left buttock. On physical examination, he has some limitation of movement into flexion, extension and left-side bend. He has local tenderness across the lower lumbar spine and left paravertebral soft tissues. Neurological testing is normal.

Based upon the evidence presented, please think about the following:
1. What type/s of exercise would you prescribe for this patient and why?
2. How would you deliver the exercise programme?
3. What dose of exercise would you advise (intensity, frequency and duration)?

knee pain (Chia et al. 2016; Peat et al. 2001a). This prevalence is likely to rise with an ageing population (Wilmoth 2000) and increasing levels of obesity (James 2008). Most knee pain in older adults is likely to be attributable to osteoarthritis (OA). Traditionally, OA was believed to be a progressive, degenerative disease, but it is now viewed as a dynamic repair process involving all joint tissues including cartilage, bone, ligament and muscle (NICE 2014; Peat et al. 2001b). X-ray changes may not correlate well with clinical symptoms of OA, making diagnosis difficult (Peat et al. 2006). This is supported by Turkiewicz et al. (2015), who found a 25% prevalence of radiographic OA in a random sample of 10,000 56- to 88-year-olds, with only 15% reporting symptoms. Recent UK national guidelines propose the following working diagnosis of peripheral joint OA: patients aged 45 and over, with persistent joint pain that is worse with use, and morning stiffness lasting no more than half an hour (NICE 2014). The evidence synthesis in this chapter focuses on exercise for knee pain generally, with the assumption that most older adults with this condition will have a clinical problem of OA, some of whom with radiographic changes.

Persistent knee pain can have a considerable impact on the individual and is one of the leading causes of disability worldwide (NICE 2014). Pain, joint stiffness, instability, swelling and muscle weakness can contribute to functional limitations, psychological distress and reduced quality of life (Bennell & Hinman 2011; Hurley 2003; Jordan et al. 2003; Neame & Doherty 2005). It has wider societal implications, with £43 million spent on community services for OA between 1999 and 2000 in the United Kingdom (NICE 2008). Each year 2 million adults visit their GP because of OA in the United Kingdom (Arthritis Research Campaign 2002).

Clinical guidelines and safety

All guidelines for optimisation of healthcare for patients with knee pain recommend exercise as frontline treatment (Zhang et al. 2007a). The most recent UK guidelines state that three core treatments should be considered first for every patient with OA: advice and education to enhance understanding of the condition; weight loss if the person is overweight or obese; and activity and exercise, including local muscle strengthening and general aerobic fitness (NICE 2014). The MOVE set of evidence-based recommendations that address specific questions about the role of exercise in knee and hip OA are provided in Table 11.1 (Roddy et al. 2005a).

The MOVE recommendations also explored safety (Roddy et al. 2005a). No direct evidence was found regarding contraindications to exercise therapy and serious adverse events were rare. Quicke et al. (2015) undertook a systematic and narrative review of 49 studies, with 8920 participants. They also concluded that exercise is a safe treatment, with no serious adverse events or radiographic evidence of OA progression. A systematic review of high-quality prospective cohort studies explored specifically whether exercise can cause knee OA and associated knee pain (Bosomworth 2009). Knee problems were found to be as common in those who exercise as those who didn't, and there was no increase in the rate of progression of knee problems in individuals who exercised compared with those who did not. Although Tveit et al. (2012) reported that OA progression to arthroplasty of the hip or knee was higher in retired male athletes compared to a matched sample group, they noted that previous trauma played a role in this, so the finding is unlikely to apply to therapeutic exercise.

Exercise for knee pain: the evidence

A large body of evidence supports the use of exercise for older adults with knee pain. Uthman et al. (2014) in a systematic review and meta-analysis concluded that as of

Table 11.1 Summary of the 10 propositions included in the exercise recommendations for hip and knee OA

Proposition	Category of evidence (1-41)	Strength of recommendation (A-D2)
Both strengthening and aerobic exercise can reduce pain and improve function and health status in patients with hip and knee OA	Knee 1B Hip 4	A C (extrapolated from knee OA)
There are few contraindications to the prescription of strengthening or aerobic exercise in patients with hip or knee OA	4	C (extrapolated from adverse event data)
Prescription of both general (aerobic fitness training) and local (strengthening) exercises is an essential, core aspect of management for every patient with hip or knee OA	4	D
Exercise therapy for OA of the hip or knee should be individualized and patient-centred, taking into account factors such as age, co-morbidity and overall mobility	4	D
To be effective, exercise programmes should include advice and education to promote a positive lifestyle change with an increase in physical activity	4* 1B	D A
Group exercise and home exercise are equally effective and patient preference should be considered	1A** 4	A D
Adherence is the principal predictor of long-term outcome from exercise in patients with hip or knee OA	4	D
Strategies to improve and maintain adherence should be adopted, e.g. long-term monitoring/review and inclusion of spouse/family in exercise	1B	A
The effectiveness of exercise is independent of the presence or severity of radiographic findings	4	Not recommended
Improvements in muscle strength and proprioception (balance) gained from exercise programmes may reduce the progression of hip and knee OA	4	D

*Category 1B evidence that advice and education can promote lifestyle change and increase physical activity. Category 4 evidence that such techniques are required for exercise programmes to be effective.

**Category 1A evidence to support both group and home exercise with no clear evidence of superiority of one over the other, therefore patient preference should be considered (category 4 evidence).

1. Categories of evidence:
1A: Meta-analysis of RCTs 1B: At least one RCT
2A: At least one clinical trial without randomization
2B: At least one type of quasi-experimental study
3:   Descriptive studies (comparative, correlation, case-control)
4:   Expert committee reports/opinions and/or clinical opinion of respected authorities
2.   Strength of recommendation
A: Directly based on category 1 evidence
B: Directly based on category 2 evidence or extrapolated recommendation from category 1 evidence
C: Directly based on category 3 evidence or extrapolated recommendation from category 1 or 2 evidence
D: Directly based on category 4 evidence or extrapolated recommendation from category 1 or 2 or 3 evidence
Reprinted from Roddy E, Zhang W, Doherty M, et al (2005) Evidence-based recommendations for the role of exercise in the management of osteoarthritis of the hip or knee - the MOVE consensus, *Rheumatology;* 44(1), with permission from Oxford University Press.

2002, there was sufficient evidence to support exercise, vs no exercise, in lower limb osteoarthritis. Additional trials are unlikely to overturn this positive result (Uthman et al. 2014; Verhagen et al. 2019). Not only has exercise been shown to improve function and reduce pain (Fransen et al. 2015; Fransen & McConnell 2008; Roddy et al. 2005a), it can also improve physical performance including walking distance and stair climbing (e.g. Foroughi et al. 2011), improve muscle strength, increase joint range of motion and walking speed (e.g. Huang et al. 2003, 2005;

Salacinski et al. 2012), increase self-efficacy (e.g. Foster et al. 2007) and reduce the risk of cardiovascular disease (Haskell et al. 2007; Nelson et al. 2007). Current evidence is summarised later, focusing on exercise type, delivery, dose and safety.

Type of exercise

Many RCTs have explored the effectiveness of exercise for older adults with knee pain including both general aerobic exercise such as walking, cycling and tai chi, local knee exercises including range of movement exercises and muscle strengthening programmes, balance and coordination programmes, and exercise incorporated into wider self-management programmes. A recent Cochrane review of 54 trials (3913 participants) demonstrated the overall beneficial effects of land-based exercise for pain and function (Fransen et al. 2015). A meta-analysis found standardised mean differences (SMDs) of 0.49 for pain and 0.52 for physical function, effect sizes similar to those found in two other meta-analyses exploring the efficacy of exercise for hip and knee pain (Fransen & McConnel 2008; Zhang et al. 2007b, 2010). Although these benefits are small to moderate, they are derived from high-quality trials and are comparable to reported estimates for current simple analgesics and nonsteroidal antiinflammatory drugs (Fransen et al. 2015).

Roddy et al. (2005b) completed a systematic review including 13 RCTs to compare the efficacy of aerobic walking and home-based quadriceps exercise in patients with knee pain. Meta-analyses for aerobic walking demonstrated a pooled effect size of 0.52 for pain and 0.46 for disability. Effect sizes for pain and disability for home-based quadriceps strengthening exercises were 0.32 and 0.32, respectively. No advantage of one form of exercise over the other was found on indirect comparison of pooled data. The researchers therefore recommended allowing patients to choose their type of exercise because of the potential to improve exercise adherence. An additional systematic review of 18 RCTs (2832 participants) investigated the effectiveness of resistance training for knee pain in older adults (Lange et al. 2008). Interventions incorporated dynamic and isotonic training, machine-based resistance training, free weights, elastic resistance bands and/ or other items around the home (e.g. chairs, stairs, etc.). The number of sets of exercises ranged from 1 to 10 (most studies prescribed three sets), repetitions of each exercise ranged from 3 to 20 per set and three training sessions per week were most commonly prescribed (range 2–7 weekly sessions). Overall 50%–75% of the studies included in the review found knee symptoms, physical function and strength to improve by clinically meaningful amounts with resistance training when compared with usual care. Specifics of the resistance training (modality, duration, volume, frequency,

intensity) did not appear to be related to patient outcomes (Lange et al. 2008).

Delivery of exercise

Interventions in RCTs have been delivered individually, in groups and in various settings, including patients' own homes, different community settings and healthcare environments. Fransen et al. (2015) explored the influence of the delivery of exercise (home vs supervised individual or class-based exercise sessions) on pain and function. Both home and supervised exercise programmes significantly improved pain and functional status in participants with knee pain. Although the home exercises had consistently lower effect sizes than supervised exercises (either on a one-to-one basis or within a group), the differences were not statistically significant, perhaps explained by some element of supervision in most home exercise programmes. Hurley et al. (2018), in a Cochrane review of 21 studies of group programmes of OA knee, concluded that participation may positively influence people's beliefs regarding exercise, reported pain (–6%, –1.25 points on visual analogue scale (VAS)), physical health (+5.6%), mental health (+2.4%) and quality of life (+7.9%). Although the improvements were arguably modest, the review supports the proposition within the MOVE exercise recommendations (see Table 11.1) that 'group exercise and home exercise are equally effective and patient preference should be considered' (Roddy et al. 2005a).

Gohir et al. (2021) investigated delivery of an internet-based exercise programme, comparing against usual self-management advice. It was reported that upon completion of the 6-week programme, which included daily exercise and informative texts, patients had seen improvements in pain levels and functional tests. The follow-up duration was short, so further study assessing long-term efficacy is required to assess this increasingly popular method of delivering care, especially since the COVID-19 pandemic.

Exercise dose

Evidence about the optimal dose of exercise for older adults with knee pain, including its frequency, intensity and duration, is currently lacking (Bennell et al. 2010; Fransen et al. 2015). A Cochrane review of the effectiveness of different exercise intensities for OA identified only one small RCT that tested the efficacy of low-intensity versus high-intensity stationary bicycling for people with knee pain. High- and low-intensity aerobic exercises were equally effective in improving function, gait, pain and aerobic capacity (Brosseau et al. 2003). An additional review of the literature identified one subsequent RCT that compared high- and low-intensity strengthening programmes for older adults with knee pain. This also concluded that both exercise intensities were beneficial but that neither was clearly superior for pain, function, walking time and muscle strength over 8 weeks (Bennell et al. 2010; Jan et al. 2008).

To the authors' knowledge, no RCTs have specifically investigated the optimal frequency and duration of exercise for older adults with knee pain. Within their Cochrane review exploring the efficacy of land-based exercise, Fransen et al. (2015) conducted sensitivity analyses to explore the effect of the number of supervised exercise sessions, dichotomised as those with less than 12 directly supervised sessions and those with 12 or more, on pain and function for older adults with knee pain. Both categories achieved significant treatment benefits in terms of pain and function, but the effect sizes for programmes with fewer than 12 supervised sessions were considered small, and the effect sizes for exercise programmes with at least 12 directly supervised sessions were moderate. This difference was statistically significant, so the authors concluded that most people with knee pain need some form of ongoing monitoring or supervision for optimal outcomes from exercise.

Short-term and long-term effects of exercise for knee pain

A systematic review explored the long-term effectiveness of exercise therapy in patients with hip and knee pain, defined as 6 months or more after the treatment period ended (Pisters et al. 2007). Eleven RCTs were included, incorporating a variety of modes of delivery of exercise and different types of exercises delivered at different doses. Overall, the small to moderate effects of exercise declined over time and finally disappeared at long-term follow-up, and there was strong evidence for no long-term effect of exercise on pain or function. However, adding booster sessions in the period after treatment had a positive influence on maintenance of long-term effects (Pisters et al. 2007). One reason for this may be the effect of booster sessions on exercise adherence over time. Pisters et al. (2010) went on to investigate this further, concluding that improved ongoing adherence and increased levels of physical activity improve the long-term efficacy of exercise programmes in people with OA hip/knee.

Summary

In summary, therapeutic exercise is a recommended core treatment for knee pain in older adults. Evidence suggests that many different types of exercise, of both high and low intensities, delivered in groups or to individuals, are effective and safe, for older adults with knee pain. Basing the prescription of exercise on the preferences of individual

patients may therefore be the optimal approach. The challenge remains to find effective ways to maintain the beneficial effects of exercise over time.

CASE STUDY 11.2

Knee pain in older adults

A patient with knee pain attends an initial appointment with you. Her history and clinical examination findings are presented here.

A 65-year-old woman has a 3-year history of left knee pain, which was of insidious onset and has gradually worsened over time. She is a retired shop manageress and usually enjoys swimming, but this has become difficult due to her knee problem. Her general health is good, despite being overweight and suffering from mild hypertension. She also has pain in both hands.

Today she rates the intensity of her knee pain as 6 out of 10. Descending stairs, bending and rising from sitting all aggravate her knee pain. She has some difficulty when walking and has started to use a stick outdoors. Her knee is stiff first thing in the morning and after staying in one position for too long. She finds some relief from an antiinflammatory gel and takes up to three 200-mg ibuprofen tablets per day.

Despite not having an X-ray she feels her problem is due to arthritis as her father suffered from this. It is her first visit to a healthcare professional and she is optimistic about its outcome. On examination, the left knee has a mild effusion and a valgus alignment. Flexion is limited and the quadriceps are weak. The joint line is tender on palpation. No other examination findings are remarkable.

Based upon the evidence presented, and the basic physiological and psychological principles of exercise training, please think about the following:

1. What type/s of exercise would you prescribe to this patient?
2. How would you deliver the exercise programme?
3. What dose of exercise would you advise (intensity, frequency and duration)?

Example 3: Exercise for hand pain in older adults

The problem

Hand pain is common (Dahaghin et al. 2005a; Mannoni et al. 2000; Oliveria et al. 1995). A large survey of older adults with MSK hand problems in North Staffordshire, UK, found 1-year prevalence of hand problems of 47% and 1-month prevalence of hand pain was estimated at 30.8% (Dziedzic et al. 2007). Severe hand-related

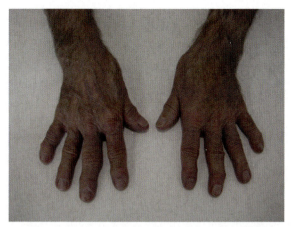

Fig. 11.2 Photograph of individual with hand osteoarthritis.

disability affected 12.3% and was significantly more common in females than in males, and it increased in prevalence to the oldest age groups (ibid). Coggon et al. (2019) investigated risk factors for wrist and hand pain in a cohort of 1373 patients. They reported that patient factors (e.g. multisite pain and psychosocial factors, job dissatisfaction and time pressure at work) and biomechanical factors (e.g. keyboard use, age (>50) and female gender) were significant risk factors.

In the United Kingdom, an estimated 4.4 million people have X-ray evidence of moderate-to-severe OA of their hands (Fig. 11.2) (Arthritis Research UK 2002; ARMA 2004). Dahaghin et al. (2005b) reported that 67% and 54.8% of females and males aged >55 had radiographic evidence of OA in at least one joint of the hand. In-depth interviews with patients identified the personal impact and loss of independence caused by OA of the hand with disruption of day-to-day activities such as washing, toileting and dressing, together with psychological and emotional distress (Hill et al. 2007, 2010). Mattap et al. (2021), in a prospective, population-based study of 519 patients, found that an increasing number of involved joints was associated with higher reported pain scores and reduced function. Despite this impact, many sufferers never seek medical advice (Dahaghin et al 2005b; Zhang et al. 2002).

Clinical guidelines

A Cochrane review of exercise for hand pain found only seven eligible studies, two of which had high dropout rates (Østerås et al. 2017). The exercise interventions lacked heterogeneity, with a wide range of content, dosage and frequency. They concluded that exercise may have a small benefit on pain symptoms, but that its impact on quality-of-life measures was unclear. The European League Against Rheumatism (EULAR) OA Task Force developed recommendations for the management of hand OA using an evidence-based format involving both a systematic review of research evidence and expert consensus (Kloppenburg et al. 2019). They arguably included a broader range of literature than the Cochrane review (Østerås et al. 2017), but also had a higher risk of bias. The EULAR guidelines recommend that the optimal management of hand OA requires a combination of non-pharmacological and pharmacological treatments, individualised to patients' requirements. Specifically, education concerning joint protection (how to avoid adverse mechanical factors) together with an exercise regimen (involving both range of motion and strengthening exercises) is recommended for all patients with hand OA. This recommendation was based mainly on expert opinion and research evidence from a trial of 40 patients with hand OA (Stamm et al. 2002). The trial compared active treatment by an occupational therapist—a 45-minute education on joint protection techniques along with 15-minute instruction on range of movement exercise with an instruction leaflet. The study outcome was at 3 months. It is difficult to ascertain the specific clinical benefit of hand exercises alone. The two elements of treatment were not directly compared, so it is not known whether the benefit was derived from the range of motion exercise, the joint protect programme or both. These questions were investigated by Dziedzic et al. (2015) in an RCT of 252 participants, which concluded that occupational therapists can support self-management of hand pain, with statistically significant differences for joint protection/exercise versus no treatment. However, the threshold for minimal important clinical difference was not met for joint protection and there was no statistically significant benefit in instructed exercise at 6 and 12 months.

Exercise for hand OA: the evidence

In addition to Cochrane and EULAR guidelines, there are six systematic reviews of nonsurgical treatments for hand OA (Beasley et al. 2019; Kjeken et al. 2011; Mahendira & Towheed 2009; Moe et al. 2009; Towheed 2005; Valdes & Marik 2010). Valdes & Marik (2010) examined the quality of the evidence regarding hand therapy interventions between 1986 and 2009. Nine studies (369 participants) examined the role of exercise in the treatment of patients with hand OA, of which eight found that subjects who performed exercises demonstrated gains in grip strength ranging from 1.94 kg to a 25% improvement over baseline. However, the studies of exercise were of moderate methodological quality and provided only limited support for exercise in increasing hand strength and decreasing pain. Due to limitations of existing studies, it is difficult to be certain of the clinical benefit of specific doses and intensities of hand exercises for hand OA.

Beasley et al. (2019) reviewed conservative management of finger OA in their systematic review. They

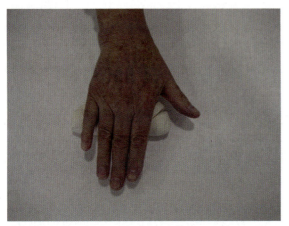

Fig. 11.3 Specific hand exercises can include dough squeezing and rolling.

reported that a range of measures could be beneficial, with moderate evidence to support strength exercise, range of motion exercises and joint protection advice. There was some evidence to support paraffin wax, balneotherapy and magnetotherapy. It is important to note that the authors cited a paucity of evidence as a significant limitation. Literature ranged from RCTs to case studies, potentially limiting generalisability to patient cohorts. New studies may provide further evidence.

Although recommendations support the use of simple, easily accessible interventions to manage hand pain, patients are not receiving this care in practice (Porcheret et al. 2007). The first approach to improve the primary care of patients with OA is the integration of and continued support for self-management strategies (Dziedzic et al. 2009). Encouraging the use of self-management strategies is particularly important for patients with mild hand OA. For the reduction of pain, improvement of activities of daily living and increase of grip strength, the use of exercise, joint protection education and heat modalities should be considered (Valdes & Marik 2010). Specific hand exercises can include dough squeezing and rolling (Fig. 11.3), and active range of movement exercises (Fig. 11.4), performed at a low pain level (ibid).

Summary

In summary, therapeutic exercise is a recommended treatment for hand pain in older adults. There is moderate evidence supporting hand exercises for pain reduction, increased grip strength, improved function and improved range of movement (Valdes & Marik 2010). Prescribing exercise alongside other self-management strategies, joint protection education and heat therapy is likely to provide additional benefits. Unfortunately, specific clinical benefit of hand exercise programmes alone are under researched at present.

CASE STUDY 11.3

Hand pain in older adults

A patient with hand pain attends an initial appointment with you. His history and clinical examination findings are presented here.

A 54-year-old farmer presents with pain radiating down his left thumb and is left handed. He has difficulty with everyday tasks, from holding a hammer to grasping a button on his shirt. He finds these difficulties very frustrating and hates asking his wife for help with simple jobs. His GP has given him topical antiinflammatory gel to rub on his thumb base and has referred him to occupational therapy for advice on joint protection and looking after his hand joints. His GP has mentioned that a steroid joint injection may be indicated but has recommended hand exercises in the first instance. On examination, there's evidence of subluxation and adduction of the carpometacarpal (CMC) joint of both hands, prominent nodes and enlargements of all interphalangeal joints, and thenar muscle wasting of the left hand. On palpation, bony changes of the left CMC joint are confirmed and there's some evidence of changes in the right CMC joint. Palpation of the left CMC joint provokes pain. There are no signs of Dupuytren's contracture, carpal tunnel syndrome or triggering of tendons on testing, so his signs and symptoms can be attributed to hand OA.

Based upon the evidence presented, please think about the following:
1. What type/s of exercise would you prescribe for this patient and why?
2. How would you deliver the exercise programme?
3. What dose of exercise would you advise (intensity, frequency and duration)?

Exercise adherence

Exercise is a core management option for those with persistent pain, so long-term adherence is important. Exercise adherence can be defined as *the extent to which a person's behaviour corresponds with agreed recommendations from a healthcare provider* (WHO 2003, from Jordan et al. 2010). The importance of adherence in determining clinical outcomes from exercise programmes for chronic MSK pain is increasingly recognised (NICE 2008; Roddy et al. 2005a, b). Studies of patients with LBP and knee pain have shown that those with higher adherence levels obtain significantly better improvements in pain and function (Ettinger et al. 1997; Petrella et al. 2000; Hayden et al. 2005b). There is some evidence of dose–response effects (Thomas et al. 2002). There is also evidence that

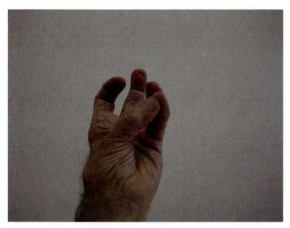

Fig. 11.4 Specific hand exercises can include active range of movement exercises.

adherence to exercise programmes and physical activity is associated with greater long-term improvements in pain, physical function and self-perceived effect after treatment period has ended (Pisters et al. 2010). It is therefore important to ensure that therapeutic exercise programmes facilitate early engagement and longer-term adherence, in ways that work for the individual in pain. In the final section of this chapter, the following questions are addressed:

1. How can exercise adherence be assessed?
2. What factors can influence exercise adherence?
3. How can adherence to exercise be enhanced?

Assessment of exercise adherence

No gold standard for assessing adherence to exercise exists (Treuth 2002) and adherence can change over time and vary per type of exercise. This makes the accurate assessment of exercise adherence challenging. Within clinical settings, when time is often limited, physiotherapists frequently report measuring exercise adherence by observing a patient's exercise technique or by relying on self report (Pisters et al. 2010). These methods have disadvantages. Self-reported exercise levels may be overreported by the patient to be viewed positively by the healthcare professional (Marks & Allegrante 2005). Exercises performed under direct observation may not reflect accurately how the exercises are performed at home (Meichenbaum & Turk 1987). Use of a daily exercise diary, an example of which can be found in Box 11.1, may overcome some of these problems. Use of a diary might have an additional positive influence on exercise adherence (Hughes et al. 2004). However, it still requires patients to be motivated to complete it accurately (Melanson & Freedson 1996). An objective assessment of exercise adherence,

e.g. a pedometer (to measure step count) or accelerometer (to measure total activity count), can reduce the biases associated with self-report data (Paul et al. 2007). Their relatively high cost, sometimes complex data interpretation requirements and inability to capture information on all domains of exercise behaviour, made these inappropriate or difficult for clinicians and researchers in the past (Myers & Midence 1998; Paul et al. 2007). However, developments in smartphone and smartwatch technology have made objective measures of adherence accessible to most people.

Factors that influence exercise adherence

Nonadherence to exercise programmes may be unintentional, e.g. the individual may forget to do the exercise, be unable to follow the recommendations or decide not to follow treatment as agreed as a result of rational decision-making (Horne 1997). Adherence behaviour is a complex phenomenon influenced by attitudes, beliefs and many other factors. The WHO (2003) propose five interacting dimensions that may influence adherence to medical regimes into patient-related factors, social and economic factors, healthcare team and system-related factors, condition-related factors, and therapy-related factors (Box 11.2). Rather than blaming patients for nonadherence, healthcare professionals need to assess how best to support them to maintain exercise and active lifestyles over the longer-term.

Strategies to enhance adherence to exercise

A Cochrane systematic review summarised interventions that can improve adherence to exercise and physical activity in adults with chronic MSK pain (Jordan et al. 2010). The review included 42 trials (8243 participants) and individual trials were grouped into five categories, based on characteristics of their interventions, that explored the effect of the following on exercise adherence: type of exercise therapy or physical activity; delivery of exercise; exercise combined with a specific adherence component; self-management programmes; and interventions based on cognitive and/or behavioural principles. Eighteen of the 42 trials indicated that the intervention improved adherence to exercise or physical activity. Strategies that positively influenced exercise adherence included:

- Adherence-enhancing strategies such as problem-solving, goal setting, systematic feedback, skills building, individualisation of exercise (e.g. choice of activity and exercise setting), reinforcement messages, exercise diaries and pedometers
- Supervision of exercise

BOX 11.1 **Example exercise diary**

Instructions

Please:

1. Try to fill your diary in regularly.

2. Every time you complete a set of exercises place a tick in the appropriate box.

3. Record how hard you felt the exercises were (using the scale on the next page).

4. There is a comments box for you to write any thoughts or feelings you have each day. For example, you could record if the exercises are becoming easier, or if you find any exercises particularly difficult.

If you did not manage to complete any exercises that day you can note why, and your physiotherapist can help you to work around any obstacles you uncover.

Below is an example of what part of a week might look like:

	Sets of each exercise completed (please tick)						How the exercises feel	Comments
	Exs. 1	Exs. 2	Exs. 3	Exs. 4	Exs. 5	Exs. 6		
Monday	✓	✓	✓	✓	✓	✓	5	*Exercise 1 was easy,*
	✓		✓	✓	✓	✓		*2 was difficult*

'How the exercises feel' scale

1. Very, very easy / no problem

2. Very easy

3. Fairly easy

4. **Moderate/**
   beginning to feel hard

5. **Fairly hard**

6. **Hard**

7. Very hard

8. Very, very hard

9. Extremely hard

10. Maximum

The exercises should feel between level 4 ("moderate/ beginning to feel hard") and level 6 ("Hard"). Below this you are not getting the maximum benefit and above this you are working harder than you need to.

REMEMBER

- It is very important to build up your exercises gradually
- Work at a level/pace that is right for you
- After exercise, it is normal to experience some discomfort around in your muscles, and this may last for a couple of days. BUT, if the discomfort is severe, or lasts for longer than this, reduce your exercises and contact your physiotherapist.

Week commencing:......./......./......./

	Sets of each exercise completed (please tick)						How the exercises feel	Comments
	Exs. 1	Exs. 2	Exs. 3	Exs. 4	Exs. 5	Exs. 6		
Monday								
Tuesday								
Wednesday								
Thursday								
Friday								
Saturday								
Sunday								

Developed by the BEEP trial team, Arthritis Research UK Primary Care Centre, Keele University, UK

Week commencing:......./......./......./

	Sets of each exercise completed (please tick)						How the exercises feel	Comments
	Exs. 1	Exs. 2	Exs. 3	Exs. 4	Exs. 5	Exs. 6		
Monday								
Tuesday								
Wednesday								
Thursday								
Friday								
Saturday								
Sunday								

BOX 11.2 **Interacting dimensions influencing adherence**

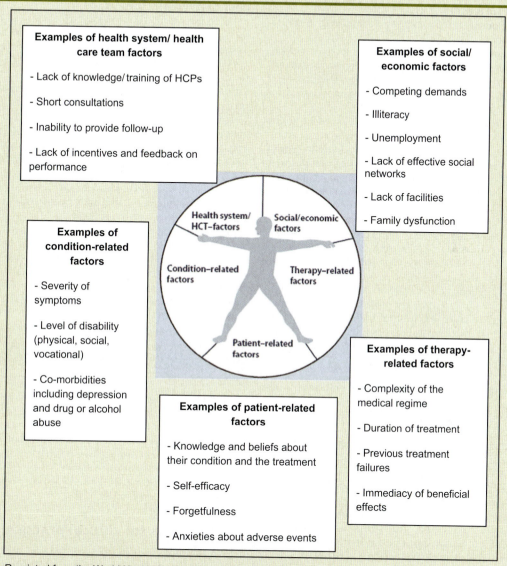

Examples of health system/ health care team factors

- Lack of knowledge/ training of HCPs

- Short consultations

- Inability to provide follow-up

- Lack of incentives and feedback on performance

Examples of social/ economic factors

- Competing demands

- Illiteracy

- Unemployment

- Lack of effective social networks

- Lack of facilities

- Family dysfunction

Examples of condition-related factors

- Severity of symptoms

- Level of disability (physical, social, vocational)

- Co-morbidities including depression and drug or alcohol abuse

Examples of therapy-related factors

- Complexity of the medical regime

- Duration of treatment

- Previous treatment failures

- Immediacy of beneficial effects

Examples of patient-related factors

- Knowledge and beliefs about their condition and the treatment

- Self-efficacy

- Forgetfulness

- Anxieties about adverse events

Health system/ HCT–factors

Social/economic factors

Condition–related factors

Therapy–related factors

Patient–related factors

Reprinted from the World Health Organization 2003, with kind permission, http://www.who.int/chp/knowledge/publications/adherence_report/en/.

HCPs: Healthcare practitioners
HCT-factors: Healthcare technology factors
Both may be either written out in full in the diagram, or added to the legend.

- Supplementing exercise programmes with refresher or booster sessions or by providing audiotapes or videotapes of exercises
- Incorporating exercise into wider self-management programmes
- Utilising behavioural graded activity programmes (increasing physical activity in a time contingent manner)

Interestingly, the type of exercise (e.g. strengthening vs aerobic exercise) did not appear to be an important factor influencing adherence.

Ezzat et al. (2015), in a systematic review of 22 studies of patients with OA, rheumatoid arthritis or mixed arthritis, concluded that there was limited evidence to suggest that adherence could be improved. The interventions were subgrouped by the authors into two main approaches: (1) knowledge-based and (2) motivational-based interventions. The knowledge-based group focused on patient education regarding the benefits of exercise, while motivational interventions focussed on behaviour change, feedback mechanisms and goal setting. Unfortunately, a lack of high-quality RCTs was the main limiting factor to drawing conclusions.

Other systematic reviews of adherence-enhancing interventions for exercise and physical activity have predominantly focused on healthy populations, but their findings may be of relevance. Foster et al. (2005) used 17 trials (6255 adults) to compare the effectiveness of different strategies to encourage sedentary, community-dwelling adults to become more physically active. Results showed that physical activity could be enhanced in the short- to mid-term, and that professional guidance and self-direction, plus ongoing professional support, are effective strategies. In a meta-analysis of 8 trials and 18 observational studies, Bravata et al. (2007) investigated the effect of pedometer use on physical activity among adults in outpatient settings. Pedometer users significantly increased their daily step count, increased their overall physical activity by 26.9% over baseline, and significantly decreased body mass index and blood pressure compared to controls. In addition, goal setting and a step diary were found to be key motivational strategies for increasing physical activity (ibid). Finally, Ogilvie et al. (2007) completed a meta-analysis of 19 randomised trials and 29 nonrandomised studies to explore how best to promote walking. Although pedometers were effective in the short term (up to 3 months), increases in steps were not sustained in the long term (at 6 or 12 months). Together, these reviews suggest that adherence to exercise and physical activity can be enhanced and that some strategies are relatively simple and inexpensive (use of diaries and pedometers, additional booster sessions with professional support in the longer term). The reviews also highlight the variable quality of previous trials, the inconsistency in measures of exercise adherence and the need for further research with long-term follow-up that explicitly addresses adherence to exercise and physical activity in adults with chronic MSK pain.

In an increasingly digital world, clinicians can deliver home exercise programmes online, with the aim of improving adherence (Bunting et al. 2021). This was arguably not the case at the time the most recent Cochrane review (Jordan et al. 2010) was undertaken. Bennell et al. (2019) undertook an RCT investigating the effect of commercially available exercise platforms for 305 participants with a range of MSK complaints. They reported that adherence was improved in the web-based exercise cohort; however, the study had a short follow-up. Bunting et al. (2021) undertook a subsequent systematic review of digital interventions to improve adherence. They highlighted the problems with the current research: only seven studies met the inclusion criteria set and study quality was generally poor. Studies in the review suggest that digital interventions can improve adherence in other health conditions such as diabetes (Schwarz et al. 2018), chronic heart disease (McLean et al. 2016), chronic lung disease (Lycett et al. 2018) and weight loss (Foley et al. 2016). However, Bunting et al. (2021) found insufficient evidence to confidently support these interventions for chronic MSK disorders, with only small beneficial effects found.

Conclusion

Therapeutic exercise is clearly a core treatment for persistent MSK pain, such as that in nonspecific LBP, knee pain and hand pain related to osteoarthritis. However, the evidence synthesis in this chapter highlights that exercise overall tends to result in small to moderate effects on pain and function, and that a key challenge is these effects most often decline over time, likely explained by poor adherence to exercise in the long term.

Implications for clinical practice

Healthcare professionals can confidently recommend and prescribe exercise for persistent MSK pain patients, such as those with nonspecific LBP, or knee or hand pain related to OA. The type of exercise does not appear to be as important as previously thought for adults with persistent pain, at least when investigated in heterogeneous groups of patients with LBP or knee pain. Patient preferences for the type of exercise may be a more useful guide for choice of interventions, with potential for maximising motivation and the likelihood of behaviour change. The characteristics of exercise programmes that appear to differentially influence clinical outcomes may be related to the way exercise is delivered. Exercise adherence is crucial if the benefits of exercise are to be realised in patients with persistent MSK pain. Simply advising patients to exercise, with little supervision and no longer-term follow-up, is unlikely to be effective for many patients with persistent MSK pain.

Implications for research

Further research is required to assist healthcare professionals to design exercise programmes and maximise the potential of exercise for patients with persistent pain. For example, it is not yet clear how exercise outcomes might be mediated by exercise type, exercise programme length, intensity or duration in MSK pain problems. We also do not know how to identify individuals who might do well with exercise versus other treatments, or who might benefit most from a particular exercise approach. Studies that test ways to better match exercise treatments to individual patients are needed, following the early examples from Hicks et al. (2005), Brennan et al. (2006) and Long et al. (2004). Moreover, the highly individual nature of preferences for different types of exercise and physical activities

means that future research should test how to incorporate these preferences into clinical decision-making. Promising early research in this area includes the development of an exercise preferences questionnaire and a trial comparing preference-based exercise with usual exercise prescription (Slade & Keating 2009). It also remains unclear whether digital tools sit within the context of the aforementioned factors. Finally, there are clear challenges to optimising patients' outcomes from exercise and physical activity in the long term and studies that develop and test ways to support patients with persistent MSK pain to adhere to long-term exercise and physical activity behaviour are needed.

Acknowledgements

The authors would like to thank the BEEP (Best Evidence for Exercise in knee Pain) trial team for providing the example exercise diary.

References

ACSM, 2021. Guidelines for Exercise Testing and Prescription, eleventh ed. Williams and Wilkins, Lippincott.

APTA (American Physical Therapy Association), 2001. Guide to physical therapist practice, second edition. American Physical Therapy Association. Phys. Ther. 81 (1), 9–746.

ARMA, 2004. Standards of Care for People With Osteoarthritis. Arthritis and Musculoskeletal Alliance, London. Available from: www.arma.uk.net.

Åsenlöf, P., Denison, E., Lindberg, P., 2009. Long-term follow-up of tailored behavioural treatment and exercise based physical therapy in persistent musculoskeletal pain: a randomized controlled trial in primary care. Eur. J. Pain. 13 (10).

Bandura, A., 1977. Self-efficacy: towards a unifying theory of behaviour change. Psychol. Rev. 84, 191–215.

Beasley, J., Ward, L., Knipper-Fisher, K., Hughes, K., Lunsford, D., Leiras, C., 2019. Conservative therapeutic interventions for osteoarthritic finger joints: a systematic review. J. Hand. Ther. 32 (2), 153–164.e2.

Bennell, K.L., Hinman, R.S., 2011. A review of the clinical evidence for exercise in osteoarthritis of the hip and knee. J. Sci. Med. Sport. 14 (1), 4–9.

Bennell, K.L., Marshall, C.J., Dobson, F., Kasza, J., Lonsdale, C., Hinman, R.S., 2019. Does a web-based exercise programming system improve home exercise adherence for people with musculoskeletal conditions? A randomized controlled Trial". Am. J. Phys. Med. Rehabil. 98 (10), 850–858.

Bosomworth, N.J., 2009. Exercise and knee osteoarthritis: benefit or hazard? Can. Fam. Physician. 55, 871–878.

Bouwmeester, W., van Enst, A., van Tulder, M., 2009. Quality of low back pain guidelines improved. Spine 34, 2562–2567.

Bravata, D.M., Smith-Spangler, C., Sundaram, V., Gienger, A.L., Lin, N., Lewis, R., et al., 2007. Using pedometers to increase physical activity and improve health: a systematic review. J. Am. Med. Assoc. 298, 2296–2304.

Brennan, G.P., Fritz, J.M., Hunter, S.J., Thackeray, A., Delitto, A., Erhard, R.E., 2006. Identifying subgroups of patients with acute/subacute "nonspecific" low back pain: results of a randomized clinical trial. Spine 31 (6), 623–631.

Brosseau, L., MacLeay, L., Robinson, V., Wells, G., Tugwell, P., 2003. Intensity of exercise for the treatment of osteoarthritis. Cochrane. Database. Syst. Rev. 2, CD004259.

Bunting, J.W., Withers, T.M., Heneghan, N.R., Greaves, C.J., 2021. "Digital interventions for promoting exercise adherence in chronic musculoskeletal pain: a systematic review and meta-analysis". Physiotherapy 111, 23–30.

Chia, Y.C., Beh, H.C., Ng, C.J., Teng, C.L., Hanafi, N.S., Choo, W.Y., et al., 2016. Ethnic differences in the prevalence of knee pain among adults of a community in a cross-sectional study, 2016. BMJ. Open 6, e011925.

Coggon, D., Ntani, G., Walker-Bone, K., Felli, V.E., Harari, F., Barrero, L.H., et al., 2019. "Determinants of international variation in the prevalence of disabling wrist and hand pain". BMC. Musculoskelet. Disord. 20 (1), 436–438.

Croft, P.R., Macfarlane, G.J., Papageorgiou, A.C., Thomas, E., Silman, A.J., 1998. Outcome of low back pain in general practice: a prospective study. Br. Med. J. 316, 1356–1359.

Dagenais, S., Tricco, A.C., Haldeman, S., 2010. Synthesis of recommendations for the assessment and management of low back pain from recent clinical practice guidelines. Spine J. 10, 514–529.

Dahaghin, S., Bierma-Zeinstra, S.M.A., Reijman, M., Pols, H.A.P., Hazes, J.M.W., Koes, B.W., 2005a. Prevalence and determinants of one month hand pain and hand related disability in the elderly (Rotterdam study). Ann. Rheum. Dis. 64, 99–104.

Dahaghin, S., Bierma-Zeinstra, S.M.A., Ginai, A.Z., Pols, H.A.P., Hazes, J.M.W., Koes, B.W., 2005b. Prevalence and pattern of radiographic hand osteoarthritis and association with pain and disability (the Rotterdam study). Ann. Rheum. Dis. 64, 682–687.

Dunn, K.M., Croft, P.R., 2005. Classification of low back pain in primary care: using "bothersomeness" to identify the most severe cases. Spine 30, 1887–1892.

Dziedzic, K., Thomas, E., Hill, S., Wilkie, R., Peat, G., Croft, P., 2007. The impact of musculoskeletal hand problems in older adults: findings from the North Staffordshire Osteoarthritis Project (NorStOP). Rheumatology. 46 (6), 963–977.

Dziedzic, K.S., Hill, J.C., Porcheret, M., Croft, P.R., 2009. New models for primary care are needed for osteoarthritis. Phys. Ther. 89 (12), 1371–1378.

Dziedzic, K., Nicholls, E., Hill, S., Hammond, A., Handy, J., Thomas, E., et al., 2015. Self-management approaches for osteoarthritis in the hand: a 2×2 factorial randomised trial. Ann. Rheum. Dis 74 (1), 108–118. https://doi.org/10.1136/annrheumdis-2013-203938. Epub 2013 Oct 9. PMID: 24107979; PMCID: PMC4283664.

Ettinger Jr., W.H., Burns, R., Messier, S.P., et al., 1997. A randomized trial comparing aerobic exercise and resistance exercise with a health education program in older adults with knee osteoarthritis. The Fitness Arthritis and Seniors Trial (FAST). Journal of American Medicine Association 277 (1), 25–31.

Ezzat, A.M., MacPherson, K., Leese, J., Li, L.C., 2015. The effects of interventions to increase exercise adherence in people with arthritis: a systematic review: exercise adherence interventions in arthritis. Muscoskel. Care. 13 (1), 1–18.

Foroughi, N., Smith, R.M., Lange, A.K., Baker, M.K., Fiatarone Singh, M.A., Vanwanseele, B., 2011. Lower limb muscle strengthening does not change frontal plane moments in women with knee osteoarthritis: a randomized controlled trial. Clinical Biomechanics 26 (2), 167–174.

Gohir, S.A., Eek, F., Kelly, A., Abhishek, A., Valdes, A.M., 2021. Effectiveness of internet-based exercises aimed at treating knee osteoarthritis: the iBEAT-OA Randomized rlinical trial. JAMA. Netw. Open 4 (2), e210012. https://doi.org/10.1001/jamanetworkopen.2021.0012. Erratum in: JAMA Netw Open. 2021 Mar 1;4(3):e216209. PMID: 33620447; PMCID: PMC7903254.

Foley, P., Steinberg, D., Levine, E., Askew, S., Batch, B.C., Puleo, E.M., et al., 2016. Track: A randomized controlled trial of a digital health obesity treatment intervention for medically vulnerable primary care patients. Contemp. Clin. Trials 48, 12–20. https://doi.org/10.1016/j.cct.2016.03.006. Epub 2016 Mar 17. PMID: 26995281; PMCID: PMC4885789.

Ferreira, M.L., Smeets, R.B.E.M., Camper, S.J., Ferreira, P.H., Machado, L.A.C., 2010. Can we explain heterogeneity among randomized clinical trials of exercise for chronic back pain? A meta-regression analysis of randomized controlled trials. Phys. Ther. 90, 1383–1403.

Foster, C., Hillsdon, M., Thorogood, M., 2005. Interventions for promoting physical activity. Cochrane. Database. Syst. Rev. 1, CD003180.

Foster, N.E., Thomas, E., Barlas, P., Hill, J.C., Young, J., Mason, E., et al., 2007. Acupuncture as an adjunct to exercise based physiotherapy for osteoarthritis of the knee: randomised controlled trial. Br. Med. J. 335, 436.

Fransen, M., McConnell, S., 2008. Exercise for osteoarthritis of the knee. Cochrane. Database. Syst. Rev. 4, CD004376.

Fransen, M., McConnell, S., Harmer, A.R., Van der Esch, M., Simic, M., Bennell, K.L., 2015. Exercise for osteoarthritis of the knee. Cochrane. Database. Syst. Rev. 1, CD004376.

Friedrich, M., Gittler, G., Arendasy, M., Friedrich, K.M., 2005. Long-term effect of a combined exercise and motivational program on the level of disability of patients with chronic low back pain. Spine. 30 (9), 995–1000.

Glynn, A., Fiddler, H., 2009. The Physiotherapist's Pocket Guide to Exercise Assessment, Prescription and Training. Elsevier, London.

Haskell, W.L., Lee, I.-M., Pate, R.R., Powell, K.E., Blair, S.N., Franklin, B.A., et al., 2007. Physical activity and public health: updated recommendation for adults from the American College of Sports Medicine and the American Heart Association. Med. Sci. Sports. Exerc. 39, 1423–1434.

Hayden, J.A., van Tulder, M.W., Malmivaara, A., 2005a. Exercise therapy for treatment of non-specific low back pain. Cochrane Database Syst. Rev. 3, CD000335.

Hayden, J.A., van Tulder, M.W., Tomlinson, G., 2005b. Systematic review: strategies for using exercise therapy to improve outcomes in chronic low back pain. Ann. Intern. Med. 142, 776–785.

Hayden, J.A., Ellis, J., Ogilvie, R., Malmivaara, A., van Tulder, M.W., 2021a. Exercise therapy for chronic low back pain. Cochrane Database Syst. Rev. 9, CD009790.

Hayden, J.A., Ellis, J., Ogilvie, R., Stewart, S.A., Bagg, M.K., Stanojevic, S., et al., 2021b. "Some types of exercise are more effective than others in people with chronic low back pain: a network meta-analysis". J. Physiother. 67 (4), 252–262.

Hestbaek, L., Leboeuf, Y.C., Manniche, C., 2003. Low back pain: what is the long-term course? A review of studies of general patient populations. Eur. Spine. J. 2, 149–165.

Hettinga, D.M., Jackson, A., Moffett, J.K., May, S., Mercer, C., Woby, S.R., 2007. A systematic review and synthesis of higher quality evidence of the effectiveness of exercise interventions for non-specific low back pain of at least 6 weeks' duration. Phys. Ther. Rev. 12, 221–232.

Hicks, G.E., Fritz, J.M., Delitto, A., McGill, S.M., 2005. Preliminary development of a clinical prediction rule for determining which patients with low back pain will respond to a stabilization exercise program. Arch. Phys. Med. Rehabil. 86 (9), 1753–1762.

Hill, S., Dziedzic, K., Thomas, E., Baker, S.R., Croft, P., 2007. The illness perceptions associated with health and behavioural outcomes in people with musculoskeletal hand problems: findings from the North Staffordshire Osteoarthritis Project (NorStOP). Rheumatology. 46 (6), 944–951.

Hill, S., Dziedzic, K.S., Ong, B.N., 2010. The functional and psychological impact of hand osteoarthritis. Chronic. Illn. 6 (2), 101–110.

Horne, R., 1997. Representation of medication and treatment: advances in theory and measurement. In: Petrie, K.J., Weinman, J.A. (Eds.), Perceptions of Health and Illness. Hardwood Academic Press, Amsterdam.

Huang, M.H., Lin, Y.S., Yang, R.C., Lee, C.L., 2003. A comparison of various therapeutic exercises on the functional status of patients with knee osteoarthritis. Semin. Arthritis. Rheum. 32, 398–406.

Huang, M.H., Lin, Y.S., Lee, C.L., Yang, R.C., 2005. Use of ultrasound to increase effectiveness of isokinetic exercise for knee osteoarthritis. Arch. Phys. Med. Rehabil. 86, 1545–1551.

Hughes, S.L., Seymour, R.B., Campbell, R., Pollak, N., Huber, G., Sharma, L., 2004. Impact of the fit and strong intervention on older adults with osteoarthritis. Gerontol. 44, 217–228.

Hurley, M.V., 2003. Muscle dysfunction and effective rehabilitation of knee osteoarthritis: what we know and what we need to find out. Arthritis. Care. Res. 49, 444–452.

Hurley, M.V., Bearne, L.M., 2009. The principles of therapeutic exercise and physical activity. Chapter 7. In: Dziedzic, K., Hammond, A. (Eds.), Rheumatology. Elsevier, Edinburgh.

Hurley, M., Dickson, K., Hallett, R., Grant, R., Hauari, H., Walsh, N., et al., 2018. Exercise interventions and patient beliefs for people with hip, knee or hip and knee osteoarthritis: a mixed methods review. Cochrane. Database. Syst. Rev. 4 (4), CD010842.

James, W.P., 2008. The epidemiology of obesity: the size of the problem. J. Intern. Med. 263, 336–352.

Jan, M., Lin, J., Liau, J., Lin, Y., Lin, D., 2008. Investigation of clinical effects of high- and low-resistance training for patients with knee osteoarthritis: a randomised controlled trial. Phys. Ther. 88, 427–435.

Jordan, K.M., Arden, N.K., Doherty, M., Bannwarth, B., Bijlsma, J.W., Dieppe, P., et al., 2003. Standing Committee for International Clinical Studies Including Therapeutic Trials ESCISIT. EULAR Recommendations 2003: an evidence based approach to the management of knee osteoarthritis: report of a task force of the standing committee for international clinical studies including therapeutic trials (ESCISIT). Ann. Rheum. Dis. 62, 1145–1155.

Jordan, J.L., Holden, M.A., Mason, E.E., Foster, N.E., 2010. Interventions to improve adherence to exercise for chronic musculoskeletal pain in adults. Cochrane. Database. Syst. Rev. 1, CD005956.

Kloppenburg, M., Kroon, F.P.B., Blanco, F.J., Doherty, M., Dziedzic, K.S., Greibrokk, E., et al., 2019. 2018 Update of the EULAR recommendations for the management of hand osteoarthritis. Ann. Rheum. Dis. 78, 16–24.

Lange, A.K., Vanwanseele, B., Singh, M.A.F., 2008. Strength training for treatment of osteoarthritis of the knee: a systematic review. Arthritis. Care. Res. 59, 1488–1494.

Long, A., Donelson, R., Fung, T., 2004. Does it matter which exercise? A randomized control trial of exercise for low back pain. Spine. 29 (23), 2593–2602.

Lycett, H.J., Raebel, E.M., Wildman, E.K., Guitart, J., Kenny, T., Sherlock, J., et al., 2018. Theory-based digital interventions to improve asthma self-management outcomes: systematic review. J. Med. Internet. Res. 20 (12), e293.

Macedo, L.G., Maher, C.G., Latimer, J., McAuley, J.H., 2009. Motor control exercise for persistent, nonspecific low back pain: a systematic review. Phys. Ther. 89, 9–25.

Macedo, L.G., Smeets, R.J., Maher, J., McAuley, J.H., 2010. Graded activity and graded exposure for persistent nonspecific low back pain: a systematic review. Phys. Ther. 90, 1538–6724.

Mahendira, D., Towheed, T.E., 2009. Systematic review of non-surgical therapies for osteoarthritis of the hand: an update. Osteoarthritis. Cartilage. 17, 1263–1268.

Maniadakis, N., Gray, A., 2000. The economic burden of back pain in the UK. Pain. 84, 95–103.

Mannoni, A., Briganti, M.P., Di Bari, M., Ferrucci, L., Serni, U., Masotti, G., et al., 2000. Prevalence of symptomatic hand osteoarthritis in community-dwelling older persons: the ICARe Dicomano study. Osteoarthritis. Cartilage. 8, S11–S13.

Marcus, B.H., Rakowski, W., Rossi, J.S., 1992. Assessing motivational readiness and decision-making for exercise. Health. Psychol. 22, 3–16.

Marks, R., Allegrante, J.P., 2005. Chronic osteoarthritis and adherence to exercise: a review of the literature. J. Aging. Phys. Act. 13, 434–460.

Mattap, S.M., Laslett, L.L., Squibb, K., Wills, K., Otahal, P., Pan, F., et al., 2021. Hand examination, ultrasound, and the association with hand pain and function in community–based older adults. Arthritis. Care. Res. 73 (3), 347–354.

McArdle, W.D., Katch, F.I., Katch, V.L., 1996. Exercise Physiology: Energy, Nutrition and Human Performance, fourth ed. Williams and Wilkins, Maryland.

McAuley, E., 1992. The role of efficacy cognitions in the prediction of exercise behaviour in middle aged adults. J. Behav. Med. 15, 65–88.

McLean, G., Band, R., Saunderson, K., Hanlon, P., Murray, E., Little, P., et al., 2016. Digital interventions to promote self-management in adults with hypertension systematic review and meta-analysis. J. Hypertens. 34 (4), 600.

Meichenbaum, D., Turk, D., 1987. Facilitating Treatment Adherence. Plenum Press, New York.

Melanson, E.L., Freedson, P.S., 1996. Physical activity assessment: a review of methods. Crit. Rev. Food Sci. Nutr. 36, 385–396.

Moe, R.H., Kjeken, I., Uhlig, T., Hagen, K.B., 2009. There is inadequate evidence to determine the effectiveness of nonpharmacological and nonsurgical interventions for hand osteoarthritis: an overview of high-quality systematic reviews. Phys. Ther. 89, 1363–1370.

Myers, L.B., Midence, K., 1998. Methodological and conceptual issues in adherence. In: Myers, L.B., Midence, K. (Eds.), Adherence to Treatment in Medical Conditions. Haywood Academic Publishers, The Netherlands.

Neame RL, Doherty M, 2005. Osteoarthritis update. Clin. Med. 5, 207–210.

Nelson, M.E., Rejeski, W.J., Blair, S.N., Duncan, P.W., Judge, J.O., King, A.C., et al., 2007. Physical activity and public health in older adults: recommendations from the American College of Sports Medicine and the American Heart Association. Med. Sci. Sports Exerc. 39, 1435–1445.

NICE (National Institute for Health and Clinical Excellence), 2014. Osteoarthritis: care and management (CG177). Available from www.nice.org.uk/guidance/cg177.

NICE (National Institute for Health and Clinical Excellence), 2021a. Chronic Pain (Primary and Secondary) in Over 16s: Assessment of all Chronic Pain and Management of Chronic Primary Pain (NG193). Available from https://www.nice.org.uk/guidance/ng193.

NICE (National Institute for Health and Clinical Excellence), 2021b. Managing Low Back Pain and Sciatica. Available from http://pathways.nice.org.uk/pathways/low-back-pain-and-sciatica (NG59https://www.nice.org.uk/guidance/ng59.

Oesch, P., Kool, J., Hagen, K.B., Bachman, S., 2010. Effectiveness of exercise on work disability in patients with non-acute non-specific low back pain: systematic review and meta-analysis of randomised controlled trials. J. Rehabil. Med. 42, 193–205.

Ogilvie, D., Foster, C.E., Rothnie, H., Cavill, N., Hamilton, V., Fitzsimons, C.F., et al., 2007. Scottish physical activity research collaboration. Interventions to promote walking: systematic review. Br. Med. J. 334, 1204–1207.

Oliveria, S.A., Felson, D.T., Reed, J.I., Cirillo, P.A., Walker, A.M., Oliveria, S.A., et al., 1995. Incidence of symptomatic hand, hip, and knee osteoarthritis among patients in a health maintenance organization. Arthritis. Rheum. 38, 1134–1141.

Østerås, N., Kjeken, I., Smedslund, G., Moe, R.H., Slatkowsky-Christensen, B., Uhlig, T., et al., 2017. Exercise for hand osteoarthritis. Cochrane. Database. Syst. Rev. 1, CD010388.

O'Connell, N.E., Cook, C.E., Wand, B.M., 2017. Clinical guidelines for low back pain: a critical review of consensus and inconsistencies across three major guidelines. Best. Pract. Res. Clin. Rheumatol. 30, 6.

Paul, D.R., Kramer, M., Moshfegh, A.J., Baer, D.J., Rumpler, W.V., 2007. Comparison of two different physical activity monitors. BMC Med. Res. Methodol. 7, 26.

Peat, G., McCarney, R., Croft, P., 2001a. Knee pain and osteoarthritis in older adults: a review of community burden and current use of primary health care. Ann. Rheum. Dis. 60, 91–97.

Peat, G., Croft, P., Hay, E., 2001b. Clinical assessment of the osteoarthritis patient. Best Practice and Research. Clin. Rheumatol. 15, 527–544.

Peat, G., Thomas, E., Wilkie, R., Croft, P., 2006. Multiple joint pain and lower extremity disability in middle and old age. Disabil. Rehabil. 28, 1543–1549.

Petrella, R.J., Bartha, C., 2000. Home based exercise therapy for older patients with knee osteoarthritis: a randomised clinical trial. J. Rheumatol. 27, 2215–2221.

Pisters, M.F., Veenhof, C., van Meeteren, Ostelo, R.W., de Bakker, D.H., Schellevis, F.G., et al., 2007. Long-term effectiveness of exercise therapy in patients with osteoarthritis of the hip or knee: a systematic review. Arthritis. Care. Res. 57, 1245–1253.

Pisters, M.F., Veenhof, C., Schellevis, F.G., Twisk, J.W., Dekker, J., De Bakker, D.H., 2010. Exercise adherence improving long-term patient outcome in patients with osteoarthritis of the hip and/or knee. Arthritis. Care. Res. 62, 1087–1094.

Porcheret, M., Jordan, K., Jinks, C., 2007. With the Primary Care Rheumatology Society. Primary care treatment of knee pain a survey in older adults. Rheumatology. 46, 1694–1700.

Quicke, J.G., Foster, N.E., Thomas, M.J., Holden, M.A., 2015. Is long-term physical activity safe for older adults with knee pain?: a systematic review. Osteoarthritis. Cartilage. 23 (9), 1445–1456.

Arthritis Research Campaign, 2002. Arthritis: The Big Picture. Arthritis research campaign, London. Available from: www.arc.org.uk.

Roddy, E., Zhang, W., Doherty, M., Arden, N.K., Barlow, J., Birrell, F., et al., 2005a. Evidence-based recommendations for the role of exercise in the management of osteoarthritis of the hip or knee – the MOVE consensus. Rheumatology. 44, 67–73.

Roddy, E., Zhang, W., Doherty, M., 2005b. Aerobic walking or strengthening exercise for osteoarthritis of the knee? A systematic review. Ann. Rheum. Dis. 64, 544–548.

Salacinski, A.J., Krohn, K., Lewis, S.F., Holland, M.L., Ireland, K., Marchetti, G., 2012. The effects of group cycling on gait and pain-related disability in individuals with mild-to-moderate knee osteoarthritis: a randomized controlled trial. J. Orthop. Sports. Phys. Ther. 42 (12), 985–995.

Schaafsma, F., Schonstein, E., Whelan, K.M., Ulvestad, E., Kenny, D.T., Verbeek, J.H., 2010. Physical conditioning programs for improving work outcomes in workers with back pain. Cochrane. Database. Syst. Rev. 1, CD001822.

Schonstein, E., Kenny, D.T., Keating, J.L., Koes, B.W., 2003. Work conditioning, work hardening and functional restoration for workers with back and neck pain. Cochrane. Database. Syst. Rev. 1, CD001822.

Schwarz, P.E.H., Timpel, P., Harst, L., Greaves, C.J., Ali, M.K., Lambert, J., et al., 2018. Blood sugar regulation for cardiovascular health promotion and disease prevention. JACC. Health. Promotion Series 72 (15), 1829–1844.

Slade, S.C., Keating, J.L., 2009. Effects of preferred-exercise prescription compared to usual exercise prescription on outcomes for people with non-specific low back pain: a randomized controlled trial [ACTRN12608000524392]. BMC Musculoskelet. Disord. 10, 14.

Stamm, T.A., Machold, K.P., Smolen, J.S., Fischer, S., Redlich, K., Graninger, W., et al., 2002. Joint protection and home hand exercises improve hand function in patients with hand osteoarthritis: a randomized controlled trial. Arthritis. Rheum. 47, 44–49.

Thomas, K.S., Muir, K.R., Doherty, M., Jones, A.C., O'Reilly, S.C., Bassey, E.J., 2002. Home based exercise programme for knee pain and knee osteoarthritis: randomised controlled trial. Br. Med. J. 325, 752.

Towheed, T.E., 2005. Systematic review of therapies for osteoarthritis of the hand. Osteoarthritis. Cartilage. 13, 455–462.

Treuth, M.S., 2002. Applying multiple methods to improve the accuracy of activity assessments. In: Welk, G.J. (Ed.), Physical Activity Assessments for Health Related Research. Human Kinetics Publishers, Champaign, Illinois.

Turkiewicz, A., De Verdier, M.G., Engström, G., Nilsson, P.M., Mellström, C., Stefan Lohmander, L., et al., 2015. "Prevalence of knee pain and knee OA in southern Sweden and the proportion that seeks medical care". Rheumatology. 54 (5), 827–838.

Tveit, M., Rosengren, B.E., Nilsson, J.Å., Karlsson, M.K., 2012. Former male elite athletes have a higher prevalence of osteoarthritis and arthroplasty in the hip and knee than expected. Am. J. Sports. Med 40 (3), 527–533. https://doi.org/10.1177/0363546511429278. Epub 2011 Nov 30. PMID: 22130474.

Uthman, O.A., van der Windt, D.A., Jordan, J.L., Dziedzic, K.S., Healey, E.L., Peat, G.M., et al., 2014. Exercise for lower limb osteoarthritis: systematic review incorporating trial sequential analysis and network meta-analysis. Br. J. Sports. Med. 48 (21), 1579.

Valdes, K., Marik Tambra, 2010. A systematic review of conservative interventions for osteoarthritis of the hand. J. Hand. Ther. 23 (4), 334–335.

Van Middelkoop, M., Rubinstein, S.M., Verhagen, A.P., Ostelo, R.W., Koes, B.W., van Tulder, M.W., 2010. Exercise therapy for chronic nonspecific low-back pain. Best. Pract. Res. Clin. Rheumatol. 24, 193–204.

Verhagen, A.P., Ferreira, M., Reijneveld, E., Teirlinck, C.H., 2019. Do we need another trial on exercise in patients with knee osteoarthritis?: No new trials on exercise in knee OA. Osteoarthritis. Cartilage. 27 (9), 1266–1269.

Waddell, G., 2004. The back pain revolution, second ed. Churchill Livingstone, Edinburgh.

Walker, B.F., 2000. The prevalence of low back pain: systematic review of the literature from 1966 to 1998. J. Spinal. Disord. 13, 205–217.

WHO, 2003. Adherence to Long-Term Therapies: Evidence for Action. World Health Organization Library.

Wilmoth, J.R., 2000. Demography of longevity: past, present and future trends. Exp. Gerontol. 35, 1111–1129.

Zhang, Y.Q., Niu, I.B., Kelly-Hayes, M., Chaisson, C.E., Aliabadi, P., Felson, D.T., 2002. Prevalence of symptomatic hand osteoarthritis and its impact on functional status among the elderly - the Framingham Study. Am. J. Epidemiol. 156, 1021–1027.

Zhang, W., Doherty, M., Leeb, B.F., Alekseeva, L., Arden, N.K., Bijlsma, J.W., et al., 2007a. EULAR evidence based recommendations for the management of hand osteoarthritis: report of a task force of the EULAR Standing Committee for International Clinical Studies Including Therapies (ESCISIT). Ann. Rheum. Dis. 66, 377–388.

Zhang, W., Moskowitz, R.W., Nuki, G., Abramson, S., Altman, R.D., Arden, N., et al., 2007b. OARSI recommendations for the management of hip and knee osteoarthritis, part I: critical appraisal of existing treatment guidelines and systematic review of current research evidence. Osteoarthritis. Cartilage. 15, 981–1000.

Zhang, W., Nuki, G., Moskowitz, R.W., Abramson, S., Altman, R.D., Arden, N.K., et al., 2010. OARSI recommendations for the management of hip and knee osteoarthritis: part III: changes in evidence following systematic cumulative update of research published through January 2009. Osteoarthritis. Cartilage. 18, 476–499.

Chapter | 12 |

Psychological management of pain

Michael Nicholas

LEARNING OBJECTIVES

At the end of this chapter, readers will understand:
1. The strategic approach to helping a complex case in which psychological and environmental factors appear to be contributing.
2. How to tailor a psychologically based intervention for a patient with disabling chronic pain.

Introduction

This chapter builds on Chapter 5, on psychological aspects of pain. In that chapter, the case was made for taking a case-formulation-based approach to pain management. This can also be described as a patient-centred approach in that treatment should be individualised and based on a biopsychosocial model of care, as recommended in the most recent guidelines from a taskforce report from the U.S. Department of Health and Human Services (2019). Those guidelines also recommended that treatments for chronic pain should focus on measurable (especially functional) outcomes that enhance the quality of life of patients and minimise adverse outcomes.

Clinicians were also encouraged to consider using a multimodal approach, involving a combination of treatment methods as it is unlikely that a single modality will be able to address all the biopsychosocial contributors to a patient's chronic pain condition and its impact on their lives.

As outlined in Chapter 5, developing a case formulation of a patient's presenting problems before embarking on an intervention requires a consideration of information gleaned from a careful, and comprehensive assessment of the patient. It was also argued that such an assessment would be consistent with the principles outlined in ICD-11 (Treede et al. 2019); namely, that the diagnostic classification of a patient's chronic pain condition should include evidence of possible biological, psychological and social/environmental contributors that may be playing a role in the presenting patient's chronic pain condition and associated mood and disability features.

In relation to psychological factors thought to be contributing, it was argued that these need to be identified, rather than being assumed in the absence of biological factors (Pincus & McCracken 2013). By taking this approach, a clinician will be better able to provide interventions that are tailored to the individual patient. Tailoring treatment to the individual patient may create a potential problem for those conducting group-based treatment programs, but this is not insurmountable, and this will be addressed as well in this chapter.

Besides the importance of identifying psychological contributors to a patient's presenting problems in order to target these in treatment, another side to psychological interventions concerns the clinicians' behaviours and the manner in which they are delivering the treatments. That is, there are psychological considerations for the application or delivery of a treatment, and this applies regardless of whether the treatment is considered 'psychological' or not. A good example here is the role of communication style and the manner in which the patient is engaged in the intervention by the clinician (e.g. Main et al. 2010; Nicholas & George 2011). These issues have also been documented by placebo researchers (Evers et al. 2021). Accordingly, this chapter will also consider this topic.

Another important issue to consider when discussing interventions in any health domain concerns different versions of treatments that may be very similar but have different names and champions. Just as exercises are generally recommended for chronic pain conditions generally, especially painful musculoskeletal conditions, it is notable that despite the plethora of types of exercise and names they are called, no specific exercise is usually recommended in evidence-informed guidelines (Ambrose & Golightly 2015). The main reason is usually that the available evidence doesn't support such distinctions and it is usually adherence to exercises that is most important (Hayden et al. 2005). Much the same pattern can be seen in the pain and mental health treatment research literature, where researchers often refer to particular brands or labels given to treatments, like cognitive-behavioural therapy (CBT) or acceptance and commitment therapy (ACT), as if they were a unitary substance. In reality, there are many different versions of both, different skill levels in the practitioners and they both have their roots in what was called behaviourism. CBT, for example, is often referred to as a family of therapies, albeit with some common features (Tang 2018). A major problem with the labelling approach is that it risks missing potentially important common features, limits our ability to identify which elements of these multicomponent treatments may be especially important and restricts our ability to improve overall treatment effectiveness (i.e. achieving better outcomes for patients).

The last two Cochrane reviews of psychological treatments for chronic pain (Williams et al. 2012, 2020) have pointed to the need for us to stop asking questions like: is CBT-based pain management better or worse than ACT-based pain management? The reasons for this call include their many features in common, the considerable variation in content and delivery within both approaches of the same label, and the evidence that any differences in outcome between them are not so substantial they merit further study and resources. Proponents of both approaches claim they are trying to achieve better health and quality-of-life outcomes for their patients, as well as functional gains, but these treatments are not a black box and pitting one against the other isn't going to tell us much of value. There is evidence that both approaches can work for a proportion of patients (no treatment works with everyone), but the gains are often small to moderate relative to usual care, so it doesn't seem worthwhile to argue about relative effectiveness of CBT versus ACT. Thus as these Cochrane reviewers say, the important questions now are more to do with what works, for whom and in

what circumstances. The question of 'what works' is, of course, very broad and the answer must depend on the context or measure being used. But in this chapter, it also refers to particular elements in these treatments. Accordingly, the approach taken in this chapter will address these sorts of questions that are more to do with the processes and how psychological interventions might help. These questions also seem well suited to a case-formulation approach and research studies that use single-case designs rather than group designs (Linton & Nicholas 2008; Maroti et al. 2011).

Taking a case-formulation approach to treatment

We will use the case study from Chapter 5 in Case Study 12.1 given below.

Before proceeding to implement any treatment with this man, it would be important to check its accuracy with him. If he agrees it is accurate then the first stage of the intervention is close to being achieved. This is what von Korff et al. (1977) described as developing a collaborative relationship with the patient, where there is a shared understanding (between the patient and the clinician) of the patient's problems. The guidelines from the U.S. Department of Health and Human Services (2019) also included this as an important element of any treatment for someone with chronic pain.

Once there is a shared understanding of the full picture of the patient's problems, then the clinician can proceed to outline possible interventions for the relevant aspects. This also enables the clinician to avoid a common trap in working with chronic pain patients and that is the traditional medical/surgical approach whereby physical treatments, like medication and/or exercises, are initiated first, and it is only if they fail or do not deliver the expected outcomes that more overtly psychological interventions are considered. This is known as the 'stepped care' model (Balderson & von Korff 2002). The stepped care model has widespread institutional support in many countries, probably as it might be considered cheaper than adding a psychological treatment into the mix when the patient might get better anyway and not need psychological care and its associated costs. A major problem is that it risks the patient being given the message that physical treatments haven't worked, so let's try psychological ones. From the patient's perspective, at least, this is close to suggesting to them that their pain is 'psychological', that is, 'in their heads'. If this occurs, it is hard to see how adherent the patient will be to any treatment that requires their taking a major role, especially if they believe the problem is in their back and not in their head and that they are worried

CASE STUDY 12.1

A 45-year-old man reports persisting low back pain following a fall at work 12 months ago. Initial radiography did not reveal any abnormalities, though a computed tomography (CT) scan subsequently revealed moderate posterior disc bulging at L4/5, but no apparent compression of neural structures. Neurological examination revealed no neurological abnormality. Heat treatment and manipulation have provided only brief relief of his pain. Simple analgesics and antiinflammatory medication provided little help. His doctor then prescribed an antidepressant to help his mood and sleep problems as well as low-dose opioids to be taken as needed, but lately he has been taking them on a daily basis without noticeable benefit and he now reports constipation. His doctor is concerned about this. His doctor referred him to a physiotherapist for exercises and advice, but he doesn't adhere to the exercise plan as he finds they aggravate his pain. But he does find the heat pack on his back comforting when sitting or lying on the couch or in bed.

He describes his pain as almost constantly present and fluctuating in severity. On average, he rates the pain as 6/10 in severity. It is aggravated by most activities and reduced by resting and heat (hot showers and a heat pack). He has been off work since his accident, and he doubts he will be able to return to his old job. His employer was sympathetic initially but now says he has had to terminate his job. He does have a workers compensation claim and has been receiving wage replacement income, but the amount is gradually being reduced. The independent insurance doctor told him he could not find anything seriously wrong with him and he should continue with exercises and return to work. He and his wife are having to rely more on her wages to cover their expenses.

Currently, he reports being unable to perform most of his normal house and yard chores as it seems everything he does aggravates his pain. His mood is often depressed, and

he reports often feeling useless and frustrated. His score on a depression symptom scale places him in the moderately depressed range for people with chronic pain. Sleep at night is disturbed and the days are marked by lethargy and tiredness. He is comfort eating and has put on over 16 kg in the last year. He reports that he and his wife are having more arguments than usual, and he avoids social engagements as they usually involve a lot of sitting. He has gradually lost touch with his old friends, and he hasn't played golf with them since his fall.

On examination, the patient appears noticeably distressed and walks slowly and spends most of the examination session standing and leaning on a chair. He is unable to touch his toes and reports tenderness in his lumbar spine (L3/4). All back movements, rotation, flexion/extension appear reduced and are accompanied by grimaces and reports of increased pain. There is no evidence of muscle wasting and no sensory loss is detected. He reports he can only stand for about 10 minutes before his pain increases and he has to change position. Walking is limited to about 12 minutes and sitting to about 10 minutes. When asked what he thinks is causing his persisting pain he says he is not sure but is concerned something is wrong with his spine and has been missed. He doesn't feel he can return to work or resume his normal life until his pain is relieved. He was asked to complete self-report questionnaires about his pain, and they indicate he has very low pain self-efficacy (i.e. low confidence in being active while in pain), and he tends to worry a lot about his pain and what it means for his future (his catastrophising score was in the high range for people with pain). Another scale indicated a high level of fear of movement when in pain.

Based on that case description, a preliminary case formulation for this man might look like as shown in Fig. 12.1.

---

something has been missed. This outcome would not be consistent with a collaborative, shared approach between patients and clinicians (Nicholas & Blyth 2016). Furthermore, if the patient has low pain self-efficacy, we also have evidence that simply giving them exercises to do or telling them to resume normal activities is unlikely to be effective (Ledingham et al. 2020).

A preferable alternative might be to better integrate the more 'physical' aspects of the treatment plan with the more 'psychological' elements. In the physiotherapy literature, this has been described as 'psychologically informed physiotherapy' (PIP) (Keefe et al. 2018; Main & George 2011). Keefe et al. point out that PIP requires the therapist to shift away from the 'traditional

biomechanical and pathology-based approaches that have been traditionally used to manage musculoskeletal pain' (p. 398), to incorporate a focus on 'the behavioral aspects of pain (i.e., peoples' responses to pain) by identifying individual expectations, beliefs, and feelings as prognostic factors for clinical and occupational outcomes indicating progression to chronicity' (p. 398). Of course, this more comprehensive biopsychosocial perspective should not be limited to physiotherapists, rather it should be relevant to all healthcare providers dealing with patients experiencing pain.

Whilst an individual healthcare provider may undertake a psychologically informed approach in their practice, the model applies equally to a multidisciplinary team

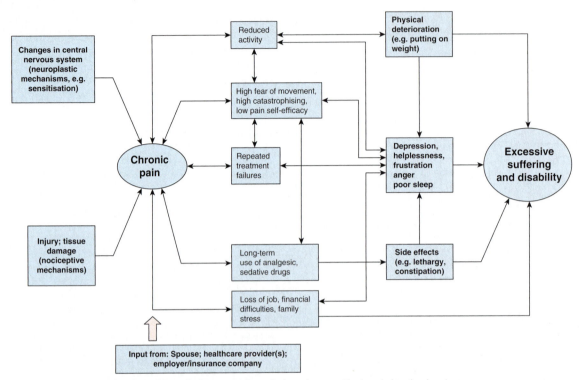

Fig. 12.1 Preliminary case formulation of man with chronic low back pain.

dealing with the same patient, each using their profession-specific skillset, but supplemented by the use of more psychological treatment principles and targets. This has been a standard feature in multidisciplinary pain management programs for over 30 years (Williams et al. 1996) and is often now referred to as interdisciplinary multimodal pain management (Nicholas et al. 2017b).

If we return to the case study, the treatment options for each identified target (distressed mood, sleep problems, reduced activity, etc.) might be expected to address a number of targets revealed by the case formulation. For example, there is evidence that resuming regular exercises can help to improve a patient's mood, as well as pain and function (Vaegter & Jones 2020). Recalling the discussion in Chapter 5 about mediating variables, it is likely that many of these targets are acting as mediators. That means the intervention plan may not need to target each element (or contributor) directly as a change in a mediator should produce a change in its effects.

A similar model was outlined by Detweiler-Bedell (2008) for patients with comorbid depression and chronic (physical) diseases, like diabetes. These authors pointed out that exercise was good for both depression and diabetes, so there was no need to have two sets of exercise (one for each condition). The same applies in the case we are

considering here where the man with chronic pain has multiple problems associated with his chronic pain condition.

Working through the options for each contributor based on the case formulation, we will consider the possible options and the evidence for them. A fuller account of how some of these strategies can be presented to patients can be found in a book for people with chronic pain by Nicholas et al. (2011). A summary of common ways in which CBT methods have been employed in treating people with chronic low back is also useful in providing an overview of these methods (Hanscom et al. 2015).

1. Pain

As there doesn't seem to be a reason for surgery in this case and analgesics have a poor long-term record with chronic low back pain (Maher et al. 2017)—consistent with this man's experience—a safer and more effective way of reducing his pain severity and its impact on his life would be to target his pain-related distress (frustration/anger, catastrophic thoughts) and avoidant behaviours (activity avoidance) as there is evidence that improvements in these domains are often associated with reductions in how troubling pain is for the patient (Nicholas et al. 2014). Initially, this could mean clarifying his understanding of his pain and, assuming his fears are not fully warranted, we could then share a more accurate perspective. This might be referred to as 'pain education', but it will be more efficient (and faster) to be more targeted in how it is applied, especially if we confirm with the patient that we have answered his concerns (Maguire & Pitceathly 2002; Main et al. 2010), as opposed to a general lecture about current pain science. A review of the topic by Edmond & Keefe (2015) described this process as relevant to the issue of validating the patient's concerns, in part as it can enhance the patient's sense that they are being taken seriously. In relation to pain education, it is generally recognised that by itself, no form of pain education is likely to be sufficient to reduce pain and disability in patients like this man (Geneen et al. 2017). Instead, Geneen et al. recommend that pain education in these types of cases is delivered in conjunction with other modalities. In this context, the results of a recent randomised controlled trial (RCT) with acute low back pain patients may be instructive. The patients in the study were identified by screening as being at risk for long-term problems with back pain and found that adding general information about pain science to usual, evidence-based care (basically exercises) by physiotherapists was no more effective than the control condition which received empathic support (plus exercises) and no education about pain (Treager et al. 2019).

A more accurate understanding of his pain and responding to his specific concerns can assist in lessening his unwarranted fears, but knowledge and 'reassurance' about one's pain, by themselves, are unlikely to be sufficient to overcome the emotional aspects of pain-related fears (Linton et al. 2005). We will need to address these aspects too. These have been successfully addressed by training the patient in various coping skills, including applied relaxation for when he starts feeling more pain and associated distress (Feldman et al. 2021; Hayes-Skelton et al. 2013), mindfulness training (Hilton et al. 2017), and training in basic cognitive coping strategies (thought management and imagery) (Linton et al. 2005). In the medium term, if he learns to pace his activities and exercises while gradually upgrading these, they can also reduce his pain severity (Nicholas et al. 2014; Vaegter & Jones 2020) and his 'as-needed' use of opioids (Andrews et al. 2016). None of these skills by themselves is likely to be sufficient, but there is evidence that they can help, providing the patient actually uses them actively (Nicholas et al. 2012, 2014).

2. Reduced activities

While avoiding activities associated with pain is a common and understandable solution for someone in this man's position, at least initially, it is well-established that

continuing in this manner is one of the high-risk factors for long-term disability (Hayden et al. 2009). For his successful recovery and rehabilitation, he should have started increasing his activity levels long before 12 months were up. This applies especially to those activities he is limiting or avoiding due to his pain. While many people seem to work this out for themselves and do not require much health service input (Blyth et al. 2005), the man described here is clearly among those who are seeking help. But patients with chronic low back pain, like this man, can still change and substantially increase their levels of functioning and reduce their levels of disability in a sustainable way (Williams et al. 1999).

In general, exercises and resumption of activity are routinely recommended (Ambrose & Golightly 2015). There is consistent evidence that increasing levels of activity generally, including exercises, although not specific exercises, are helpful for people living with chronic pain generally. A comprehensive narrative review by Ambrose & Golightly (2015) provides a useful summary of the available evidence for the benefits of being active for people living with chronic pain. These authors also confirmed that the benefits of sustained activity and exercise could extend well beyond levels of fitness and function; they also appear to promote better sleep and mood. However, lest exercises/activities be thought of as a panacea, while a Cochrane systematic review by Geneen et al. (2017) was generally supportive of the conclusions drawn by Ambrose & Golightly, Geneen et al. did caution that the evidence was variable and the effects were only small to moderate. They also noted a slightly higher dropout rate from exercises than controls in the studies reviewed, and in a majority of studies, adherence to exercises wasn't mentioned.

Despite the supporting evidence for exercises and activities, the obvious challenge in cases like the man in this case study is that he has found this difficult due to his persisting pain and increased pain when he does try to exercise or be more active. These experiences have probably led to his avoidance of recommended exercises, at least when his pain levels are high, or he fears they will get worse when he exercises. The case formulation described in Fig 12.1 illustrates the problem for him, with the consequences of both avoiding and embarking on activities ending up in a vicious cycle of deteriorating well-being. Clearly, there is a need to find a method for helping him to overcome his fears about worse pain while increasing his activity levels, including exercises, without aggravating his pain so much that he retreats into old habits of basing his activities on his levels of pain. These patterns of behaviour have been referred to as 'pain-dependent behaviour', or an 'activity-rest cycle', where the patient tends to do less when pain is more severe, then does much more when the pain is less, thereby aggravating their pain leading to more rest until the pain flare-up settles and the cycle is repeated

(Gil et al. 1988). Others have referred to it as a pattern of 'overdoing and underdoing' (Andrews et al. 2012). In other words, it has commonly been observed by different clinicians and researchers.

Overcoming this challenge was a major part of the operant behavioural methods described by Fordyce (1976). Central to Fordyce's solution to this cycle was to engage the patient in setting themselves goal activities that would be important enough to motivate them to work towards these goals (e.g. walking a set distance within a set time). Fordyce described a step-by-step approach of setting activity-specific (and small) quotas (e.g. an extra 1–2 minutes of walking every second or third day) a patient could use to gradually upgrade their activities over several days or weeks. This method (or versions of it) was subsequently referred to as activity pacing. Since those pioneering days, goal setting and graduated upgrading of activities and exercises have been a standard feature of psychologically based pain management programs (e.g. Williams et al. 1996; Nicholas et al. 2012).

Goal setting has not been subject to nearly as much scrutiny in the research literature, and it features prominently in the two main theory-based approaches, CBT and ACT, for managing chronic pain, but activity pacing has been the subject of recurring debate for some time. It seems this is largely because of different definitions of pacing and the difficulties inherent in measuring it accurately (Andrews et al. 2012). For some researchers, and in some measures, activity pacing has been confused with avoidance due, in part, to the advice given to patients that they should stop activities frequently when in pain (McCracken & Samuel 2007). However, others have defined it as a means of gradually upgrading activities and exercises, usually according to preset quotas, despite pain but in a way that does not excessively aggravate pain. For example, Williams et al. (1996) used the method described by Gil et al. (1988).

While studies of complex, multifaceted treatments like interdisciplinary pain management (or rehabilitation) programs have often featured activity pacing as one of their methods, they cannot identify its precise contribution as they were not designed to answer that question. However, we do have evidence that adding these psychological and behavioural strategies to exercises is more effective in improving outcomes than exercises alone (Nicholas et al. 2017a; Sterling et al. 2019).

There are other indications of the usefulness of both these strategies for increasing activity levels. A qualitative study of activity pacing among patients with chronic pain has reported they found pacing to be very acceptable and useful as a practical way of managing their pain (Antcliff et al. 2021) and a Delphi study of researchers and clinicians found activity pacing and goal setting among the highest ranked in the necessary and desirable categories of pain management strategies for chronic pain (Sharpe et al. 2020). Data from two studies reported by Nicholas et al. (with different samples) have also indicated that when adherence to activity pacing (and other self-management strategies) was assessed by a combination of patient self-report and staff observations in a 3-week pain management program, those who adhered strongly were much more likely to have less pain and disability at the end of the program (Nicholas et al. 2012) and at 1-year follow-up (Nicholas et al. 2014).

In summary, if we are to help the man under review here to increase his activity levels and limit his avoidance of activities likely to aggravate his pain, the approach based on these accounts of goal setting and activity pacing would include the healthcare providers (individually or as members of a multidisciplinary team) working with the patient to identify his preferred functional goals (e.g. resuming his previous duties at home, and golf with his friends, as well as returning to work). In turn, he would need to specify what activities or behaviours he needs to increase to achieve these goals. These might include standing, sitting, walking, driving his car, swinging a golf club, etc. To pace these up to his goal levels, he would need to calculate what he can manage in each of these activities now, then set his initial quotas for each activity (ideally, starting a little below what he thinks he can do so it's well within his capacity and likely to be successful, thereby reinforcing his efforts). These quotas would be gradually raised, usually every second or third day, through discussions with his healthcare team. An important consideration would be to encourage him to set these quotas in advance rather than wait to see how his pain levels are each day, as that would risk his relapsing into his old pain-dependent behaviour patterns and the associated reliance on passive forms of treatment (e.g. rest and medications). To make his activity and exercise upgrading as sustainable as possible, he should also be helped to establish a weekly activity timetable that will provide him with a daily structure of planned tasks. In turn, this can help him move away from basing his activities each day on his pain levels.

3. Increased weight

The exercise program and increased activity levels should be helpful here, but some education about his diet and alternatives found for his use of food as a comfort when feeling distressed would be beneficial. This is an example of how improving his mood by learning and applying more adaptive cognitive strategies should help. There is certainly widespread evidence that obesity is a risk factor for disability, and poor health outcomes generally (Janek & Kozak 2012).

There is also a growing body of evidence that a combination of dietary changes and exercises can lead to better outcomes in patients with chronic painful conditions (Bell et al. 2012). The RCT reported by Messier et al. (2013) illustrated this with overweight and obese patients with painful knees due to osteoarthritis who were helped to improve pain, weight loss, functional activities and quality-of-life outcomes following a trial of combined dietary changes and exercises vs the same interventions offered separately.

4. High fear of movement

Education about his pain and answering his questions about the chances of further injury if he moves is very important—not only for its information value but also for its more subtle message that the therapy team has listened to his concerns and takes them seriously. This process has also been called validation and has been found to be associated with adherence to treatment regimens (Edmond & Keefe 2015; Linton et al. 2011). Simple reassurance that all will be fine is not advised, even though often mentioned in treatment guidelines for acute back pain, as this can make anxious people worse (Linton et al. 2011). The gradual upgrading and reduced avoidance of painful activities will also help to overcome this fear as the patient is encouraged to gradually confront the feared situation and is able to experience for themselves that their worst fears are not realised and that they can manage. This, in turn, can assist the strengthening of self-efficacy beliefs that they can do this activity despite their pain. It is easy to see that the activity pacing approach to upgrading activities mentioned earlier can assist in this process. This approach, often called exposure therapy in the CBT literature where it is usually described in terms of a series of brief behavioural experiments designed to allow the patient to test and deny their fears in daily life (Bennett-Levy et al. 2004), has strong support from studies on anxieties and phobias (Roth & Fonagy 2005). In the pain field, while seldom tested in isolation, this approach is a well-established component of multimodal and multidisciplinary pain management programs (Boersma et al. 2004; de Jong et al. 2012; Woods & Asmundson 2012).

5. High catastrophising

Providing accurate information about his concerns regarding long-term outcomes of pain would be useful, together with training in thought management (recognising these thoughts as unhelpful and developing and practising more helpful responses), as well as applied relaxation to reduce his level of alarm. Problem-solving training could also help him to develop practical options

for implementing whenever he starts to engage in these worrying thoughts.

There is good evidence that a number of strategies can help to reduce catastrophic types of thinking about pain (Schütze et al. 2018), and their reduction is typically associated with improvements in mood, pain levels and function (Hanscom et al. 2015; Moore et al. 2016; Nicholas et al. 2014). However, there is also evidence that these benefits are mainly seen in those in the higher catastrophising category (Burns et al. 2012).

6. Low pain self-efficacy

Bandura (1977) identified three main ways in which self-efficacy beliefs might be improved—by gradually engaging in activities/exercises the person is not confident to perform (e.g. starting with small steps, as in activity pacing), watching others like himself perform the same tasks (usually in a group format), and by verbal persuasion by authoritative and experienced healthcare providers (e.g. occupational therapist, physiotherapist, general practitioner or specialist medical practitioner). Each of these options is likely to exist in a multidisciplinary pain management program.

Not surprisingly, several researchers have found links between pain self-efficacy beliefs and fear-avoidance beliefs about pain. An early cross-sectional study with low back pain patients by Woby et al. (2007), for example, found that self-efficacy mediated the relationship between pain-related fear and pain intensity and between pain-related fear and disability. The authors concluded from their findings that when self-efficacy is high, elevated pain-related fear might not lead to greater pain and disability. However, where self-efficacy is low, elevated pain-related fear is likely to lead to greater pain and disability. This suggests that pain self-efficacy is likely to have a greater influence on outcomes than pain-related fear. Mansell et al. (2013) also reported evidence suggesting a mediating role for self-efficacy beliefs and catastrophising thought patterns in pain management outcomes. A recent study has found results consistent with this. Van Hoof et al. (2021) found that after a 2-week multidisciplinary pain management program, posttreatment pain self-efficacy levels, rather than the so-called 'dysfunctional' cognitions (catastrophising and fear of movement) were the best predictor of functional levels a year later.

Even so, numerous studies of multidisciplinary pain management programs with disabled chronic pain patients have reported significant improvements in mood, depression, disability and the likely mediators of pain self-efficacy, fear-avoidance beliefs and pain-related catastrophic beliefs (Nicholas et al. 1992, 2012, 2014; Williams et al. 1996, 1999). Interestingly, in these studies, these improvements were not always associated with significant improvements in pain levels, suggesting that pain reductions are not necessary in order for functional gains to be achieved.

7. Repeated treatment failure

Education about the limitations of treatments for chronic pain may provide some perspective on this, but a copy of the case formulation could also help the patient to see that any treatment will need to address multiple targets and that makes it unlikely a single intervention (also called unimodal treatment) would be unlikely to help significantly. This should be confirmed by referring to his experiences to date. Some reflection on how he was left feeling after each treatment failure may also be helpful to understand that while each attempted treatment might be accompanied by hope, it also carries the risk of failure and that has consequences too. This might be an area that pain education could address too.

A 2018 systematic review found moderate evidence that the addition of pain neuroscience education (PNE) to usual physiotherapy intervention in patients with chronic low back pain (CLBP) improved disability in the short term, but not the longer term (Woods & Hendrick 2012). However, it is interesting to note that another systematic review of pain education for patients found the education delivered by physicians was significantly more reassuring than that delivered by other primary care practitioners (e.g. physiotherapist or nurse). It also found there was moderate-quality evidence that patient education reduces low back pain–related primary care visits more than usual care/control education over a 12-month follow-up. Even so, the number needed to treat to prevent 1 low back pain–related visit to primary care in the following year was 17, suggesting it is unlikely to be sufficient by itself.

8. Continuing use of ineffective medication

As medication for pain is one of the most common treatments patients with chronic pain will try, an opportunity to learn more about the nature of medication for chronic pain and their limitations is important for ensuring the patient is an informed consumer and can decide for themselves. As withdrawing from unhelpful medication is a common aspect of pain management, it is a standard practice to have a plan prepared to address the patient's likely concerns and questions. A flexible approach was outlined by Ziadni et al. (2020) and this is now being evaluated in a large US trial (Darnell et al. 2020). One essential element for clinicians engaged in this process is to ensure the patient understands that rather than simply ceasing a medication the plan will be to replace the need for the medication by learning a range of pain self-management

skills. This is normally a gradual process, often referred to as tapering.

In cases of resistance to ceasing medication, which is understandable, a problem-solving approach can be worthwhile. This would entail weighing up the costs and benefits of the different options and it might be acceptable for the patient to see gradual withdrawal from their medication as a trial process while they learn the pain self-management strategies. They might also be more willing to try this if they understand they can always resume the medication being ceased if the alternatives do not work out. Despite the likely obstacles for tapering opioids and other medications used for patients with chronic disabling pain, there is consistent evidence that such patients can successfully cease their regular use of the agents and maintain those changes for at least a year posttreatment (Nicholas et al. 2020; Williams et al. 1999).

In the case of the man under discussion here, although he does not appear to be taking high doses of opioids, he does seem to be taking more than his prescribing doctor recommended. This is a concern, and it would be appropriate to develop an opioid tapering plan with the patient to be managed by that doctor.

9. Side effects of medication

This is related to the previous section and can be highlighted in discussion with the patient in relation to the benefits of tapering off the current opioid use. However, preparation for the withdrawal process is strongly advised as this can be quite unpleasant. In practice, it is usually recommended that the withdrawal/tapering program is managed by a single prescriber and a consistent contact person, like a clinic nurse, skilled in drug-withdrawal management (Ziadni et al. 2020).

10. Depressed mood

As the patient starts to become more active working towards his goal activities and exercising daily his mood should benefit (Ambrose & Golightly 2015), but some additional strategies can help as well. These include thought management, problem-solving, pleasant activity scheduling and self-regulation strategies.

Thought management strategies are the cognitive part of CBT. These may include learning to recognise unhelpful thoughts and responses to pain and other stressors, and then responding to them in ways that either allow the unhelpful thoughts to be acknowledged as just thoughts that do not need to be attended to while he continues with his goal pursuits (as described in accounts of mindfulness and ACT) or by developing another, more helpful perspective and response to the trigger stimuli for the unhelpful thoughts. Both approaches involve recognising thoughts or ways of thinking or responding as unhelpful and choosing to respond differently (Kabat-Zinn et al. 1985; Tang 2018). The net effect of these strategies is expected to be shown in reduced catastrophic types of thinking, which to the extent that they act as a mediator for depressed mood, should and often does appear to be associated with reduced levels of depression (Feldman et al. 2021; Schütze et al. 2018). However, direct modification of catastrophising thought patterns is not essential as other interventions can improve mood as well (Ambrose & Golightly 2015).

Training in using problem-solving strategies to come up with ways of managing challenging situations has also been used to improve mood and function, including return to work (Pierce 2012; van den Hout et al. 2003).

11. Frustration/anger

Sullivan et al. (2014) pointed to the negative impact on treatment outcomes of a sense of injustice among patients with chronic pain conditions. These researchers noted that frustration and anger, often directed towards others thought to be responsible for their pain and associated difficulties, were also particularly difficult to change. Not surprisingly, improving reactions like anger and frustration is likely to be enhanced by the ways in which the clinicians interact with the patient. Vangronsveld & Linton (2011), for example, found that the use of validating communications was associated with greater improvements in anger and frustration than invalidating styles of communicating with nurses experiencing low back pain. Practising the recognition of these emotions and responses and using thought management strategies like those mentioned for depressed mood, as well as practising applied relaxation in the stressful situations, can also help (Feldman et al. 2021; Hanscom et al. 2015).

These strategies can facilitate clearer thinking and problem solving in these situations.

In the case of the man under discussion here, the available evidence suggests that a combination of a validating communication style, applied relaxation training and thought management strategies would be worth instituting.

12. Poor sleep

Addressing this usually requires a combination of monitoring current sleep patterns (using a diary) and habits just before sleep, as well as usual waking times and responses when he wakes through the night. Attention to the bedroom and time to bed in the evening should also be undertaken. There are basic sleep hygiene habits that have been found helpful. These include ensuring, as much as possible, the bedroom is mainly used for sleep

and not watching TV/videos, or working on a computer as well. The bedroom at night should be kept as dark as possible and as quiet and cool as possible. Learning to use a relaxation technique while waiting to go to sleep is recommended, as well as a plan to get up again if not asleep within about 20 to 30 minutes and sitting in a chair in another room, if possible, doing something quiet (e.g. reading, listening to soft music, relaxing) then returning to bed to try falling asleep again. If the patient is finding worries are keeping him awake, then he will need to develop a thought management plan to deal with those as well. There is a burgeoning empirical literature on CBT methods for insomnia, which is often called CBTi (Tang et al. 2015; Trauer et al. 2015). A systematic review and meta-analysis by Tang et al. (2015), for example, found that nonpharmacological sleep treatments, like CBTi, in chronic pain patients were associated with a large improvement in sleep quality, a small reduction in pain and moderate improvement in fatigue at posttreatment. The effects on sleep quality and fatigue were maintained at follow-up (up to 1 year), along with a moderate reduction in depression. Interestingly, both cancer and noncancer pain patients benefited from these strategies.

In the case of the man under discussion here, a sleep management plan using CBTi principles would seem warranted. This process might be aided by the use of one of the numerous free Apps that are available online.

13. Loss of job and role in the workplace

People with chronic pain conditions are particularly vulnerable to loss of employment due to their functional limitations, often accompanied by uncertainty over how to manage them when they do return to work (Franche et al. 2005). At the same time, it is well-established that the longer an injured worker is away from work, the less chance they will have of a successful return to work outcome (Johnson & Fry 2002). It is also increasingly clear that achieving a sustainable return to work after the development of persisting pain by an injured worker is best done through a collaboration between the treatment providers, the workplace and other agencies, such as insurance companies (Cullen et al. 2018). In the case of the patient under consideration in this chapter, the fact that he has lost his job is likely to be a major obstacle for his successful return to work as he has no employer to relate to and applying to a new employer at this stage is likely to end in rejection. Accordingly, his best chance of a successful return to work outcome may be to regain as much functionality in his daily life as possible, along with improved mood, before he starts working with a rehabilitation provider to assess his work capacity and skill set. However, his ultimate success in returning to work may depend on the support for this outcome provided by the society in which he lives, as different countries have quite different support systems operating for people like this case (Main & Shaw 2016; Peterson et al. 2018).

14. Home stress and input from the spouse/family

While commonly overlooked in more biomedical approaches to chronic pain which focus on the person in pain, especially their body, a biopsychosocial approach entails assessment of the possible contributions to the presenting case by their significant others, and well as their local context. Even if these are not amenable to change, just being aware of their contributions can enable the healthcare providers to take these into account when designing their treatment plan.

In this case, the issues identified from the initial assessment include financial pressures, conflict with his wife, becoming isolated from his social networks, and possibly a sense of guilt on the patient's part that he is not doing his share of the household duties. The treatment plan already includes activity upgrading with exercises and home-related chores and these would be expected to help him resume the household duties expected of him, and eventually the social activities that have been dropped. If he were able to return to some form of paid employment that would assist in reducing the financial pressures and his interactions with his wife, and her support for the self-management program should be amenable to change as well. There is growing evidence to support the involvement of spouses, and even families when children are involved, in pain self-management programs. Their involvement should also be expected to facilitate sustainable behavioural changes by the person living with chronic pain.

Keefe and colleagues (1999) were one of the first groups to show the potential benefits of using spouses in their psychologically based pain management programs. These programs involved dyadic sessions that teach couples communication skills and use mutual goal setting to assist the patients to acquire, maintain and implement their new pain-coping skills. Keefe et al. (2004) in an RCT with patients experiencing chronic osteoarthritic knee pain found that spouse-assisted coping skills training and exercise training could improve physical fitness, strength, pain coping and self-efficacy in their study cohort relative to those in the exercise-only comparison group.

More recent evidence supporting the role of spouse involvement in the management of a range of chronic illnesses was reported by Martire et al. (2019) from a systematic review and meta-analysis that found that couple interventions had significant (though small) effects on patients' depressive symptoms, marital functioning and pain. These interventions were also more efficacious than either patient psychosocial intervention or usual care.

In the case of the man under discussion here, it would seem worthwhile to explore the willingness of his wife to attend some sessions at the clinic with the patient to develop a home management plan they are prepared to undertake.

15. Input from other healthcare providers

A recurring challenge for healthcare providers in working with patients with chronic pain is the high risk of these patients receiving mixed and inconsistent messages from other healthcare providers they may also be seeing. This situation is not only likely to be confusing to the patient but also to potentially undermine the effectiveness of their interventions. In multidisciplinary teams, it has long been recognised that the contribution by each team member to the treatment program needs to consistent across the whole team. But when patients are seen in the community, the members of a team of healthcare providers are often working separately and not in the same room or building at the same time. This creates a risk for the coherence of the intervention and to the patient it may feel like they are dealing with people working in a series of silos, each working independently.

Accordingly, the importance of consistency in the language and terminology used by healthcare providers is repeatedly emphasised when addressing patients' beliefs about their pain (Main et al. 2010). One possible indicator of the problem of inconsistency within a team may be seen in the study by Williams & Potts (2010) which found that periods of high staff turnover were significantly related to poorer outcomes on pain self-efficacy and distance walked at the end of an intensive multidisciplinary pain management program. Periods of high staff turnover would be expected to be when inconsistency in program delivery between members of the team would be most likely.

In the rehabilitation of injured workers, a systematic review by Cullen et al. (2018) of the occupational rehabilitation literature and return to work (RTW) outcomes after injury concluded that the best RTW outcomes were associated with treatments that included engagement with the workplace. This review found that cognitive behavioural treatments were more effective, in RTW terms, when workplace engagement was part of the treatment plan. This conclusion indicates that RTW after pain treatments is possible, but less likely without ensuring there is consistent follow-through from the treatment providers to the workplace.

In the case of the man under discussion here, this evidence would suggest that in order to achieve the outcomes sought by the patient, it would be important to liaise with his doctor and the insurance company covering his claim to obtain agreement with the pain management plan and a rehabilitation plan for the period following the program. As he no longer has an employer, this is likely to require the appointment of a rehabilitation provider who can assist with helping the patient to ready himself for a graduated return to suitable work.

Could we use online methods to deliver these interventions?

With advances in technology and the impetus from the COVID-19 pandemic restrictions, online pain management options have flourished. The potential benefits for patients have been readily apparent, including ease of attendance at treatment sessions, and reduced costs and stress associated with travelling to and from clinic appointments. Many researchers had already been evaluating so-called e-health options before the arrival of COVID-19 (e.g. Eccleston et al. 2014), but at that time, these treatment modalities were relatively rare and limited to trials. But a review of the state of the art in 2020 highlighted the rapid expansion in these forms of treatment delivery and the research opportunities they represented (Eccleston et al. 2020). A series of studies of online pain self-management programs had demonstrated impressive results, especially with very large samples of patients relative to the usual numbers enrolling in psychological treatments for chronic pain (Dear et al. 2015, 2018; Hadjistavropoulos et al. 2018). Dear et al. (2018) also reported a high degree of maintenance of changes in key outcome domains over 12 to 24 months posttreatment.

While these outcomes have been impressive, and a considerable improvement over those reported in a systematic review by Eccleston et al. (2014), it is important to note that the samples being treated in some studies appear to differ from those typically seen in face-to-face tertiary pain services, with much higher proportions reporting high levels of formal education (46% had a university education in Dear et al. 2015) and employment. Some studies have also reported quite large dropout rates or nonadherence (or nonattendance) rates (e.g. Palermo et al. 2020) and these have been associated with reduced effectiveness. Other researchers, however, have reported relatively low dropout rates (e.g. Dear et al. 2018). Overall, these findings are encouraging, though it is not yet clear if the

detailed case-formulation-based intervention described in this chapter for more complex patients will fare as well in the online format. It may be easier to develop an approach that incorporates a bit of both in-person and online delivery of such programs. Tauber et al. (2020) identified several additional challenges for those contemplating e-health interventions for chronic pain, including the problem of assessing a patient initially, especially by physiotherapists and medical practitioners, who are generally reluctant to diagnose a patient without physically examining them. Tauber et al. also identified the regulatory and funding framework for pain services in many countries as potential major obstacles for the widespread implementation of e-health services for patients with chronic pain.

Building an interdisciplinary pain management program based on psychological principles

It will always be tempting, and often, expedient to add in whatever options are available in a multidisciplinary clinic. But it must be kept in mind that the fundamental purpose of these programs is to help patients with disabling chronic pain to change their behaviour, as needed, towards a sustainable self-management lifestyle with low disability, low distress and manageable pain. That means we need to consider how might any proposed ingredients contribute to this purpose, whether singly or in combination with other modalities. For example, if we know that a medial branch nerve block by local anaesthetic injection is likely to have only transient effects, at best, we should consider how might that promote a patient's ability to learn pain self-management strategies? Some have argued that even if such pain relief were only transient, it might provide the patient with an opportunity for 'capitalising on improved analgesia by an increase in physical and psychosocial functioning' (p. 140) (Collett 2001). Leaving aside the lack of evidence for this approach with chronic pain patients, the obvious question is what would the patient learn regarding managing their pain? There must be a high chance they would learn, or have reinforced, the common belief that they need their pain relieved before they will engage in rehabilitation. Unfortunately, as such effective pain relief is not on offer for the vast majority of patients with chronic pain, this is likely to reinforce what Eccleston & Crombez (2007) called misdirected problem-solving.

Similar arguments can be made about combining analgesic medication with pain self-management, where attributions for any improvement might reinforce a patient's belief that any improvement was due to the drug and not to their own efforts. This would appear contradictory to the evidence for pain self-efficacy (see van Hoof et al. 2021). That doesn't mean medication should not be included in the mix, but rather in a comprehensive multimodal approach, ideally medication should be prescribed in the context of specific preparation of the patient for this approach, whereby the role and use of medication should be clearly understood by the patient, along with the importance of their adherence to the self-management strategies being taught. One example of this is a study by Holroyd et al. (2001) who found that the combinations of medication plus stress management training were more effective for reducing headache activity than either alone. In another study with patients diagnosed with recent onset (less than 2 years) seropositive rheumatoid arthritis, while all participants received routine medical management (with medication), the half who were randomly allocated to receive an adjunctive psychological (CBT) intervention had significantly fewer depressive symptoms at posttreatment and 6-month follow-up. Significant improvements in joint involvement at 6-month follow-up were found for the CBT group, but not for the standard care group.

Many researchers have explicitly utilised behaviour change theories to build the components of their multimodal pain management program. Carnes et al. (2013), for example, described a feasibility study in which they used social learning theory and cognitive behavioural approaches to inform the content of their program. This included understanding and accepting pain, mood and pain, unhelpful thoughts and behaviour, problem solving, goal setting, action planning, movement, relaxation and social integration/reactivation. Similarly, Porcheret et al. (2014) described a case study to illustrate the systematic selection and use of theory to develop a behaviour change intervention to implement GP delivery of enhanced self-management support for people with osteoarthritis (OA) in primary care.

At a practical level, if the goal of a complex interdisciplinary pain management program is to foster greater functional independence by patients, then we need to consider how the components of the program might contribute to that goal. Ideally, this would be aimed at promoting a synergistic relationship between the various components, where the whole might be greater than the sum of the parts (e.g. Turk 2001). In the examples provided in this chapter, a focus has been on identifying and overcoming barriers to increased function in daily life. As we have seen this might involve not just an activity and exercise upgrading plan, but also training for the patients in performing the exercises and strategies, like pacing, as well as training in ways of overcoming unhelpful beliefs

and fears that may limit a patient's willingness to perform activities that could aggravate pain.

In sum, when deciding on which components to incorporate in a complex, multimodal treatment like an interdisciplinary pain management program, care needs to be taken to ensure they are a good 'fit' for the purpose of the program and that they are likely to enhance each other's effects.

Conclusion

Consistent with current guidelines for a patient-centred approach to the management of patients with chronic pain conditions, the case-formulation-based approach presented in this chapter on the psychological management of pain requires that each person is treated on their own merits. This means that before commencing any intervention, a careful assessment within a biopsychosocial framework should be conducted to identify the likely contributors to the presenting case. This should not only assist in making a diagnosis with the likely contributors, as per ICD-11 (Treede et al. 2019), but also it will enable the clinicians involved to develop a comprehensive case formulation, and in turn, a treatment plan that can be tailored to the individual patient.

It may seem that such complex interventions would be limited to working with patients individually, but this is not necessarily so. Given the changes across multiple dimensions by individual patients reported by studies with group-based programs, it is clearly possible to achieve outcomes relevant to individual patients within a group setting (e.g. Kamper et al. 2014; Nicholas et al. 2012, 2014; Williams et al. 1999). Even so, for this to be reliably achieved, healthcare providers staffing these group-based programs are likely to require adequate training in order to achieve competence in group delivery of individualised interventions (Gatchel et al. 2014). Williams &Potts (2010), for example, found that high periods of staff turnover from an inpatient pain management program were significantly related to poorer outcomes on some measures, suggesting that high-quality outcomes, even in established programs, are dependent on highly trained staff. But the patients treated in these programs must also be considered. Williams and colleagues (2012, 2020) have repeatedly encouraged researchers and clinicians to go beyond the limited confines of RCTs that compare two or more interventions and instead to focus more on more granular questions, such as what works, for which patients, and under what conditions.

This chapter has attempted to provide a closer examination than usual of complex psychologically based multidisciplinary pain management programs for patients with chronic disabling pain. In this instance, a case study was employed to illustrate how a case formulation of the problems presented by an individual patient could be used to build a complex treatment that addressed the contributing factors identified in the initial assessment. The case formulation represents a hypothesis that can then be tested and modified in light of initial results, but it does provide a rationale for the different treatment components and allows the clinicians to engage the patient in the process. This is critical as the ultimate goal for these types of intervention is to achieve self-management of pain by the patient (Nicholas & Blyth 2016).

Review questions Q

1. What do we know about attributions patients often make to account for their improvement after self-management intervention?
2. How might we help patients to maintain their improvements following a self-management program, especially given the dominance of advertising for biomedical treatments?
3. If you were writing a training curriculum for health professionals learning about pain self-management, what might you include?
4. Are different psychological approaches to pain self-management likely to end up with similar outcomes, regardless of their theoretical differences?

References

Ambrose, K.R., Golightly, Y.M., 2015. Physical exercise as non-pharmacological treatment of chronic pain: why and when. Best Pract. Res. Clin. Rheumatol. 29, 120–130.

Andrews, N.E., Strong, J., Meredith, P., 2012. Activity pacing, avoidance, endurance, and associations with patient functioning in chronic pain: a systematic review and meta-analysis. Arch. Phys. Med. Rehabil. 93, 2109–2212.

Andrews, N.E., Strong, J., Meredith, P.J., Fleming, J.A., 2016. The relationship between overactivity and opioid use in chronic pain, a 5-day observational study. Pain 157, 466–474.

Antcliff, D., Keenan, A.M., Keeley, P., Woby, S., McGowan L. 2021Testing a newly developed activity pacing framework for chronic pain/fatigue: a feasibility study. BMJ Open 11:e045398. doi:10.1136/bmjopen-2020-045398

Balderson, B.H.K., Von Korff, M., 2002. The stepped care approach to chronic back pain. In: Linton, S.J. (Ed.), New Avenues for the Prevention of Chronic Musculoskeletal Pain and Disability. 1. Elsevier, Amsterdam, pp. 237–243.

Bandura, A., 1977. Self-efficacy: toward a unifying theory of behavioural change. Psychol. Rev. 84, 191–215.

Bell, R.F., Borzan, J., Kalso, E., Simonnet, G., 2012. Food, pain, and drugs: does it matter what pain patients eat? Pain 153, 1993 1996.

Bennett-Levy, J.E., Butler, G.E., Fennell, M.E., Hackman, A.E., Mueller, M.E., Westbrook, D.E., 2004. Oxford Guide to Behavioural Experiments in Cognitive Therapy. Oxford University Press, Oxford.

Blyth, F.M., March, L.M., Nicholas, M.K., Cousins, M.J., 2005. Self-management of chronic pain, a population-based study. Pain 113 (3), 285–292.

Boersma, K., Linton, S., Overmeer, T., Jansson, M., Vlaeyen, J., de Jong, J., 2004. Lowering fear-avoidance and enhancing function through exposure in vivo, a multiple baseline study across six patients with back pain. Pain 108 (1), 8–16.

Burns, J.W., Day, M.A., Thorn, B.E., 2012. Is reduction in pain catastrophizing a therapeutic mechanism specific to cognitive-behavioral therapy for chronic pain? Translat. Behav. Med. 2, 22–29.

Carnes, D., Homer, K., Underwood, M., Pincus, T., Rahman, A., Taylor, S.J.C., 2013. Pain management for chronic musculoskeletal conditions, the development of an evidence-based and theory informed pain self-management course. BMJ Open 3, e003534.

Collett, B.J., 2001. Chronic opioid therapy for noncancer pain. Br. J. Anaesth. 87, 133–144.

Cullen, K.L., Irvin, E., Collie, A., F Clay, Gensby, U., Jennings, P.A., et al., 2018. Effectiveness of workplace interventions in return-to-work for musculoskeletal, pain-related and mental health conditions: an update of the evidence and messages for practitioners. J. Occup. Rehabil. 28, 1–15.

Darnell, B., Mackey, S.C., Lorig, K., Kao, M.-C., Mardian, A., Stieg, R., et al., 2020. Comparative effectiveness of cognitive behavioral therapy for chronic pain and chronic pain self-management within the context of voluntary patient-centered prescription opioid tapering: the EMPOWER study protocol. Pain Med. 21 (8), 1523–1531.

de Jong, J.R., Vlaeyen, J.W., van Eijsden, M., Loo, C., Onghena, P., 2012. Reduction of pain related fear and increased function and participation in work-related upper extremity pain (WRUEP), effects of exposure in vivo. Pain 153 (10), 2109–2118.

Dear, B.F., Gandy, M., Karin, E., Staples, L.G., Johnston, L., Fogliati, V.J., et al., 2015. The pain course, a randomised controlled trial examining an internet-delivered pain management program when provided with different levels of clinician support. Pain 156, 1920–1935.

Dear, B.F., Gandy, M., Karin, E., Fogliati, R., Fogliati, V.J., Staples, L.G., et al., 2018. The pain course: 12- and 24-month outcomes from a randomized controlled trial of an Internet-delivered pain management program provided with different levels of clinician support. J. Pain. 19 (12), 1491–1503.

Detweiler-Bedell, J.B., Friedman, M.A., Leventhal, H., Miller, I.W., Leventhal, E.A., 2008. Integrating co-morbid depression and chronic physical disease management. Identifying and resolving failures in self-regulation. Clin. Psychol. Rev. 28, 1426–1446.

Eccleston, C., Crombez, G., 2007. Worry and chronic pain: a misdirected problem solving model. Pain 132, 233–236.

Eccleston, C., Fisher, E., Craig, L., Duggan, G.B., Rosser, B.A., Keogh, E., 2014. Psychological therapies (internet-delivered) for the management of chronic pain in adults. Cochrane Database Syst Rev. CD010152.

Eccleston, C., Blyth, F.M., Dear, B.F., Fisher, E.A., Keefe, F.J., Lynch, M.E., et al., 2020. Managing patients with chronic pain during the COVID-19 outbreak: considerations for the rapid introduction of remotely supported (eHealth) pain management services. Pain 161, 889–893.

Edmond, S.N., Keefe, F.J., 2015. Validating pain communication, current state of the science. Pain 156, 215–219.

Evers, A.W.M., Colloca, L., Blease, C., et al., 2021. What should clinicians tell patients about placebo and nocebo effects? Practical considerations based on expert consensus. Psychother. Psychosom. 90, 49–56.

Feldmann, M., Hein, H.J., Voderholzer, U., et al., 2021. Cognitive change and relaxation as key mechanisms of treatment outcome in chronic pain: evidence from routine care. Front. Psychiatry 12, 617–871 2021.

Fordyce, W.E., 1976. Behavioural Methods for Chronic Pain and Illness. Mosby, St. Louis.

Franche, R.-L., Baril, R., Shaw, W., Nicholas, M., Loisel, P., 2005. Workplace-based return-to-work interventions: optimizing the role of stakeholders in implementation and research. J. Occup. Rehabil. 15, 525–542.

Gatchel, R.J., McGeary, D.D., McGeary, C.A., Lippe, B., 2014. Interdisciplinary chronic pain management: past, present, and future. Am. Psychol. 69 (2), 119–130.

Geneen, L.J., Moore, R.A., Clarke, C., Martin, D., Colvin, L.A., Smith, B.H., 2017. Physical activity and exercise for chronic pain in adults: an overview of Cochrane Reviews. Cochrane Database Syst. Rev. 4, CD011279.

Gil, K.M., Ross, S.L., Keefe, F.J., 1988. Behavioral treatment of chronic pain, four pain management protocols. In: France, R.D., Krishnan, K.D.D. (Eds.), Chronic Pain. American Psychiatric Press, Washington, pp. 376–413. 1988.

Hadjistavropoulos, H.D., Schneide, L.H., Hadjistavropoulos, T., Titov, N., Dear, B.F., 2018. Effectiveness, acceptability and feasibility of an Internet-delivered cognitive behavioral pain management program in a routine online therapy clinic in Canada. Can. J. Pain. 2 (1), 62–73.

Hanscom, D.A., Brox, J.I., Bunnage, R., 2015. Defining the role of cognitive behavioral therapy in treating chronic low back pain: an overview. Global Spine J. 5, 496–504.

Hayden, J.A., van Tulder, M.W., Tomlinson, G., 2005. Systematic review: strategies for using exercise therapy to improve outcomes in chronic low back pain. Ann. Intern. Med. 142, 776–785.

Hayden, J.A., Chou, R., Hogg-Johnson, S., Bombardier, C., 2009. Systematic reviews of low back pain prognosis had variable methods and results: guidance for future prognosis reviews. J. Clin. Epidemiol. 62, 781 96.e1.

Hayes-Skelton, S., Roemer, E., Orsillo, S.M., Borkovec, T.D., 2013. A contemporary view of applied relaxation for generalized anxiety disorder. Cognit. Behav. Ther. 42 (4), 292–302.

Hilton, L., Hempel, S., Ewing, B.A., Apaydin, E., et al., 2017. Mindfulness meditation for chronic pain: systematic review and meta-analysis. Ann. Behav. Med. 51, 199–213.

Holroyd, K.A., O'Donnell, F.J., Stenland, M., et al., 2001. Management of chronic tension-type headache with tricyclic antidepressant medication, stress management therapy, and their combination—a randomized controlled trial. JAMA. 285, 2208–2217.

Janke, E.A., Kozak, A.T., 2012. The more pain I have, the more I want to eat. Obesity in the Context of Chronic Pain. Obesity 20, 2027–2034.

Johnson, D., Fry, T., 2002. Factors Affecting Return to Work after Injury: A Study for the Victorian WorkCover Authority. Melbourne Institute of Applied Economic and Social Research Melbourne.

Kabat-Zinn, J., Lipworth, L., Burney, R., 1985. The clinical use of mindfulness meditation for the self-regulation of chronic pain. J. Behav. Med. 8 (2), 163–190.

Kamper, S.J., Apeldoorn, A.T., Chiarotto, A., Smeets, R.J., et al., 2014. Multidisciplinary biopsychosocial rehabilitation for chronic low back pain. Cochrane Database Syst. Rev. 9 CD000963.

Keefe, F.J., Caldwell, D.S., Baucom, D., Salley, A., et al., 1999. Spouse-assisted coping skills training in the management of knee pain in osteoarthritis: long-term follow-up results. Arthritis Care Res. 12, 101–111.

Keefe, F., Blumenthal, J., Baucom, D., Affleck, G., et al., 2004. Effects of spouse-assisted coping skills training and exercise training in patients with osteoarthritic knee pain, a randomized controlled study. Pain 110, 539–549.

Keefe, F.J., Main, C.J., George, S.Z., 2018. Advancing psychologically informed practice (PiP) for patients with persistent musculoskeletal pain: promise, pitfalls and solutions. Phys. Ther. 98, 398–407.

Ledingham, A., Cohn, E., Baker, K., Keysor, J., 2020. Exercise adherence, beliefs of adults with knee osteoarthritis over 2 years. Physiother. Theory Pract. 36 (12), 1363–1378.

Linton, S., Nicholas, M.K., 2008. After assessment: then what? Integrating findings for successful case formulation and treatment tailoring. In: Rice, A., Warfield, C., Justins, D., Eccleston, C. (Eds.), Textbook of Clinical Pain Management, second ed. , pp. 95–106.

Linton, S.L., Boersma, K., Jansson, M., Svärd, L., Botvalde, M., 2005. The effects of cognitive-behavioral and physical therapy preventive interventions on pain-related sick leave. Clin. J. Pain. 21, 109–119.

Linton, S.J., Boersma, K., Vangronsveld, K.L.H., Fruzzetti, A.E., 2011. Painfully reassuring? The effects of validation on emotions and adherence in a pain test. Eur. J. Pain. 16, 592–599.

Maguire, P., Pitceathly, C., 2002. Key communication skills and how to acquire them. Br. Med. J. 325, 697–7002002.

Maher, C., Underwood, M., Buchbinder, R., 2017. Non-specific low back pain. Lancet 389, 736–747.

Main, C.J., George, S.Z., 2011. Psychologically informed practice for management of low back pain, future directions in practice and research. Phys. Ther. 91, 820–824.

Main, C.J., Shaw, W.S., 2016. The Hopkinton Conference Working Group on Workplace Disability Prevention. Employer policies and practices to manage and prevent disability, conclusion to the special issue. J. Occup. Rehabil. 26, 490–498.

Main, C.J., Buchbinder, R., Porcheret, M., Foster, N., 2010. Addressing patient beliefs and expectations in the consultation. Best Pract. Res. Clin. Rheumatol. 24 (2), 219–225.

Mansell, G., Kamper, S.J., Kent, P., 2013. Why and how back pain interventions work, what can we do to find out? Best Pract. Res. Clin. Rheumatol. 27, 685–697.

Maroti, D., Folkeson, P., Jansson-Fröjmark, M., Linton, S.J., 2011. Does treating insomnia with cognitive–behavioural therapy influence comorbid anxiety and depression? An exploratory multiple baseline design with four patients. Behav. Change 28 (4), 195–205.

Martire, L.,M.,, Zhaoyangm, R., Marini, C.M., Nah, S., Darnel, B.D., 2019. Daily and bidirectional linkages between pain catastrophizing and spouse responses. Pain 60, 2841–2847.

McCracken, L.M., Samuel, V.M., 2007. The role of avoidance, pacing, and other activity patterns in chronic pain. Pain 130, 119–125.

Messier, S.P., Mihalko, S.L., Legault, C., Miller, C.D., et al., 2013. Effects of intensive diet and exercise on knee joint loads, inflammation, and clinical outcomes among overweight and obese adults with knee osteoarthritis: the IDEA Randomized Clinical Trial. JAMA 310 (12), 1263–1273.

Moore, E., Thibault, P., Adams, H., Sullivan, M.J.L., 2016. Catastrophizing and pain-related fear predict failure to maintain treatment gains following participation in a pain rehabilitation program. Pain Rep. 1–6 2016 e567.

Nicholas, M.K., George, S., 2011. Psychologically informed interventions for physical therapists. Phys. Ther. 91, 765–776.

Nicholas, M.K., Wilson, P.H., Goyen, J., 1992. Comparison of cognitive behavioural group treatment and an alternative non-psychological treatment for chronic low back pain. Pain 48, 339–347.

Nicholas, M.K., Linton, S.J., Watson, P.J., Main, C.J., 2011. The early identification and management of psychological risk factors (Yellow Flags) in patients with low back pain: a reappraisal. Phys. Ther. 91 (5), 737–753.

Nicholas, M.K., Asghari, A., Corbett, M., Smeets, R.J., Wood, B.M., Overton, S., et al., 2012. Is adherence to pain self-management strategies associated with improved pain, depression and disability in those with disabling chronic pain? Eur. J. Pain 16, 93–104.

Nicholas, M.K., Asghari, A., Sharpe, L., Brnabic, A., Wood, B.M., Overton, S., et al., 2014. Cognitive exposure versus avoidance in patients with chronic pain: adherence matters. Eur. J. Pain 18, 424–437.

Nicholas, M.K., Blyth, F.M., 2016. Are self-management strategies effective in chronic pain treatment? Pain Manage 6, 75–88.

Nicholas, M.K., Asghari, A., Blyth, F.M., Wood, B.M., Murray, R., McCabe, R., et al., 2017a. Long-term outcomes from training in self-management of chronic pain in an elderly population: a randomised controlled trial. Pain 158, 86–95.

Nicholas, M., Ushida, T., Wallace, M., Williams, A., Wittink, H., Edwards, R., et al., 2017b. Task force on multimodal pain treatment defines terms for chronic pain care. IASP. Available from: https://www.iasp-pain.org/PublicationsNews/NewsDetail.aspx?ItemNumber56981.

Nicholas, M.K., Asghari, A., Sharpe, L., Beeston, L., et al., 2020. Reducing the use of opioids by patients with chronic pain: an effectiveness study with long-term follow-up. Pain 161, 509–519.

Palermo, T., 2020. Pain prevention and management must begin in childhood: the key role of psychological interventions. Pain 161 (Suppl. l), S114–S121.

Peterson, K., Anderson, J., Bourne, D., Mackey, K., Helfand, M., 2018. Effectiveness of models used to deliver multimodal care for chronic musculoskeletal pain: a rapid evidence review. J. Gen. Intern. Med. 33 (S1), S71–S81.

Pierce, D., 2012. Problem solving therapy, Use and effectiveness in general practice. Aust. Fam. Physician. 41 (9), 676–678.

Pincus, T., McCracken, L., 2013. Psychological factors and treatment opportunities in low back pain. Best Pract. Res. Clin. Rheumatol. 27, 625–635.

Porcheret, M., Main, C., Croft, P., et al., 2014. Development of a behaviour change interventioncase study on the practical application of theory. Implement. Sci. 9, 42. http://www.implementationscience.com/content/9/1/42.

Roth, A., Fonagy, P., 2005. Anxiety disorders I, specific phobia, social phobia, generalized anxiety disorder, and pain disorder with and without agoraphobia. In: What Works for Whom, Critical Review of Psychotherapy Research, second ed. The Guilford Press, London, pp. 150–197.

Schütze, R., Rees, C., Smith, A., Slater, H., Campbell, J.M., O'Sullivan, P., 2018. How can we best reduce pain catastrophizing in adults with chronic noncancer pain? A Systematic Review and Meta-Analysis. J. Pain 19 (3), 233–256.

Sharpe, L., Jones, E., Ashton-James, C.E., Nicholas, M.K., Refshauge, K., 2020. Necessary components of psychological treatment in pain management programs: a Delphi study. Eur. J. Pain. 24, 1160–1168.

Sterling, M., Smeets, R., Keijzers, G., Warren, J., Kenardy, J., 2019. Physiotherapist delivered stress inoculation training integrated with exercise versus physiotherapy exercise alone for acute whiplash-associated disorder (StressModex), a randomised controlled trial of a combined psychological/physical intervention. Br. J. Sports Med. 53, 1240–1247.

Sullivan, M.J., Yakobov, E., Scott, W., Tait, R., 2014. Perceived injustice and adverse recovery outcomes. Psychol. Inj. and Law. 7, 325–334.

Tang, N.K.Y., 2018. Cognitive behavioural therapy in pain and psychological disorders: towards a hybrid future. Prog Neuro-Psychopharmacology & Biol Psychiatry. 87, 281–289.

Tang, N.K.Y., Lereya, S.T., Boulton, H., Miller, M.A., et al., 2015. Nonpharmacological treatments of insomnia for long-term painful conditions: a systematic review and meta-analysis of patient-reported outcomes in randomized controlled trials. Sleep 38 (11), 1751–1764.

Tauben, D.J., Langford, D.J., Sturgeon, J.A., Rundell, S.D., Towle, C., Bockman, C., et al., 2020. Optimizing telehealth pain care after COVID-19. Pain 161, 2437–2445.

Treede, R.D., Rief, W., Barke, A., Aziz, Q., Bennett, M.I., Benoliel, R., et al., 2019. Chronic pain as a symptom and a disease, the IASP classification of chronic pain for the international classification of diseases ICD-11. Pain 160, 19–27.

Trauer, J.,M., Qian, M.,Y., Doyle, J.S., Rajaratnam, S.M.W., et al., 2015. Cognitive behavioral therapy for chronic insomnia: a systematic review and meta-analysis. Ann. Intern. Med. 163, 191–204.

Treager, A.C., Lee, H., Hübscher, M., et al., 2019. Effect of intensive patient education vs placebo patient education on outcomes in patients with acute low back pain a randomized clinical trial. JAMA Neurol. 76, 161–169.

Turk, D.,C., 2001. Combining somatic and psychosocial treatment for chronic pain patients, perhaps 1 + 1 does = 3. Clin. J. Pain. 17, 281–283.

U.S. Department of Health and Human Services, 2019. Pain Management Best Practices Inter-Agency Task Force Report: Updates, Gaps, Inconsistencies, and Recommendations. Retrieved from U. S. Department of Health and Human Services website: https://www.hhs.gov/ash/advisory-committees/pain/reports/index.html.

Vaegter, H.B., Jones, M.D., 2020. Exercise-induced hypoalgesia after acute and regular exercise, experimental and clinical manifestations and possible mechanisms in individuals with and without pain. Pain Reports 9, e823, 2020.

van den Hout, J.H.C., Vlaeyen, J.W.S., Heuts, P.H.T.G., Zijlema, J.H.L., Wijnen, J.A.G., 2003. Secondary prevention of work-related disability in nonspecific low back pain: does problem-solving therapy help? A randomized clinical trial. Clin. J. Pain. 19, 87–96.

van Hoof, M., Vriezekolk, J.E., Kroeze, R.J., O'Dowd, J.K., van Limbeek, J., Spruit, M., 2021. Targeting self-efficacy more important than dysfunctional behavioral cognitions in patients with longstanding chronic low back pain: a longitudinal study. BMC Muscoskel. Disord. 22, 824, 2021.

Vangronsveld, K.L.H., Linton, S.J., 2011. The effect of validating and invalidating communication on satisfaction, pain and affect in nurses suffering from low back pain during a semi-structured interview. Eur. J. Pain. 16, 239–246. 2011.

Von Korff, M., Gruman, J., Schaefer, J., Curry, S., Wagner, E.H., 1997. Collaborative management of chronic illness. Ann. Intern. Med. 127 (12), 1097–1102.

Williams, A.C. de C., Potts, H.H.W., 2010. Group membership and staff turnover affect outcomes in group CBT for persistent pain. Pain 148, 481–486.

Williams, A.C. de C., Richardson, P.H., Nicholas, M.K., et al., 1996. Inpatient versus outpatient pain management: results of a randomised controlled trial. Pain 66, 13–22.

Williams, A.C. de C., Nicholas, M.K., Richardson, P.H., et al., 1999. Does randomisation affect the generality of findings from a controlled trial? The effects of patient preference versus randomisation on inpatient versus outpatient chronic pain management. Pain 83, 57–65.

Williams, A.C.D.C., Eccleston, C., Morley, S., 2012. Psychological therapies for the management of chronic pain (excluding headache) in adults. Cochrane Database Syst. Rev. 11 CD007407.

Williams, A.C.D.C., Fisher, E., Hearn, L., Eccleston, C., 2020. Psychological therapies for the management of chronic pain (excluding headache) in adults. Cochrane Database Syst. Rev. 8, CD007407.

Woby, S.R., Urmston, M., Watson, P.J., 2007. Self-efficacy mediates the relation between pain-related fear and outcome in chronic low back pain patients. Eur. J. Pain. 11, 711–718.

Wood, L., Hendrick, P.A., 2012. A systematic review and meta–analysis of pain neuroscience education for chronic low back pain: short–and long–term outcomes of pain and disability. Eur. J. Pain. 23, 234–249 2019.

Woods, M.P., Asmundson, G.J., 2012. Evaluating the efficacy of graded in vivo exposure for the treatment of fear in patients with chronic back pain: a randomized controlled clinical trial. Pain 136 (3), 271–280.

Ziadni, M., Chen, A.L., Krishnamurthy, P., Flood, P., Stieg, R.L., Darnall, B.D., 2020. Patient-centered prescription opioid tapering in community outpatients with chronic pain: 2- to 3-year follow-up in a subset of patients. Pain Reports 1–4 PR9 5, e851.

Chapter | 13 |

Neuropathic pain and complex regional pain syndrome

Nicola Cook, Hubert van Griensven, and Tom Jesson

LEARNING OBJECTIVES

At the end of this chapter, readers will understand the:
1. Pathophysiological mechanisms underlying neuropathic pain and complex regional pain syndrome.
2. Symptoms that alert the clinician to the possible presence of these conditions.
3. Current diagnostic criteria and their limitations.
4. Methodical approach to examination and treatment, based on current international evidence and guidelines.

Overview

This chapter covers two types of pain which have confused and frustrated patients and clinicians alike. Neuropathic pain (NP) can mimic other pain conditions and

frequently lacks any response to normal pain-relieving modalities. Complex regional pain syndrome (CRPS) is equally enigmatic by its dramatic response to a minor injury. It is called type 2 if it coincides with neuropathy and type 1 if it doesn't.

This chapter was written with particular attention to information which is relevant to clinicians. It first discusses neuropathic and neurogenic pain, starting with clinical characteristics, examination techniques and clinical reasoning. It ends with a review of therapeutic recommendations and practical advice. The second section of the chapter is devoted to CRPS. It discusses modern diagnostic criteria and their application in the examination and diagnosis of CRPS, followed by detailed recommendations for treatment and management.

Section 1. Neuropathic pain

Introduction

Neuropathic pain is defined as 'pain caused by a lesion or disease of the somatosensory nervous system' (International Association for the Study of Pain 2011).

NP can have its origin in the central or peripheral nervous system and can have a number of causes (Table 13.1). Its diagnosis is not straightforward, because it can mimic other painful conditions and present with seemingly contradictory signs and symptoms. This is further complicated by the fact that pain may have a nociceptive as well as a neurogenic component, requiring careful examination and possibly multimodal treatment.

Selecting the most efficient treatment can be even more difficult, as presentation and responses are extremely variable, even within one type of NP. This has led to the suggestion

Table 13.1 Conditions possibly associated with neuropathy
Central
Stroke
Multiple sclerosis (MS)
Spinal cord injury
Syringomyelia or syringobulbia
Epilepsy
Space-occupying lesions
Peripheral
Mononeuropathies
Trauma, including surgery
Nerve entrapment (see Table 13.2)
Postherpatic neuralgia
Trigeminal and glossopharyngeal neuralgia
Ischemia
Inflammatory or infectious
Spinal nerve root pathology, e.g. as a result of a intervertebral disc lesion
Plexus injury, e.g. brachial plexus avulsion
Other plexopathy, e.g. following viral syndrome
Tumour
Nerve damage induced by radiation or chemotherapy
Polyneuropathies
Metabolic, e.g. diabetic
Toxic, e.g. misuse of alcohol or other drugs
Nutritional, e.g. vitamin B deficiency
Amyloidosis
Vasculitis
Note: phantom pain is not included here because of its complex pain genesis
Based on Hansson et al. (2002) and Ross (2004).

that treatments should be based on underlying mechanisms instead of aetiological categories (Woolf & Max 2001).

Mechanisms of neuropathic pain

'When a telephone cable is cut, the phone falls silent. Damaged nerves behave differently'.

—Marshall Devor

NP is caused by a lesion or disease of the somatosensory system (Finnerup et al. 2016). It is typically felt in the sensory distribution of the affected nerves and presents with a wide array of sensations (positive or added features) such as burning, shooting, prickling, pins and needles, hot and cold sensations, and abnormal sensitivity to touch. It may be accompanied by negative features through loss of nerve function, including impaired sensation, muscle power and reflexes.

Broadly speaking, peripheral NP is caused by hyperexcitability of injured peripheral sensory neurons and central nervous system (CNS) circuits, as well as reduced central inhibition (see later). Peripheral sensory neurons are cells that create electrical impulses from external and internal stimuli and carry those impulses proximally to the spinal cord. This process relies on ion channels, which are embedded in the cell membrane. Changes in the function and expression of these ion channels may make neurons hyperexcitable, generate impulse generating sites along the neurons and drive peripheral NP.

Ion channel changes

After nerve injury, the production of neuronal ion channels is altered (Finnerup et al. 2020). As a consequence, ion channels may become more numerous and more sensitive to stimuli, and create more electrical impulses. This explains why drugs that inhibit ion channel function, e.g. gabapentin, may reduce NP (Attal & Bouhassira 2015). By contrast, genetic variations that enhance ion channel function may increase NP (Colloca et al. 2017). Some NP conditions called channelopathies may be caused solely by a genetic gain of function in sodium ion channels (Spillane et al. 2016).

Another aspect of NP is ion channel expression. Under normal conditions, ion channels are distributed evenly along an unmyelinated axon or concentrated at the Nodes of Ranvier of a myelinated axon. After nerve injury, an abnormal concentration of ion channels can form around the injury site (Devor 2006). As a consequence, this site may become hyperexcitable and create its own (i.e. ectopic) impulses. Peripheral nerve blocks, which interrupt ectopic impulses by preventing membrane depolarisation, temporarily reduce peripheral NP (Meacham et al. 2017).

Ion channels may concentrate in parts of the axon because of transection or degeneration of the axon. The affected part effectively becomes a new nerve ending with an overconcentration of ion channels (Finnerup et al. 2020). A nerve entrapment injury, e.g. carpal tunnel syndrome or radicular pain, may also demyelinate the neuron. Ion channels can accumulate in the demyelinated patch of the neuron. Finally, an injury may inflame the neuron (Dilley et al. 2013). This impedes the normal axonal transport of ion channels, causing them to accumulate at the inflammation site.

Ectopic impulse generating sites

High concentrations of ion channels can generate ectopic electrical impulses in response to a variety of stimuli. This includes internal and external temperature, which partly accounts for increased pain in response to cold in some people with NP (Devor 2013). Mechanical stimuli like stretch and pressure account for a positive Tinel's test (Costigan et al. 2009). New ion channels may create a responsiveness to such as an increase of circulating noradrenaline, so NP may be more prominent in stressful situations (Devor 2013). Other potential triggers include ischaemia and hypoglycemia (Finnerup et al. 2020). Spontaneous ectopic impulses account for paraesthesia and dysaesthesia (Devor 2013). The particular quality of an individual's neuropathic symptoms may depend on the types of neurone and the pattern of the ectopic impulses (Finnerup et al. 2020).

The role of the immune system

The immune system helps to determine how the nervous system responds to injury. There are three key features of this response. White blood cells are attracted to the area, infiltrate neurons through the blood-nerve barrier and break down nervous tissue (Ellis & Bennett 2013). Glial cells, i.e. Schwann cells in the peripheral nervous system (PNS), and microglia and astrocytes in the CNS, become activated (Ji et al. 2016). They sustain the inflammatory response through the release of inflammatory mediators (ibid), which sensitise and excite nociceptors, and enhance synaptic transmission (Calvo et al. 2012).

Neuroinflammatory changes may spread to sites in the nervous system remote from the original nerve injury (Albrecht et al. 2018; Xanthos & Sandkühler 2014). The extent of spread depends partly on the severity of the inciting injury. In animal studies, severe transection causes neuroinflammatory changes in the CNS, whereas the neuroinflammatory changes associated with mild constriction injuries may be more limited to the peripheral nerve (Schmid et al. 2013). Of note, neuroinflammatory changes are often observed in the dorsal root ganglion, even after distal nerve injuries (Calvo et al. 2012). This may account for the way in which peripheral NP can spread beyond its innervation territory (Furman & Johnson 2019; Nora et al. 2004). This neuroinflammatory response may seem undesirable, but it helps to clear up damaged cells and debris and restore homeostasis. It concludes with a resolution phase, in which the immune system releases antiinflammatory mediators and other substances (Ji et al. 2011). Ongoing NP might be due in part to a failure of this resolution phase (ibid).

Nervi nervorum

The epineurium is innervated by nervi nervorum—the 'nerves of the nerve', which may in part be nociceptive (Bove & Light 1997; Teixeira et al. 2016). Inflammation may sensitise these nervi nervorum, which may generate aching pain which is worse when the nerve is stretched or pressed. An element of peripheral NP may therefore be nociceptive in nature (Schmid et al. 2020).

Central changes

Central changes (see Chapter 7) may be particularly marked in NP and are partly responsible for key features such as hyperalgesia, allodynia and gradual temporal summation (Bannister et al. 2020). Neuropathy can lead to the development of central sensitisation, reinforced by reduced spinal and descending control (Dickenson & Bee 2008).

Changes in the somatosensory cortex of the brain have been determined both in response to ongoing pain (Flor et al. 1997) and in response to injury to peripheral nerves (Jensen 2002; Lundborg & Rosen 2007; Rosen et al. 2003). Cortical changes following peripheral nerve injury (traumatic and nontraumatic) occur immediately and continue throughout the reconstructive and rehabilitation phases (Osborne et al. 2018). Lack of a sensory input not only alters the cortical circuitry subserving the deprived sense, but also produces compensatory changes in the functionality of other sensory modalities (Hassan-zadeh & Esfahani 2012).

Distortion of the cortical map can contribute to an inaccurate prediction of the sensory consequences of a movement (*sensorimotor mismatch*) (Lewis et al. 2011). In those with high levels of pain and neural insult, sensory discrimination is poor and there are reduced levels of activity in the sensory maps (ibid). Neuroplasticity research has confirmed and continues to unravel the interplay between CNS and PNS, with several studies confirming that injury to the peripheral nerve causes functional and structural changes in the brain (Osborne et al. 2018). CNS changes include organisational degradation of the somatosensory cortex and loss of dendritic input of up to 50% on the motor neuron (Walsh 2012). A nerve injury in the upper extremity is followed by profound functional reorganisational changes in the somatosensory cortex (Lundborg & Rosen 2007).

Conclusion

The etiologies, mechanisms and manifestations of NP are diverse (Schmid et al. 2020). The same mechanisms may cause different symptoms in different people (Woolf & Mannion 1999). Conversely, the same symptom can be caused by different mechanisms in different people (ibid). Epistemic humility is therefore warranted when interpreting NP in clinical practice. That said, an understanding of the mechanisms of NP is important for diagnosis, patient education and treatment selection.

Clinical examination

The clinical characteristics of neuropathy may include a mixture of sensory, autonomic and motor changes, as well as NP. Treatment of NP is a priority because of its correlation with decreased function (Quintal et al. 2021).

Sensory changes include increased or decreased sensation or pain, allodynia, paraesthesia, dysaesthesia, spatial changes, and temporal changes such as latency, aftersensation and summation (Hansson & Kinnman 1996). Neuropathies may present with different combinations of signs and symptoms, with large variations between individuals and conditions. Symptoms are often continuous, may include spontaneous pain and pain that lingers after an evoking stimulus has ended (hyperpathia) (Walsh 2012). Classic descriptions include burning and electrical pains as well as paraesthesia and numbness, but these are not always present, nor does their absence exclude neuropathy. Signs may be paradoxical, such as intense pain

felt in a cutaneous region which is numb to the touch. Hypoaesthesia, hyperaesthesia and dysesthesia are all sensory alterations which may exist simultaneously with the cutaneous surface of a single functional unit of the body (Packham et al. 2018). Finally, neuropathies may mimic, and occur alongside, other conditions (Table 13.2). It is for these reasons that careful subjective and objective clinical examination is essential. A diagnostic grading system is provided in Fig. 13.1. If there is any doubt about the diagnosis, a referral should be made to a neurologist or pain specialist (Dworkin et al. 2007).

Comprehensive evaluation should include physical measures and subjective reports, using valid and reliable

Table 13.2 Entrapment neuropathies of the extremities

Nerve	Entrapment site	Symptoms	May masquerade as
Radial	Lateral elbow	Pain and sensory changes, radial distribution	Tennis elbow, De Quervain's
Radial	Wartenberg's point, under brachioradialis	Pain and sensory changes, radial distribution	De Quervain's
Median	Carpal tunnel	Paraesthesia and pain in hand	
Median	Pronator teres Lacertus fibrosus	Pain in median distribution	Carpal tunnel syndrome
Ulnar	Cubital tunnel	Pain and sensory changes ulnar distribution	
	Tunnel of Guyon	Pain and sensory changes ulnar distribution	
Lateral femoral cutaneous	Inguinal ligament	Pain and sensory changes antero-lateral thigh	L3 nerve root entrapment
Saphenus	Medial knee	Medial knee and calf pain	
Common peroneal	Proximal fibular head	Pain and sensory changes antero-lateral lower leg and dorsum foot	L4-5 nerve root entrapment
Superficial peroneal	Lateral lower leg	Pain and sensory changes dorsum foot and first four toes	L5 nerve root entrapment
Deep peroneal	Metatarsal 1	Pain first and second toe	
Tibial	Medial ankle (tarsal tunnel)	Pain heel, sole and toes	Plantar faciitis, tibialis posterior tendonitis, tarsal tunnel syndrome
Medial and lateral plantar	Medial calcaneum	Pain sole and toes	Plantar faciitis, tibialis posterior tendonitis, tarsal tunnel syndrome
Digital pedal	Between metatarsal heads	Pain in toe, typically 3rd or 4th	

Based on van Griensven (2005), with permission.

measurement tools (Novak 2018). Careful history taking is the cornerstone of every examination. This may start with a body chart, and it may be advantageous to ask the patient to do this themselves. The exact signs and symptoms, and the way they developed, may suggest what the pathology and aetiology are. Concomitant diseases can also give an indication (see Table 13.1) and may require their own tests. Spontaneous as well as evoked signs and symptoms must be explored, as well as their exact localisation on the body. Patients may be concerned that they may not be believed because of the nature of the symptoms. It is essential to reassure them that what they report is understandable and not uncommon. It is recommended that clinicians give patients a chance to formulate their own descriptions of symptoms without attempting to step in. At the end of history taking, the clinician should have at least one hypothesis regarding the underlying pathology.

A number of validated screening tools based on common features can aid the diagnosis (Table 13.3). They include questions about the most common neuropathic symptoms such as tingling, electrical and burning sensations. The inclusion of other sensations or numbness varies per questionnaire. The Leeds Assessment of Neuropathic Symptoms and Signs (LANSS) and Douleur Neuropathique 4 (DN4) have the advantage of including basic sensory tests.

Sensory impairments provide complex challenges and require tools to evaluate and monitor them and to quantify outcomes of treatment (Packham et al. 2018). (Box 13.1).

Signs and symptoms are likely to follow a distribution which is anatomically consistent with a peripheral nerve, spinal nerve root, plexus, or a structure in the CNS. The objective examination is aimed at testing the hypothetical cause of the symptoms. If pain is a prominent feature, testing other modalities such as motor function and reflexes first is advisable in order not to sensitise the nervous system.

Sensory testing is the final part of the examination and aims to map out the exact distribution of sensory changes. Ideally several tests are done because neuropathies do not always affect all sensory modalities, but basic tests include light touch, pinprick and proprioception. Abnormal sensory function may include two-point discrimination

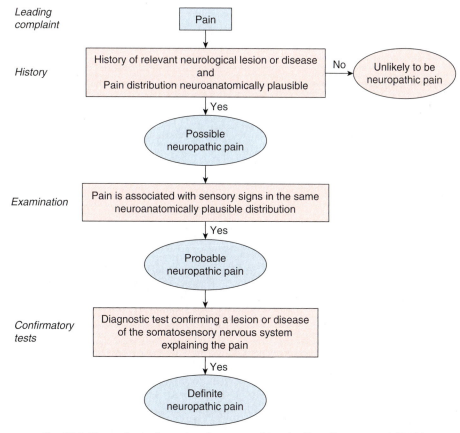

Fig. 13.1 Diagnostic grading system for neuropathic pain. (From Finnerup et al. 2016.)

Table 13.3 Neuropathic screening tools

Comparison of items within five neuropathic pain screening tools (*shaded boxes highlight features shared by two or more tools*)

	LANSS[a]	DN4[a]	NPQ	PainDETECT	ID pain
Symptoms					
Pricking, tingling, pins and needles	•	•	•	•	•
Electric shocks or shooting	•	•	•	•	•
Hot or burning	•	•	•	•	•
Numbness		•		•	
Pain evoked by light touching	•		•		
Painful cold or freezing pain		•			
Pain evoked by mild pressure				•	
Pain evoked by heat or cold				•	
Pain evoked by changes in weather			•		
Pain limited to joints[b]					∘
Itching		•			
Temporal patterns				•	
Radiation of pain				•	
Autonomic changes	•				
Clinical examination					
Brush allodynia	•	•			
Raised soft touch threshold		•			
Raised pin prick threshold	•	•			

[a] Tools that involve clinical examination.
[b] Used to identify non-neuropathic pain.
DN4, Douleur Neuropathique 4; *LANSS*, Leeds Assessment of Neuropathic Symptoms and Signs; *NPQ*, Neuropathic Pain Questionnaire.

From Bennett et al. (2007). This table has been reproduced with permission of the International Association for the Study of Pain (IASP). The table may not be reproduced for any other purpose without permission.

BOX 13.1 Outcome measures for NP in the clinical setting

Numerical Rating Scale (NRS) and Visual Analogue Scale (VAS)
Radboud Evaluation of Sensitivity, English version (RES-E)
Patient Rated Wrist and Hand Evaluation (PRWHE)
The TenTest
Grip Strength/Dynamometry
Disabilities of the Arm, Shoulder, and Hand (DASH)
Michigan Hand Outcomes Questionnaire (MHQ)
Boston Questionnaire for Carpal Tunnel Syndrome
Neuropathic Pain Scale (NPS)
Cold Induced Sensitivity Score (CISS)
Patient Specific Functional Scale (PSFS)
Brief Pain Inventory (BPI)
McGill Pain Questionnaire

From Novak & von der Heyde 2013; Packham et al. 2018; Quintal et al. 2021; Valdes et al. 2014; Walsh 2012.

Table 13.4 Sensory modalities and testing methods

Threshold sensation	Semmes–Weinstein monofilaments
Vibration threshold	Tuning fork
Tactile discrimination	Two-point discrimination (2PD) Discriminator
Sensory function of the hand	STI and Sollerman hand test
Cold intolerance	Self-report or cold stress test

(2PD), vibration, mechanical stimuli and warmth/cold, as well as decreased fine motor skills (Osborne et al. 2018).

Sensory tests are briefly summarised in Table 13.4; for extensive examples refer to Valdes et al. 2014 (Table 13.3, p. 281). In the presence of positive features such as hyperaesthesia and allodynia, testing from outside the affected area towards its perimeter is recommended.

Changes in allodynia severity can be measured using a selection of Semmes-Weinstein Mono-Filaments (SWMF) recording the most severe allodynia elicited by a smaller mono-filament (Quintal et al. 2021). In cases with negative features, i.e. reduced sensation, sensory function may be best tested from inside the zone going outwards. The most commonly used and simple to apply are SWMF and 2PD (Hassan-zadeh & Esfahani 2012; Lundborg and Rosen 2007; Miller et al. 2012; Saleem et al. 2015). Saleem et al. (2015) suggest applying each SWMF 3 times, plus the Moberg Method for 2PD applying enough pressure to blanch the skin and getting 7 out of 10 correct.

Once a diagnosis of neuropathy has been established, a clear explanation to the patient is required. A treatment strategy may be discussed, although often the aim of further action is management and not a cure (British Pain Society 2008). If diagnosis or further management cannot be determined from the examination, specialised diagnostic techniques such as imaging, neurophysiological testing, quantitative sensory testing (QST), thermography or diagnostic nerve block may be required (Hansson et al. 2002, 2007).

Treatment and management of neuropathic pain

There is little correspondence between disease or injury and specific mechanisms of neuropathy. Over recent years, QST has yielded promising results when comparing patients with controls (Maier et al. 2010). However, these profiles have been called into question by a recent study that showed no clear difference between patients with painful and pain-free neuropathy (Forstenpointner et al. 2021).

Treatment objectives can be summarised as follows (Schlereth 2020):
- Pain relief of at least 30%.
- Improved quality of life and sleep.
- Maintaining work, relationships and other social activities.
- Improvement in function.

Medication

Multidisciplinary care is recommended at all stages of treatment (Bates et al. 2019). It may be trialled without medication or interventions for up to 8 weeks, or combined with first-line medication (see later; ibid). The following staged process is based on the available evidence and a review of international guidelines (ibid):
- First line, 4- to 6-week trial of:
  - Tricyclic antidepressants (TCAs; amitriptyline or nortriptyline).
  - Gabapentin or pregabalin.
  - Serotonin and noradrenaline reuptake inhibitors (SNRIs).
  - Topical treatment for localised NP, for instance with lidocaine patches or capsaicin cream.
- Second line, 4- to 6-week trial, in case of insufficient pain relief or worsening symptoms:
  - Combination of first-line therapies. Although there is empirical evidence that this can be effective as long as side effects are acceptable, there is insufficient evidence for specific approaches to polypharmacy (Cruccu & Truini 2017).
  - Tramadol.
- Third line, in case of insufficient pain relief or worsening symptoms:
  - Referral to a specialist for consideration of specialist medications or invasive treatments. These options are beyond the scope of this chapter.

A detailed review of evidence-based medication options for NP is provided by (Schlereth 2020).

Therapy intervention

Sensory rehabilitation has been described as the gradual and progressive process of reprogramming the brain through the use of cognitive learning techniques such as visualisation and verbalisation, the use of alternate senses such as vision or hearing and the use of graded tactile stimuli designed to maintain and/or restore sensory areas affected by nerve injury or compression to improve tactile gnosis (Miller et al. 2012).

Tactile stimulation: desensitisation and somatosensory rehabilitation method

Desensitisation programs are commonly recommended for the treatment of hyperaesthesia, hyperalgesia and allodynia after nerve injury (Novak 2018). Desensitisation is used to address responses to tactile, thermal, conflict and vibrational stimuli. The aim is to normalise sensation over the abnormal territory, thus reducing the intensity and topographical area of pain (Lewis et al. 2011). Treatment parameters are set to not increase pain or as tolerated (Lewis 2011; Packham et al. 2018; Quintal et al. 2021; Rosen & Lundborg 2005). Patients with NP may have a visceral reaction to tactile stimulation and a deep nauseating feeling is not uncommon. The health professional must support and educate the patient to understand that touch is not something to be scared of. They should work within comfortable boundaries and not cause distressing symptoms. It is worth noting that in the presence of a neuroma, pain is worsened by desensitisation, even when applied carefully.

Desensitisation utilises progressive exercises to challenge the sensory responses and relearn interpretation of tactile stimuli as nonpainful (Novak 2018). It requires a texture, particle, temperature or vibration that is tolerated in the painful area. Stimuli may be applied to the skin through stroking, placing an object or immersion. The patient should give the area sustained visual attention, provide a silent conscious description of what is touching the skin and perform the task in a quiet environment. Once suitable tactile stimuli have been chosen, the patient can carry out the desensitisation as a home programme. Desensitisation is based on theories of neuroplasticity, so frequent sessions of short duration while viewing the affected limb are recommended (Lewis et al. 2011), i.e.

1 to 10 minutes, for at least 3 to 4 times, up to 12 times per day. The duration of the session should be increased based on the patient's response (tolerable symptoms or no increase in pain) (Quintal et al. 2021). Traditionally desensitisation moved from smooth to rough, but it is more important to work from stimuli that are tolerated to those that are less tolerated—see Waylett-Rendall (1995) for examples.

Some patients cannot tolerate any stimulation directly to the body part because of pain. Options available to initiate desensitisation include visual feedback using a mirror (Novak 2018; Rosen & Lundborg 2005) and Somatosensory Rehabilitation Method (SRM) (Nedelec et al. 2016; Packham et al. 2018; Packham 2017; Quintal et al. 2021). Mirror visual feedback (MVF) is suggested for treatment of severe hyperaesthesia or allodynia (Rosen & Lundborg 2005). The affected limb is obscured from view behind a mirror. The unaffected side is reflected in the mirror. The stimuli are applied in a graded way as in traditional desensitisation, but in this case to the unaffected side with attention on the reflection in the mirror. This provides a visual and perceptual illusion of stimulating the affected side, which allows a progressive sensory desensitisation effect (Novak 2018; Rosen & Lundborg 2005). It is still important to select a stimulus that is tolerated and does not increase pain.

In SRM, patients are asked to use comfortable somatosensory stimulation (like rubbing or stroking with soft fur or silk) on an area of skin related to the same nerve, but **away** from the injury, so the sensations are normal (Packham 2017). The area of allodynia may reduce and reveal numbness, which is then treated with usual sensory reeducation techniques (Packham et al. 2017, 2018; Quintal et al. 2021). The method of evaluation to determine the affected area (which should not be stimulated) is very detailed and includes allodynography and the rainbow pain scale, see Packham (2017, 2018).

Sensory reeducation

Sensory reeducation (SR) is used to improve sensibility and decrease pain, allodynia and hyperalgesia (Novak & von der Heyde 2013). Most SR has followed the basic principles of classic training principles for SR (Dellon 1981; Wynn-Parry & Salter 1976). Initially touch is performed, with and without sight of the body part, with a variety of textures/particles/sensations (Box 13.2). This way vision assists the training and improves the deficient sense (sensation) (Lundborg & Rosen 2007).

As sensibility improves, exercises are progressed to include challenges such as localisation of touch; identifying shapes, textures and different objects; and having eyes open or closed. The aim is to further *challenge the sensory system, and optimize cortical remapping and normal movement patterns* (Novak & von der Heyde 2013) (Box 13.3).

BOX 13.2 Items to use for desensitisation and sensory reeducation

Textures can be used for light touch or light massage. Examples are cotton wool, velvet, fur, fleece, terry towelling, wool, soft Velcro, felt, soft and hard paint brushes, hedgehog balls, foam, hard Velcro, leather, carpet, plastic, silk, eraser end of a pencil, various coarseness's of sandpaper.

Particles such as rice, pasta, sand, foam pieces, popcorn, chickpeas, beans, lentils and sago can be used for immersion.

Temperatures include warm or cool water, paraffin wax, hydrotherapy, holding a cold or warm cup of water, getting in or out of a shower or bath, holding a frozen item.

Other modalities are air from a fan, running water, percussion/tapping, vibration and functional tasks. Vibration is often the form of stimulation which is tolerated earliest in this process.

BOX 13.3 Additional resources for use in SR

Sensory reeducation:
Temperature, weights, shapes, objects—behind a curtain
Braille
Matching dominoes
Matching coins, beads, buttons
Eraser on the end of a pencil
Touch localisation
Soft and hard
Rough and smooth
Wood and metal
Shapes of large wooden blocks
Small metal objects
Objects disguised in a container of beans or rice

From Bellugou et al. 1991; Miller et al. 2012; Nedelec et al. 2016; Packham 2017.

Classic SR is commenced once reinnervation of the hand has occurred and is measured by touch/pressure of 4.56 using SWMF testing, Tinel's sign or perception of vibration (Hassan-zadeh & Esfahani 2012; Lundborg & Rosen 2007; Miller et al. 2012).

As mentioned, it is important to perform SR in a quiet, undisturbed environment with sustained concentration. The time the patient is able to sustain focused concentration determines the duration of their home exercise sessions. Focused attention on the affected body part may enhance SR (Moseley et al. 2008). This may be done watching the affected limb or the opposite body part in a mirror (Moseley & Weich 2009).

The tasks should relate to the function of the affected body part. In the upper limb, dexterity, stereognosis, manipulation, grip, etc. are especially important, while the lower limb requires tolerance to, e.g. weight-bearing and balance. See Wynn-Parry (1980, p. 226) for detailed training programmes for the upper limb.

Evidence suggests that SR may prevent or reverse changes in the somatosensory cortex induced by deafferentation and loss of sensory input following peripheral nerve injury (Miller et al. 2012; Novak & von der Heyde 2013). These changes present as altered sensations such as allodynia, hyperaesthesia and dysaesthesia. Using SR in isolation has shown disappointing results (Rosen et al. 2003), so Lundborg & Rosen (2007) proposed a two-phased approach. Phase 1 addresses cortical reorganisation of the somatosensory cortex and aims to maintain cortical hand representation before the skin is reinnervated. It does so by using other senses (Miller et al. 2012). Phase 1 uses visuo-tactile and audio-tactile interaction, as well as mirror imagery. It can be used either when complete paraesthesia is present, or with any type of altered sensory feedback. This phase is helpful for all patients who have a possibility of sensory cortex remapping.

Phase 2 explores novel principles to enhance the effects of classic sensory training using *temporary deafferentiation* (TD). It uses classic SR with an additional cutaneous deafferentation technique. Like classic SR, TD can be used when reinnervation of the body part has begun. Anaesthetic cream is applied to areas with normal sensation to temporarily block sensory signals from that region and allow the cortical representation of the injured area to 'expand' (Lundborg & Rosen 2007). The technique uses the concept of guided plasticity of the CNS and has a rapid effect on the organisation of the primary somatosensory cortex (S1) by unmasking existing synapses and increasing intra-cortical inhibition (Saleem et al. 2015).

TD combined with intensive SR may be useful in rehabilitation of nerve injuries and neuropathies (Miller et al. 2012; Petoe et al. 2013; Rosen et al. 2006; Saleem et al. 2015). Research for the hand suggests that application of 10 g of EMLA cream to the volar forearm, 10 mm proximal to the wrist crease over 15 cm by 5 cm, for 60 minutes under an occlusive bandage, is optimal to produce a clinical improvement in sensibility in adjacent areas (Petoe et al. 2013; Rosen et al. 2006; Saleem 2015). A frequency of twice a week for 2 weeks is recommended (Lundborg & Rosen 2007). The practitioner must remember the possibility of side effects of medication application and to work closely with the medical team. See Saleem et al. (2015), Petoe et al. (2013) or Rosen et al. (2006) for details regarding and Novak (2011) and Jerosch-Herold (2011) for a detailed summary and consensus regarding SR (Box 13.4).

Sensorimotor training

The sensorimotor system integrates the neurosensory and neuromuscular processes responsible for coordination and dynamic stability (Valdes et al. 2014). These processes are adversely influenced by NP and injury, as well as joint stiffness, pain and loss of mechanoreceptor feedback (ibid).

Phase 1 SR activities

- Motor Imagery (Lacourse et al. 2004). (1) received motor imagery instruction, (2) performed motor imagery practice, (3) observation of a model performing the named task.
- Reading or listening to 'action words' relating to activities involving the body part.
- Observed tactile stimulation. The patient observes their affected limb being touched by the therapist, optionally amplified by using MVF (Rosen & Lundborg 2005). Observing limbs being touched activates visual as well as somatosensory areas in the cortex (Keysers et al. 2004; Lundborg 2008).
- Mirror therapy—the nerve-injured limb is hidden and the healthy limb observed in the reflection, providing an illusion of touching the nerve-injured limb by combining the mirror illusion with the true touch of the healthy limb (Lundborg & Rosen 2007).
- Auditory feedback—the original research used a sensor glove system (SGS) (Rosen & Lundborg 2007) using a glove that gives auditory feedback from microphones mounted at the fingertip. Texture rods that are rubbed while being held close to the ear can make the specific sounds of touch audible (Svens & Rosen 2009). Hassan-zadeh & Esfahani (2012) trained a patient with denervated fingers with texture rods, resulting in significantly improved sensory outcomes compared with the control. Their *Audiovisual Tactile* makes it possible to touch textures with the denervated finger and hear different sounds.

BOX 13.4 **Sensory reeducation**

1. Touch the body part or hold an object with eyes open.
2. Aim to identify the surface/texture/object/temperature.
3. Compare these feelings to the normal side.
4. Concentrate thoughts on the shape, texture, temperature of the item. e.g. a marble table is flat, smooth, shiny, cold. A tennis ball is fuzzy/soft, warmer to touch, round, slightly rough.
5. Once this can be achieved with eyes open, progress to repeating all steps with eyes closed or with vision obscured, e.g. behind a curtain.
6. Add sustained visual attention towards the affected side, MVF, or cutaneous deafferentation (as detailed in this section) to enhance the effects of sensory reeducation techniques.

Sensorimotor training (ST) educates patients through the application of sensorimotor activities to attend to sensory cues, so that the brain can generate more appropriate motor commands, sensory information is interpreted correctly and sensorimotor control is promoted (ibid).

Therapeutic ST strategies

- Mirror visual feedback (MVF)—see CRPS later.
- Motor imagery/imagined movements—The motor control system interacts with the autonomic nervous system and rehearsal of movements may provide therapeutic benefit for those with chronic pain (Lewis et al. 2011). See CRPS later.
- Graded motor imagery—Aims to improve cortical organisation through activation of the brain's motor networks (Osborne et al. 2018). See CRPS later.
- Gyroscope—stimulates proprioception in the wrist (Balan & Garcia-Elias 2008).
- Resistance exercises, fine motor tasks, ADLS, arts and crafts (Pleger et al. 2005).
- Multitextural and temperature sensory discrimination (see desensitisation earlier).
- EMLA cream—see SR Phase 2 earlier.
- Mental rehearsal (Fourkas et al. 2008).
- Proprioception exercises—relating to the senses of limb position and limb movement (Brun et al. 2018). Early conscious appreciation of proprioception is likely to stimulate cortical areas connected to sensorimotor joint control, and may diminish reorganizational changes in the cortex after nerve injury (Hagert 2010). See CRPS later.

Valdes et al. (2014, Table 13.4, p. 282) provide a range of sensorimotor interventions that can easily be incorporated into clinical practice.

Neural mobilisations

Limitations of neural excursion have been demonstrated in compressive neuropathies and tension within the nerve can affect intraneural blood flow and nerve function (Walsh 2012). Neural mobilisation and neurodynamic evaluation, nerve mobilisation or gliding in isolation, and a combination of nerve and tendon gliding have reported benefits in decreasing the need for surgery, decreasing the incidence of cumulative trauma, and increasing a more rapid reduction of pain along with greater functional movement (Walsh 2012).

Aids and adaptations

Maintaining function of the affected body part is an important component of treatment. Cold sensitivity is common, so aids that can be utilised long term include warm clothing, e.g. gloves and heated devices (Novak

2018). To optimise function of the lower limb, walking aids or orthoses may be considered. Upper-limb aids are many and varied and can assist with personal or domestic activities of daily living. Other examples include adapted knives, can openers and aides to assist with fastening clothes or shoes. It is worthwhile liaising with the local occupational therapy department for details of suppliers or a comprehensive assessment of the patient's needs.

A range of techniques can be utilised to improve a person's experience of NP. Active and conscious use of the limb in activities of daily life, combined with high motivation by the patient, are of great importance for return of functional sensibility, as are patient education and compliance with therapy interventions (Lundborg & Rosen 2007).

Section 2. Complex regional pain syndrome

Introduction

Characteristics of CRPS were described by S. Weir Mitchell (1872), and years of hypotheses and names for the condition followed (Table 13.5). It often develops in response to often minor trauma to the limbs (Table 13.6). The term CRPS was introduced in 1994 by the IASP (Merskey & Bogduk 1994; Stanton-Hicks et al. 1995). It was chosen for the following reasons:

- *Complex* expresses the varying clinical features (Hayek & Mekhail 2004; Stanton-Hicks et al. 1995, 1998).
- *Regional* emphasises that in the majority of cases it involves a region of the body, usually an extremity (Hayek & Mekhail 2004; Stanton-Hicks et al. 1998).
- *Pain* is the *sine qua non* for diagnosis (Hayek & Mekhail 2004; Stanton-Hicks et al. 1995). In rare conditions resembling CRPS, pain may be minimal or absent.

The Budapest Criteria developed to have four clinical subgroups (sensory, motor/trophic, sudomotor/oedema, and vasomotor) (Bruehl et al. 1999; Harden et al. 1999; Harden & Bruehl 2005) (Table 13.7). For clinical work, these *Budapest criteria* provide excellent sensitivity (0.99) and greatly improved specificity (0.68) (Harden et al. 2010). They have been incorporated in current guidelines (Goebel et al. 2018; Goebel et al. 2019).

Clinical characteristics of CRPS

Clinicians may first suspect CRPS from initial observation. Application of the four subgroups of the Budapest

Table 13.5 Terms used for CRPS

Algo(neuro)dystrophy
Causalgia
Chronic traumatic oedema
Complex regional pain disorder
Neurodystrophy
Pain-dysfunction syndrome
Posttraumatic oedema
Posttraumatic osteoporosis
Posttraumatic pain syndrome
Posttraumatic spreading neuralgia
Reflex (sympathetic) dystrophy
Shoulder-hand syndrome
Südeck's atrophy
Sympathalgia
Sympathetic overdrive syndrome
Traumatic arthritis

CRPS, Complex regional pain syndrome.
After Abram (1990) and Wilson (1990). The length of the list reflects the confusion over the interpretation of CRPS.

Table 13.6 Initiating events of CRPS

The results of four studies have been pooled for a total of 778 patients (Abram 1990).

Trauma	
Blunt	32%
Laceration	11%
Fracture	21%
Sprain	2%
Nerve injury	1%
Total trauma	67%
Postoperative	
Carpal tunnel	6%
Dupuytren's	4%
Ganglion cyst	2%
Other	2%
Unspecified	5%
Total postop	21%
Burns	
Thermal	1%
Electrical	1%
Total burns	2%
Other	
MI	2%
Cerebral disease	1%
Spinal cord injury	<1%
Other/unknown	5%

Criteria is strongly recommended to maximise the chance of correct diagnosis and treatment. The traditional view that CRPS progresses in specific stages has been discredited (Bruehl 2015; Bruehl et al. 2002). For more detailed information about CRPS clinical characteristics, see Goebel et al. (2019), Bharwani et al. (2017), Birklein & Dimova (2017), Bruehl (2015) and Harden et al. (2013).

Pain and sensory changes

In CRPS these are characterised by hyperpathia, allodynia, hyperalgesia and hyperaesthesia. Typical subjective descriptors include aching, burning, pricking or shooting, deep, spontaneous, superficial, throbbing and sharp. Sensory changes may include decreased temperature sensation and decreased sensitivity to pinprick. Patients may report feeling that their body part feels distorted or no longer belongs to them (Birklein & Dimova 2017).

Allodynia may present in response to one or more stimuli. There is a positive correlation between the degree of somatosensory reorganisation, level of allodynia and chronicity of pain in CRPS (Lewis et al. 2011). Temperature allodynia is produced in response to warm or cool stimuli. Mechanical allodynia may be either static (sensitivity to light touch or pressure) or dynamic (sensitivity to brushing or stroking of the skin). Vibration allodynia may be provoked by travelling in a car or touching a vibrating object. Spatial allodynia is underreported but common; some patients describe an increase in pain when someone or something approaches the affected area. Patients must be asked about this because they may be reluctant to report symptoms without tactile cause.

Motor and trophic changes

These changes were grouped together because of statistical significance. Motor changes include motor neglect, limitation of range of movement, weakness, tremor, dystonia, motor dysfunction, myoclonus and reduced or altered muscle power. Patients may not use the affected limb in daily tasks, feel that it is not readily available for use, or experience lack of coordination.

Trophic changes affect the appearance of skin, hair and nails. They can be observed during assessment (sign) or be intermittent (symptom). Skin changes are typically

Table 13.7 The Budapest Criteria for CRPS

General definition of the syndrome

CRPS describes an array of painful conditions that are characterised by a continuing (spontaneous and/or evoked) regional pain that is seemingly disproportional in time or degree to the usual course of any known trauma or other lesion. The pain is regional (not in a specific nerve territory or dermatome) and usually has a distal predominance of abnormal sensory, motor, sudomotor, vasomotor and/or trophic findings. The syndrome shows variable progression over time.

There are two versions of the proposed diagnostic criteria: a clinical version meant to maximise diagnostic sensitivity with adequate specificity and a research version meant to more equally balance optimal sensitivity and specificity.

Proposed modified clinical diagnostic criteria for CRPS

1. Continuing pain, which is disproportionate to any inciting event.
2. Must report at least one symptom in three of the four following categories:
Sensory: Reports of hyperesthesia and/or allodynia.
Vasomotor: Reports of temperature asymmetry and/or skin colour changes and/or skin colour asymmetry.
Sudomotor/oedema: Reports of oedema and/or sweating changes and/or sweating asymmetry.
Motor/trophic: Reports of decreased range of motion and/or motor dysfunction (weakness, tremor, dystonia) and/or trophic changes (hair, nails, skin).
3. Must display at least one sign* at time of evaluation in **two or more** of the following categories:
Sensory: Evidence of hyperalgesia (to pinprick) and/or allodynia (to light touch and/or deep somatic pressure and/or joint movement).
Vasomotor: Evidence of temperature asymmetry and/or skin colour changes and/or asymmetry.
Sudomotor/oedema: Evidence of oedema and/or sweating changes and/or sweating asymmetry.
Motor/trophic: Evidence of decreased range of motion and/or motor dysfunction (weakness, tremor, dystonia) and/or trophic changes (hair, nails, skin).
4. There is no other diagnosis that better explains the signs and symptoms.
Proposed modified research diagnostic criteria for CRPS
1. Continuing pain, which is disproportionate to any inciting event.
2. Must report at least one symptom in **each of the four** following categories:
Sensory: Reports of hyperesthesia and/or allodynia.
Vasomotor: Reports of temperature asymmetry and/or skin colour changes and/or skin colour asymmetry.
Sudomotor/oedema: Reports of oedema and/or sweating changes and/or sweating asymmetry.
Motor/trophic: Reports of decreased range of motion and/or motor dysfunction (weakness, tremor, dystonia) and/or trophic changes (hair, nails, skin).
3. Must display at least one sign* at the time of evaluation in **two or more** of the following categories:
Sensory: Evidence of hyperalgesia (to pinprick) and/or allodynia (to light touch and/or deep somatic pressure and/or joint movement).
Vasomotor: Evidence of temperature asymmetry and/or skin colour changes and/or asymmetry.
Sudomotor/oedema: Evidence of oedema and/or sweating changes and/or sweating asymmetry.
Motor/trophic: Evidence of decreased range of motion and/or motor dysfunction (weakness, tremor, dystonia) and/or trophic changes (hair, nails, skin).
4. There is no other diagnosis that better explains the signs and symptoms.

SUMMARY OF SENSITIVITY AND SPECIFICITY OF THE PROPOSED CLINICAL AND RESEARCH CRITERIA

Criterion type	Symptoms required for diagnosis	Signs required for diagnosis	Sensitivity	Specificity
Clinical	3	2	0.85	0.69
Research	4	2	0.70	0.96

*A sign is counted only if observed at the time of diagnosis.
From Harden & Bruehl (2005). This table has been reproduced with permission of the International Association for the Study of Pain (IASP). The table may not be reproduced for any other purpose without permission.

fibrosis, hyperkeratosis and thin glossy skin (Stanton-Hicks et al. 2002). Patients will have skin that is flaky, thick, thin, fragile or shiny. Hair may be absent, but more frequently grows thicker and darker. Nails may grow thick and strong or become flaky and brittle.

Vasomotor changes

Patients may present with changes or asymmetry in temperature and skin colour. These are often intermittent, and very noticeable when they occur. Skin may be very red, very pale or mottled—blotchy purple and white. Temperature can be either very hot or very cold and may fluctuate between the two. In winter, CRPS patients often need to wear gloves when outdoors.

Sudomotor changes and oedema

These include changes or asymmetries in sweating and swelling or oedema. Oedema is common after trauma, but excessively so in CRPS. The swelling often fluctuates and may be exacerbated by simple function or even imagined movements (Moseley 2004). Changes in sweating can present as hyperhydrosis or anhydrosis (Stanton-Hicks et al. 2002). Excessive sweating may present in response to activities. Anhydrosis is most limiting functionally, especially in the hand, as the fine layer of moisture on the palms gives significant assistance to grip.

Mechanisms of CRPS

Understanding of what causes or maintains the diverse range of signs and symptoms associated with CRPS is still far from complete. There are no absolute diagnostic tests; diagnosis is by exclusion of other conditions and the presence of variable signs and symptoms. Research studies may therefore include participants who present with similar signs and symptoms, but who have different underlying pathologies. A unifying theory continues to elude scientists and clinicians. This section discusses aspects of the syndrome which have been identified.

Inflammation and autoimmune responses

Limbs with CRPS display classic characteristics of inflammation such as redness, raised temperature and swelling, especially in the early stages. Tissue fluid from the affected area has a heightened concentration of proinflammatory cytokines (Huygen et al. 2002). Most of these changes normalise within 6 months of symptomatic treatment (Lenz et al. 2013). The origin of the inflammation may be

at least partially neurogenic, i.e. facilitated by the release of neuropeptides including Substance P (SP) and calcitonin gene-related peptide (CGRP) from the terminals of nociceptive fibres (Birklein & Schmelz 2008). These neuropeptides contribute to vasodilation, extravasation of plasma and local sensitisation (ibid). There is support for this mechanism from research in which CRPS patients showed a much stronger vasodilation response and enhanced protein extravasation in response to strong transcutaneous nerve stimulation, compared with healthy participants (Weber et al. 2001).

Relatively recent hypotheses for CRPS are autoinflammation and autoimmunity, in which the immune system targets the body's own tissues, similar to ankylosing spondylitis and psoriasis (Clark et al. 2018). Supporting evidence includes changes in levels of proinflammatory cytokines in CRPS patients and preclinical changes in immune responses (ibid). It is unclear whether autoinflammation and autoimmunity are viable explanations for the physiology for CRPS (Chang et al. 2021).

Pain and sensory changes

The local processes discussed previously account for local pain and sensitisation. Hypothetically, CRPS type 1 resulting from trauma including surgery may also be the result of local small-fibre neuropathy in some patients (Oaklander & Fields 2009; Oaklander et al. 2006). This might account for the fact that CRPS patients experience negative sensory changes such as hypoaesthesia (Veldman et al. 1993a, b). However, no consistent relationship between QST and small-fibre changes has been found and the relevance of minor neuropathies is disputed (Jänig & Baron 2006; Kharkar et al. 2012).

Pain in CRPS is also likely to be due to changes in the CNS. Sensory changes may spread beyond the affected tissues and even to the contralateral side (Rommel et al. 1999). Interestingly, the most common general changes were *hypo*aesthesia and *hypo*algesia, while mechanical hyperalgesia was found in the affected limb of 10 out of 24 patients (ibid). Psychological disorders could not account for changes beyond the affected area (Rommel et al. 2001). However, considerable reorganisation of the cortical representation, correlated with pain and sensory change, has been found in patients with CRPS of the upper limb (Maihöfner et al. 2003). Cortical representation may normalise as pain improves (Maihöfner et al. 2004). A heightened cortical response to mechanical stimulation and altered cortical representation have also been demonstrated in patients with CRPS (Juottonen et al. 2002).

Autonomic involvement

CRPS has features suggestive of involvement of the sympathetic nervous system. Changes in tissue temperature and colour can be observed in over 90% of patients (Veldman et al. 1993). A patient's CRPS-related pain may or may not have a sympathetically maintained component, so they can be subcategorised as having sympathetically maintained or sympathetically independent pain (SMP or SIP) (Harden & Bruehl 2005).

There is preclinical evidence for sympathetic–sensory interaction, for example in the form of neuronal coupling in the dorsal root ganglion (Gibbs et al. 2008). An alternative mechanism may be sympathetic activity leading to release of chemicals such as SP or histamine, thus activating or sensitising nociceptive nerve endings (ibid). Finally, in posttraumatic CRPS, nerve damage may lead to responsiveness of nociceptive neurones to local noradrenaline or sympathetic activation (Sato & Perl 1991).

Increased sensitivity to NA and circulating adrenaline may also develop in blood vessels and sweat glands (Sandroni & Wilson 2005; Wasner & Baron 2005). It has been attributed to increased expression of adrenergic receptors in the afferent neurones innervating these tissues (Sandroni & Wilson 2005). This *adrenergic supersensitivity* can also develop in the smooth muscle in blood vessels. Supersensitivity may be an adaptive response to a reduction in sympathetic output in the early stages of CRPS, for example due to an initial disruption of tissue innervation. Its consequence is that normal or even lowered concentrations of (nor)adrenaline have an abnormal vascular and sudomotor response.

Motor changes

Tremor and lack of coordination may be found in around 50% of CRPS patients (Veldman et al. 1993). In persistent CRPS, muscle spasm may develop in 25% and weakness in 95% of patients (ibid). The exact reasons for these symptoms are yet to be explained and are likely to vary between individuals; see van Hilten et al. (2005) for a review. A period of immobility, for instance after an injury or operation, may itself engender a lack of motor control. Tissue swelling is likely to make a limb more difficult to control, similar to wearing a boxing glove or thick stocking. This combined with pain is likely to distort proprioceptive feedback and alter motor control. CRPS patients may also have an altered response of the motor cortex (Juottonen et al. 2002). This may explain the success of motor imagery strategies in some patients (Moseley 2004; Moseley et al. 2008).

Psychological factors

Anecdotally, clinicians have reported that some patients display a 'CRPS personality'. To date, the weight of evidence is against such a claim. For example, Ciccone et al. (1997) compared a group of CRPS sufferers with patients with either low back pain or local NP. A range of measures assessing symptom reporting, illness behaviour and psychological distress failed to find a significant difference between the groups. There was also no greater incidence of childhood trauma. Similarly, a review of the literature found no evidence of CRPS as a psychogenic disorder (Covington 1996). Patients who develop CRPS following a wrist fracture are psychologically indistinguishable from those who don't (Puchalski & Zyluk 2005). Even patients with severe CRPS and dystonia do not have a distinct psychological profile (Reedijk et al. 2008). Despite reporting higher levels of pain, patients with CRPS have a psychological profile similar to those with other persistent pain conditions (Park et al. 2020).

The strongest predictor of the development of CRPS may be pain intensity (Moseley et al. 2014). A pain score of ≥5 in the first week after fracture should be considered a *red flag* for CRPS (Moseley et al. 2014). However, recent research suggests that a large proportion of patients may have symptoms of posttraumatic stress disorder before they develop CRPS (Speck et al. 2016). The therapeutic implications of this finding are as yet undetermined.

Covington (1996) suggests that severe pain may be the cause of suffering rather than vice versa. In this sense, CRPS is no different from other painful conditions. However, anxiety, pain-related fear and self-perceived disability may be associated with reduced improvements in pain in CRPS (Bean et al. 2015), suggesting that early assessment of these aspects may be prudent. Psychological factors must be addressed as part of the overall management strategy for any pain patient (see Chapters 5 and 12).

Clinical examination

A positive diagnosis of CRPS requires that at the time of clinical assessment the patient has a reported symptom in *three* of the four categories and a displayed physical sign in *two* of the four categories of the Budapest Criteria (Harden et al. 2010). There must also be no other diagnosis that better explains the signs and symptoms. The diagnosis should be established as soon as possible, in order to start early interdisciplinary treatment (Atkins 2003; Bharwani et al. 2017; Birklein & Dimova 2017; Bruehl 2015; Goebel et al. 2019; Harden et al. 2013; Rho et al. 2002; Stanton-Hicks et al. 2002; Thomas & Degnan 2005; Zhongyu et al. 2005).

Subjective assessment

This is no different from other painful conditions and should include a body chart filled out by the patient, and at least the 11-point NRS for pain intensity (Bear-Lehman & Abreu

1989). The assessment should include signs and symptoms, but also individual functional goals, current limitations and barriers to therapy (Packham & Holly 2018). CRPS patients are often embarrassed about their symptoms and may feel that they are too odd to report, so it is important to ask specific questions about each of the diagnostic criteria.

Objective assessment

Physical examination is guided by an accurate subjective history. It may take more than one session to assess all aspects fully. At least one assessment measure must be taken from each of the four diagnostic subsections; each individual diagnostic component is reasonably sensitive, but not as specific as the combination of all components (Harden et al. 2010). Early instigation of treatment is essential so the initial consult should always include some treatment, typically at least patient education, empathy and support, and a home exercise programme.

Given the labile nature of the disease, assessment and tracking of changes in CRPS status is challenging (Harden et al. 2017). The CRPS Severity Score (CSS, http://links.lww.com/PAIN/A419) was developed to create a continuous index of CRPS severity and allow the practitioner to track changes. It has been validated to demonstrate real change in a patient's CRPS, is responsive to changes in CRPS severity over time, and demonstrates good discrimination between CRPS and non-CRPS patients (Harden et al. 2017). Clinicians who may see patients with CRPS are advised to have the Budapest Criteria and CSS to hand. See Moseley (2014) or a user-friendly version of the diagnostic criteria.

Sensory changes

Particular attention should be paid to allodynia and hyperalgesia. Threshold sensation and mechanical allodynia may be measured by Semmes–Weinstein monofilaments and 2PD (Bahm et al. 2018; Bear-Lehman et al. 1989; Prosser & Conolly 2003; Li et al. 2005; Seftchick et al. 2011; Lewis et al. 2011) or von Frey hairs (Tichelaar et al. 2006). Light palpation of the affected limb (Li et al. 2005; Prosser & Conolly 2003) should be carried out to assess hyperalgesia or hyperpathia (Atkins 2003). Vibration and weight bearing (ideally using a force-plate) may be included in a comprehensive assessment. It may be useful to determine a subjective pain rating elicited by each type of physical stimulation.

Vasomotor changes

Temperature and colour changes in a general clinical setting are assessed through palpation and observation. Thermography gives greater objectivity (Bruehl et al. 1996; Uematsu et al. 1981), but tends to be reserved for research.

Sudomotor changes and oedema

Oedema can be measured using a volumeter (Bear-Lehman & Abreu 1989; Li et al. 2005; Prosser & Conolly 2003; Seftchick et al. 2011) or a tape measure referring to anatomical landmarks (Bear-Lehman & Abreu 1989; Hunter et al. 1995; Prosser & Conolly 2003; Li et al. 2005). Atrophy on the affected side can skew the accuracy of circumferential measurements. Changes or asymmetry in sweat production is determined through palpation.

Motor and trophic changes

It is essential to measure range of motion (ROM) using goniometry. Reliability and validity of goniometry are greatest using an agreed standardised protocol and the same examiner (Burr et al. 2003; Bear-Lehman et al. 1989; Pratt & Burr 2001; Seftchick et al. 2011). Quality of movement and any motor dysfunction must be noted. Assessment of strength may be limited by pain and should be judged per individual, but a baseline strength measurement using Medical Research Council standards (MacAvoy & Green 2007) or with dynamometry for grip strength (Massy-Westropp et al. 2004; Coldham et al. 2006; Seftchick et al. 2011) is preferable. However, strength assessment is best deferred if it is likely to significantly increase symptoms. Changes to skin, hair and nails are assessed through observation and palpation, and should be recorded.

Treatment of CRPS

The overall aims for treatment of CRPS are to:
- maximise function
- relieve pain
- improve quality of life.

Due to the complex nature of CRPS, multifaceted and usually multidisciplinary care is essential. Chronic CRPS is a challenging and complex biopsychosocial condition (Bruehl 2015), so therapy intervention should be part of a *well-structured* integrated clinical pathway (Birklein & Dimova 2017; Harden et al. 2013; Rho et al. 2002; Stanton-Hicks et al. 1998, 2002). It should be offered as soon as possible (Goebel et al. 2019). The primary goal of treatment is functional restoration (Harden et al. 2013; Stanton-Hicks et al. 2002). Invasive therapies such as regional sympathetic blocks or sympathetic blocks may be considered in extreme cases (Birklein & Dimova 2017; Bruehl 2015), but are not discussed here.

Therapy intervention for CRPS

Therapy intervention is the mainstay of treatment (Rho et al. 2002; Stanton-Hicks et al. 2002) and has been shown to reduce pain and improve function in patients with CRPS

(Bharwani et al. 2017). Intervention may be provided by physical and/or occupational therapists. Immediate or early access to this treatment may shorten the disease course and preserve limb function (Goebel et al. 2018). Moreover, early assessment of anxiety, pain-related fear and self-perceived disability may be prudent, because they are associated with reduced improvements in pain (Bean et al. 2015). There is a disappointing lack of high-quality clinical trials of therapy management of CRPS (Birklein & Dimova 2017; Dommerholt 2004), so best guidance is consensus-based guidelines (Harden et al. 2013; Stanton-Hicks et al. 1998 2002) and systematic reviews (Daly & Bialocerkowski 2008). Fig. 13.2 shows the IASP treatment algorithm for CRPS (Stanton-Hicks et al. 2002). Patients who do not respond to treatment by 12 to 16 weeks should be given a trial of interventional therapies (Stanton-Hicks et al. 2002).

Fig. 13.3. [Harden et al. 2013, p. 8, Fig. 1] shows the most recent treatment algorithm for CRPS (Harden et al. 2013). The recommendations are based on functional restoration with the addition of medication, psychotherapy or interventional therapies as needed to engage in the rehab programme.

It is imperative to agree specific, measureable, achievable, realistic and time-related (SMART) goals with the patient and use functional gains as a measure of progress. Therapy should be based on best practice *and* tailored to the individual patient (Lewis et al. 2011; Stanton-Hicks et al. 1998). Therapy interventions, while challenging the patient's abilities, must be graded to prevent an exacerbation of their signs or symptoms.

Education

Adequate analgesia, encouragement and education are essential (Stanton-Hicks et al. 2002). This includes explanation that signs and symptoms all come under one umbrella of CRPS. It is essential that patients understand that CPRS is not their fault, made up or exaggerated by them, and that they can be treated. Education about the importance of full participation in therapy alongside pain management and possibly psychological treatments is essential to facilitate optimal recovery. The patient should be encouraged to engage the body part in normal functional activities where possible, while avoiding exacerbation of symptoms. Pacing of activities should be discussed.

Motivation is an integral part of the recovery process. It is achieved through positive reinforcement, encouragement, education and SMART goal setting. Goals can be broken down into smaller subsections as required.

Management of pain

It is important to explain that concurrent medication, taken regularly and not as needed, facilitates

rehabilitation and recovery. If there is any doubt, liaison with the treating doctor or pain management team is recommended, especially if the therapist is the first-line practitioner. There may be locally agreed pathways of care.

Transcutaneous electrical nerve stimulation (TENS) can be a useful pain-relieving adjunct to therapy—see Chapter 16. Although empirically some patients gain great benefit from TENS (Stanton Hicks et al. 1998, 2002), Daly & Bialocerkowski (2008) state that there is no formal research evidence to support this.

Medication

Medication is used to support the therapy approach and control symptoms, especially pain (Goebel et al. 2018; Palmer 2015). CRPS is multifactorial and its manifestations vary per individual, so it is advisable to target the mechanism that is thought to be most prominent (Bharwani et al. 2017):

- Pain—treated with analgesics and possibly adjuvant medication typically used for NP, such as tricyclics, gabapentin and pregabalin.
- Inflammation—antiinflammatory drugs, including bisphosphonates. This is particularly relevant in the acute phase (Birklein & Dimova 2017).
- Vascular constriction (cold, pale tissues)—vasodilators.
- Motor disorders—muscle relaxants or spasmolytics.
- Prevention—vitamin C taken immediately following surgery or injury may help prevent CRPS (Aim et al. 2017). As mentioned, high levels of pain ≥5 in the first week after fracture may be an indicator of risk (Moseley et al. 2014).

Prescription of a single drug is preferable but often not sufficient (Harden et al. 2013). Unfortunately high-quality evidence to support clinical decision making is lacking (Bruehl 2015).

Desensitisation

Desensitisation can use any form of nonnoxious sensory stimulation, but its effectiveness is specific to the somatosensory modality utilised (Allen et al. 2004). The aim is to help restore normal sensory processing (Stanton-Hicks et al. 1998). In CRPS with high levels of pain, sensory discrimination is poor and there are reduced levels of activity in the sensory maps (Lewis et al. 2011). The process of desensitisation is described earlier in this chapter (NP). Allodynia has been identified as a predictor of negative outcomes in CRPS and a barrier to participation in rehabilitation (Packham &Holly 2018), so it should be addressed as a priority. *Graded exposure* is a form of functional desensitisation which has been used in the treatment of chronic CRPS.

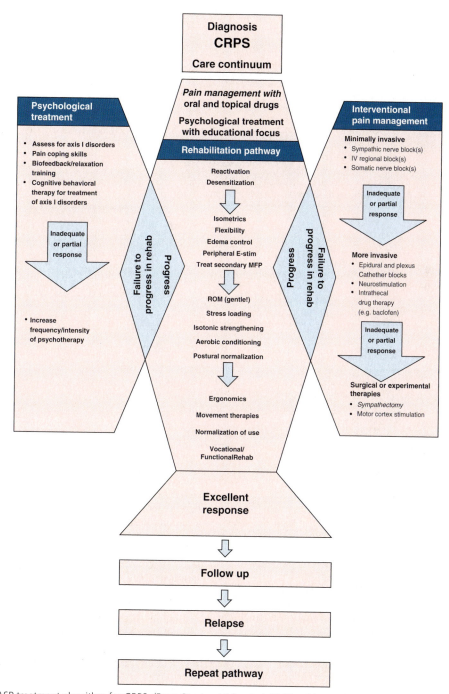

Fig. 13.2 IASP treatment algorithm for CRPS. (From Stanton-Hicks et al. 2002, with permission.) *MFP,* myofascial pain; *ROM,* range of motion.

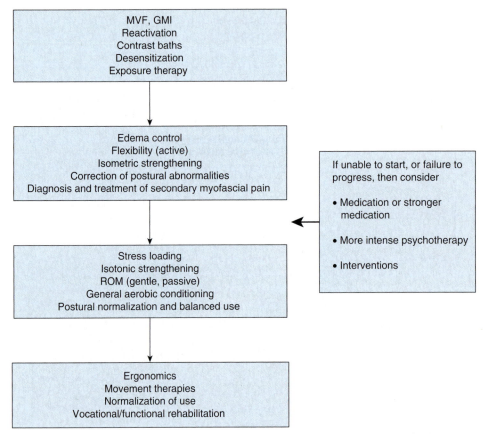

Fig. 13.3 Treatment algorithm. (Harden et al. 2013). *GMI,* Graded motor imagery; *MVF,* mirror visual feedback; *ROM,* range of motion.

Oedema management

Oedema can be managed in a number of ways, often using a range of modalities (Boscheinen-Morrin & Conolly 2001; Clemens & Foss-Campbell 1993; Harden et al. 2013; Hunter et al. 1995; Palmada et al. 1999; Prosser & Conolly 2003; Li et al. 2005, Stanton-Hicks et al. 2002; Rho et al. 2002; Villeco 2011).

- *Elevation* increases venous and lymphatic flow.
- *Retrograde massage* increases venous and lymphatic return. It must be performed softly, harmoniously, rhythmically and with supple hands (Villeco 2011). Massage for oedema should never be painful and should always go towards the regional lymph nodes. Pressures above 60 mmHg can cause mechanical occlusion of the capillaries and are counterproductive to fluid reabsorption.
- *Compression* can be provided in the form of gloves, bandages or pneumatic compression. It works by reinforcing body tissue hydrostatic pressure (HP).
- *Active exercise* stimulates the muscle pump. It increases blood flow and creates soft tissue movement.

- *Contrast baths.* The application of alternating hot and cold therapy alters afferent input resulting in a decrease in pain and increase in HP. Thermal allodynia may be a contraindication. Hot water should be like a comfortable bath and cool water not cold.
- *Splinting* can aid reduction of oedema in the hand through optimal placement of joints and soft tissues. Position of safe immobilisation (POSI) splinting maintains soft tissue length and can prevent or help treatment of joint contractures. If the patient is at risk of developing contractures, splinting can be used prophylactically at rest times. Splinting should not be used full time so as not to limit functional integration.
- *Kinesiotaping.* Application of kinesiotape specifically for oedema can be defined as *wavy application of thin kinesiotape stripes converging at lymphatic drainage centres* (Hörmann et al. 2020). In a systematic review, Hörmann et al. (2020) found positive evidence for kinesiotape application for the reduction of swelling and beneficial effects on secondary outcome parameters such as pain and patient satisfaction.

Addressing cortical changes

Techniques available to specifically address cortical changes associated with CRPS are based mainly on mirror therapy, graded motor imagery (GMI) and observed tactile discrimination. Desensitisation, sensory reeducation and sensorimotor rehabilitation are discussed earlier. Inclusion of proprioceptive rehabilitation activities is also important for maintaining or recovering the cortical map of the injured body part.

Graded motor imagery

GMI is a specific programme for the cortical retraining of rehabilitation activities. The mechanism is thought to be the sequential activation of premotor and motor networks, followed by reconciliation of sensory feedback and motor output through mirror movements. Moseley (2005) researched the components in varying orders and reached the following conclusions:

- Laterality training decreases NP scores irrespective of its place in GMI.
- The order of mirror therapy and imagined movements is important:
  - Imagined movements only have effect when they follow laterality training.
  - Mirror therapy only has an effect when it follows imagined movements.

For further reading, see Moseley (2004, 2006) and www.gradedmotorimagery.com.

GMI has good efficacy for the treatment of CRPS (Daly & Bialocerkowski 2008), is recommended in the first stage of the CRPS treatment algorithm (see Fig. 13.3) and is the current evidence-based treatment of choice for CRPS (Lewis et al. 2011).

Practical application of graded motor imagery

GMI consists of three stages (Moseley 2004, 2005, 2006). In studies, each stage has been performed for 2 weeks, but optimal frequency and duration for clinical practice have not been established.

1. Recognition of hand laterality activates the premotor cortices. The patient can use laterality training in different ways. They can use hands pictured on cards, photographs on a database, photos in newspapers or magazines, or left/right photos uploaded into specific computer programs (Recognise) or Smartphone Apps (Recognise or Orientate). The original method was to use a pack of 56 cards (www.noigroup.com) showing hands in random orientations. The Recognise app has a useful scoring tool and has a number of levels of progression available.
2. Imagined hand movements (explicit motor imagery) activate the primary motor cortex and similar parts of the brain as when a patient actually moves. There are many ways to apply imagined movements. The patient can imagine themselves adopting particular positions or movements, or they may imagine functional or recreational tasks in graded levels of difficulty. All movements must be purely imaginary. Care should be taken not to increase pain and motor imagery used should be at a 'movement' level that is achievable for the patient at that time. It may be useful to maintain hand laterality exercises during this time.
3. Mirror movements have many forms. The patient may use the mirror box to perform bilateral tasks according to the hand position shown in pictures from the 56-card pack. They adopt the postures on each picture slowly and smoothly. GMI authors (www.gradedmotorimagery.com) suggest starting with exercises involving little or no movement. They caution that mirror therapy offers potent brain stimulation and is the *final* part of the GMI process.

The clinician is advised to agree on a programme with the patient, emphasising the importance of frequency of activity. As with mirror therapy, a treatment regime of 5 minutes, 5 times a day is likely to have great benefit.

Observed tactile discrimination

In CRPS, decreased tactile acuity is related to reorganisation of the primary sensory cortex and pain (Moseley & Weich 2009). Discrimination of the location and diameter of tactile stimuli applied to the affected limb of patients with unilateral CRPS can decrease pain and 2PD thresholds, whereas tactile stimulation alone does not (Moseley et al. 2008). Focusing attention on the stimulated area can increase S1 response to touch and improves tactile performance (ibid). Moseley & Weich (2009) further demonstrated that a single 30-minute tactile discrimination session led to a sustained improvement in tactile acuity if the CRPS patients looked towards the affected limb during the training, while watching the skin of the opposite body part in a mirror.

Mirror feedback therapy (MFT)

MFT was developed by Ramachandran (1998) in the treatment of phantom limb pain. It has been used for CRPS to correct a presumed disruption of normal interaction between motor intention and sensory feedback (Lewis et al. 2011; McCabe et al. 2003). MFT has been found to be effective only in the treatment of acute CRPS. It has been investigated most robustly by McCabe (2003) and Moseley (2004, 2005, 2008). MFT may be more effective as part of GMI than in isolation (Moseley et al. 2008).

Principles of MVF

MVF involves placing the affected limb behind a mirror that is freestanding and large enough to obscure the affected body part, or inside a mirror box. The unaffected limb is placed in front of the mirror, creating an image as if it is the affected limb. The patient is asked to concentrate fully on the reflection in the mirror and to perform active range of movement exercises, rehabilitation activities or functional tasks with both limbs simultaneously. The movements should be based on the patient's individual needs, interests and capabilities.

General principles are:

- Use of the mirror must not provoke pain.
- Bilateral movements, rehabilitation activities or functional tasks performed using the mirror must be SYMMETRICAL.
- The unaffected body part should look as similar to the affected side as possible. Remove jewellery, watches, etc. and cover major distinguishing features if possible.
- MFT requires focused concentration from the individual, so short duration performed frequently is recommended. McCabe (2011) suggests 5 to 6 times a day until concentration is lost, but no more than 5 minutes.
- If pain is elicited, unilateral unaffected limb activities can be tried. GMI should be used if this still causes pain or an increase in other signs or symptoms.

Range of movement and exercise

Harden et al. (2013) emphasise the importance of functional restoration and suggest that the initial stages of movement and exercise should begin with progressive activation of sensorimotor cortices through GMI and MFT. The treatment pathway then moves to gentle but progressive ROM and strengthening. This requires adequate analgesia. If the patient is unable to start or progress medication, psychological help may be needed alongside physical treatment.

The efficacy of active range of motion (AROM) exercises is well documented (Boscheinen-Morrin & Conolly 2001; Hunter et al. 1995; Li et al. 2005; Prosser & Conolly 2003). ROM exercises are performed to maintain tendon gliding and supple joints and to minimise adhesions and contractures (Birklein & Dimova 2017; Clemens & Foss-Campbell 1993). The exercise programme must

be tailored to the individual and not exacerbate pain (Atkins 2003; Harden et al. 2013; Li et al. 2005). In the early stages, isometric exercises alongside AROM are recommended (Harden et al. 2013; Rho 2002; Stanton-Hicks et al. 1998, 2002). It is important to avoid aggressive or strong passive ROM treatment (Harden et al. 2013; Stanton-Hicks et al. 1998).

The consensus guidelines (Harden et al. 2013; Rho 2002; Stanton-Hicks et al. 1998, 2002) describe a gradual progression of AROM and isometrics, followed by stretching and isotonic strengthening, stress loading (see later), postural normalisation and general aerobic conditioning. The exercise programme provided should be individualised and address all joints with active or passive limitation, while maintaining a focus on functional movements. Progression should occur once the patient can comfortably achieve exercise tasks at their current level. If trauma is the initiating event, the exercises initiated should be appropriate for the stage of tissue healing.

Muscle strengthening starts with isometric exercises. Traditional strengthening equipment can be used to progress to isotonic exercise. Functional strengthening tasks and vocationally related training activities should be considered. Aerobic conditioning and core muscle training can promote general well-being and function, assist with feelings of low mood and promote strength and stability.

Hydrotherapy can be very useful. In the early stages, the water can assist exercise and promote weightbearing, while also acting to reduce oedema (Hall et al. 2008; Packham & Holly 2018). Later water can be used to resist movement, exercise aerobically and promote strength and stability.

Stress loading, also known as *scrub and carry*, is a process of active traction and compression exercises without joint motion (Watson & Carlson 1987). It was developed as a regime of *scrubbing* plywood with a bristle brush for 3 minutes, 3 times a day in four-point kneeling or on a table with the shoulder directly above the hand, and *carrying* a purse or briefcase of 1 to 5 lb in weight (as tolerated by the patient) whenever standing or walking. To progress the treatment, duration of scrubbing and the weight being carried are gradually increased. Other modalities were introduced as the pain subsides (Watson & Carlson 1987).

The stress loading regime tends to be used as an adjunct to other therapies. Stress loading is recommended as part of the package of care and as a progression of treatment rather than a starting point (Harden et al. 2013; Stanton-Hicks et al. 2002; Rho et al. 2002).

Proprioception

People with CRPS have deficits in proprioception, so their conscious and unconscious sense of limb position and movement is altered (Bank et al. 2013; Bean et al. 2016;

Brun et al. 2018). There may be a correlation between deficits in proprioception and pain severity (Brun et al. 2018). Rehabilitation of proprioception requires sequential activation of the sensorimotor system.

Six-stage proprioception programme (Hagert 2010)

1. Basic rehabilitation—oedema and pain control, promote range of motion.
2. Proprioception awareness—promote conscious joint control—mirror therapy (stimulate activity in the somatosensory cortex to enhance functional proprioception reeducation).
3. Joint position sense—ability to replicate a predetermined joint angle—passive and active reproduction of joint angle.
4. Kinesthesia—ability to sense joint position without audiovisual clues—motion detection using manual passive motion.
5. Conscious neuromuscular rehabilitation—strengthening of specific muscles to enhance joint stability—isometric training, eccentric training, isokinetic training, co-activation.
6. Unconscious neuromuscular rehabilitation—reactive muscle activation—powerball exercises, plyometric training.

Functional tasks and workshop activities

A functional activity programme aids return to work, sport or simple domestic tasks (Prosser & Conolly 2003). Functional, goal-orientated tasks increase motivation and can enhance self-esteem (Palmada et al. 1999) and facilitate sensorimotor integration. The clinician should agree functional, SMART goals with the patient, and grade them as appropriate.

Aids and adaptations, used with due consideration, can be helpful to promote independence—see Section 1. Neuropathic Pain. Workshop activities can engage a patient and promote functional use of the affected limb. Activities relating to a patient's hobbies or work tasks should be a priority, together with work hardening (Harden et al. 2013; Stanton-Hicks et al. 1998). It is valuable to liaise with the patient's workplace.

Novel concepts

Treating without pain, wedges and more. Allison Taylor developed a number of novel treatment ideas. The aim is

to calm the superficial sensory nervous system, facilitate functional movement and reeducate movement patterns with less pain, see https://www.handtherapyed.com/wedges-and-more.html#/.

Microbiota. There has been a recent surge of interest in the potential role of gut microbiota in pain (Crock & Baldridge 2020). Clinical studies suggest that decreased bacterial diversity or dysbiosis of the human gut microbiome may be associated with painful conditions such as visceral pain, fibromyalgia and arthritic knee pain. In preclinical models, microbiota are known to change production of short-chain fatty acids, butyrate, serum glutamate; alter microglial activity; change the ability to mount an appropriate inflammatory response, autoantibody production, humoral immunity and immune regulation (Crock & Baldridge 2020). This suggests a variety of ways in which the microbiota might contribute to the development or maintenance of CRPS. It is an active research area, still in the preclinical stages, which may provide treatment strategies in the future.

Conclusion

NP and CRPS can be difficult to diagnose and even harder to treat. Armed with an understanding of possible underlying mechanisms and a systematic approach to assessment and reasoning, clinicians can avoid some of the pitfalls of diagnosing these conditions. The diagnosis, a range of therapeutic options and a flexible mind can make a real difference to patients.

Review questions   Q

1. Why could the presentation of neuropathy be paradoxical?
2. Name three ways to clinically decide whether a pain is likely to be nociceptive or neuropathic.
3. Name three ways to manage or treat NP.
4. Are CRPS symptoms considered proportionate to the inciting event?
5. What are the four main subgroups for diagnosis of CRPS?
6. Describe two forms of objective assessment for each of the four subgroups.
7. Name three types of motor or trophic changes in CRPS.

References

Abram, S., 1990. Incidence-hypothesis-epidemiology. In: Stanton-Hicks, M. (Ed.), Pain and the Sympathetic Nervous System. Kluwer, Boston, pp. 1–16.

Aim F, Klouche S, Frison A, Bauer T, Hardy P (2017) Efficacy of vitamin C in preventing complex regional pain syndrome after wrist fracture: A systematic review and meta-analysis. Orthopaedics and Traumatology: Surgery & Research.103: 465-470.

Albrecht, D.S., Ahmed, S.U., Kettner, N.W., Borra, R.J.H., Cohen-Adad, J., Deng, H., et al., 2018. Neuroinflammation of the spinal cord and nerve roots in chronic radicular pain patients. Pain 159 (5), 968–977.

Allen, R.J., Wu, C., Horiuchi, G., Friends, J.W., Campbell, K.R., 2004. Pressure desensitization effects on pressure tolerance and function in patients with complex regional pain syndrome. Ortho. Phy. Ther. Prac 16 (4), 13–16.

Atkins, R.M., 2003. Aspects of current management: complex regional pain syndrome. J. Bone. Joint. Surg. 85-B, 1100–1106.

Attal, N., Bouhassira, D., 2015. Pharmacotherapy of neuropathic pain: which drugs, which treatment algorithms? Pain 156, S104–S114.

Bahm, J., Winkel, R., Zyluk, A., 2018. Neuropathic pain: we need more interdisciplinary and holistic treatment. Neurol. Psychiatr. Brain. Res. 28, 24–28.

Balan, S.A., Garcia-Elias, M., 2008. Utility of the Powerball® in the invigoration of the musculature of the forearm. Hand. Surg. 13 (2), 79–83.

Bank, P.J., Peper, C.L., Marinus, J., Beek, P.J., van Hilten, J.J., 2013. Motor dysfunction of complex regional pain syndrome is related to impaired central processing of proprioceptive information. J. Pain 14, 1460–1474.

Bannister, K., Sachau, J., Baron, R., Dickenson, A.H., 2020. Neuropathic pain: mechanism-based therapeutics. Annu. Rev. Pharmacol. Toxicol. 60 (1), 257–274.

Bates, D., Schultheis, B., Hanes, M., Jolly, S., Chakravarthy, K., Deer, T., et al., 2019. A comprehensive algorithm for management of neuropathic pain. Pain. Med. 20, S2–S12.

Bean, D., Johnson, M., Heiss-Dunlop, W., Lee, A., Kydd, R., 2015. Do psychological factors influence recovery from complex regional pain syndrome type 1? A prospective study. Pain 156, 2310–2318.

Bean, D.J., Johnson, M.H., Heiss-Dunlop, W., Kydd, R.R., 2016. Extent of recovery in the first 12 months of complex regional pain syndrome type-1: a prospective study. Eur. J. Pain 20, 884–894.

Bear-Lehman, J., Abreu, B.C., 1989. Evaluating the hand: issues in reliability and validity. Phys. Ther. 69, 1025–1033.

Bellugou, M., Allieu, Y., de Godebout, J., Thaury, M.N., Ster, J.F., 1991. "Desensitization" technique in the rehabilitation of the painful hand]. Ann. Hand. Up. Limb. Surg. 10, 59–67.

Bennett, M., Attal, N., Backonja, M., Baron, R., Bouhassira, D., Freynhagen, R., et al., 2007. Using screening tools to identify neuropathic pain. Pain 127 (3), 199–203.

Bharwani, K., Dirckx, M., Huygen, F., 2017. Complex regional pain syndrome: diagnosis and treatment. BJA. Edu 17 (8), 262–268.

Birklein, F., Dimova, V., 2017. Complex regional pain syndrome–up-to-date. Pain. Clin. Update 2, e624.

Birklein, F., Schmelz, M., 2008. Neuropeptides, neurogenic inflammation and complex regional pain syndrome (CRPS). Neurosci. Lett. 437, 199–202.

Boscheinen-Morrin, J., Conolly, W.B., 2001. The Hand: Fundamentals of Therapy, third ed. Butterworth-Heinemann, Oxford.

Bove, G.M., Light, A.R., 1997. The nervi nervorum: missing link for neuropathic pain? Pain. Forum 6 (3), 181–190.

British Pain Society, 2008. A Case of Neuropathic Pain. British Pain Society; Royal College of General Practitioners, London.

Bruehl, S., 2015. Complex regional pain syndrome. Br. Med. J. 350, h2730.

Bruehl, S., Lubenow, T.R., Nath, H., Ikanovich, O., 1996. Validation of thermography in the diagnosis of reflex sympathetic dystrophy. Clin. J. Pain 12, 316–325.

Bruehl, S., Harden, R.N., Galer, B.S., Saltz, S., Bertram, M., Backonja, M., et al., 1999. External validation of IASP diagnostic criteria for complex regional pain syndrome and proposed research diagnostic criteria. Pain 81, 147–154.

Bruehl, S., Harden, R., Galer, B., Saltz, S., Backonja, M., Stanton-Hicks, M., 2002. Complex regional pain syndrome: are there distinct subtypes and sequential stages of the syndrome? Pain 95 (1–2), 11–124.

Brun, C., Giorgi, N., Pinard, A.-M., Gagne, M., McCabe, C.S., Mercier, C., 2018. Exploring the relationships between altered body perception, limb position sense, and limb movement sense in complex regional pain syndrome. J. Pain 20 (1), 17–27.

Burr, N., Pratt, A.L., Stott, D., 2003. Inter-rater and intra-rater reliability when measuring interphalangeal joints: comparison between three hand-held goniometers. Physiotherapy 89 (11), 641–652.

Calvo, M., Dawes, J.M., Bennett, D.L., 2012. The role of the immune system in the generation of neuropathic pain. Lancet. Neurol. 11 (7), 629–642.

Chang, C., McDonnell, P., Gershwin, M., 2021. Complex regional pain syndrome—autoimmune or functional neurologic syndrome. J. Tran. Auto 4, 100080.

Ciccone, D., Bandilla, E., Wu, W., 1997. Psychological dysfunction in patients with reflex sympathetic dystrophy. Pain 71, 323–333.

Clark, J., Tawfik, V., Tajerian, M., Kingery, W., 2018. Autoinflammatory and autoimmune contributions to complex regional pain syndrome. Mol. Pain 14, 1–13.

Clemens, S., Foss-Campbell, B., 1993. Rehabilitation following traumatic hand injury: hand therapist's perspective. Part 1: acute phase of hand rehabilitation. Plast. Surg. Nurs. 13 (3), 129–134.

Coldham, F., Lewis, J., Lee, H., 2006. The reliability of one vs. three grip trials in symptomatic and asymptomatic subjects. J. Hand Ther. 19 (3), 318–327.

Colloca, L., Ludman, T., Bouhassira, D., Baron, R., Dickenson, A.H., Yarnitsky, D., et al., 2017. Neuropathic pain. Nat. Rev. Dis. Prim. 3, 17002.

Costigan, M., Scholz, J., Woolf, C.J., 2009. Neuropathic pain: a maladaptive response of the nervous system to damage. Annu. Rev. Neurosci. 32 (1), 1–32.

Covington, E., 1996. Psychological issues in reflex sympathetic dystrophy. In: Stanton-Hicks, M., Jänig, W. (Eds.), Reflex Sympathetic Dystrophy: A Reappraisal. 6. IASP Press, Seattle, pp. 191–216.

Crock, L.W., Baldridge, M.T., 2020. A role for the microbiota in complex regional pain syndrome? Neurobiol. Pain 8, 100054.

Cruccu, G., Truini, A., 2017. A review of neuropathic pain: from guidelines to clinical practice. Pain. Ther 6 (Suppl. 1), S35–S42.

Daly, A.E., Bialocerkowski, A.E., 2008. "Does evidence support physiotherapy management of adult complex regional pain syndrome type one? A systematic review. Eur. J. Pain 13, 339–353.

Dellon, A., 1981. Evaluation of Sensibility and Re-education of Sensation in the Hand. Williams & Wilkins, Baltimore, MD.

Devor, M., 2006. Response of nerves to injury in relation to neuropathic pain. In: McMahon, S., Koltzenburg, M. (Eds.), Wall & Melzack's Textbook of Pain, fifth ed. Churchill Livingstone, Edinburgh, pp. 905–928.

Devor, M., 2013. Neuropathic pain: pathophysiological response of nerves to injury. In: McMahon, S.B., Koltzenburg, M., Tracey, I., Turk, D.C. (Eds.), Wall and Melzack's Textbook of Pain, sixth ed. Elsevier/Saunders. 2013.

Dickenson, A., Bee, L., 2008. Neurobiological mechanisms of neuropathic pain and its treatment. In: Castro-Lopes, J., Raja, S., Schmelz, M. (Eds.), Pain 2008. An Updated Review. IASP Press, Seattle, pp. 277–286.

Dilley, A., Richards, N., Pulman, K.G., Bove, G.M., 2013. Disruption of fast axonal transport in the rat induces behavioral changes consistent with neuropathic pain. J. Pain 14 (11), 1437–1449.

Dommerholt, J., 2004. Clinical management: CRPS. Complex Regional Pain Syndrome – 2: physical therapy management. J. Bodyw. Mov. Ther. 8 (4), 241–248.

Dworkin, R., O'Connor, A., Backonja, M., Farrar, J., Finnerup, N., Jensen, T., et al., 2007. Pharmacologic managemen of neuropathic pain: evidence based recommendations. Pain 132, 237–251.

Ellis, A., Bennett, D.L.H., 2013. Neuroinflammation and the generation of neuropathic pain. Br. J. Anaesth. 111 (1), 26–37.

Finnerup, N.B., Haroutounian, S., Kamerman, P., Baron, R., Bennett, D.L.H., Bouhassira, D., et al., 2016. Neuropathic pain: an updated grading system for research and clinical practice. Pain 157 (8), 1599–1606.

Finnerup, N.B., Kuner, R., Jensen, T.S., 2020. Neuropathic pain: from mechanisms to treatment. Physiol. Rev. Vol. 101, Issue 1, January 2021, 259–301.

Flor, H., Braun, C., Elbert, T., Birbaumer, N., 1997. Extensive reorganisation of primary somatosensory cortex in chronic back pain patients. Neurosci. Lett. 224, 5–8.

Forstenpointner, J., Ruscheweyh, R., Attal, N., Baron, R., Bouhassira, D., Enax-Krumova, E., et al., 2021. No pain, still gain (of function): the relation between sensory profiles and the presence or absence of self-reported pain in a large multicenter cohort of patients with neuropathy. Pain 162 (3), 718–727.

Fourkas, A.D., Bonavolanta, V., Avenanti, A., Aglioti, S.M., 2008. Kinaesthetic imagery and tool-specific modulation of corticospinal representations in expert tennis players. Cerebr. Cortex 18, 2382–2390.

Furman, M.B., Johnson, S.C., 2019. Induced lumbosacral radicular symptom referral patterns: a descriptive study. Spine. J. 19 (1), 163–170.

Gibbs, G., Drummond, P., Finch, P., Phillips, J., 2008. Unravelling the pathophysiology of complex regional pain syndrome: focus on sympathetically maintained pain. Clin. Exp. Pharmacol. Physiol. 35, 717–724.

Goebel, A., Barker, C., Turner-Stokes, L., et al., 2018. Complex Regional Pain Syndrome in Adults: UK Guidelines for Diagnosis, Referral and Management in Primary and Secondary Care. Royal College of Physicians, London.

Goebel, A., Barker, C., Birklein, F., Brunner, F., Casale, R., Eccleston, C., et al., 2019. Standards for the diagnosis and management of complex regional pain syndrome: results of a European Pain Federation task force. Eur. J. Pain 23, 641–651.

Hagert, E., 2010. Proprioception of the wrist joint: a review of current concepts and possible implications on the rehabilitation of the wrist. J. Hand. Ther. 23, 2–17.

Hall, J., Swinkels, A., Briddon, J., McCabe, C.S., 2008. Does aquatic exercise relieve pain in adults with neurologic or musculoskeletal disease? A systematic review and meta-analysis of randomized controlled trials. Arch. Phys. Med. Rehabil. 89 (5), 873–883

Hansson, P., Kinnman, E., 1996. Unmasking mechanisms of peripheral neuropathic pain in a clinical perspective. Pain. Rev. 3 (4), 272–292.

Hansson, P., Lacerenza, M., Marchettini, P., 2002. Aspects of clinical and experimental neuropathic pain: the clinical perspective. In: Hansson, P., et al (Eds.), Neuropathic Pain: Pathophysiology and Treatment. IASP Press, Seattle, pp. 1–18.

Hansson, P., Backonja, M., Bouhassira, D., 2007. Usefulness and limitations of quantitative sensory testing: clinical and research application in neuropathic pain states. Pain 129 (3), 256–259.

Harden, R., Bruehl, S., 2005. Diagnostic criteria: the statistical derivation of the four criterion factors. In: Wilson, P., Stanton-Hicks, M., Harden, R. (Eds.), CRPS: Current Diagnosis and Therapy. IASP Press, Seattle, pp. 45–58.

Harden, R.N., Bruehl, S., Galer, B.S., Saltz, S., Bertram, M., Backonja, M., et al., 1999. Complex Regional Pain Syndrome: are the diagnostic criteria valid and sufficiently comprehensive? Pain 83, 211–219.

Harden, R., Bruehl, S., Perez, R., Birklein, F., Marinus, J., Maihöfner, C., et al., 2010. Validation of proposed diagnostic criteria (the "Budapest Criteria") for complex regional pain syndrome. Pain 150 (2), 268–274.

Harden, R., Oaklander, A., Burton, A., Perez, R., Richardson, K., Swan, M., et al., 2013. Complex regional pain syndrome: practical diagnostic and treatment guidelines, 4th edition. Pain. Med. 14 (2), 180–229.

Harden, R.N., Maihofner, C., Abousaad, E., Vatine, J.-J., Kirsling, A., Perex, R.S.G.M., et al., 2017. A prospective, multisite, international validation of the complex regional pain syndrome severity score. Pain 158, 1430–1436.

Hassan-zadeh, R., Esfahani, A.R.R., 2012. The effect of use of the audiovisual tactile on sensory recovery following hand replantation: a case report. Procedia. Soc. Behav. Sci 32, 421–424.

Hayek, S.M., Mekhail, N.A., 2004. Complex regional pain syndrome: redefining reflex sympathetic dystrophy and causalgia. Phys. Sportsmed. 32, 5.

Hörmann, 2020. Kinesiotaping for postoperative oedema – what is the evidence? A systematic review. BMC. Sport. Sci. Med. Rehabil 12, 1–14.

Hunter, J.M., Mackin, E.J., Callahan, A.D., 1995. Rehabilitation of the Hand. Surgery and Therapy, fourth ed. Mosby, St Louis.

Huygen, F., de Bruijn, A., de Bruin, M., Groeneweg, G., Klein, H., Zijlstra, F., 2002. Evidence for local inflammation in complex regional pain syndrome type 1. Mediat. Inflamm. 11, 47–51.

International Association for the Study of Pain, 2011. IASP Taxonomy. Available from: http://www.iasp-pain.org/Content/NavigationMenu/GeneralResourceLinks/PainDefinitions/default.htm.

Jänig, W., Baron, R., 2006. Is CRPS 1 a neuropathic pain syndrome? Pain 120 (3), 227–229.

Jensen, T.S., 2002. An improved understanding of neuropathic pain. Eur. J. Pain 6 (Suppl. B), 3–11.

Jerosch-Herold, C., 2011. Sensory relearning in peripheral nerve disorders of the hand: a web-based survey and Delphi consensus method. J. Hand. Ther. 24, 292–299.

Ji, R.-R., Xu, Z.-Z., Strichartz, G., Serhan, C.N., 2011. Emerging roles of resolvins in the resolution of inflammation and pain. Trends. Neurosci. 34 (11), 599–609.

Ji, R.-R., Chamessian, A., Zhang, Y.-Q., 2016. Pain regulation by non-neuronal cells and inflammation. Science. (New York, N.Y.) 354 (6312), 572–577.

Juottonen, K., Gockel, M., Silen, T., Hurri, H., Hari, R., Forss, N., 2002. Altered central sensorimotor processing in patients with complex regional pain syndrome. Pain 98 (3), 315–323.

Keysers, C., Wicker, B., Gazzola, V., Anton, J.L., Fogassi, L., Gallese, V., 2004. A touching sight: SII/PV activation during the observation and experience of touch. Neuron 42, 335–346.

Kharkar, S., Venkatesh, Y., Grothusen, J., Rojas, I., Schwartzman, R., 2012. Skin biopsy in complex regional pain syndrome: case series and literature review. Pain. Phy 15, 255–266.

Lacourse, M.G., Turner, J.A., Randolf-Orr, E., Schandler, S.L., Cohen, M.J., 2004. Cerebral and cerebellar sensorimotor plasticity following motor imagery-based mental practice of sequential movement. J. Rehabil. Res. Dev. 41, 505–524.

Lenz, M., Üçeyler, N., Frettlöh, J., Höffken, O., Krumova, E., Lissek, S., et al., 2013. Local cytokine changes in complex regional pain syndrome type I (CRPS I) resolve after 6 months. Pain 154, 2142–2149.

Lewis, J.S., Coales, K., Hall, J., McCabe, C.S., 2011. "Now you see it, now you do not": sensory-motor re-education in complex regional pain syndrome. Hand. Ther. 16 (2), 29–38.

Li, Z., Paterson-Smith, B., Smith, T.L., Koman, L.A., 2005. Diagnosis and management of complex regional pain syndrome complicating upper extremity recovery. J. Hand. Ther. 18 (2), 270–277.

Lundborg, G., 2008. Lund University Faculty of Medicine. Available from: http://www.med.lu.se/klinvetmalmo/hand_surgery/clinical_projects/enhanced_sensory_relearning.

Lundborg, G., Rosen, B., 2007. Hand function after nerve repair. Acta. Physiol. 189, 207–217.

MacAvoy, M.C., Green, D.P., 2007. Critical reappraisal of Medical Research Council muscle testing for elbow flexion. J. Hand. Surg. 32A, 149–153.

Maier, C., Baron, R., Tölle, T., Binder, A., Birbaumer, N., Birklein, F., et al., 2010. Quantitative sensory testing in the German Research Network on Neuropathic Pain (DNFS): somatosensory abnormalities in 1236 patients with different neuropathic pain syndromes. Pain 150 (3), 439–450.

Maihöfner, C., Handwerker, H., Neundorfer, B., Birklein, F., 2003. Patterns of cortical reorganisation in complex regional pain syndrome. Neurology 61, 1707–1715.

Maihöfner, C., Handwerker, H., Neundorfer, B., Birklein, F., 2004. Cortical reorganization during recovery from complex regional pain syndrome. Neurology 63, 693–701.

Massy-Westropp, N., Rankin, W., Ahern, M., Krishnan, J., Hearn, T.C., 2004. Measuring grip strength in normal adults: reference ranges and a comparison of electronic and hydraulic instruments. J. Hand. Surg. 29 (3), 514–519.

McCabe, C., 2011. Mirror visual feedback therapy. A practical approach. J. Hand. Ther. 24, 170–179.

McCabe, C.S., Haigh, R.C., Ring, E.F.J., Halligan, R.W., Wall, P.D., Blake, D.R., 2003. A controlled pilot study of the utility of visual feedback in the treatment of complex regional pain syndrome (type 1). Rheumatology 42, 97–101.

Meacham, K., Shepherd, A., Mohapatra, D.P., Haroutounian, S., 2017. Neuropathic pain: central vs. peripheral mechanisms. Curr. Pain. Headache. Rep. 21 (6), 28.

Merskey, H., Lindblom, U., Mumford, J., Nathan, P., Sunderland, S., 1994. Pain terms, a current list with definitions and notes on usage. In: Merskey, H., Bogduk, N. (Eds.), Classification of Chronic Pain. IASP Press, Seattle, pp. 207–214.

Miller, L.K., Chester, R., Jerosch-Herold, C., 2012. Effects of sensory re-education programs on functional hand sensibility after median and ulnar repair: a systematic review. J. Hand. Ther. 25, 297–307.

Moseley, G.L., 2004. Imagined movements cause pain and swelling in a patient with complex regional pain syndrome. Neurology 62, 1644.

Moseley, G.L., 2005. "Is successful rehabilitation of complex regional pain syndrome due to sustained attention to the affected limb? A randomised clinical trial. Pain 114, 54–61.

Moseley, G.L., 2006. Graded motor imagery for pathologic pain: a randomized controlled trial. Neurology 67 (12), 2129–2134.

Moseley, G.L., Weich, K., 2009. The effect of tactile discrimination training is enhanced when patients watch the reflected image of their unaffected limb during training. Pain 144, 314–319.

Moseley, G., Gallace, A., Spence, C., 2008. Is mirror therapy all it is cracked up to be? Current evidence and future directions. Pain 138 (1), 7–10.

Moseley, G.L., Herbert, R.D., Parsons, T., Lucas, S., Van Hilten, J.J., Marinus, J., 2014. Intense pain soon after wrist fracture strongly predicts who will develop complex regional pain syndrome: prospective cohort study. J. Pain 15 (1), 16–23.

Nedelec, B., Calva, V., Chouinard, A., Couture, M.-A., Godbout, E., de Oliveira, A., LaSalle, L., 2016. Somatosensory rehabilitation for neuropathic pain in burn survivors: a case series. J. Burn. Care. Res. 37, 37–46.

Nora, D.B., Becker, J., Ehlers, J.A., Gomes, I., 2004. Clinical features of 1039 patients with neurophysiological diagnosis of carpal tunnel syndrome. Clin. Neurol. Neurosurg. 107 (1), 64–69.

Novak, C.B., 2011. Clinical commentary in response to: sensory relearning in peripheral nerve disorders of the hand: a web-based survey and Delphi consensus method. J. Hand. Ther. 24, 300–302.

Novak, C.B., 2018. Cold intolerance after nerve injury. J. Hand. Ther. 31, 195–200.

Novak, C.B., von der Heyde, R.L., 2013. Evidence and techniques in rehabilitation following nerve injuries. Hand. Clin. 29, 383–392.

Oaklander, A., Fields, H., 2009. Is reflex sympathetic dystrophy/complex regional pain syndrome type I a small-fibre neuropathy? Ann. Neurol. 65, 629–638.

Oaklander, A., Rissmiller, J., Gelman, L., Zheng, L., Chang, Y., Gott, R., 2006. Evidence of focal small-fibre axonal degeneration in complex regional pain syndrome-I (reflex sympathetic dystrophy). Pain 120 (3), 235–243.

Osborne, N.R., Anastakis, D.J., Davis, K.D., 2018. Peripheral nerve injuries, pain, and neuroplasticity. J. Hand. Ther. 31, 184–194.

Packham, 2017. Using Somatosensory Rehabilitation to Treat Allodynia. Blog Available from: https://rsds.org/somatosensory-rehabilitation-allodynia/.

Packham, T., Holly, J., 2018. Mechanism-specific rehabilitation management of complex regional pain syndrome: proposed recommendations from evidence synthesis. J. Hand. Ther. 31, 238–249.

Packham, T., Spicher, C.J., MacDermid, J.C., Michlovitz, S., Buckley, D.N., 2018. Somatosensory rehabilitation for allodynia in complex regional pain syndrome of the upper limb: a retrospective cohort study. J. Hand. Ther. 31, 10–19.

Palmada, M., Shah, S., O'Hare, K., 1999. Hand oedema: pathophysiology and treatment. Br. J. Hand. Ther. 4 (1), 26–32.

Palmer, G., 2015. Complex regional pain syndrome. Aust. Prescr. 38 (3), 82–86.

Park, H., Jang, Y., Oh, S., Lee, P., 2020. Psychological characteristics in patients with chronic complex regional pain syndrome: comparisons with patients with major depressive disorder and other types of chronic pain. J. Pain. Res. 13, 389–398.

Petoe, M.A., Molina Jacque, F.A., Byblow, W.D., Stinear, C.M., 2013. Cutaneous anaesthesia of the forearm enhances sensorimotor function of the hand. J. Neurophysiol. 109, 1091–1096.

Pleger, B., Tegenthoff, M., Ragert, P., Förster, A.-F., Dinse, H.R., Schwenkreis, P., et al., 2005. Sensorimotor retuning [corrected] in complex regional pain syndrome parallels pain reduction. Ann. Neurol. 57 (3), 425–429.

Pratt, A.L., Burr, N., 2001. A review of goniometry use within current hand therapy practice. Br. J. Hand. Ther. 6 (2), 45–49.

Prosser, R., Conolly, W.B., 2003. Rehabilitation of the Hand and Upper Limb. Butterworth-Heinemann, Oxford.

Puchalski, P., Zyluk, A., 2005. Complex regional pain syndrome type 1 after fractures of the distal radius: a prospective study of the role of psychological factors. J. Hand. Surg. 30 (6), 574–580.

Quintal, I., Carrier, A., Packham, T., Bourbonnais, D., Dyer, J.-O., 2021. Tactile stimulation programs in patients with hand dysesthesia after a peripheral nerve injury: a systematic review. J. Hand. Ther. 34, 3–17.

Ramachandran, V., 1998. Phantoms in the Brain. Fourth Estate Limited, London.

Reedijk, W., van Rijn, M., Roelofs, K., Tuijl, J., Marinus, J., van Hilten, J., 2008. Psychological features of patients with complex regional pain syndrome type I related dystonia. Mov. Disord. 23 (11), 1551–1559.

Ref Type: Pamphlet

Rho, R.H., Brewer, R.P., Lamer, T.J., Wilson, P.R., 2002. Complex regional pain syndrome. Mayo. Clin. Proc. 77, 174–180.

Rommel, O., Gehling, M., Dertwinkel, R., Witscher, K., Zenz, M., Malin, J., et al., 1999. Hemisensory impairment in patients with complex regional pain syndrome. Pain 80 (1,2), 95–101.

Rommel, O., Malin, J., Zenz, M., Jänig, W., 2001. Quantitative sensory testing, neurophysiological and psychological examination in patients with complex regional pain syndrome and hemisensory deficits. Pain 2001, 279–293.

Rosen, B., Lundborg, G., 2005. Training with a mirror in rehabilitation of the hand. Scan. J. Plast. Reconstr. Surg. Hand. Surg 39, 104–108.

Rosen, B., Lundborg, G., 2007. Enhanced sensory recovery after median nerve repair using cortical audio-tactile interaction. A randomised multicentre study. J. Hand. Surg. Eur 32 (1), 31–37.

Rosen, B., Balkenius, C., Lundborg, G., 2003. Sensory re-education today and tomorrow: a review of evolving concepts. Br. J. Hand. Ther. 8 (2), 48–56.

Rosen, B., Bjorkman, A., Lundborg, G., 2006. Improved sensory relearning after nerve repair induced by selective temporary anaesthesia – a new concept in hand rehabilitation. J. Hand. Surg. 31B, 126–132.

Ross, E., 2004. Peripheral neuropathy. In: Ross, E. (Ed.), Pain Management. Hanley & Belfus, Philadelphia, pp. 81–89.

Saleem, S., Rosen, B., Engblom, J., Bjorkman, A., 2015. Improvement of hand sensibility resulting from application of anaesthetic cream on the forearm: importance of dose and time. Hand. Ther. 20 (4), 109–114.

Sandroni, P., Wilson, P., 2005. Sudomotor changes and edema - pathophysiology and measurement. In: Wilson, P., Stanton-Hicks, M., Harden, R. (Eds.), CRPS: Current Diagnosis and Therapy, vol. 32. IASP Press, Seattle, pp. 107–118.

Sato, J., Perl, E., 1991. Adrenergic excitation of cutaneous pain receptors induced by peripheral nerve injury. Science 251 (5001), 1608–1610.

Schlereth, T., 2020. Guideline "diagnosis and non interventional therapy of neuropathic pain" of the German Society of Neurology (Deutsche Gesellschaft für Neurologie). Neurol. Res. Pract. 2 (16).

Schmid, A.B., Coppieters, M.W., Ruitenberg, M.J., McLachlan, E.M., 2013. Local and remote immune-mediated inflammation after mild peripheral nerve compression in rats. J. Neuropathol. Exp. Neurol. 72 (7), 662–680.

Schmid, A.B., Fundaun, J., Tampin, B., 2020. Entrapment neuropathies: a contemporary approach to pathophysiology, clinical assessment, and management. Pain. Rep. 5 (4), e829.

Seftchick, J.L., Detullio, L.M., Fedorczyk, J.M., Aulicino, P.L., 2011. Clinical examination of the hand. In: Skirven, T., Osterman, A.L., Fedorczyk, J.M., Amadio, P.C. (Eds.), Rehabilitation of the Hand and Upper Extremity, sixth ed. Elsevier, Philadelphia, pp. 55–71. 2011.

Speck, V., Schlereth, T., Birklein, F., Maihöfner, C., 2016. Increased prevalence of posttraumatic stress disorder in CRPS. Eur. J. Pain 21, 466–473.

Spillane, J., Kullmann, D.M., Hanna, M.G., 2016. Genetic neurological channelopathies: molecular genetics and clinical phenotypes. J. Neurol. Neurosurg. Psychiatry 87 (1), 37–48.

Stanton-Hicks, M.D., Burton, A.W., Bruehl, S.P., Carr, D.B., Harden, R.N., Hassenbusch, S.J., et al., 2002. An updated interdisciplinary clinical pathway for CRPS: report of an expert panel. Pain. Pract. 2 (1), 1–16.

Stanton-Hicks, M., Janig, W., Hassenbuch, S., Haddox, J.D., Boas, R., Wilson, P., 1995. Reflex sympathetic dystrophy: changing concepts and taxonomy. Pain 63, 127–133.

Stanton-Hicks, M.D., Baron, R., Boas, R., Gordh, T., Harden, N., Hendler, N., et al., 1998. Complex regional pain syndromes: guidelines for therapy (consensus report). Clin. J. Pain 14 (2), 155–166.

Svens, B., Rosen, B., 2009. Early sensory re-learning after median nerve repair using mirror training and sense substitution. Hand. Ther. 14 (3), 75–82.

Teixeira, M.J., Almeida, D.B., Yeng, L.T., 2016. Concept of acute neuropathic pain. The role of nervi nervorum in the distinction between acute nociceptive and neuropathic pain. Revista. Dor 17.

Thomas, R.J., Degnan, G.G., 2005. Managing complex regional pain syndrome. J. Muscoskel. Med. 22, 514–526.

...V., Geertzen, J.H.B., Keizer, D., van Wilgen, C.P., ...rror box therapy added to cognitive behavioural therapy in three chronic complex regional pain syndrome type I patients: a pilot study." Int. J. Rehab. Res. 30, 181–188.

Uematsu, S., Hendler, N., Hungerford, D., Long, D., Ono, N., 1981. Thermography and electromyography in the differential diagnosis of chronic pain syndromes and reflex sympathetic dystrophy. Electromyogr. Clin. Neurophysiol. 2, 165–182.

Valdes, K., Naughton, N., Algar, L., 2014. S Sensorimotor interventions and assessments for the hand and wrist: a scoping review. J. Hand. Ther. 27, 272–286.

van Griensven, H., 2005. Pain in Practice. Theory and Treatment Strategies for Manual Therapists. Copyright Elsevier, Butterworth Heinemann, Oxford, p. 49.

van Hilten, J., Blumberg, H., Schwartzman, R., 2005. Factor IV: movement disorders and dystrophy - pathophysiology and measurement. In: Wilson, P., Stanton-Hicks, M., Harden, R. (Eds.), CRPS: Current Diagnosis and Therapy. IASP Press, Seattle, pp. 119–137.

Veldman, P., Reynen, H., Arntz, I., Goris, R., 1993a. Signs and symptoms of reflex sympathetic dystrophy: prospective study of 829 patients. Lancet 342 (8878), 1012–1016.

Veldman, P., Reynen, H., Arntz, I., Goris, R., 1993b. Signs and symptoms of reflex sympathetic dystrophy: prospective study of 829 patients. Lancet 342 (8878), 1012–1016.

Villeco, J.P., 2011. Edema: therapist's management. In: Skirven, T., Osterman, A.L., Fedorczyk, J.M., Amadio, P.C. (Eds.), Rehabilitation of the Hand and Upper Extremity, sixth ed. Elsevier, Philadelphia, pp. 55–71. 2011.

Walsh, M.T., 2012. Interventions in the disturbances in the motor and sensory environment. J. Hand. Ther. 25, 202–219.

Wasner, G., Baron, R., 2005. Factor II: vasomotor changes - pathophysiology and measurement. In: Wilson, P., Stanton-Hicks, M., Harden, R. (Eds.), CRPS: Current Diagnosis and Therapy. IASP Press, Seattle, pp. 81–106.

Watson, H.K., Carlson, L., 1987. Treatment of reflex sympathetic dystrophy of the hand with an active "stress loading" program. J. Hand. Surg. 12 (5, part 1), 779–785.

Waylett-Rendall, J., 1995. Desensitisation of the traumatised hand. In: Hunter, J., Mackin, E., Callahan, A. (Eds.), Rehabilitation of the Hand: Surgery and Therapy, fourth ed. Mosebyn, St Louis, pp. 693–700.

Weber, M., Birklein, F., Neundorfer, B., Schmelz, M., 2001. Facilitated neurogenic inflammation in complex regional pain syndrome. Pain 91 (3), 251–257.

Weir Mitchell, S., 1872. Gunshot Wounds and Other Injuries of Nerves. Lippincott, Philadelphia.

Wilson, P., 1990. Sympathetically maintained pain: diagnosis, measurement, and efficacy of treatment. In: Stanton-Hicks, M. (Ed.), Pain and the Sympathetic Nervous System. Kluwer Academic Publishers, Boston, pp. 91–123.

Woolf, C.J., Mannion, R.J., 1999. Neuropathic pain: aetiology, symptoms, mechanisms, and management. Lancet 353 (9168), 1959–1964.

Woolf, C., Max, M., 2001. Mechanism-based pain diagnosis: issues for analgesic drug development. Anesthesiology 95 (1), 241–249.

Wynn-Parry, C.B., 1980. Sensory rehabilitation of the hand. Aust. N. Z. J. Surg. 50 (3), 224–227.

Wynn-Parry, C.B., Salter, M., 1976. Sensory re-education after median nerve lesions. Hand 8 (3), 250–257.

Xanthos, D.N., Sandkühler, J., 2014. Neurogenic neuroinflammation: inflammatory CNS reactions in response to neuronal activity. Nat. Rev. Neurosci. 15 (1), 43–53.

Zhongyu, L., Paterson-Smith, B., Smith, T.L., Koman, L.A., 2005. Diagnosis and management of complex regional pain syndrome complicating upper extremity recovery. J. Hand. Ther. 18, 270–277.

Chapter | 14 |

Manual therapy and influence on pain perception

Chris McCarthy

LEARNING OBJECTIVES

At the end of this chapter, readers will understand:

1. MT in the context of biopsychosocial management of MSK pain.
2. The effects of MT on local tissue, spinal and supraspinal pain mechanisms.
3. The effects of pleasant touch on pain.
4. The effects of treatment-related pain on pain perception.
5. The effects of MT on motor control.
6. How MT may be applied in practice.

Introduction

Manual therapy (MT) is a complex intervention from a clinical trials perspective (Dieppe 2004), so it is difficult to design methodologies that evaluate the specific effects, actions and interactions of the process. Although MT has nonspecific effects, including placebo, it has a sound physiological basis to support its undoubted clinical and cost effectiveness (Hoving et al. 2006; UK BEAM 2004a). In spinal joint dysfunction, there is evidence from systematic reviews of moderate benefit for spinal MT in neck disorders (Bronfort et al. 2004; Gross et al. 2004; 2015) with an effect size similar to exercise (Fredin & Lorås 2017), cervicogenic headache (Bronfort et al. 2001) and acute low back pain.

In the same way that movement is universal to the human condition, manually applied touch has an impact at every level of our physiology. Manually guided or passively produced movement influences local tissue healing, selectively influences afferent neurological stimulus, influences spinal and supraspinal moderation of afferent information, provides an experience of pain or pleasure, conveys an emotional context to physical sensation and signals actual or perceived threat. Consequently, establishing the precise elements of interventions that will target our patients' specific needs and expectations is a combination of intuition, expert knowledge and refined communication. This highly attuned work means that MT can never be applied as a 'one-size-fits-all' approach, which may account for the varying results in research trials.

This chapter describes the underlying principles and treatment of MT for readers who do not necessarily practice it. Physiological evidence for how MT may reduce pain and improve function in musculoskeletal (MSK) pain patients will be presented and the interactions between mechanisms discussed.

The rationale of manual therapy

Manual therapies could conceivably boast the longest tradition in analgesic history, being reportedly undertaken in the earliest writings on medicine (Mattick & Wyatt 2000). Although the magnitude of analgesic effect of MT may be less than, for instance, surgery or pharmaceutical opiates, it is a ubiquitous approach to MSK pain that can offer immediate pain relief (Wright 1995), improvements in tissue healing (Zusman 2010), reductions in anxiety and fear of movement (George & Zeppieri 2009; Gifford 2000), pleasurable and rewarding tactile stimulation (Leknes & Tracey 2008), increased motivation to replicate pain-relieving movement (Schultz 2002) and a window of opportunity to relearn pain-free movement memories through repetition and active involvement in the rehabilitation process (Zusman 2004, 2005). MT is associated with minor adverse events (treatment soreness, which in fact may be a component of its effect), but major adverse events are rare (Carnes et al. 2010) and clinical and cost effectiveness are acceptable (UK BEAM 2004b). Existing trials assessing MT treatment for low back pain (where it is commonly utilised) tend to show small to moderate benefits when MT is compared to other conservative interventions or sham treatments. Not all trial evidence is consistent in demonstrating benefits from MT (NICE 2016; Paige et al. 2017), so clinical guidelines mostly recommend MT as an option for people with nonspecific low back pain. Recent clinical guidelines for low back pain in the United Kingdom and Unites States have recommended consideration of MT treatment (Bernstein et al. 2017; Qaseem et al. 2017). The UK NICE clinical guideline only recommends MT as part of a broader treatment approach that includes exercise (Bernstein et al. 2017), in recognition of the fact that MT should not be delivered or construed as a passive monotherapy but in the context of a biopsychosocial package of care. The modest evidence of benefit is at odds with manual therapists' experience of the large improvements and high levels of satisfaction delivering care to people with back pain.

Manual therapy in a biopsychosocial context

We all move, and to move is to change place, position or posture. The positions we adopt to allow full function are three-dimensional and continuously adapting to the functional demands placed on us. Naturally, the body cannot always immediately change to accommodate these demands, so short- and long-term dysfunction can result. In a system that continuously changes position and demands the acquisition of new and challenging positions, integrated control of movement can be compromised. When movement has become dysfunctional, the body receives prompts to that effect (pain, restriction). The brain registers that we are not moving efficiently, assesses

the value of this information and adopts strategies to address the situation (cessation, adaptation). We can learn to reduce the pain by changing some aspects of the way we move, and with time, new movement patterns occur. If we have been unable to improve our movement and pain, we may seek assistance from an expert in movement dysfunction such as a manual therapist (McCarthy 2010).

Movement dysfunction is a complex situation that must be considered in a biopsychosocial context. Our bodies are continuously moving from one starting position of movement to another. The point at which this process is considered dysfunctional is dependent on the perception of the individual (Pincus & Morley 2001). The psychological perspective of the individual and societal influences has an important effect on just when function is considered to have become dysfunctional. Thus the presentation of MSK dysfunction is incredibly variable.

Patients are people who have a perception that something is problematic, so they must be assessed from a biopsychosocial perspective. Each patient presents with a biopsychosocial profile that needs to be carefully interpreted to produce a tailored intervention. In other words, a clinician cannot afford to look at a patient from only one perspective. The ability of the clinical examination to weigh the relative value of each domain of a patient's biomechanical, physiological, psychological and social profile is essential (McCarthy 2010).

The necessity of considering the psychological and social influences on patients with pain can be seen in the following example. The patient has restricted movement of their lumbar spine, with this physiological impairment leading to the symptom of pain in the back. A manual therapist should recognise this association and evaluate the psychosocial influences on the perception, cause and maintenance of symptoms before instigating a strategy to change the symptoms. If the patient has had an excellent response to previous MT, has low levels of fear of movement and appropriate beliefs regarding causality, has a social environment encouraging recovery and has no maladaptive coping strategies, the priority for treatment would be to address the biomechanical stressors and physiological impairment of the region. The techniques and explanations used would teach the patient that the local movement restriction was indeed minor as it responded to just a few seconds of stretching. The patient would learn that a simple stretch could reduce pain and limitation and learn how to replicate this stretch as required. Fear of movement would be reduced, and self-efficacy facilitated. However, if there were important psychological and social influences on the patient, merely treating the biomechanical stressors and physiological impairment would be likely to have an unpredictable, possibly deleterious, effect on symptoms.

The predictability of the effects of MT increases once maladaptive psychosocial influences have been addressed.

Conversely, addressing the physiological impairments in the absence of an appreciation of the patient's psychosocial influences on perception may lead to unpredictable responses. Similarly, simply addressing the psychosocial influence on symptom perception without considering the physiological impairment of MSK dysfunction may also lead to unpredictable responses. Establishing how we accurately weigh and target the predominant barriers to recovery in our patient's profile is one of the main challenges for the future of diagnostic practice (Billis et al. 2007a,b, 2010; Foster et al. 2013; McCarthy & Cairns 2005; McCarthy et al. 2004, 2006).

Many MSK presentations suggest that a mechanically focused intervention may be the optimal strategy for treatment, for instance, when a dysfunction has a strong relationship to the positions the body is held or moved into. The quest to identify who is most suited to MT as opposed to other conservative therapies is currently being undertaken by researchers around the world (Childs et al. 2004; Cleland et al. 2010; Flynn et al. 2002; Foster et al. 2013; Fritz et al. 2007).

People have expectations of how their symptoms should respond, based on previous experience and information from social contacts, healthcare professionals and the media (Plank et al. 2021). If a person's strategies to reduce their pain have proven unsuccessful, they may seek assistance from healthcare professionals. An expectation that MT will be of benefit may prompt a consultation with a healthcare practitioner (an active adaptive coping style). MT is therefore more than a passive treatment which does not foster a maladaptive passive coping style in patients. It is essential that the manual therapist recognises maladaptive passive coping styles; reduces anxiety, fear of movement and catastrophising; and encourages self-efficacy. Not doing so may reduce the effectiveness of MT or even be counterproductive.

Patients tend to seek the intervention from manual therapists when their strategies for ameliorating pain and dysfunction have not met their own expectations, sometime after their painful dysfunction has first been perceived. The nervous system and therefore MSK systems are likely to have adapted physiologically to the painful afferent stimuli (DeLeo 2006; Ren & Dubner 1999). MT therefore aims to influence the higher centres of the central nervous system as well as MSK function (Gyer et al. 2019).

Mechanisms of pain relief through manual therapy

The underlying hypothesis of MT is that the specific position, direction and quality with which movements are performed and learned have a superior effect on pain and dysfunction, compared with movement in a random fashion. If a position or movement is strongly related to the patient's pain and dysfunction, then interventions are chosen which utilise these features. Specific assessment and specific correction of movement dysfunction are therefore paramount.

In conjunction with a detailed examination of the specific biomechanical and physiological impairments of an MSK dysfunction, the manual therapist has several ways to alter the perception of pain (Table 14.1).

TABLE 14.1 Theoretical processes in pain relief with manual therapy

Selective afferent stimulation

Selective stimulation of fast adapting afferents (light touch and stroking) of the skin

Selective stimulation of slow adapting skin afferents (deep pressure/pain sensation)

Stimulation of high-threshold (type III) joint and muscle afferents (stretch/pain sensation)

Stimulation of C-tactile afferents with slow, light, stroking touch

Reduced local tissue afferent barrage

Reduced tonic activity in muscle, skin and joint afferents following 'lengthening' manoeuvres

Mechanical perturbation inducing fibroblastic tissue healing

Down-regulation of local inflammatory cytokines

Gate control

Stimulation of Aβ fibres (mechanoreceptive afferent information) modulates perception of Aδ and C fibre afferent information

Descending pain inhibition

Mechanoreceptive afferent (type III) stimulation of PAG–RVM centres inhibits perception of nociceptive pain

---

TABLE 14.1 Theoretical processes in pain relief with manual therapy—*cont'd*

Inhibition of dorsal horn sensitisation in response to type III afferent information (deep stretch, pressure stimulus)

Distant noxious inhibitory control
Pain evoked remotely reduces the relative attention to pre-existing pain

Pleasure/pain tactile mechanisms
Pleasant touch causes phasic release of dopamine to reduce attention to pain and increase motivation to repeat the movement that induced the hypoalgesic reward

Deep pressure/stretch and tactile pain stimulate pleasure centres in the orbitofrontal cortex that reduce the perception of pain

Somatosensory influences
Localisation

Tactile discrimination and acuity

Ablation of painful movement memories
Reduction in pain perception facilitates the relearning of pain-free memories

Learning of pain-free movement memories
Correction of physiological impairment allows fearless, pain-free movement that facilitates the relearning of pain-free memories of movement

Distraction
Reduction in attention on the painful function to focus on other afferent information (stretch, pleasant touch, control with reward for mastery)

Production of deep, pressure, stretching tactile pain averts attention from distressing pain

Habituation
Plastic changes in the central nervous system, in response to repetition of pain-free stimulus, reduce the sensitivity to nociceptive afferents in a process of long-term potentiation

Nonspecific effects
Placebo effects negatively influenced by anxiety, low mood, fear of pain and movement and positively influenced by expectation, conditioning and positive communication

---

PAG, Periaqueductal grey; *RVM,* rostral ventromedial medulla.

The somatosensory system

Skin, joints and muscles are supplied with receptors to allow the interpretation of movement and nociceptive stimuli (Fig. 14.1). Skin mechanoreceptors can be categorised based on the type of stimulation to which the receptor responds, the speed with which they adapt to stimulus and the size of their field of reception (Box 14.1). The neuroanatomy of skin, the first contact receptor for tactile stimulus, allows a clear distinction between deep and superficial stimuli.

Joints and ligaments also have mechanoreceptors (Table 14.2). Type I receptors, found infrequently in ligaments, are slowly adapting receptors with a low threshold and continuous firing, even at rest. Type II receptors are dynamic with rapid adaptation and a low threshold to stimulus; thus they convey information at the beginning of joint motion. Type III receptors are also dynamic-type receptors with a high threshold and slow adaptation providing sensation at the extremes of movement. These fibres can also transmit some nociceptive stimuli at extremes of deformation (Wyke 1972). Type IV receptors are free nerve endings in the tissues and are responsible for the majority of nociceptive sensation (Michelson & Hutchins 1995). Placement of a joint towards the end of its range of motion during MT therefore influences specific skin, joint capsule and ligament receptors which are not activated in a neutral (loose-packed) position.

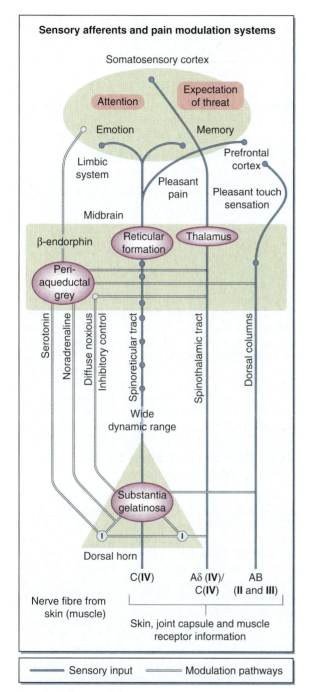

Sensory afferents and pain modulation systems

Somatosensory cortex

Attention

Expectation of threat

Emotion

Memory

Limbic system

Prefrontal cortex

β-endorphin

Pleasant pain

Pleasant touch sensation

Midbrain

Reticular formation

Thalamus

Peri-aqueductal grey

Serotonin

Noradrenaline

Diffuse noxious inhibitory control

Spinoreticular tract

Spinothalamic tract

Dorsal columns

Wide dynamic range

Substantia gelatinosa

Dorsal horn

C(**IV**)

Aδ (**IV**)/ C(**IV**)

AB (**II and III**)

Nerve fibre from skin (muscle)

Skin, joint capsule and muscle receptor information

——— Sensory input   ═══ Modulation pathways

Fig. 14.1 Diagram of the somatosensory systems.

Muscles are richly innervated with mechanoreceptors, classified as above (Mense 2003). Muscle spindles (types Ia and II) are extremely sensitive to length changes

BOX 14.1 **Mechanical cutaneous stimulation is detected by a combination of receptors**

- Meissner corpuscles (FA1): light stroking and fast vibration; fast acting, local specific stimulation.
- Pacinian corpuscles (FA2): deep, quick touch; fast and large field, thus poor spatial resolution.
- Ruffini endings (SA2): slow acting with a large receptive field; respond to slow direction-specific stretch; poor spatial resolution.
- Merkel cell neurite complexes (SA1): slow acting; better special resolution (Macefield 2005).
- Pleasant touch can activate receptors on C fibres (see 'The somatosensory system'). Thus sensations on the skin are generated by distinctly different receptors, enabling us to accurately appreciate the type, depth and direction of cutaneous stimulation.

in the muscle and have an efferent innervation (gamma motor neurons), allowing them to dynamically respond to changes in muscle length. In contrast, Golgi tendon organs have a high threshold and are therefore insensitive to small muscle length changes, but they do respond to forceful muscle contraction and extreme stretch stimulation (Mense 2003).

Aβ afferents transmitting mechanoreceptive information terminate mainly in laminae III to V, which is projected to the primary (S1) and secondary somatosensory (S2) cortex via the dorsal-medial lemniscal pathway (see Chapter 6). In addition, pleasant touch (slow, light stroking of the skin, distinct to discriminatory touch) is transmitted in unmyelinated, slow C fibres known as *C-tactile afferents* (Liu et al. 2007). This afferent information projects to the limbic system. While it does not provide discriminative information, it does facilitate the evaluation of the emotional attachment to touch (Andrew 2010). 'Valuation' of this tactile afferent information occurs predominantly in the orbitofrontal cortex, an area that processes sexual and affective components of pain/pleasure sensations (Leknes & Tracey 2008). Finally, excessive mechanical as well as chemical and thermal stimuli activate nociceptive C and Aδ fibres.

Localised sensations, such as fine touch, vibration, two-point discrimination and proprioception from the skin, muscles and joints, are transmitted from the body to the somatosensory cortex corresponding to stimulated body segments through the posterior column medial lemniscal pathway (Roudaut et al. 2012). This ascending information helps in the formation of the 'map' of the human body (homunculus) in the sensory and motor cortices. Tactile acuity deficits coincide with the disruption of body image (Louw et al. 2015), and current studies postulate a vicious cycle involving

TABLE 14.2 Mechanoreceptors in joint capsules and ligaments

Type	Morphology	Parent nerve	Physiology
I	Thinly encapsulated globular corpuscles in clusters of 3 to 6	Small, myelinated	Low-threshold, slow adapting static and dynamic
II	Thickly encapsulated corpuscles in clusters of 2 to 4	Medium, myelinated	Low-threshold, rapidly adapting dynamic
III	Thinly encapsulated fusiform corpuscles	Large, myelinated	High-threshold, slowly adapting dynamic
IV	Plexuses and free nerve endings	Very small, myelinated	High-threshold pain receptors

Reprinted from Wyke, B., 1972. Articular neurology. Physiotherapy, 58 (3), 94–99, with permission from Elsevier.

altered homunculus organisation, limited movement and increased pain (Bray & Moseley 2011; Louw et al. 2015; Luomajoki & Moseley 2011). Luomajoki & Moseley (2011) have described a significant difference of two-point discrimination threshold between participants with and without nonspecific low back pain, while Bray & Moseley (2011) have reported that patient groups with chronic low back pain have significantly lower accuracy in trunk rotation tasks compared to controlled groups.

Localisation, that is, tactile stimulus training without physical movement (Louw et al. 2015), has been shown to have a positive influence on movement, with lumbar touch and localisation training leading to reduction in the pain during flexion and an increase in active flexion range (Louw et al. 2015). The authors suggest that training to improve tactile discrimination can 'sharpen' or 'refocus' the homunculus and lead to greater certainty in movement, with concomitant increase in range (Bray & Moseley 2011; Louw et al. 2015; Luomajoki & Moseley 2011). Puentedura & Flynn (2016) have suggested that MT interventions (incorporating localised touch effects) can reduce the viscous cycle of homunculus disorganisation, movement uncertainty and concomitant pain, as evidenced by the observation that movement-based interventions, including localised passive touch (MT), reduce spinal pain and typically improve quality and range of movement. It is highly likely that the delivery of MT, which is classically considered to be a bottom-up hands-on approach, could in fact reorganise and sharpen the homunculus and improve mobility (Puentedura & Flynn 2016; Serino & Haggard 2010).

The gate control theory

The gate control theory (Melzack & Wall 1965) proposed that the information transmitted in Aβ afferents can reduce the passage of nociceptive information conveyed by Aδ and C fibres at the level of the dorsal horn. This mechanism was found to be mediated by inhibitory interneurons, which can exert a suppressing influence on the firing thresholds of postsynaptic second-order cells (Giordano 2005; also see Chapter 7).

Small-diameter afferents may be excited with stimulation of Aβ receptors (Schweinhardt et al. 2006), particularly in the presence of substance P and other sensitising chemicals (see Chapter 6). As a consequence, movement within the normal range of a joint or muscle may stimulate sensitised (previously silent) small-diameter joint nociceptors (type IV) under certain circumstances (Wright et al. 2002). Thus the gate control theory may explain some of the immediate pain-relieving effects from mechanoreceptor stimulation (Mancini et al. 2015), but it does not fully cover the pain modulation commonly observed as an effect of MT.

Hypoalgesia mediated by the central inhibition

Over the last 30 years, there has been significant investigation of the effects of MT-induced mechanoreceptive afferent barrage on the perception of nociceptive pain (Schmid et al. 2008). Several authors have demonstrated MT-induced hypoalgesia concurrent to up-regulation of noradrenergic *fight or flight* system responses. There has been a strong assertion that descending pain mechanisms associated with the noradrenergic/serotinergic systems result in immediate as well as longer lasting reduction in pain perception (Gyer et al. 2019; Lascurain-Aguirrebeña et al. 2016; Schmid et al. 2008; Sterling et al. 2001; Vicenzino et al. 1998; Wirth et al. 2019; Wright 1999).

With regard to MT-induced hypoalgesia, the periaqueductal grey (PAG) and rostroventromedial medullary (RVM) centres of the brain stem may play an important role as centres of descending pain inhibition (Close et al. 2009; Schmid et al. 2008; Sterling et al. 2001; Vicenzino et al. 1998; Wright 1999; see Chapter 6). There are distinct areas within the PAG that mediate transmission of nociceptive information. Afferent stimulation of the dorsal PAG elicits a fight or flight reaction, with sympatho-excitation leading to a modulation of pain that is effectively instantaneous (Gyer et al. 2019; Lascurain-Aguirrebeña et al. 2016; Wirth et al. 2019). The dorsal PAG mediates a noradrenergic mechanism, which specifically influences cortical perception of nociceptive pain and induces an inhibition of substance P release from the terminals of nociceptive fibres at the peripheral source of pain (Pertovaara 2006). The ventral PAG on the other hand, facilitates recuperative behaviour through an opioid/serotinergic-mediated pathway. Typically, this response is observed 20 to 45 minutes after MT treatment (Close et al. 2009; Gyer et al. 2019; Schmid et al. 2008; Sterling et al. 2001; Lascurain-Aguirrebeña et al. 2016; Wirth et al. 2019).

Descending pain inhibitory systems have been shown to be bidirectional, so they are able to inhibit or facilitate nociception in response to the importance of the stimuli (Close et al. 2009; Heinricher et al. 2009). These responses are mediated by ON cells and OFF cells in the RVM (ibid). For example, nociceptive thresholds can be raised (reducing pain perception) during feeding and micturition (via OFF cell activation) and lowered in the presence of acute inflammation (via ON cell activation) allowing attention to be focused towards the most functionally important stimulus.

High-threshold mechanoreceptive afferent input, be it from the spine (Bretischwerdt et al. 2010; George et al. 2006; Ruiz-Saez et al. 2007), peripheral joints (Slater et al. 2006; Vicenzino et al. 2001), muscles (Bretischwerdt et al. 2010) or nerves (Beneciuk et al. 2009), can result in clinically meaningful reductions in nociception (Schmid et al. 2008). This reduction in pain perception has been measured both locally to and remote from the site of MT (Bretischwerdt et al. 2010; Cleland et al. 2005).

Recent work has suggested that MT may have a greater influence on mechanical rather than thermal nociception (Beneciuk et al. 2009; George et al. 2006; Willett et al. 2010). Greater hypoalgesia has been demonstrated closer to the site of MT stimulation compared with distant sites (Perry & Green 2008; Willett et al. 2010). These effects are likely to be influenced by higher cerebral centres, as they appear to be more pronounced in the presence of the expectation that MT will be effective, while negative expectations reduce hypoalgesic effects (Bialosky et al. 2008).

The potential of MT to selectively inhibit C-fibre afferent information has been identified in recent studies measuring the effect of MT on temporal summation of nociceptive stimulation. Temporal summation can be measured in the laboratory through increases in reported pain intensity in response to repeated noxious stimulation of constant intensity at an application frequency higher than 0.3 Hz (Mendell 1966). The degree of temporal summation is thought to correlate to the extent of dorsal horn wind-up (see Chapter 6). One study investigated the effect of spinal MT on asymptomatic subjects' temporal summation to repeated thermal stimulus (George et al. 2006), while the other investigated the effect of upper limb neural tension testing (see Elvey 1997 for details of this test) on afferent nociception and temporal summation (Bialosky et al. 2009). Both studies demonstrated a greater inhibition of temporal summation with MT than with the comparative interventions (sham MT, extension exercise or exercise bicycle), suggesting that MT may reduce dorsal horn sensitisation. Aδ fibre activity appeared to be influenced less than C fibre activity, which may be consistent with the more acute protective role of Aδ fibres. This is consistent with observations that simple deep pressure sensations mediated by Aδ fibres appear to have less limbic and cortical moderation en route to the somatosensory cortex, perhaps reflecting limited need for interpretation of its value (Rolls et al. 1983).

Interestingly, previous work has demonstrated that a greater magnitude of temporal summation is evoked by frequent stimulation of deep tissue nociceptors than by stimulating receptors in the skin (Nie et al. 2005). The fact that these recent studies have suggested that brief MT stimuli to the deeper tissues can reduce the magnitude of subsequent temporal summation suggests that certain sensory stimuli may be more effective than others in evoking changes in pain.

Diffuse noxious inhibitory control

Diffuse noxious inhibitory control (DNIC), the inhibition of activity in wide-dynamic range (WDR) spinal neurons triggered by a separate, spatially distant noxious stimulus, is considered to be the underlying mechanism of counter-irritation theory, where 'one pain masks another' (Jinks et al. 2003; see Chapter 6). DNIC is thought to provide a surrounding inhibition that heightens the contrast in importance between the noxious stimulation and the pre-existing pain (Pinto-Ribeiro et al. 2008).

MT techniques may produce mild pain from deep pressure and stretch during application, stimulating type III and IV fibres. A recent review of minor adverse reactions to MT treatment reveals that approximately 50% of patients report some transient treatment soreness during or posttreatment (Carnes et al. 2010). Manual therapists may therefore have to accept that some techniques will induce and perhaps require a little 'therapeutic pain'. It is likely that the infliction of mild pain, in the context of a therapeutic setting, is modulated by the patient's pain modulation systems without being associated with the degree of distress or sensitisation of a traumatising injury.

The pleasure and pain of manual therapy

There has been recent interest in human processing of painful and pleasant afferent information and the beginnings of an understanding of their interactions. Avoiding pain and seeking pleasure are key concepts for survival (Leknes & Tracey 2008). Relief from severe pain is considered more rewarding than relief when in less pain (Leknes & Tracey 2008). In Fields' motivation-decision model of pain, any activity that reduces a threat to survival exerts an antinociceptive influence (Fields 2007). In this model, a long distance runner may perceive pain during the race as being less important than the reward of completing/winning, leading to down-regulation of their pain during the race. Similarly, while the tactile stretch and pressure of some MT techniques may induce some pain, the post-treatment reward will be perceived by the brain as more important than the treatment discomfort. Thus post-MT hypoalgesia might be viewed as the reward following the uncomfortable process of generating it.

Induced hypoalgesia, particularly if the magnitude of relief is unexpectedly high, also evoked a phasic release of the neurotransmitter dopamine (Schultz 2002). Phasic bursts of dopamine release increase the motivation to seek the reward that has just precipitated its release, but not the degree of enjoyment of the reward (Leknes & Tracey 2008). However, dopamine release does produce corresponding increases in opioid levels, which in turn enhance the enjoyment of the reward (ibid). The magnitude of the phasic dopamine response is related to unexpectedness and the size of the reward experienced (Schultz 2002). Responses to repeated constant stimuli will lead to a lowering of the level of phasic dopamine release and thus a reduction in the motivation to repeat the stimulus. Unexpectedly large pain relief will intensify the motivation to repeat the behaviour that caused the relief. Interestingly, low motivation to adopt changes in pain behaviour in chronic pain patients has been related to low tonic dopamine levels (Wood et al. 2007).

MT-induced hypoalgesia may facilitate change in patients, mediated by phasic release of dopamine in response to an unpredicted reward (reduction in pain). When responses to treatment become predictable, there is an associated reduction in dopamine-driven motivation (Schultz 2002). A change in eliciting stimulus is required to restore motivation to change (ibid). MT treatment progression typically involves changing intensity, position, direction, velocity and other features of stimulus. The impact of MT techniques on dopamine-mediated motivation to change and perception of pain may underpin the way MT's approach to progression of treatment has evolved over the years (McCarthy & Rivett 2019).

Not all MT treatment induces pain (Maitland 1966). Massage, gentle stretching, manually controlled muscle contractions and stroking of the skin are all pleasant tactile sensations. Human beings are very accurate in interpreting the emotional content of touch (Hertenstein et al. 2006), with touch sensations being interpreted in the limbic system and in multiple centres through the cortex, particularly the orbitofrontal cortex (OFC) (Rolls et al. 2003). The more affective aspects of touch (pleasant touch and distressing pain) appear to be assessed in the OFC, while stronger Aδ-mediated pressure/stretch is processed more immediately in the somatosensory cortex (Rolls et al. 2003).

The OFC is involved in the judgement of the value of reward and threat of stimuli (Schultz 2002). It is vital in motivation and learning (ibid). Light touch and slow stroking motions provide afferent information that is processed as conveying a pleasant emotional message (Ellingsen et al. 2016; Hertenstein et al. 2006). Thus pleasant tactile sensation is likely to be processed in areas of the brain that weigh up the value of the reward of MT against its current pain. In response to pleasant empathetic touch that is considered pleasurable and pain relieving, the reward includes supraspinal facilitation of the hypoalgesic descending pain mechanisms (Leknes & Tracey 2008). It is therefore credible that pleasurable MT can reduce pain by tipping the homeostatic pain balance from pain towards pleasure through limbic and cortical mediation in the brain.

Taken together, current theories suggest that there are physiological mechanisms that may explain the changes in pain perception in response to MT, whether MT stimulus is pleasant or uncomfortable (Ellingsen et al. 2016; Schmid et al. 2008). The coming years will no doubt see the development of a better understanding of these mechanisms, allowing further refinement of MT.

Manual therapy as an aid to motor control

Restoration of movement and control of movement are key objectives of MT. A recent review on the effects of spinal mobilisation on motor control and muscle function concluded that passive joint mobilisations can alter muscle function immediately. Moderate level evidence suggests that joint mobilisation causes an immediate decrease in the activation of superficial muscles during low load conditions in symptomatic individuals. This may reflect increased deep muscle recruitment and an improved motor pattern. With regard to the ability to alter maximum muscle strength, low-level evidence indicates that joint mobilisation can improve maximum muscle strength in asymptomatic individuals, but very low-level evidence suggests that this does not happen in symptomatic individuals (Pfluegler et al. 2020). Aberrant movement associated with chronic pain can be considered maladaptive, which may in itself maintain pain. It has been suggested that pain diverts attention away from processing movement performance (Price 2000; Price & Gilden 2000), and pain has been associated with reductions in proprioceptive ability (Gill & Callaghan 1998). In addition, fear of movement associated with pain has been shown to influence the recruitment, strength and endurance of paraspinal muscles (Watson et al. 1997). These findings suggest that MT treatment should aim to reduce pain and improve proprioception (Hodges 2003; Hodges et al. 2003).

By reducing pain and subsequently encouraging patients to actively move into functional positions they could not previously achieve, maladaptative movement control can be corrected. The expectation is that following MT, there is improved attention to movement performance, fear of movement is reduced and muscles are recruited and controlled more efficiently and accurately due to improved proprioception. In addition, graded exposure to previously painful movements is thought to lead to a reduction in activation of postsynaptic spinal neurons, due to habituation of presynaptic nerve calcium ion channels and the neuroplastic depression of spinal neurons (Boal & Gillette 2004). Habituation to pain has been referred to as 'pain boredom' (Gifford 2000) which may underpin the effectiveness of techniques such as repeated movements (McKenzie 1987) or oscillatory mobilisation (Maitland 1966; Robson & Gifford 2006). These approaches may stimulate the formation of fearless painless movement memories (Robson & Gifford 2006), which in turn can lead to extinction of maladaptive pain memories (Zusman 2004).

Effects of manual therapy on local tissue

Over 30 years ago, Zusman argued that stretching joints with oscillatory mobilisations reduces intraarticular pressure and lengthens joint capsules and ligaments, leading to a temporary reduction in nociceptive afferent barrage (Zusman 1986). Years later, Zusman (2010) suggested that local tissue mobilisation may facilitate fibroblastic and myofibroblastic tissue repair. He proposed that MT could provide the specific external mechanical influence needed to promote structural and biochemical events associated with optimal tissue repair and growth (Zusman 2010). Early evidence suggests that movement can induce growth hormones and either provoke inflammatory mediators with excessive loading or reduce inflammatory mediators with gentle motion (Langevin et al. 2005). Thus fascial

and ligament biomechanical and intracellular health may adapt in response to motion stimulus applied to the tissues. The time required to evoke these changes appears to be at least a few minutes and is likely to be dose respondent. (Langevin et al. 2005; Leong et al. 2011; Parravicini & Bergna 2017). Movement, such as at least 1 hour daily of cyclical motion such as walking or cycling, has been shown to provide an important mechanical stimulus for both joint capsule and cartilage nutrition, growth and apoptosis (cell death, which promotes new cell synthesis) (Leong et al. 2011).

Recent research has shown a down-regulation of proinflammatory cytokines in response to the application of MT (Teodorczyk-Injeyan et al. 2006). The investigators assessed levels of inflammatory cytokines, either in response to a single spinal manipulative thrust to a clinically dysfunctional spinal segment of the thoracic spine or a sham procedure for a control condition (venipuncture). However, the available evidence for the capacity of MT to trigger a significant systemic immune-endocrine response is mixed, so its clinical relevance remains to be established (Colombi & Testa 2019).

Nonspecific effects of specific movement/manual therapy

The magnitude of treatment effects of interventions for pain is dependent on the context in which they are provided. Every intervention involves an interaction between the patient and provider, a context which involves the social and physical environment, as well as the beliefs of patient and provider and the language that is used. Contextual mechanisms resulting from these interactions are part of the effectiveness of any intervention. This effectiveness results from engagement of complex supraspinal regions broadly studied as the mechanisms of placebo (improvement) and nocebo (worsening). Placebo is therefore a contributing mechanism through which rehabilitation interventions alter MSK pain, rather than an inert intervention. The magnitude of placebo is dependent upon factors related to negative mood (Vase et al. 2005), expectation (Pollo et al. 2001) and conditioning (Voudouris et al. 1985). Consequently, manual therapists should maximise the placebo effect within their interventions. The placebo effect is lessened with negative moods such as greater desire for pain relief (Vase et al. 2005), fear of pain (Lyby et al. 2010) and anxiety (Morton et al. 2009). Placebo-related hypoalgesia corresponds to improvements in these measures (Morton et al. 2009). Manual therapists may therefore wish to address factors related to negative effects such as fear of pain and anxiety. Positive expectation is associated with both a greater magnitude of placebo-related hypoalgesia (Vase et al. 2005) and clinical outcomes in patients presenting with MSK pain (Myers et al. 2008). Clinicians could therefore assess and even enhance patient expectation for MT interventions (within ethical limits) in order to maximise clinical outcomes. This includes providing patients with their treatment of choice, because patient preferences can have a positive influence on treatment outcome in patients with low back pain (Kalauokalani et al. 2001). Moreover, matching the 'patients' beliefs with a manipulation adds to the perception of a successful treatment (Plank et al. 2021). Allowing patient preference and beliefs to influence the treatment of choice sits within a framework of evidence-based practice (Sackett et al. 1996). 'Patients' expectations and beliefs are often related to their previous experience (Thompson & Sunol 1995), and therefore listening to patients' experience of previous treatment should influence treatment choice.

A model of the mechanisms of manual therapy

Bialosky et al. (2009, 2018) have proposed a comprehensive model which integrates the mechanisms of MT (Fig. 14.2). Briefly, the model suggests that a mechanical stimulus initiates a number of potential neurophysiological effects which produce the clinical outcomes associated with MT in the management of MSK pain.

Manual therapy case study

The clinical reasoning process underpinning the application of MT can be difficult to access and understand. The following case study of a typical MT approach to a common MSK pain syndrome may therefore be helpful. It describes a presentation, examination process

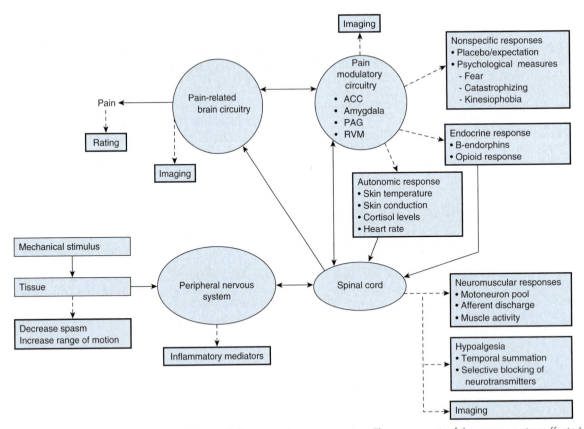

Fig. 14.2 A mechanistic model of manual therapy's influence on the nervous system. The components of the nervous system affected by manual therapy and their interactions. *ACC*, Anterior cingulate cortex; *PAG*, periaqueductal grey; *RVM*, rostroventromedial medullary. (Bialosky et al. 2009, 2018.)

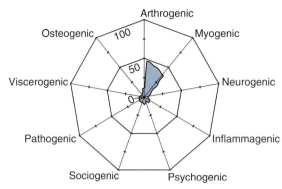

Fig. 14.3 Radar plot of problem components (%).

and treatment following a *combined movement* paradigm (McCarthy 2001, 2010). This concept was developed by Dr Brian Edwards and has been updated and developed in subsequent years (McCarthy 2010, 2019). Combined movement theory advocates the use of specific starting positions for passive mobilisation, manipulation or muscle contractions, which may be familiar from the writings of Maitland (1966).

Initial interview
Symptomology

A 29-year-old male presented with pain in the right lower cervical spine, referring to the right shoulder. The pain was not radicular in quality but severe (8/10). There was no suggestion of an upper motor neuron lesion or other red flags, no features suggestive of segmental cervical instability or shoulder derangement and no headaches. There was no history of cervical locking, catching or weakness. No significant barriers to recovery, for example, attitude to pain, pain behaviour, financial compensation, dilemmas over diagnosis, emotional problems, family history of pain or blue/black flags (Main & Williams 2002).

Relevant history

Symptoms developed over a 6-day period following a mild rear shunt, whiplash injury, 3 weeks ago.

Behaviour of symptoms

Pain was reproduced with low cervical flexion and left lateral flexion. Sitting in this position reproduced symptoms within 2 minutes. Symptoms were eased immediately by positioning the lower cervical spine in extension and right lateral flexion.

Diurnal pattern

No stiffness in the cervical spine in the morning. Neck and shoulder pain developed in the evening. Sleep was not disturbed.

Special questions

General health was good. No weight loss, dizziness, dysphagia, dysarthria or diplopia, no raised blood pressure or symptoms of cervical artery dysfunction. Radiographs of the cervical spine were normal. The patient was not taking any anticoagulants or steroid therapy and had received no benefit from antiinflammatory medication.

Clinical reasoning

Pain worsened with increased mechanical afferent stimulation of tissues and lessened with reduced stimulation. There was nothing to suggest widespread central sensitivity or a neurogenic driver to the pain. This suggested a predominantly nociceptive pain mechanism and was therefore labelled a mechanical presentation (See Fig. 14.3).

Interpretation

There is strong evidence for the hypoalgesic effect of MT on afferent nociceptive perception, so MT was appropriate as an analgesic treatment.

Physical examination
Observation

No atrophy of the cervical musculature was observed. Increased muscle activity of the right sternocleidomastoid, upper fibres of trapezius, levator scapulae and right scalenes.

Active movement

Pain reproduced earliest in range of left lateral flexion (the most painful movement is termed the *prime movement*). Pain also reproduced with flexion but further into range. Restriction was most obvious in the mid-cervical region. Proprioceptive ability was reduced slightly when testing repositioning of the head with eyes closed (Jull et al. 2007).

Passive physiological intervertebral movement

Because of the severity, the examination was undertaken in right lateral flexion and extension, minimising stimulation of nocigenic structures and establishing the position that most reduced pain and dysfunction. Right lateral

217

flexion induced greatest increase in movement and reduction in muscle tone.

Effect of trial of brief passive treatment

Treatment using right lateral flexion of the mid-cervical spine reduced the pain from the functional demonstration by 10%.

Passive accessory intervertebral movement

As before, examination was undertaken in right lateral flexion and extension to establish the movement that most reduced pain and dysfunction. Antero-posterior (AP) pressure on C5 induced greatest increase in movement and reduction in muscle tone (greater than induced by AP movement of C4 or C6).

Effect of trial of brief passive treatment

Treatment using this accessory movement reduced the pain from functional demonstration by 40%.

Muscular assessment

In right lateral flexion and extension, palpation of musculature revealed hypertonicity of deep paraspinals and the region's phasic muscles. No trigger points were detected.

Effect of trial of brief passive treatment

Palpation and length assessment of sternocleidomastoid, upper fibres of trapezius, levator scapulae and right scalenes did not alter on functional demonstration.

First treatment

Position: right lateral flexion, extension
Technique: Unilateral AP glide of C5 on C6, Grade III, 1 ×
    1 minute
Outcome: 40% reduction in pain

Clinical reasoning. This treatment was based on the greatest observed change in the patient's dysfunction. The starting position for the technique allowed the production of specific passive movement at the site of pain generation. Pain relief was rapid, and within seconds, the therapist was able to detect a reduction in paraspinal hypertonicity and a concurrent increase in compliance to passive movement. This occurred after 1 minute of mobilisation, and thus the technique was stopped to allow reassessment of the patients' demonstration of dysfunction.

Hypothetical mechanisms. In response to the stimulation of tactile C fibres with type II and III afferent fibres, modulation of nociceptive transmission occurred at spinal and supraspinal levels. Changes in excitability at the dorsal root ganglion and dorsal horn reduced release of substance P, reduced motor neuron pool activity and lessened paraspinal muscle spasm. Thus nociceptive pain drivers were reduced. Immediate and unexpectedly large improvements in pain stimulated a phasic release of dopamine, facilitating opioid release and motivating the patient to repeat the process. Threat and anxiety associated with the painful movement were reduced, producing a stress-free, fearless environment to relearn efficient motor control. Localised touch facilitated somatosensory cortical change, thus 'refocusing' the sensory homunculus, and improving proprioceptive and motor function.

Second treatment

Position: identical starting position
Technique: identical technique
Outcome: no improvement

Clinical reasoning. The previous beneficial treatment technique was repeated, but the therapist perceived less change in muscle tone and mobility.

Hypothetical mechanisms. The previous treatment had led to a reduction in local nociceptive activity already and the effect was less unexpected (reduced phasic dopamine release). Previously experienced dramatic reductions in pain may have reduced the impact of smaller reductions. A change in afferent stimulus might maintain the improvement in pain perception.

Third treatment

Position: right side flexion, flexion
Technique: unilateral PA glide of C5 on C6, Grade III, 1 ×
    1 minute
Outcome: 25% reduction in pain

Clinical reasoning. The dysfunction was less severe and so a new afferent stimulus and mechanical stretch could be introduced. This starting position induced more stretch on posterior structures than the previous technique, while the starting position avoided the patient's prime movement. The patient's prime movement was left lateral flexion, hence the progression of stretch into flexion (counterclockwise around the box) rather than left lateral flexion (clockwise around the box).

Hypothetical mechanisms. The descending inhibitory effects evoked by stimulation of the anterior tissues (unlikely to be a nociceptive source) had plateaued, so now posterior tissues received a graded exposure to stimulation. By gradually introducing an exposure to tension posterior to the spine, a process of habituation of nociceptors occurred (progressive reduction in afferent barrage and hypoalgesic adaptations in dorsal horn, spinal cord and supraspinal centres had ensued, in response to repeated exposure to submaximal stimulus of the 'trigger' nociceptors) (Boal & Gillette 2004). This change of stimulus was new to the system, so phasic dopamine was produced in higher volumes. Specific lengthening of the tissues containing the nociceptive 'trigger' had increased the resting length of the tissue and thus reduced their firing (Zusman 1986).

Fourth treatment

Position: identical starting position
Technique: identical technique
Outcome: no improvement

Clinical reasoning. As the previous treatment technique had been so beneficial, it was repeated.

Hypothetical mechanisms. Posterior structures had been desensitised maximally for the stimulus. Previous lengthening of tissues had already led to a reduction in local afferent barrage. There was a reduced element of surprise. An increase in afferent stimulus might be required to maintain the process of habituation.

Fifth treatment

Position: left lateral flexion, flexion
Technique: unilateral PA glide of C5 on C6, Grade III, 1 × 1 minute
Outcome: pain free, repositioning tests improved but still impaired

Clinical reasoning. It was necessary to progress the starting position for mobilisation into the prime combination (the position of functional pain). The technique stretched the posterior structures maximally and evoked maximal afferent barrage from mechanoreceptors stimulated to their maximum tension. A degree of nonthreatening 'stretch pain' was induced.

Interpretation. Habituation to the gradual exposure to tension reduced nociceptive pain perception. The lengthening of nocigenic tissues reduced the afferent stimulus after stretch. Movement of healing tissue had facilitated mechanosensitive tissue healing processes (Zusman 2010)

and reduced sensitivity at the dorsal horn (Boal & Gillette 2004). Stimulation of mechanoreceptive afferents inhibited nociception and the 'pleasantly uncomfortable' sensations of stretch stimulated pleasure centres in the OFC. Phasic dopamine release facilitated the desire to repeat the movement into the previously painful range of movement and facilitation of pain-free movement memories began. Motor control became easier to regain with reduced pain, while proprioceptive control improved with repetition of movement through increased control demands of movement tasks (Jull et al. 2007).

Sixth treatment

Provision of a 'mimicking' home stretching/exercise programme

Clinical reasoning. It was important to explain to the patient the mechanisms of the treatment effect and reinforce the message of the dysfunction as a simple 'mechanical fault'. Emphasising the benign mechanical aspect of the painful dysfunction reduced anxiety and fear avoidance. It was imperative that the patient was educated about the importance of a home stretching programme that mimicked the treatment. This reinforced active involvement in managing the dysfunction and maintained gains in motor control.

Interpretation. Regular movement into previously painful ranges created periods of hypoalgesia. This led to reduced fear of moving into these positions, reduced pain memories and the generation of pain-free memories of movement onto this area. Regular perturbation and stretching of tissue aided the mechanosensitive aspects of the healing and tissue remodelling process over the subsequent weeks.

Conclusion

MT is a common way of managing MSK pain that offers immediate pain relief (Wright 1995), improvements in tissue healing (Zusman 2010), reductions in anxiety and fear of movement (Gifford 2000), pleasurable and rewarding tactile stimulation (Leknes & Tracey 2008), increased motivation to replicate pain-relieving movement (Schultz 2002) and a window of opportunity to relearn pain-free movement memories (Zusman 2004) through repetition and active involvement in the rehabilitation process (Zusman 2002). MT is associated with minor adverse events such as treatment soreness, which may in fact be a component of its effect, while major adverse events are rare (Carnes et al. 2010). The clinical and cost effectiveness are considered to be acceptable to the Western society, so MT is widely recommended in the management of MSK dysfunction (NICE 2016; Savigny et al. 2009). Although MT often involves simple, specific strategies to regain normal movement, it encompasses the biopsychosocial aspects of pain and is a complex intervention. For a model of the mechanisms of MT integrating biopsychosocial interactions, see Bialosky et al. (2018). Our understanding of MT's impact on health will deepen if we accept that MT needs complex, mixed-method research designs and interpretation over the coming years.

Review questions Q

1. What is the biggest challenge for the future of diagnostic practice?
   A: Establishing how we accurately weight and target the predominant barriers to recovery in our patient's profile.
2. What do C-tactile afferents convey?
   A: Slow, light stroking of the skin, distinct to discriminatory touch.
3. What does the gate control theory propose?
   A: Information transmitted in the larger/faster Aβ afferents would impede the afferent passage of information conveyed by Aδ and C fibres at the level of the dorsal root ganglion and dorsal horn.
4. What does the PAG do?
   A: Afferent stimulation of the dorsal PAG elicits a 'fight or flight' reaction, with sympatho-excitation leading to a modulation of pain that is effectively instantaneous. The dorsal PAG mediates a nonopioid or noradrenergic mechanism.
5. What is dorsal horn wind-up and how does MT affect it?
   A: Dorsal horn wind-up is a process of dorsal horn sensitisation that results from tonic (C-fibre transmitted) nociceptive barrage and has been observed in chronic MSK pain conditions. MT selectively inhibits this process.
6. What is DNIC?
   A: Diffuse noxious inhibitory control (DNIC) describes the inhibition of activity in wide-dynamic range nociceptive spinal neurons that is triggered by a separate, spatially distant noxious stimulus.
7. What does the phasic release of dopamine, in response to MT do?
   A: Phasic bursts of dopamine release increase the motivation to seek the reward that has just precipitated its release, but not actually the degree of enjoyment of the reward. However, dopamine release does produce corresponding increases in opioid levels, which in turn enhance the enjoyment of the reward.
8. Where are judgements of reward to pleasant sensation made?
   A: Orbitofrontal cortex
9. How does pain reduce motor control?
   A: According to (Hodges (2003)), it diverts attention away from processing movement performance. Fear of movement reduces the recruitment, strength and endurance of paraspinal muscles. Pain reduces proprioceptive ability.
10. How do local tissue changes reduce pain perception?
    A: Stretching joints with oscillatory mobilisations will reduce intraarticular pressure and lengthen joint capsules and ligaments, and as a consequence, there will be a temporary reduction in nociceptive afferent barrage. MT in addition to upregulating fibroblastic and myofibroblastic activity may also induce a complimentary reduction in inflammatory chemicals within target tissues.

References

Andrew, D., 2010. Quantitative characterization of low-threshold mechanoreceptor inputs to lamina I spinoparabrachial neurons in the rat. J. Physiol. 588 (Pt 1), 117–124.

Beneciuk, J.M., Bishop, M.D., George, S.Z., 2009. Effects of upper extremity neural mobilization on thermal pain sensitivity: a sham-controlled study in asymptomatic participants. J. Orthop. Sports. Phys. Ther. 39 (6), 428–438.

Bernstein, I.A., Malik, Q., Carville, S., Ward, S., 2017. Low back pain and sciatica: summary of NICE guidance. BMJ 356, i6748.

Bialosky, J.E., Bishop, M.D., Robinson, M.E., et al., 2008. The influence of expectation on spinal manipulation induced hypoalgesia: an experimental study in normal subjects. BMC. Musculoskelet. Disord. 9, 19.

Bialosky, J.E., Bishop, M.D., Price, D.D., et al., 2009. The mechanisms of manual therapy in the treatment of musculoskeletal pain: a comprehensive model. Man. Ther. 14 (5), 531–538.

Bialosky, J.E., Beneciuk, J.M., Bishop, M.D., Coronado, R.A., Penza, C.W., Simon, C.B., et al., 2018. Unraveling the mechanisms of manual therapy: modeling an approach. J. Orthop. Sports. Phys. Ther. 48 (1), 8–18.

Billis, E.V., McCarthy, C.J., Oldham, J.A., 2007a. Subclassification of low back pain: a cross-country comparison. Eur. Spine. J. 16 (7), 865–879.

Billis, E.V., McCarthy, C.J., Stathopoulos, I., et al., 2007b. The clinical and cultural factors in classifying low back pain patients within Greece: a qualitative exploration of Greek health professionals. J. Eval. Clin. Pract. 13 (3), 337–345.

Billis, E., McCarthy, C.J., Gliatis, J., et al., 2010. Which are the most important discriminatory items for subclassifying non-specific low back pain? A Delphi study among Greek health professionals. J. Eval. Clin. Pract. 16 (3), 542–549.

Boal, R.W., Gillette, R.G., 2004. Central neuronal plasticity, low back pain and spinal manipulative therapy. J. Manip. Physiol. Ther. 27, 314–326.

Bray, H., Moseley, G.L., 2011. Disrupted working body schema of the trunk in people with back pain. Br. J. Sports. Med. 45 (3), 168–173.

Bretischwerdt, C., Rivas-Cano, L., Palomeque-del-Cerro, L., et al., 2010. Immediate effects of hamstring muscle stretching on pressure pain sensitivity and active mouth opening in healthy subjects. J. Manip. Physiol. Ther. 33 (1), 42–47.

Carnes, D., Mars, T.S., Mullinger, B., et al., 2010. Adverse events and manual therapy: a systematic review. Man. Ther. 15 (4), 355–363.

Childs, J.D., Fritz, J.M., Flynn, T.W., et al., 2004. A clinical prediction rule to identify patients with low back pain most likely to benefit from spinal manipulation: a validation study. Ann. Intern. Med. 141 (12), 920–928.

Cleland, J.A., Childs, J.D., McRae, M., et al., 2005. Immediate effects of thoracic manipulation in patients with neck pain: a randomized clinical trial. Man. Ther. 10 (2), 127–135.

Cleland, J.A., Mintken, P.E., Carpenter, K., et al., 2010. Examination of a clinical prediction rule to identify patients with neck pain likely to benefit from thoracic spine thrust manipulation and a general cervical range of motion exercise: multi-center randomized clinical trial. Phys. Ther. 90 (9), 1239–1250.

Close, L.N., Cetas, J.S., Heinricher, M.M., et al., 2009. Purinergic receptor immunoreactivity in the rostral ventromedial medulla. Neuroscience 158 (2), 915–921.

Colombi, A., Testa, M., 2019. The effects induced by spinal manipulative therapy on the immune and endocrine systems. Medicina (Kaunas). 55 (8), 448.

DeLeo, J.A., 2006. Basic science of pain. J. Bone. Joint. Surg. Am. 88 (Suppl 2), 58–62.

Dieppe, P., 2004. Complex interventions. Muscoskel. Care. 2 (3), 180–186.

Ellingsen, D.-M., Leknes, S., Løseth, G., Wessberg, J., Olausson, H., 2016. The neurobiology shaping affective touch: expectation, motivation, and meaning in the multisensory context. Front. Psychol. 6, 1986.

Elvey, R.L., 1997. Physical evaluation of the peripheral nervous system in disorders of pain and dysfunction. J. Hand. Ther. 10 (2), 122–129.

Fields, H.L., 2007. Understanding how opioids contribute to reward and analgesia. Reg. Anesth. Pain. Med. 32 (3), 242–246.

Flynn, T., Fritz, J., Whitman, J., et al., 2002. A clinical prediction rule for classifying patients with low back pain who demonstrate short-term improvement with spinal manipulation. Spine 27 (24), 2835–2843.

Foster, N.E., Hill, J.C., O'Sullivan, P., Hancock, M., 2013. Stratified models of care. Best. Pract. Res. Clin. Rheumatol. 27 (5), 649–661.

Fredin, K., Lorås, H., 2017. Manual therapy, exercise therapy or combined treatment in the management of adult neck pain - a systematic review and meta-analysis. Musculoskelet Sci. Pract. 62–71.

Fritz, J.M., Lindsay, W., Matheson, J.W., et al., 2007. Is there a subgroup of patients with low back pain likely to benefit from mechanical traction? Results of a randomized clinical trial and subgrouping analysis. Spine 32 (26), E793–E800.

George, S.Z., Bishop, M.D., Bialosky, J.E., et al., 2006. Immediate effects of spinal manipulation on thermal pain sensitivity: an experimental study. BMC. Musculoskelet. Disord. 7, 68.

George, S.Z., Zeppieri, G., 2009. Physical therapy utilization of graded exposure for patients with low back pain. J. Orthop. Sports. Phys. Ther. 39 (7), 496–505.

Gifford, L., 2000. The patient in front of us: from genes to environment. In: Gifford, L. (Ed.), Biopsychosocial Assessment and Management. Relationships and Pain, Topical Issues in Pain. CNS Press.

Gill, K.P., Callaghan, M.J., 1998. The measurement of lumbar proprioception in individuals with and without low back pain. Spine 23 (3), 371–377.

Giordano, J., 2005. The neurobiology of nociceptive and anti-nociceptive systems. Pain. Physician. 8 (3), 277–290.

Gyer, G., Michael, J., Inklebarger, J., Tedla, J.S., 2019. Spinal manipulation therapy: is it all about the brain? A current review of the neurophysiological effects of manipulation. J. Integr. Med. 17 (5), 328–337.

Heinricher, M.M., Tavares, I., Leith, J.L., et al., 2009. Descending control of nociception: specificity, recruitment and plasticity. Brain. Res. Rev. 60 (1), 214–225.

Hertenstein, M.J., Keltner, D., App, B., et al., 2006. Touch communicates distinct emotions. Emotion 6 (3), 528–533.

Hodges, P.W., 2003. Core stability exercise in chronic low back pain. Orthop. Clin. North. Am. 34 (2), 245–254.

Hodges, P.W., Moseley, G.L., Gabrielsson, A., et al., 2003. Experimental muscle pain changes feedforward postural responses of the trunk muscles. Exp. Brain. Res. 151 (2), 262–271.

Hoving, J.L., de Vet, H.C., Koes, B.W., et al., 2006. Manual therapy, physical therapy, or continued care by the general practitioner for patients with neck pain: long-term results from a pragmatic randomized clinical trial. Clin. J. Pain. 22 (4), 370–377.

Jinks, S.L., Martin, J.T., Carstens, E., et al., 2003. Peri-MAC depression of a nociceptive withdrawal reflex is accompanied by reduced dorsal horn activity with halothane but not isoflurane. Anesthesiology 98 (5), 1128–1138.

Jull, G., Falla, D., Treleaven, J., et al., 2007. Retraining cervical joint position sense: the effect of two exercise regimes. J. Orthop. Res. 25 (3), 404–412.

Kalauokalani, D., Cherkin, D., Sherman, K., et al., 2001. Lessons from a trial of acupuncture and massage for low back pain. Spine 26, 1418–1424.

Langevin, H.M., Bouffard, N.A., Badger, G.J., Iatridis, J.C., Howe, A.K., 2005. Dynamic fibroblast cytoskeletal response to subcutaneous tissue stretch ex vivo and in vivo. Am. J. Physiol. Cell. Physiol. 288 (3), C747–C756.

Lascurain-Aguirrebeña, I., Newham, D., Critchley, D.J., 2016. Mechanism of action of spinal mobilizations: a systematic review. Spine 41 (2), 159–172.

Leknes, S., Tracey, I., 2008. A common neurobiology for pain and pleasure. Nat. Rev. Neurosci. 9 (4), 314–320.

Leong, D.J., Hardin, J.A., Cobelli, N.J., Sun, H.B., 2011. Mechano-transduction and cartilage integrity. Ann. N. Y. Acad. Sci. 1240, 32–37.

Liu, Q., Vrontou, S., Rice, F.L., et al., 2007. Molecular genetic visualization of a rare subset of unmyelinated sensory neurons that may detect gentle touch. Nat. Neurosci. 10 (8), 946–948.

Louw, A., Farrell, K., Wettach, L., Uhl, J., Majkowski, K., Wedling, M., 2015. Immediate effects of sensory discrimination for chronic low back pain: a case series. N. Z. J. Physiother. 43 (2), 58–63.

Luomajoki, H., Moseley, G.L., 2011. Tactile acuity and lumbopelvic motor control in patients with back pain and healthy controls. Br. J. Sports. Med. 45 (5), 437–440.

Lyby, P.S., Aslaksen, P.M., Flaten, M.A., 2010. Is fear of pain related to placebo analgesia? J. Psychosom. Res. 68, 369–377.

Macefield, V.G., 2005. Physiological characteristics of low-threshold mechanoreceptors in joints, muscle and skin in human subjects. Clin. Exp. Pharmacol. Physiol. 32 (1–2), 135–144.

Main, C.J., Williams, A., 2002. Musculoskeletal pain. BMJ 325 (7363), 534–537.

Maitland, G.D., 1966. Manipulation–mobilisation. Physiotherapy 52 (11), 382–385.

Mancini, F., Beaumont, A.L., Hu, L., Haggard, P., Iannetti, G.D.D., 2015. Touch inhibits subcortical and cortical nociceptive responses. Pain 156 (10), 1936–1944.

Mattick, A., Wyatt, J.P., 2000. From Hippocrates to the Eskimo – a history of techniques used to reduce anterior dislocation of the shoulder. J. R. Coll. Surg. Edinb. 45 (5), 312–316.

McCarthy, C.J., 2001. Spinal manipulative thrust technique using combined movement theory. Man. Ther. 6 (4), 197–204.

McCarthy, C.J., 2010. Combined Movement Theory: A Rational Approach to Mobilisation and Manipulation of the Vertebral Column. Elsevier, Oxford.

McCarthy, C.J., Cairns, M.C., 2005. Why is the recent research regarding non-specific pain so non-specific? Man. Ther. 10 (4), 239–241.

McCarthy, C.J., Arnall, F.A., Strimpakos, N., et al., 2004. The bio-psycho-social classification of non- specific low back pain: a systematic review. Phys. Ther. Rev. 9, 17–30.

McCarthy, C.J., Rushton, A., Billis, V., et al., 2006. Development of a clinical examination in non-specific low back pain: a Delphi technique. J. Rehabil. Med. 38 (4), 263–267.

McCarthy, C., Rivett, D., 2019. Thoracic spine pain in a soccer player: a combined movement theory approach. In: Jones, M., Rivett, D. (Eds.), Clinical Reasoning in Musculoskeletal Practice, second ed. Elsevier. Chapter 24.

McKenzie, R., 1987. Low back pain. N. Z. Med. J. 100 (827), 428–429.

Melzack, R., Wall, P.D., 1965. Pain mechanisms: a new theory. Science 150 (699), 971–979.

Mendell, L.M., 1966. Physiological properties of unmyelinated fiber projection to the spinal cord. Exp. Neurol. 16 (3), 316–332.

Mense, S., 2003. The pathogenesis of muscle pain. Curr. Pain. Headache. Rep. 7 (6), 419–425.

Michelson, J.D., Hutchins, C., 1995. Mechanoreceptors in human ankle ligaments. J. Bone. Joint. Surg. Br. 77 (2), 219–224.

Morton, D.L., Watson, A., El-Deredy, W., Jones, A.K., 2009. Reproducibility of placebo analgesia: effect of dispositional optimism. Pain 146, 194–198.

Myers, S.S., Phillips, R.S., Davis, R.B., Cherkin, D.C., Legedza, A., Kaptchuk, T.J., et al., 2008. Patient expectations as predictors of outcome in patients with acute low back pain. J. Gen. Intern. Med. 23, 148–153.

NICE, 2016. Low Back Pain and Sciatica in over 16s. NG59. National Institute for Health and Care Excellence, London. Available from https://www.nice.org.uk/guidance/ng59.

Nie, H., Rendt-Nielsen, L., Andersen, H., et al., 2005. Temporal summation of pain evoked by mechanical stimulation in deep and superficial tissue. J. Pain. 6 (6), 348–355.

Olausson, H., Lamarre, Y., Backlund, H., et al., 2002. Unmyelinated tactile afferents signal touch and project to insular cortex. Nat. Neurosci. 5 (9), 900–904.

Paige, N.M., Miake-Lye, I.M., Booth, M.S., Beroes, J.M., Mardian, A.S., Dougherty, P., et al., 2017. Association of spinal manipulative therapy with clinical benefit and harm for acute low back pain: systematic review and meta-analysis. J. Am. Med. Assoc. 317 (14), 1451–1460.

Parravicini, G., Bergna, A., 2017. Biological effects of direct and indirect manipulation of the fascial system. Narrative review. J. Bodyw. Mov. Ther. 21 (2), 435–445.

Perry, J., Green, A., 2008. An investigation into the effects of a unilaterally applied lumbar mobilisation technique on peripheral sympathetic nervous system activity in the lower limbs. Man. Ther. 13 (6), 492–499.

Pertovaara, A., 2006. Noradrenergic pain modulation. Prog. Neurobiol. 80 (2), 53–83.

Pfluegler, G., Kasper, J., Luedtke, K., 2020. The immediate effects of passive joint mobilisation on local muscle function. A systematic review of the literature. Musculoskelet. Sci. Pract. 45, 102106.

Pincus, T., Morley, S., 2001. Cognitive-processing bias in chronic pain: a review and integration. Psychol. Bull. 127 (5), 599–617.

Pinto-Ribeiro, F., Ansah, O.B., Almeida, A., et al., 2008. Influence of arthritis on descending modulation of nociception from the paraventricular nucleus of the hypothalamus. Brain. Res. 1197, 63–75.

Plank, A., Rushton, A., Ping, Y., Mei, R., Falla, D., Heneghan, N.R., 2021. Exploring expectations and perceptions of different manual therapy techniques in chronic low back pain: a qualitative study. BMC. Musculoskelet. Disord. 22 (1), 444.

Pollo, A., Amanzio, M., Arslanian, A., Casadio, C., Maggi, G., Benedetti, F., 2001. Response expectancies in placebo analgesia and their clinical relevance. Pain 93, 77–84.

Price, D.D., 2000. Psychological and neural mechanisms of the affective dimension of pain. Science 288 (5472), 1769–1772.

Price, C.M., Gilden, D.L., 2000. Representations of motion and direction. J. Exp. Psychol. Hum. Percept. Perform. 26 (1), 18–30.

Puentedura, E.J., Flynn, T., 2016. Combining manual therapy with pain neuroscience education in the treatment of chronic low back pain: a narrative review of the literature. Physiother. Theory. Pract. 32 (5), 408–414.

Qaseem, A., Wilt, T.J., McLean, R.M., Forciea, M.A., 2017. Noninvasive treatments for acute, subacute, and chronic low back pain: a clinical practice guideline from the American College of Physicians. Ann. Intern. Med. 166 (7), 514–530.

Ren, K., Dubner, R., 1999. Central nervous system plasticity and persistent pain. J. Orofac. Pain. 13 (3), 155–163.

Robson, S., Gifford, L., 2006. Manual therapy in the 21st century. In: Gifford, L. (Ed.), Topical Issues in Pain: Treatment Communication Return to Work Cognitive Behavioural Pathophysiology. CNS Press.

Rolls, E.T., Rolls, B.J., Rowe, E.A., 1983. Sensory-specific and motivation-specific satiety for the sight and taste of food and water in man. Physiol. Behav. 30 (2), 185–192.

Rolls, E.T., O'Doherty, J., Kringelbach, M.L., et al., 2003. Representations of pleasant and painful touch in the human orbitofrontal and cingulate cortices. Cereb. Cortex. 13 (3), 308–317.

Roudaut, Y., Lonigro, A., Coste, B., Hao, J., Delmas, P., Crest, M., 2012. Touch sense: functional organization and molecular determinants of mechanosensitive receptors. Channels 6 (4), 234–245.

Ruiz-Saez, M., Fernandez-de-las-Penas, C., Blanco, C.R., et al., 2007. Changes in pressure pain sensitivity in latent myofascial trigger points in the upper trapezius muscle after a cervical spine manipulation in pain-free subjects. J. Manip. Physiol. Ther. 30 (8), 578–583.

Sackett, D., Rosenberg, W., Gray, J., 1996. Evidence based medicine: what it is and what it isn't – it's about integrating clinical expertise and best external evidence. Br. Med. J. 312, 71–72.

Savigny, P., Watson, P., Underwood, M., 2009. Early management of persistent non-specific low back pain: summary of NICE guidance. BMJ 338, b1805.

Schmid, A., Brunner, F., Wright, A., et al., 2008. Paradigm shift in manual therapy? Evidence for a central nervous system component in the response to passive cervical joint mobilisation. Man. Ther. 13 (5), 387–396.

Schultz, W., 2002. Getting formal with dopamine and reward. Neuron 36 (2), 241–263.

Schweinhardt, P., Glynn, C., Brooks, J., et al., 2006. An fMRI study of cerebral processing of brush-evoked allodynia in neuropathic pain patients. Neuroimage 32 (1), 256–265.

Serino, A., Haggard, P., 2010. Touch and the body. Neurosci. Biobehav. Rev. 34 (2), 224–236.

Slater, H., Rendt-Nielsen, L., Wright, A., et al., 2006. Effects of a manual therapy technique in experimental lateral epicondylalgia. Man. Ther. 11 (2), 107–117.

Sterling, M., Jull, G., Wright, A., 2001. Cervical mobilisation: concurrent effects on pain, sympathetic nervous system activity and motor activity. Man. Ther. 6 (2), 72–81.

Teodorczyk-Injeyan, J.A., Injeyan, H.S., Ruegg, R., 2006. Spinal manipulative therapy reduces inflammatory cytokines but not substance P production in normal subjects. J. Manip. Physiol. Ther. 29 (1), 14–21.

Thompson, A., Sunol, R., 1995. Expectations as determinants of patient satisfaction: concepts, theory and evidence. Int. J. Qual. Health. Care. 7, 127–141.

UK, B.E.A.M., 2004a. United Kingdom back pain exercise and manipulation (UK BEAM) randomised trial: effectiveness of physical treatments for back pain in primary care. BMJ 329 (7479), 1377.

UK, B.E.A.M., 2004b. United Kingdom back pain exercise and manipulation (UK BEAM) randomised trial: cost effectiveness of physical treatments for back pain in primary care. BMJ 329 (7479), 1381.

Vase, L., Robinson, M.E., Verne, G.N., Price, D.D., 2005. Increased placebo analgesia over time in irritable bowel syndrome (IBS) patients is associated with desire and expectation but not endogenous opioid mechanisms. Pain 115, 338–347.

Vicenzino, B., Collins, D., Benson, H., et al., 1998. An investigation of the interrelationship between manipulative therapy-induced hypoalgesia and sympathoexcitation. J. Manip. Physiol. Ther. 21 (7), 448–453.

Vicenzino, B., Paungmali, A., Buratowski, S., et al., 2001. Specific manipulative therapy treatment for chronic lateral epicondylalgia produces uniquely characteristic hypoalgesia. Man. Ther. 6 (4), 205–212.

Voudouris, N.J., Peck, C.L., Coleman, G., 1985. Conditioned placebo responses. J. Pers. Soc. Psychol. 48, 47–53.

Watson, P.J., Booker, C.K., Main, C.J., et al., 1997. Surface electromyography in the identification of chronic low back pain patients: the development of the flexion relaxation ratio. Clin. Biomech. 12 (3), 165–171.

Willett, E., Hebron, C., Krouwel, O., 2010. The initial effects of different rates of lumbar mobilisations on pressure pain thresholds in asymptomatic subjects. Man. Ther. 15 (2), 173–178.

Wirth, B., Gassner, A., de Bruin, E.D., Axén, I., Swanenburg, J., Humphreys, B.K., et al., 2019. Neurophysiological effects of high velocity and low amplitude spinal manipulation in symptomatic and asymptomatic humans: a systematic literature review. Spine 44 (15), E914–E926 1.

Wood, P.B., Schweinhardt, P., Jaeger, E., et al., 2007. Fibromyalgia patients show an abnormal dopamine response to pain. Eur. J. Neurosci. 25 (12), 3576–3582.

Wright, A., 1995. Hypoalgesia post-manipulative therapy: a review of a potential neurophysiological mechanism. Man. Ther. 1 (1), 11–16.

Wright, A., 1999. Recent concepts in the neurophysiology of pain. Man. Ther. 4 (4), 196–202.

Wright, A., Graven-Nielsen, T., Davies, I.I., et al., 2002. Temporal summation of pain from skin, muscle and joint following nociceptive ultrasonic stimulation in humans. Exp. Brain. Res. 144 (4), 475–482.

Wyke, B., 1972. Articular neurology – a review. Physiotherapy 58 (3), 94–99.

Zusman, M., 1986. Spinal manipulative therapy: review of some proposed mechanisms and a new hypothesis. Aus. J. Physiotherapy. 32 (2), 89–99.

Zusman, M., 2002. Forebrain-mediated sensitization of central pain pathways: 'non-specific' pain and a new image for MT. Man. Ther. 7 (2), 80–88.

Zusman, M., 2004. Mechanisms of musculoskeletal physiotherapy. Phys. Ther. Rev. 9, 39–49.

Zusman, M., 2005. Cognitive-behavioural components of musculoskeletal physiotherapy: the role of control. Phys. Ther. Rev. 10, 89–98.

Zusman, M., 2010. There's something about passive movement. Med. Hypotheses. 75 (1), 106–110.

Chapter | 15 |

Pain pharmacology and the pharmacological management of pain

Maree T. Smith and Arjun Muralidharan

LEARNING OBJECTIVES

After reading this chapter, readers will be able to:
- Understand the goals for the pharmacological treatment of clinical pain.
- Understand the various ways that pain may be classified.
- Gain insight on various mechanisms that contribute to the pathobiology of peripheral and central sensitisation that underpin various types of chronic pain.
- Understand the goals for the pharmacological treatment of pain.
- Gain knowledge on the various types of analgesics and adjuvant agents used for the pharmacological management of pain.
- Gain knowledge on the efficacy and side effects of various analgesics and adjuvant agents for the pharmacological treatment of pain types and severity.
- Gain knowledge of more invasive procedures used for alleviation of severe pain.

Overview

In the general population, the sensation of pain is generally perceived in a negative connotation because of its association with physical damage to the body and its unpleasant affective quality (Apkarian 2008). This perception is reinforced by the International Association for the Study of Pain (IASP) definition of pain as 'an unpleasant sensory and emotional experience associated with, or resembling that associated with, actual or potential tissue damage' (Raja et al. 2020).

Pain detection and signalling involve a complex cascade of events. Nociceptors are free nerve endings that detect potentially damaging mechanical, electrical, thermal and chemical stimuli, resulting in the generation of action potentials (Woolf & Ma 2007). These action potentials are transmitted predominantly via first-order neurons (Aδ and C fibres) to laminae I and II of the dorsal horn of the spinal cord, from where they are relayed by second-order neurons via spinothalamic tracts to higher centres in the brain (Sherrington 1906). This nociceptive input may in turn activate descending inhibitory pathways to reduce the severity of the perceived pain (Sherrington 1906). Levels of pain reported by patients comprise nociception and interpretation of its emotional significance by the anterior cingulate cortex (Rainville et al. 1997).

It is well understood that the pathobiology of human pain encompasses a mosaic of biological and psychological phenotypes that are underpinned by multiple contributing factors (Diatchenko et al. 2006). However, despite great advances in our collective understanding of the neurobiology of chronic pain over the last three decades, with the identification of a vast array of receptors, ion channels and enzymes as potential novel drug targets, translation of

TABLE 15.1 Pain classifications and definitions

Based on duration	Based on type	Based on severity
Acute pain The IASP has defined acute pain as 'pain of recent onset and probable limited duration; it usually has an identifiable temporal and causal relationship to injury or disease' (Merskey & Bogduk 1994). Acute pain generally comprises two phases: the first phase alerts the individual to potentially dangerous stimuli and the second phase is regarded as a 'protective' mechanism characterised by 'guarding' of the injured tissue as a means of promoting healing and recovery (Merskey & Bogduk 1994). Chronic pain Chronic pain is defined as pain lasting for a long period of time. It commonly persists beyond the time of healing of an injury (Merskey & Bogduk 1994). Persistent pain is often regarded as a maladaptive response that confers no physiological advantage, such that the pain state itself has become the 'disease' requiring treatment (Cousins 2007).	Nociceptive pain Nociceptive pain is caused by ongoing activation of Aδ and C nociceptors in response to a noxious stimulation of somatic or visceral structures such as that associated with trauma, surgery or heart attack. Inflammatory pain Inflammatory pain that associated with chronic inflammation occurs in patients with arthritis, chronic visceral pain or temporomandibular joint disorders. Neuropathic pain Neuropathic pain is defined as 'pain arising as a direct consequence of a lesion or disease affecting the somatosensory system'.	1. Mild pain 2. Moderate pain 3. Severe pain Using the pain numeric rating scale (NRS), patients report their pain intensity on a 10-point scale: from 0 (no pain) to 10 (worst possible pain). On the basis of pain NRS scores, pain has been categorised as mild, moderate or severe pain with score ranges 1–3, 4–6 and 7–10, respectively (Serlin et al. 1995).

IASP, International Association for the Study of Pain.

this knowledge into new pain medicines for clinical use has been painstakingly slow. For this reason, the medications currently available for prescribing by frontline clinicians for the pharmacological treatment of pain in patients are similar to those available a decade ago.

Hence, in the following sections of this chapter, we provide a brief overview of receptors, ion channels and enzymes identified over the past three decades as potential novel targets for the development of the next generation of pain therapeutics. This is followed by a description of analgesic and adjuvant agents that are currently used in the clinical setting for the pharmacological treatment of pain.

Pain classification

Pain may be classified according to a number of different criteria, including duration (acute and chronic), type (nociceptive, inflammatory and neuropathic) and severity (mild, moderate and severe); the corresponding definitions are given in Table 15.1.

Nociceptive pain

Physiological or nociceptive pain is part of an early warning system that has evolved to instruct motor neurons of the central nervous system (CNS) to produce actions that minimise further injury after detection of physical harm (Zhuo 2007). Examples of acute nociceptive pain include

postoperative pain and pain following trauma with pain resolving as healing takes place.

Inflammatory pain

Inflammatory pain occurs in response to tissue injury and sensitisation of nociceptors by a range of proinflammatory mediators that are released at the injury site. For acute inflammatory conditions, inflammatory pain resolves once the initial tissue injury heals (Reichling & Levine 2009). However, in chronic inflammatory disorders such as rheumatoid arthritis and visceral pain conditions such as chronic pancreatitis, the pain persists while inflammation is active (Michaud et al. 2007).

Neuropathic pain

Neuropathic pain is a type of pain that occurs after injury to either peripheral nerves or the sensory pathways in the spinal cord or brain. It resembles inflammatory pain in that spontaneous pain and hypersensitivity are usually present, but the underlying disease pathology is in the nervous tissue (Meacham et al. 2017).

Put simply, acute nociceptive and inflammatory pains may be considered part of an alarm system warning of injury to limit movement that would otherwise exacerbate the injury and delay healing. By contrast, persistent neuropathic pain could be considered as having a defective

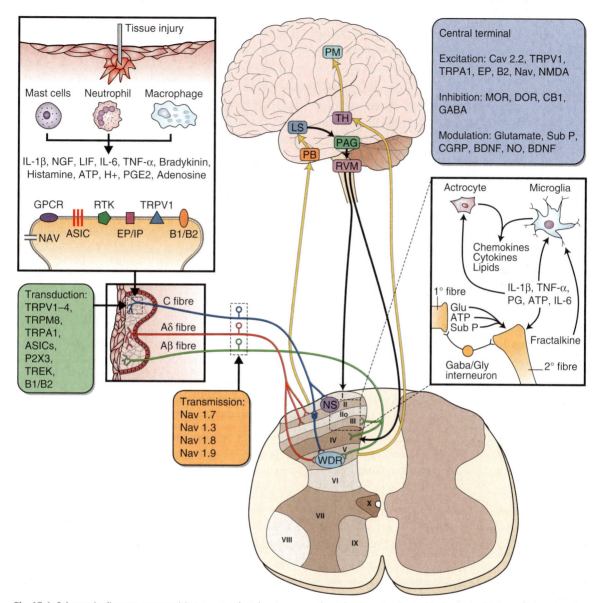

Fig 15.1 Schematic diagram summarising neuronal and non-neuronal mechanisms implicated in the pathobiology of chronic pain.

alarm system, resulting in the sending of false alerts that are nevertheless interpreted as painful signals.

Peripheral sensitisation

Following tissue and/or peripheral nerve injury, multiple chemical mediators are released, forming an 'inflammatory soup' comprising cytokines, growth factors, kinins, hydrogen ions, adenosine triphosphate (ATP), serotonin, histamine, neuropeptides and prostaglandins. This results in an inflammatory response and sensitisation of various components of the somatosensory system (Fig. 15.1) (Thacker et al. 2007). Following peripheral sensitisation, there is neuronal hyperexcitability, resulting in ectopic discharge of primary afferents and the development of so-called 'central sensitisation' in the spinal cord. The net result is that innocuous stimuli are detected as painful (allodynia) and/or there is a heightened response to painful stimuli either at the site of injury (primary hyperalgesia) or extending into the surrounding uninjured tissue (secondary hyperalgesia) (Luongo et al. 2015).

Multiple receptors and ion channels have been identified on the peripheral terminals of primary afferent nerve fibres, including receptors for serotonin (5-HT), bradykinin (B1 and B2), histamine, nerve growth factor (TrK$_A$), ATP (purinergic), epinephrine, prostaglandin E$_2$ (PGE$_2$), tumour necrosis factor-alpha (TNF-α) and interleukins (ILs) as well as sodium channels, acid-sensing ion channels (ASICs), Piezo channels and vanilloid (TRPV1) receptors (Basbaum et al. 2009; Fernandes et al. 2018; Luongo et al. 2015; Meacham et al. 2017; Zhang et al. 2019). Nociceptor hyperexcitability develops after exposure to the 'proinflammatory soup' of chemical mediators released from damaged blood vessels, nerve terminals and immune cells that accumulate at the site of injury. This in turn results in activation of multiple receptors and ion channels to induce and maintain peripheral sensitisation (Reichling & Levine 2009). Enhanced excitability of peripheral nerves with lowered activation thresholds and/or increased action potential frequency secondary to inflammation-induced peripheral sensitisation is transduced intracellularly by kinase pathways, including mitogen-activated protein kinase (MAPK) such as p38 MAPK and extracellular signal-related kinase (ERK) (Crown et al. 2008; Ji 2004), protein kinase A (PKA) (Bhave et al. 2002) and protein kinase C (PKC) (Bhave et al. 2003). Activated kinases contribute to peripheral sensitisation through phosphorylation and activation of multiple receptors and ion channels (Reichling & Levine 2009).

As neuropathic pain persists after ganglionectomy involving removal of the injured afferent soma, it is clear that maintenance of neuropathic pain is not dependent solely on changes that occur in injured afferents (Sheth et al. 2002). A hallmark of neuropathic pain is ectopic activity in damaged primary afferents underpinned by accumulation and dysregulated function of voltage-gated sodium channels after peripheral nerve injury (Costigan et al. 2009). This aberrant activity spreads rapidly to the cell bodies in the dorsal root ganglia (DRG) to generate ectopic activity in adjacent undamaged sensory afferents (ephaptic transmission), which in turn leads to an expansion of the perceived painful area (receptive field). Furthermore, sympathetic efferents have been shown to activate sensory afferents via α-adrenoceptors, with these interactions between adjacent sensory and autonomic afferents and ganglion cells providing a mechanism for the spread of ectopic discharge between nerve fibre types (Zhang & Strong 2008).

Satellite glial cells (SGCs), which form complete sheath-like structures around sensory neurones in the DRG, have been shown to respond to proinflammatory agents including ATP, nitric oxide and bradykinin (Hanani 2005). SGCs are implicated in nociceptive signalling as they express a broad range of transmitter molecules (e.g. somatostatin, NGF, BDNF, GDNF and IL-6), as well as receptors (e.g. trkA, bradykinin B2 receptors, orexin-1, somatostatin, TNF-α type-1, IL-1 and peripheral benzodiazepine receptor) and

ion channels (e.g. inwardly rectifying K$^+$ channels) (Takeda et al. 2009). Hence, SGCs are proposed to have a chemosensory role and contribute to sensory neurotransmission after tissue or peripheral nerve injury (Hanani 2005; Ohara et al. 2009; Takeda et al. 2009).

Central sensitisation

The so-called central sensitisation that develops at spinal and supraspinal levels of the CNS secondary to persistent inflammation or nerve injury is underpinned by multiple factors (Latremoliere & Woolf 2009). These include increased responsiveness of nociceptive neurons to normal or subthreshold afferent input; changes in the expression of receptors, ion channels and enzymes; changes in the properties of inhibitory interneurons; and activation of descending inhibitory as well as opposing descending facilitatory mechanisms (see Fig. 15.1) (Latremoliere & Woolf 2009; Vanegas & Schaible 2004). Furthermore, research implicates activated nonneuronal cells in the development and maintenance of the central sensitisation of neurons in the CNS (Vallejo et al. 2010; Watkins et al. 2007).

Mechanisms underpinning central sensitisation include persistent activation of the N-methyl-D-aspartate (NMDA)-nitric oxide synthase (NOS)-nitric oxide (NO) signalling cascade, upregulation of sodium channels and ASICs, as well as TRPV1, TRPM8 and α-receptors (Baron 2009; Costigan et al. 2009; Harvey & Dickenson 2008). Other mechanisms include enhanced dynorphin signalling at supraspinal levels of the CNS (Lai et al. 2001) as well as degeneration of inhibitory GABAergic interneurons in the spinal cord to cause disinhibition and increase sensitivity (Scholz et al. 2005).

Under normal homeostatic conditions, nonneuronal cells such as microglia and astrocytes have important 'house-keeper' roles to support the ongoing function and survival of neurons in the CNS. Microglia comprise 5%–10% of glia in the CNS (Watkins et al. 2007) and their major function is immune surveillance (Raivich 2005). Astrocytes comprise 40%–50% of all glial cells in the CNS to provide trophic support, energy and neurotransmitter precursors to neurons, regulation of extracellular concentrations of various ions and neurotransmitters, as well as neurite outgrowth, formation of synapses, neuronal differentiation and survival (Perea & Araque 2005). However, following activation, microglia and astrocytes release a range of pronociceptive substances, including cytokines, chemokines, neurotrophic factors, ATP, excitatory amino acids and nitric oxide, that enhance pain by increasing the excitability of nearby neurons (see Fig. 15.1) (Vallejo et al. 2010). Research also implicates a role for activated microglia and astrocytes in the development of analgesic tolerance and opioid-induced hyperalgesia that may develop following chronic morphine administration (Wang et al. 2010).

Bearing in mind the contribution of nonneuronal cells to central sensitisation, it follows that the optimal pharmacological management of chronic pain may require pharmacotherapeutic agents directed at both neuronal and nonneuronal targets at spinal and supraspinal sites of the CNS.

Nociceptive neurotransmitters and their target receptors

Factors contributing to the pathophysiology of persistent pain include proinflammatory mediators released in response to nerve injury, transcriptional changes at the level of the DRG, phenotypic changes in neural pathways, activation of glial cells in the nervous system, structural modifications including nerve sprouting and neurodegeneration of GABAergic neurons in the CNS, resulting in a hyperexcitable nervous system (Basbaum et al. 2009). Specific molecular interactions that drive the aforementioned changes in neuronal excitability may differ according to the specific injury and the consequent chemical environments that are created (Basbaum et al. 2009). The molecular interactions involve all major families of regulatory proteins, including G-protein-coupled receptors (GPCRs), ion channels, enzymes, neurotrophins, kinases, excitatory and inhibitory amino acids, thereby offering an abundance of potential analgesic targets and therapeutic opportunities (Stone & Molliver 2009). Examples include glutamate (Traynelis et al. 2010), GABAergic (Goudet et al. 2009), neurokinin (Seybold 2009), calcitonin gene–related peptide (Seybold 2009), bradykinin (Dray 1997), prostanoid (Zeilhofer 2007), purinergic (Teixeira et al. 2010), protease (Vergnolle et al. 2003), neurotrophin (Heitz et al. 2009), opioid (Wang 2019), cannabinoid (Brown 2007), cytokine (Uceyler et al. 2009), chemokine (Jiang et al. 2020) and transient receptor potential vanilloid receptors (Broad et al. 2009), as well as sodium (Alcantara Montero & Sanchez Carnerero 2021), calcium (Yaksh 2006), potassium (Busserolles et al. 2016), piezo (Zhang et al. 2019) and ASICs (Wemmie et al. 2013).

Despite the aforementioned large number of receptors and ion channels serving as potential targets for the development of a range of novel pain therapeutics, these are yet to reach the clinic. Hence, pain will continue to be managed with the currently available medications according to the principles succinctly encapsulated by the World Health Organization's three-step Analgesic Ladder (World Health Organization 1986).

Major goals for the pharmacological treatment of clinical pain

1. Increase inhibitory neurotransmission to provide analgesia by decoupling the response between an acute

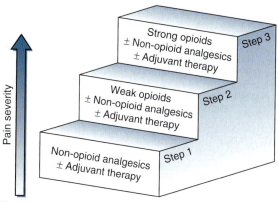

Fig 15.2 WHO three-step analgesic ladder (World Health Organization, 1986. Cancer Pain Relief. WHO, Geneva.)

noxious stimulus (e.g. postsurgery or trauma) and the painful sensation that would normally be evoked (Doubell et al. 1999).

2. Prevent development of peripheral or central sensitisation under circumstances where this would normally occur (Doubell et al. 1999).

3. Restore the normal responsiveness of the nociceptive signalling system in patients suffering from states of either hypo- or hypersensitivity so that responses to defined low- or high-intensity stimuli are perceived correctly as innocuous or painful sensations, respectively (Doubell et al. 1999).

Pharmacological treatment of pain

WHO analgesic ladder

More than three decades after its introduction in 1986 to guide the pharmacological management of chronic cancer pain, the WHO three-step analgesic ladder (Fig. 15.2) is now widely used to more broadly guide the pharmacological treatment of both acute and chronic pain.

According to step 1 of the analgesic ladder, nonopioid analgesics, including paracetamol (acetaminophen), nonsteroidal antiinflammatory drugs (NSAIDs, e.g. aspirin and ibuprofen) and coxibs (e.g. celecoxib), are recommended for the treatment of mild pain. Adjuvants (e.g. tricyclic antidepressants (TCAs), anticonvulsants and antiarrhythmics) may be co-administered if pain has a neuropathic component. When mild pain progresses to moderate pain (step 2), weak opioid analgesics such as codeine, tramadol and dextropropoxyphene are added to nonopioids with adjuvants co-administered for pain with a neuropathic component. For moderate-to-severe pain (step 3), strong opioid analgesics, including morphine,

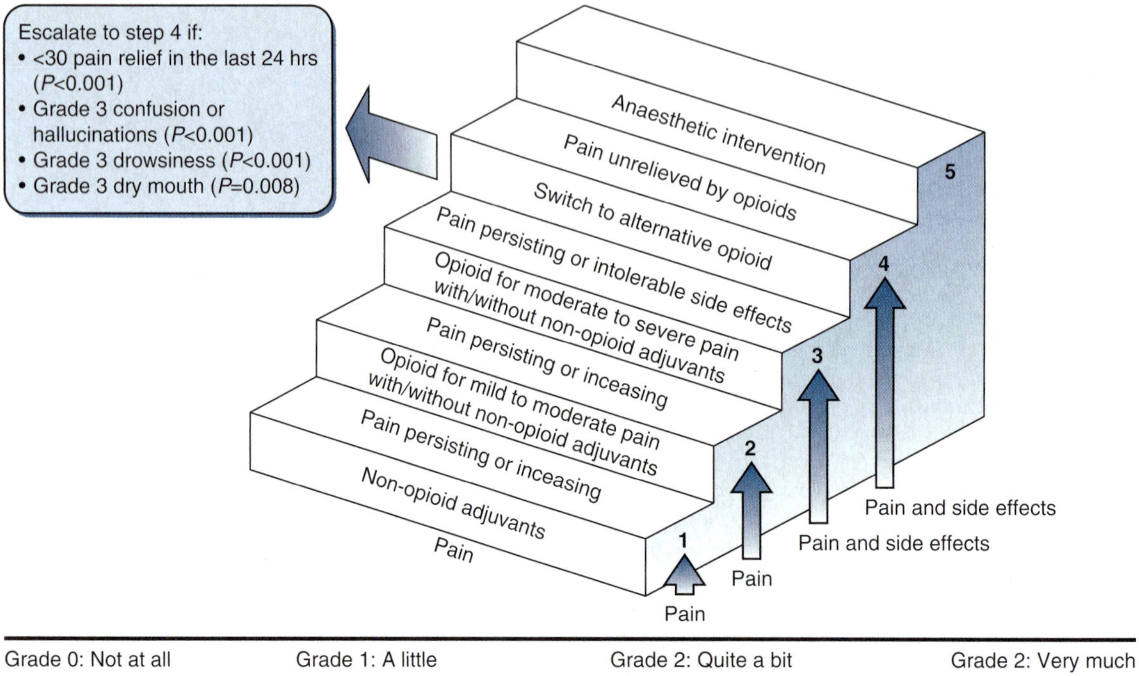

Escalate to step 4 if:
• <30 pain relief in the last 24 hrs (*P*<0.001)
• Grade 3 confusion or hallucinations (*P*<0.001)
• Grade 3 drowsiness (*P*<0.001)
• Grade 3 dry mouth (*P*=0.008)

Anaesthetic intervention
Pain unrelieved by opioids
Switch to alternative opioid
Pain persisting or intolerable side effects
Opioid for moderate to severe pain with/without non-opioid adjuvants
Pain persisting or inceasing
Opioid for mild to moderate pain with/without non-opioid adjuvants
Pain persisting or inceasing
Non-opioid adjuvants
Pain

5
4
3
2
1

Pain and side effects
Pain and side effects
Pain
Pain

Grade 0: Not at all   Grade 1: A little   Grade 2: Quite a bit   Grade 2: Very much

Fig 15.3 Overview of proposed five-step WHO analgesic and side-effect ladder. Reprinted from Riley, J., Ross, J. R., Gretton, S. K., A'hern, R., Du Bois, R., Welsh, K., Thick, M. 2007. Proposed 5-step World Health Organization analgesic and side effect ladder. *European Journal of Pain Supplements*, 1, 23-30.

oxycodone, hydromorphone, fentanyl and tapentadol, are recommended. Morphine is recommended by the WHO as the strong opioid analgesic of choice due to its worldwide availability at low cost. Strong opioid analgesics may be co-administered with nonopioids and/or adjuvants, as required (World Health Organization 1986).

The WHO guidelines also recommend that patients receive individualised dose titration to ensure an adequate dosage of the selected analgesic and/or adjuvant with drug treatment administered on a scheduled 'round the clock' basis rather than 'as required' (World Health Organization 1986). Controlled-release and sustained-release formulations of opioid analgesics allow the convenience of once or twice daily dosing, which improves patient compliance and analgesic outcomes. For the treatment of breakthrough pain, such as that which occurs during dressing changes or due to incident pain upon mobilisation, additional bolus doses of immediate-release opioid analgesic formulations may be administered on an 'as-required' basis.

While the oral dosing route is preferred for most patients, it is not practical during labour or in the immediate postoperative period due to impaired gastrointestinal transit. In circumstances where more rapid pain relief is required or there is inadequate pain relief and intolerable side effects, such as severe vomiting, severe dysphagia or bowel obstruction, changing the route of administration to parenteral (e.g. intravenous (IV), subcutaneous, intramuscular), rectal, buccal, sublingual, transdermal or spinal (epidural, intrathecal) may restore adequate analgesia with tolerable adverse effects (Walsh 2005). Another strategy for restoring satisfactory analgesia with tolerable side effects involves 'opioid rotation' by switching from the first opioid to another (Walsh 2005).

Over the years, modifications to the original WHO analgesic ladder have been proposed. For example, Eisenberg et al. suggested that invasive procedures such as neurolytic blocks should be considered for patients experiencing inadequate pain relief or intolerable side effects as an adjunct or alternative to pharmacotherapy (Riley et al. 2007). In other work, Riley et al. proposed the addition of two steps to the original WHO three-step analgesic ladder (Fig. 15.3), with the fourth step recommending use of 'opioid rotation' for patients experiencing inadequate pain relief and intolerable side effects;

TABLE 15.2 Clinically available nonopioid analgesics and their dosing schedules

Drug name	Brand name	Dose/formulation available
Paracetamol (acetaminophen)	Tylenol, Panadol	325 mg, 500 mg
Oral NSAIDs (nonprescription)		
Aspirin	Bayer	325 mg
	Ecotrin	325 mg EC
Ibuprofen	Advil	200 mg
Naproxen	Aleve	220 mg
Topical agents		
Capsaicin	Qutenza	60 g tube (0.025%) 60 g tube (0.075%) Patch (8%)
Traditional NSAIDs (prescription)		
Diclofenac	Cataflam	75 mg bid
	Voltaren	50 mg bid, 100 mg ER daily
Etodolac	Lodine	400 mg bid, 400 mg tid
Ibuprofen	Motrin	400 mg tid, 800 mg tid
Indomethacin	Indocin	50 mg tid, 75 mg SR bid
Ketoprofen	Oruvail	75 mg tid, 200 mg ER daily
Meloxicam	Mobic	7.5 mg daily, 15 mg daily
Nabumetone	Relafen	1000 mg daily, 1500 mg daily
Naproxen	Anaprox	250 mg tid
	Naprelan	500 mg bid
	Naprosyn	500 mg tid
Piroxicam	Feldene	20 mg daily
COX-2 inhibitor (coxib)		
Celecoxib	Celebrex	100 mg bid, 200 mg bid, 400 mg bid

bid, Twice a day; *EC,* Enteric coated; *ER,* extended release; *NSAID,* nonsteroidal antiinflammatory drug; *SR,* sustained release; *tid,* three times a day.
Adapted from AHRQ (2009).

if opioid rotation fails, progress to a fifth step involving use of anaesthetic intervention is recommended (Riley et al. 2007). More recently, Cuomo et al. proposed a 'multimodal trolley approach', which incorporates multimodal pharmacological and other treatments applicable to various pain conditions. This 'trolley' analgesic model takes into account the pain intensity, factors affecting the pathophysiology of pain, the complexity of symptoms, the presence of comorbidities and the social context (Cuomo et al. 2019).

Analgesic agents

Pharmacotherapy with analgesic and adjuvant agents underpins the pharmacological management of pain across all age groups from neonates to older persons. An overview of currently available analgesic agents for clinical use is provided in the following sections.

Nonopioid analgesics

A summary of commonly used nonopioid analgesics and their dosing schedules is provided in Table 15.2.

Paracetamol (acetaminophen) is a nonopioid analgesic that is widely utilised for the symptomatic relief of fever, headaches and minor aches and pains (Remy et al. 2006). Paracetamol is an active ingredient in a large number of pharmaceutical preparations, including over-the-counter cold and flu products as well as prescription medicines (Munir et al. 2007). Paracetamol produces pain relief and antipyretic actions after oral administration of usual adult doses of 1 g three or four times daily but not exceeding a total daily dose of 4 g (Myers & LaPorte 2009). In contrast to NSAIDs, paracetamol does not inhibit platelet aggregation and does not damage the gastric mucosa (Munir et al. 2007; Remy et al. 2006). A systematic review concluded that single 1 g doses of paracetamol provide effective analgesia for up to 4 hours in ~50% of patients with acute postoperative pain. In addition, patients reported few, mainly mild, adverse effects whose severity and frequency were similar to those reported by patients administered placebo (Toms et al. 2008). In other work, the combination of paracetamol and an NSAID, in particular ibuprofen, was more effective in adults after major surgery than either paracetamol or NSAID alone (Martinez et al. 2017).

Although paracetamol readily crosses the blood–brain barrier, the mechanism through which it produces its analgesic and antipyretic effects is unclear. Proposed mechanisms include modulation of serotoninergic signalling, inhibition of prostaglandin synthesis and even a cannabinoid-mediated mechanism (Pickering et al. 2006; Przybyla et al. 2020; Saliba et al. 2017). The poor ability of paracetamol to inhibit COX-1 and COX-2 and its central model of action likely underpin its lack of antiinflammatory efficacy (Lee et al. 2004).

Paracetamol adverse effects

The most serious adverse effect of paracetamol is potentially fatal liver toxicity, which may occur if therapeutic doses are exceeded. Hepatotoxicity is mediated by a reactive metabolite, N-acetyl-p-benzoquinoneimine (NAPQI), which normally accounts for only 5%–8% of a therapeutic dose of paracetamol and is detoxified by conjugation with glutathione in the liver (Larson et al. 2005; Whitcomb & Block 1994). However, if the amount of NAPQI formed exceeds liver stores of glutathione, then hepatotoxicity will occur, potentially resulting in liver failure. At therapeutic doses of paracetamol (i.e. up to 4 g/day), there is no evidence that patients with glutathione depletion due to starvation or alcohol abuse are at increased risk of hepatotoxicity (Caparrotta et al. 2018; Rumack et al. 2012).

If a patient seeks medical attention soon after paracetamol overdose, activated charcoal can be used to decrease paracetamol absorption. However, the mainstay of treatment involves administration of acetylcysteine (oral or IV), a precursor for glutathione in an endeavour to increase glutathione production sufficiently to prevent liver failure (Green et al. 2013). However, if liver damage is severe, then a liver transplant will be required. In the United States alone, ~30,000 patients are hospitalised every year for paracetamol overdose, of which 17% experience hepatotoxicity (Blieden et al. 2014).

Oral NSAIDs

NSAIDs are chemically diverse compounds that have analgesic, antipyretic and antiinflammatory properties, and are among the most widely prescribed drug products globally (Dugowson & Gnanashanmugam 2006). There are multiple chemical classes of NSAIDs, including salicylates (aspirin, methyl salicylate, diflunisal), arylalkanoic acids (indomethacin, sulindac, diclofenac), the 'profens' or 2-arylpropionic acids (ibuprofen, naproxen, ketoprofen, ketorolac) and oxicams (piroxicam, meloxicam).

NSAIDs inhibit the synthesis of prostaglandins, endogenous molecules that have diverse paracrine effects, including pronociceptive signalling, as well as modulation of inflammation and temperature

regulation in the hypothalamus (Zeilhofer 2007). With the exception of aspirin, NSAIDs produce their antiinflammatory and analgesic effects by competitive inhibition of the two isoforms of the enzyme cyclooxygenase, COX-1 and COX-2, to inhibit the formation of prostaglandins and thromboxane from arachidonic acid (Vane 1971).

COX-1 is constitutively expressed in platelets, the gastrointestinal tract and the kidneys, whereas COX-2 is inducible and found in the kidneys and the CNS (Zeilhofer 2007). The desired antiinflammatory action of NSAIDs is largely due to inhibition of COX-2, whereas aspirin irreversibly acylates both COX-1 and COX-2 (Dugowson & Gnanashanmugam 2006). Although classified as mild analgesics, NSAIDs are effective for the treatment of pain involving peripheral tissue sensitisation (Burke & Fitzgerald 2006), and they have opioid-sparing effects to reduce postoperative opioid consumption, resulting in reduced opioid-related adverse events (Marret et al. 2005).

PGE_2 release in the hypothalamus is responsible for triggering an increase in body temperature during inflammation (Zeilhofer 2007) and so NSAIDs produce their antipyretic effects secondary to inhibition of PGE_2 formation in the hypothalamus. At doses as low as 30 mg/day, aspirin irreversibly inhibits COX-1-dependent formation of thromboxane A2 in platelets to inhibit platelet aggregation with an 8- to 12-day duration of action, that is, the turnover time of platelets; it is this action that underpins the cardioprotective effects of aspirin (Munir et al. 2007).

Adverse effects of NSAIDs

The most common adverse effects of NSAIDs are gastrointestinal, renal and respiratory. All NSAIDs, including coxibs, can cause or aggravate hypertension, congestive heart failure, oedema and kidney problems (McDonagh et al. 2020).

Prostaglandins, whose synthesis is catalysed by COX-1, have a cytoprotective effect in the gastric mucosa and so NSAID-induced inhibition of COX-1 may result in dyspepsia, gastric irritation, ulceration and bleeding as well as diarrhoea (McDonagh et al. 2020). Although most NSAIDs show little selectivity between COX-1 and COX-2, selectivity is seen at low doses for some agents. For example, at relatively low doses such as 7.5 mg daily, meloxicam is a preferential inhibitor of COX-2 (Munir et al. 2007).

Prostaglandins have an important role in maintaining normal glomerular perfusion and filtration rates through their vasodilatory effects on *afferent arterioles* of the *glomeruli* (McDonagh et al. 2020). In renal failure, where the kidney is trying to maintain renal perfusion pressure by elevated angiotensin II levels that constrict the afferent arteriole into the glomerulus in addition to the efferent arteriole, prostaglandins have a protective effect on the afferent arteriole (McDonagh et al. 2020). If this is blocked by NSAID administration, there is decreased renal perfusion pressure, resulting in renal toxicity (McDonagh et al. 2020).

It is important to also be aware that aspirin-exacerbated respiratory disease presenting as rhinitis and asthma occurs in ~10% of the general population and in ~21% of adults when determined by oral provocation testing (Dugowson & Gnanashanmugam 2006). Hence, NSAIDs should be avoided in patients with known aspirin sensitivity.

In terms of NSAID-induced adverse effects, it is important to recognise the following (McDonagh et al. 2020):

1. NSAIDs increase the risk of gastrointestinal bleeding at higher doses; people older than 80 years have the highest risk.
2. NSAIDs should be avoided in people receiving anticoagulant therapy.
3. Consider using paracetamol instead as it is associated with a lower risk of gastrointestinal bleeding.
4. Co-administration of the PGE_1 analogue misoprostol or proton pump inhibitors in conjunction with NSAIDs can prevent duodenal and gastric ulceration (Rostom et al. 2002).
5. Celecoxib, ibuprofen at doses of 800 mg three times a day and diclofenac (75 mg twice a day) have increased risk of myocardial infarction. Naproxen does not increase the risk of myocardial infarction even at a dose of 500 mg twice a day.

Topical NSAIDs

Topical NSAIDs are often used to treat acute musculoskeletal conditions due to the potential of this delivery route to provide pain relief while minimising the incidence of systemic adverse events (Massey et al. 2010). Clinical trials show that topical NSAIDs are effective and relatively safe for the treatment of osteoarthritic pain with fewer systemic side effects compared with oral NSAIDs (Altman et al. 2009; Barthel et al. 2009; Simon et al. 2009). In a systematic review of 47 clinical studies that compared various topical NSAIDs in a range of formulations, including sprays, gels and creams, for the treatment of acute pain relative to the corresponding placebo preparations, the number needed to treat (NNT) for clinical success (50% pain relief) was 4.5 for treatment periods in the range 6 to 14 days (Massey et al. 2010). Topical preparations of

ibuprofen, diclofenac, ketoprofen and piroxicam were of similar efficacy but indomethacin and benzydamine were not significantly better than placebo. There were very few systemic adverse events and adverse-event-related withdrawals (Massey et al. 2010). In other work by Moore and colleagues that involved analyses of 39 Cochrane reviews of randomised trials (~n = 460), they examined the analgesic efficacy of individual drug interventions for the relief of acute postoperative pain. In short, they concluded that NSAIDs were efficacious for the treatment of pain after surgery (Moore et al. 2015).

Coxibs

Coxibs are selective COX-2 inhibitors that were developed to avoid the gastric irritation of NSAIDs due to their COX-1 inhibitory effects, while retaining equivalent analgesic properties to NSAIDs (Dugowson & Gnanashanmugam 2006). In 1999, celecoxib was the first coxib to be approved for the relief of pain and inflammation in patients with osteoarthritis, rheumatoid arthritis and primary dysmenorrhoea (Patrono et al. 2001). It was quickly followed by rofecoxib, etoricoxib, valdecoxib, parecoxib and lumiracoxib (Capone et al. 2005; Cheer & Goa 2001; Fenton et al. 2004; Wittenberg et al. 2006). Coxibs are as effective as NSAIDs in the treatment of postoperative pain, osteoarthritis and chronic low back pain (Chung et al. 2013; Moore et al. 2015; Smith et al. 2016). However, chronic administration of rofecoxib and valdecoxib (longer than 12 months) significantly increased the risk of untoward cardiovascular events, resulting in withdrawal of these medications from the market (Munir et al. 2007).

Opioid analgesics

Opioid analgesics may be classified on the basis of their (1) WHO Analgesic Ladder classification as 'weak' or 'strong', (2) chemical structure or (3) pharmacodynamic profiles as agonists, partial agonists or antagonists at opioid receptors (Krenzischek et al. 2008; Trescot et al. 2008). The various opioid receptor types/subtypes, the effects transduced and their respective endogenous ligands are summarised in Table 15.3.

Strong opioid analgesics are recommended by the WHO as the drugs of choice for the management of moderate-to-severe pain, whereas weak opioid analgesics are used in patients with mild-to-moderate pain, particularly when there are contradictions for NSAID usage (Krenzischek et al. 2008). A comparison of

TABLE 15.3 Opioid receptor types, effects transduced and endogenous ligands

Opioid receptor types[a]		Effects[b]	Endogenous ligands[c]
μ, mu or MOP	μ1	Supraspinal analgesia, dependence, withdrawal, analgesic tolerance, euphoria, emesis, sedation, prolactin release, increased feeding behaviour, immune suppression, possibly pruritus	β-endorphin (nonselective) Enkephalins (nonselective) Endomorphin-1 Endomorphin-2
	μ2	Spinal analgesia, respiratory depression, decreased gastrointestinal motility, decreased growth hormone release	
δ, delta or DOP	δ1	Supraspinal analgesia, stimulates feeding, growth hormone release	Enkephalins (nonselective) β-endorphin (nonselective)
	δ2	Supraspinal and spinal analgesia	
κ, kappa or KOP	κ1	Dysphoric responses	Dynorphin A Dynorphin B α-neoendorphin
	κ2	Decreased gastrointestinal transit, sedation, feeding behaviour	
	κ3	Supraspinal analgesia	
NOP		Analgesia and morphine tolerance	Nociception/orphanin FQ (N/OFQ)

[a]Names per current NC-IUPHAR recommended nomenclature.
[b]Adapted from Maher & Chaiyakul (2003).
[c]Adapted from International Union of Basic and Clinical Pharmacology (IUPHAR) database.

equianalgesic doses of clinically utilised opioid analgesics is shown in Table 15.4 and common starting doses for a range of orally administered opioids are listed in Table 15.5.

Apart from pain relief, opioid analgesics produce a range of adverse effects, including nausea, vomiting, sedation, pruritus, respiratory depression, constipation, thermoregulatory effects, immunomodulation, tolerance, physical dependence and addiction liability (Zollner & Stein 2007). Although it is widely believed that the analgesic and other effects produced by opioid analgesics are evoked by activation of the μ-opioid (MOP) receptor, it is widely appreciated by frontline clinicians that there are intraindividual between-opioid differences in terms of both analgesic and tolerability profiles (Smith 2008). However, the precise mechanistic basis underpinning these observations is poorly understood at present.

Guidelines recommended by The Centers for Disease Control and Prevention (CDC) (Dowell et al. 2016) for prescribing opioids for chronic pain (outside of active cancer, palliative and end-of-life care) include:

1. Before starting opioid therapy, clinicians should establish treatment goals with all patients, including realistic goals for pain and function, and discuss the known

TABLE 15.4 Total daily oral morphine equivalent conversion table (The Australian and New Zealand College of Anaesthetists 2021)

Opioid analgesic	CONVERSION FACTOR	
	Oral	IV
Pethidine	0.125	0.4
Hydromorphone	5	15
Oxycodone	1.5	3
Buprenorphine	40	—
Codeine	0.13	0.25
Dextropropoxyphene	0.1	—
Morphine	1	3
Tramadol	0.2	—
Tapentadol	0.3	—
Fentanyl	—	0.2
Sufentanil	—	2

IV, Intravenous.

TABLE 15.5 Starting doses of selected opioids (Argoff & Silvershein 2009)

Opioid	ORAL ADMINISTRATION			Plasma half-life (h)
	Dose	Frequency (h)	Duration of effect (h)	
Codeine	15–60 mg	3–6	4–6	3
Fentanyl	100–200 μg	6[a]	0.5–1 (IV), 72 (TD), 2–4 (TM)	3.7
Hydrocodone	2.5–10 mg	3–6	4–8	2.5–4
Hydromorphone	2–4 mg	3–4	4–5	2–3
Levorphanol	2–4 mg	6–8	6–8	12–16
Methadone	5–10 mg	6–8	4–6	24
Morphine	15–30 mg (IR)	3–4 (IR)	3–6	2–3.5
Oxycodone	10 mg (CR), 5–10 mg (IR)	12 (CR), 3–6 (IR)	8–12 (CR), 3–4 (IR)	2.5–3
Oxymorphone	10 mg (IR), 5–10 mg (ER)	4–6 (IR), 12 (ER)	3–6	7–9.5
Propoxyphene	65–100 mg	4	4–6	6–12
Tramadol	50–100 mg (IR), 100 mg (ER)	4–6 (IR), 24 (ER)	4–6 (IR), 24 (ER)	5–7

[a]Not more than four doses per day.
CR, Controlled-release; *ER*, extended-release; *IR*, immediate-release; *IV*, intravenous; *TD*, transdermal; *TM*, transmucosal.

risks and realistic benefits of opioid therapy with patients.

2. Clinicians should establish management plan strategies to mitigate risk, including considering offering naloxone when factors that increase risk for opioid overdose, such as history of overdose, history of substance use disorder, higher opioid dosages (≥50 MME/d) or concurrent benzodiazepine use are present.

3. Clinicians should review the patient's history of controlled substance prescriptions using state prescription drug monitoring programme data and review every 3 months during opioid therapy.

4. Clinicians should use urine drug testing before starting opioid therapy and consider urine drug testing at least annually to assess for prescribed medications as well as other controlled prescription drugs and illicit drugs.

5. Clinicians should consider opioid therapy only if expected benefits for both pain and function are anticipated to outweigh risks to the patient. Opioids should be combined with nonpharmacological therapy and nonopioid pharmacological therapy.

6. When starting opioid therapy, clinicians should prescribe the lowest effective dosage and immediate-release opioids instead of extended-release/long-acting (ER/LA) opioids.

7. Caution should be exercised when increasing dosage to 50 morphine milligram equivalents (MME) or more per day, and should avoid increasing dosage to 90 MME or more per day or carefully justify a decision to titrate dosage to 90 MME or more per day.

8. Clinicians should evaluate benefits and harms with patients within 1 to 4 weeks of starting opioid therapy for chronic pain or of dose escalation. Clinicians should evaluate benefits and harms of continued therapy with patients every 3 months or more frequently.

9. Clinicians should avoid prescribing opioid pain medication and benzodiazepines concurrently whenever possible.

10. Clinicians should offer or arrange evidence-based treatment for patients with opioid use disorder.

Weak opioid analgesics

Codeine

Codeine is a weak opioid analgesic that has low affinity for the MOP receptor. It is generally considered to be a prodrug for morphine, metabolised by the cytochrome P450 2D6 (CYP2D6) isoenzyme, with approximately 10% of an orally administered dose being metabolised to morphine (Zollner & Stein 2007). Codeine is susceptible to metabolic drug–drug interactions via either inhibition (e.g. bupropion, celecoxib, cimetidine) or induction (e.g. dexamethasone, rifampin) of its metabolism. Codeine may be administered as an oral tablet or intramuscularly or coformulated with paracetamol or an NSAID in tablet form. Doses of codeine generally do not exceed 60 mg (Trescot et al. 2008).

Meperidine

Meperidine (also known as pethidine) is a synthetic weak MOP agonist whose analgesic potency is ~10% that of morphine. Meperidine is metabolised to normeperidine (Gilman et al. 1980), which may accumulate in patients with decreased renal function and in those receiving multiple doses, resulting in myoclonus (Marinella 1997). The consensus is that use of meperidine should be discouraged in favour of other opioids in both adults and in the paediatric setting (Benner & Durham 2011; Latta et al. 2002).

Tramadol

Tramadol has been used for the treatment of mild-to-moderate pain in Germany for the past four decades and in the United Kingdom, United States and elsewhere since the mid-1990s (Bravo et al. 2017). After IV administration, the potency of tramadol is similar to that of meperidine, that is, ~ 10% that of morphine (Bravo et al. 2017). After oral administration, the bioavailability of tramadol is high, approximately 70% (Bravo et al. 2017). The starting dose of tramadol is 50 mg once or twice daily, which may be increased gradually to a maximum of 400 mg/day (100 mg, four times daily) in patients without renal or hepatic dysfunction or 300 mg/day in older patients (>75 years) (O'Connor & Dworkin 2009). For the treatment of neuropathic pain, tramadol has an NNT of 4.7 (3.6–6.7) (Finnerup et al. 2015).

The analgesic effects of tramadol are mediated via multiple mechanisms in the CNS, including activation of the descending noradrenergic and serotoninergic inhibitory system as well as weak MOP agonist activity (Bravo et al. 2017). Tramadol is metabolised in the liver to a potent MOP agonist metabolite known as M1, which also contributes to its analgesic actions. Because of the complexity of its analgesic profile, the Food and Drug Administration has classified tramadol as a nontraditional, centrally acting analgesic (Bravo et al. 2017).

Tramadol has a low incidence of adverse effects, particularly respiratory depression and constipation (Bravo et al. 2017). Although withdrawal from tramadol is uncommon, gradual tapering is recommended with lorazepam and clonidine (Miotto et al. 2017). However, convulsions have been reported when doses of tramadol exceed the recommended limits (Shadnia et al. 2012). In addition, the risk of seizures in patients taking other medications that lower the seizure threshold, such as selective serotonin-reuptake inhibitors (SSRIs), TCAs and antipsychotic drugs, is potentially increased by tramadol (Nelson & Philbrick 2012).

Strong opioid analgesics

Morphine

Morphine is an opioid alkaloid found in high abundance in opium, the dried exudate of the unripe seed capsule of the opium poppy, *Papaver somniferum* (Boerner 1975). It was first isolated by the German pharmacist Freidrich Sertürner, and named 'morphium' after Morpheus the Greek God of Dreams (Milne et al. 1996). Morphine remains the 'gold standard' opioid analgesic recommended by the WHO (1986) for the relief of moderate-to-severe chronic cancer pain. Morphine is also widely utilised for the management of acute moderate-to-severe pain such as that which occurs following trauma or heart attack and postoperatively (Bovill 1987).

The oral bioavailability of morphine is low at ~20% due to extensive first-pass metabolism in the gastrointestinal mucosa and the liver to form two major active metabolites, namely the analgesically active morphine-6-glucuronide (M6G) and the analgesically inactive morphine-3-glucuronide (M3G), which account for ~10% and >50% of the dose, respectively (Smith 2000). In patients with renal impairment, these two glucuronide metabolites may accumulate, resulting in respiratory depression and/or neuro-excitation (Klimas & Mikus 2014).

Morphine is available in a range of formulations, including oral tablets, capsules and mixtures, rectal suppositories and parenteral formulations for administration by the intramuscular, IV, subcutaneous, epidural and intrathecal routes. Oral morphine dosage forms include both immediate-release and sustained-release formulations, with the latter enabling the convenience of once or twice daily dosing (Argoff & Silvershein 2009). There is also an extended-release epidural formulation of morphine available, which utilises a proprietary liposomal carrier, DepoFoam, to provide prolonged analgesia (up to 48 hours) without the need for an indwelling catheter (Viscusi et al. 2005).

Oxycodone

Oxycodone is a semisynthetic derivative of thebaine, a naturally occurring alkaloid in the opium poppy (Kalso 2005). The analgesic potency of oxycodone is ~1.5 times that of morphine following IV injection for the relief of postoperative pain (Lenz et al. 2009) and after administration of oral controlled-release tablet formulations for the management of cancer-related pain (Bruera et al. 1998).

The oral bioavailability of oxycodone is high at 60%–87% in healthy subjects and patients with cancer (Leow et al. 1992). In humans, oxycodone is principally metabolised to its analgesically inactive, N-demethylated metabolite, noroxycodone (Lalovic et al. 2006; Poyhia et al. 1992). Although up to 10% of an oxycodone dose is metabolised to its O-demethylated metabolite oxymorphone, a potent MOP agonist, it is rapidly further metabolised to its glucuronide metabolite, resulting in very low circulating plasma concentrations of oxymorphone (Lalovic et al. 2006; Poyhia et al. 1991, 1992). Hence, the pharmacodynamic effects of oxycodone are generally attributed to the parent drug alone (Lalovic et al. 2006).

Like morphine, oxycodone is available in a range of formulations, including oral tablets, capsules and mixtures, rectal suppositories, and parenteral formulations for IV administration. Oral oxycodone dosage forms include oral mixture, immediate-release tablets and controlled-release tablets that allow twice daily dosing (Argoff & Silvershein 2009). A combination of oxycodone and naloxone (Targin) is also available to treat moderate-to-severe chronic pain, with the aim of conferring abuse-deterrent properties (Colucci et al. 2014).

Methadone

Methadone is a synthetic MOP agonist that is a racemic mixture of two enantiomers, the dextrorotatory (S-methadone) and laevorotatory (R-methadone) stereoisomers. S-methadone produces analgesia via activation of descending serotoninergic and noradrenergic inhibitory mechanisms and it also has antitussive activity (Codd et al. 1995). R-methadone produces analgesia through its activity as an agonist at MOP receptors (Leppert 2009). Both enantiomers also have antagonist activity at NMDA receptors (Gorman et al. 1997). Methadone is available in oral and rectal preparations and in ampoules for parenteral administration (Manfredi et al. 2003). For patients with an addiction to opioids, methadone is commonly utilised as maintenance treatment and it is also used in patients with chronic pain (Lugo et al. 2005).

Following administration of high doses of methadone (>60 mg per day) in combination with TCAs or other drugs that inhibit its metabolism, there is a lengthening of the QTc interval, thereby initiating torsades de pointes (Ehret et al. 2007; Krantz et al. 2002). Unfortunately, a lack of awareness of the long and highly variable elimination half-life (12–150 hours) of methadone and its many metabolic drug–drug interactions resulted in a dramatic increase in deaths associated with this opioid (Trescot et al. 2008). Thus its use as an analgesic in general requires caution and specific guidelines have been published by the American College of Medical Toxicology (2016).

Hydromorphone

Hydromorphone is a semisynthetic morphine analogue that is an MOP agonist with a parenteral potency approximately five times that of morphine for the relief of moderate-to-severe acute pain (Horn & Nesbit 2004; Quigley 2002). For the relief of chronic cancer pain, hydromorphone is equivalent to morphine in terms of pain relief and adverse event profiles (Murray & Hagen 2005). After oral administration, hydromorphone undergoes extensive first-pass metabolism with more than 50% of every dose metabolised to hydromorphone-3-glucuronide (H3G). Hydromorphone is available in immediate-release and controlled-release oral formulations as well as parenteral preparations that can be administered by either the epidural or intrathecal routes (Hagen et al. 1995; Hays et al. 1994).

Although H3G is an analgesically inactive metabolite, it can accumulate in renal failure and produce neuroexcitatory side effects (Davison & Mayo 2008; Smith 2000). There is insufficient evidence to assess the efficacy of hydromorphone in neuropathic pain (Stannard et al. 2016), but the efficacy of hydromorphone is similar to that of morphine and oxycodone in the treatment of cancer pain (Bao et al. 2016).

Buprenorphine

Buprenorphine is a semisynthetic derivative of thebaine that is a partial MOP agonist, a κ-opioid (KOP) antagonist, and it also binds to the nociceptin (ORL-1) receptor (Johnson et al. 2005; Pick et al. 1997). It is thought that the slow dissociation of buprenorphine from the MOP receptor is responsible for its slow onset and long duration of action, whereas its KOP antagonist properties are thought to underpin its limited spinal analgesia, dysphoria and psychotomimetic effects (Johnson et al. 2005). Buprenorphine is ~25 to 50 times more potent than morphine (Evans & Easthope 2003) with a ceiling effect for analgesia thought to be related to its partial MOP agonist activity (Davis 2005).

Following oral administration, the bioavailability of buprenorphine is low at ~14% due to extensive first-pass metabolism (Picard et al. 2005), whereas after buccal, sublingual, intranasal and transdermal administration, the bioavailability of buprenorphine is increased to 30%–60% as these dosing routes avoid first-pass metabolism (Davis 2005; Evans & Easthope 2003; Johnson et al. 2005). Because of its long half-life (~26 hours), buprenorphine is a suitable alternative to methadone for opioid maintenance therapy in opioid-dependent individuals

(Johnson et al. 2005; Robinson 2002). A combination product (Suboxone) containing buprenorphine and the opioid antagonist naloxone in a 4:1 ratio, respectively, has been developed to deter illicit conversion of buprenorphine tablets to parenteral routes (Harris et al. 2004).

Fentanyl

Fentanyl is a semisynthetic MOP agonist that has a rapid onset of action (1–5 minutes) but short duration (<1 hour) (Stanley 2005). Although fentanyl is structurally related to meperidine, it is ~80- to 100-fold more potent than parenteral morphine (Pasero 2005). To compensate for its short duration of action, several transdermal patch formulations of fentanyl have been developed (Davis 2006; Hair et al. 2008; Heitz et al. 2009; Herndon 2007; Hoy & Keating 2008; Marier et al. 2006; Portenoy & Lesage 1999). Fentanyl has been used clinically for ~50 years in the field of pain management (Pasero 2005; Stanley 2005).

For postoperative pain relief, fentanyl may be administered by the intraspinal route, whereas for procedural or breakthrough pain administration by the IV, oral transmucosal, intranasal or inhaled routes is preferred (Hair et al. 2008; Peng & Sandler 1999). There is insufficient evidence to assess the efficacy of fentanyl in neuropathic pain (Derry et al. 2016). Fentanyl is metabolised primarily to norfentanyl, a pharmacologically inactive metabolite (Horn & Nesbit 2004).

Tapentadol

Tapentadol is a centrally acting oral analgesic whose activity is attributed to its moderate affinity at MOP receptors as well as its inhibition of norepinephrine reuptake in the CNS to activate descending inhibitory mechanisms (Tzschentke et al. 2014). This latter action has been proposed to provide an 'opioid-sparing' effect resulting in an overall improvement in tolerability compared with other MOP analgesics (Tzschentke et al. 2006). The oral bioavailability of tapentadol is reportedly 32% due to first-pass metabolism, primarily to tapentadol-O-glucuronide (Kneip et al. 2008).

At present, the immediate-release formulation (50, 75 and 100 mg tablets) of tapentadol is approved for the relief of moderate-to-severe acute pain in adult patients (Frampton 2010). The analgesic benefits of tapentadol have been demonstrated in patients with neuropathic pain (Niesters et al. 2014; Vinik et al. 2014) and cancer pain (Mercadante 2017). In acute pain settings, tapentadol (50–100 mg every 4–6 hours) provided similar analgesia to oxycodone (10 or 15 mg every 4–6 hours) with a superior gastrointestinal adverse effect profile (Hartrick 2010; Xiao et al. 2017). Despite its lack of serotonin-reuptake

inhibition, spontaneous adverse drug events consistent with serotonin syndrome have been reported (Abeyaratne et al. 2018).

Ultra-short-acting opioid analgesics

Remifentanil

Remifentanil, a 4-anilinopiperidine derivative of fentanyl, is an ultra-short-acting MOP agonist indicated for the relief of postoperative pain (Kucukemre et al. 2005). The primary metabolite, remifentanil acid, has negligible activity compared with remifentanil (Battershill & Keating 2006). Parenteral remifentanil has a rapid onset of action (~1 minute) and a rapid offset of action following discontinuation (~3–10 minutes) (Battershill & Keating 2006).

Other ultra-short-acting structural analogues of fentanyl for use in anaesthesia include alfentanil, sufentanil and remifentanil. The ultra-short-acting agents are preferred in patients with cardiovascular instability (Horn & Nesbit 2004).

Opioid antagonists for improving constipation

To date, six peripherally selective MOP receptor antagonists, viz. naloxegol, naloxone, axelopran, naldemedine, alvimopan and methylnaltrexone, are available for improving opioid-induced constipation. While the effects of these opioid antagonists are similar, a network meta-analysis identified methylnaltrexone and alvimopan as being more effective in treating opioid-induced constipation (Sridharan & Sivaramakrishnan 2018). Oral alvimopan is approved for use in adult patients who have undergone partial small or large bowel resection (limited use: 15 doses, up to 7 days only) (Nee et al. 2018). Methylnaltrexone, a quaternary derivative of naltrexone, is available for subcutaneous injection and is indicated in patients with advanced and late-stage illness requiring chronic opioid therapy but experiencing opioid-induced constipation (Rao & Go 2010). The recommended methylnaltrexone doses are based on patient weight as follows: 8 mg (for 38–62 kg), 12 mg (for 62–114 kg) and 0.15 mg/kg for patients falling outside this weight range (Wyeth Pharmaceuticals 2009).

Adjuvant medications

Antidepressants

TCAs are recommended as first-line agents for the management of neuropathic pain with an NNT of 3.6 (Finnerup et al. 2015). TCAs produce their analgesic actions through inhibition of the reuptake of norepinephrine to augment descending inhibition (Jann & Slade 2007). TCAs also modulate other signalling pathways, including histaminergic, cholinergic and glutaminergic neurotransmission (Sindrup et al. 2005). Recent evidence suggests that they may also block Na$^+$ channels (Dick et al. 2007).

TCAs produce numerous side effects, including CNS (sedation, tremor, insomnia, convulsion), anticholinergic (dry mouth, blurred vision, constipation) and cardiovascular (orthostatic hypotension, cardiac arrhythmias) effects (Attal et al. 2006). To minimise the impact of these adverse effects, TCAs should be started at low dosages, administered at night and titrated slowly. An adequate trial of a TCA can take 6 to 8 weeks, including 2 weeks at the maximum tolerated dosage (Dworkin et al. 2007).

Although the newer classes of antidepressants such as the SSRIs, serotonin norepinephrine reuptake inhibitors (SNRIs) and bupropion (dopamine and norepinephrine reuptake inhibitor) produce few side effects, there is variable efficacy for the relief of neuropathic pain (Saarto & Wiffen 2005). SSRIs such as citalopram and paroxetine have limited efficacy for the treatment of neuropathic pain (Otto et al. 2008). By contrast, SNRIs such as duloxetine (NNT = 5.8) and venlafaxine appear to have efficacy for the relief of neuropathic pain (Dworkin et al. 2007; Sultan et al. 2008).

Anticonvulsants

Gabapentin and its structural analogue pregabalin are second-generation anticonvulsants that interact with the $\alpha_2\delta$ subunit of voltage-gated calcium channels to reduce Ca^{2+} influx into the presynaptic nerve terminal and reduce release of pronociceptive neurotransmitters such as glutamate and substance P (Dickenson & Ghandehari 2007). Multiple randomised controlled trials have shown that these agents are efficacious for the relief of a variety of neuropathic pain states (NNT = 6.3), including painful diabetic neuropathy (PDN), postherpetic neuralgia, phantom limb pain and mixed neuropathic pain (Dworkin et al. 2007; Finnerup et al. 2005, 2015).

After oral dosing, gabapentin exhibits dose-dependent pharmacokinetics, and its oral bioavailability decreases as the dose increases across the therapeutic dose range, commencing at 1200 mg per day in three divided doses up to a maximum dose of 3600 mg per day (Finnerup et al. 2015). The more recently developed pregabalin (NNT = 7.7) is an improvement on gabapentin in that it exhibits linear pharmacokinetics and it is approximately six times more potent than gabapentin (Gidal 2006). Starting doses of pregabalin are 150 mg per day administered in two or three divided doses with up-titration to 600 mg per day (Finnerup et al. 2015). The dosages of gabapentin and pregabalin should be reduced in patients with significant renal impairment as

these agents are eliminated by renal mechanisms (Tassone et al. 2007). The most commonly reported adverse events for gabapentin and pregabalin are dizziness, somnolence and peripheral oedema. Although gabapentin/pregabalin and the TCAs appear to have similar efficacy for the alleviation of PDN, gabapentin/pregabalin have a superior safety profile (Gidal 2006; Tassone et al. 2007).

Lamotrigine is a sodium channel blocker and inhibitor of Na$^+$ influx-mediated release of excitatory neurotransmitters. Although it appeared to show efficacy in small cross-over clinical trials for the treatment of trigeminal neuralgia, PDN and poststroke pain at doses exceeding 200 mg per day (Finnerup et al. 2005), systematic analysis of 12 randomised controlled studies failed to show efficacy (Wiffen et al. 2013). Currently, lamotrigine is not recommended for the treatment of neuropathic pain of any aetiology, but can be considered for off-label use.

Phenytoin and carbamazepine were the first anticonvulsants shown to have efficacy for the alleviation of neuropathic pain (Gilron et al. 2006; Jensen 2002). However, as these agents have a significant spectrum of unpleasant side effects, their use is limited. Although carbamazepine is an effective and commonly prescribed agent for the relief of trigeminal neuralgia (Wiffen et al. 2005), its more widespread use for the alleviation of neuropathic pain is restricted by adverse effects, including dyslipidaemia, decreased serum sodium levels, changes in sex hormone concentrations, increased body weight and multiple metabolic drug–drug interactions as it is a potent inducer of hepatic cytochrome P450 enzymes (Gilron et al. 2006; McCleane 2003). Additionally, carbamazepine has been linked to rare cases of liver toxicity, necessitating regular blood tests to monitor liver enzymes (Wiffen et al. 2005). Carbamazepine can also lead to reversible decreases in white cell count distinct from aplastic anaemia that requires monitoring (Wiffen et al. 2005).

NMDA receptor antagonists

The role of NMDA receptors in the induction and maintenance of central sensitisation is well documented (D'Mello & Dickenson 2008). Hence, a number of studies have investigated the potential efficacy of clinically available NMDA receptor antagonists such as amantadine, magnesium, ketamine, memantine and dextromethorphan for the relief of neuropathic pain and/or for potential opioid-sparing effects (Kreutzwiser & Tawfic 2019).

Ketamine, an analogue of phencyclidine, is a noncompetitive NMDA receptor antagonist with a history of use as a general dissociative anaesthetic (Chizh & Headley 2005). A significant drawback of ketamine is that it produces hallucinations and ataxia at doses only slightly larger than those needed to produce analgesia (Childers & Baudy 2007). However, in subanaesthetic doses, ketamine has been shown to have analgesic properties (Kronenberg 2002). Ketamine may be used as a co-analgesic for its opioid-sparing effects (Bell et al. 2006; Kronenberg 2002). When ketamine is administered in subanaesthetic doses, most reports are of no or mild psychotomimetic effects (Kronenberg 2002). The analgesic potential of ketamine has been demonstrated in patients with neuropathic pain and refractory cancer pain (Aiyer et al. 2018; Bredlau et al. 2013). Ketamine is available as a racemic mixture in Australia and New Zealand, and the more potent S-ketamine enantiomeric form, which has twice the analgesic potency, is also available in other countries (Mion & Villevieille 2013).

Dextromethorphan, a noncompetitive NMDA receptor antagonist and an antagonist at α3β4 neuronal nicotinic receptors, is found in many over-the-counter cough and cold preparations as an antitussive agent (Damaj et al. 2005). Despite its low affinity antagonism at NMDA receptors (Chizh & Headley 2005), studies have shown benefit for dextromethorphan in patients with phantom limb pain, neuropathic pain and postoperative pain (Aiyer et al. 2018; Alviar et al. 2016; King et al. 2016).

Magnesium is regarded as an NMDA receptor antagonist. However, its antinociceptive actions may also be mediated via inhibition of calcium channels, modulation of potassium channels and activation of nitric oxide pathways (Srebro et al. 2017). Although the analgesic benefits of magnesium have been shown to relieve postoperative pain (McKeown et al. 2017; Peng et al. 2018), there is a lack of evidence for its use in the treatment of neuropathic pain and cancer pain (Baaklini et al. 2017; Pickering et al. 2011)

Cannabinoids

Evidence from animal studies and clinical observations indicates that cannabinoids have some analgesic properties. However, CNS depression seems to be the predominant limiting adverse effect. Currently, there is no evidence for a role of cannabinoids in the management of acute pain (Stevens & Higgins 2017). A recent meta-analysis that evaluated 47 randomised controlled trials and 57 observational studies found a lack of efficacy of cannabis and cannabinoids in the treatment of chronic noncancer pain (Stockings et al. 2018). NeuPSIG (The Neuropathic Pain Special Interest Group of the International Association for the Study of Pain) recommends the use of cannabinoids as an off-label therapy within a multimodal therapy concept in the event of failure of other pain therapies (Finnerup et al. 2015). Sativex (GW Pharmaceuticals, Salisbury, Wiltshire, UK), a cannabis plant-based prescription pharmaceutical product administered as an oromucosal spray delivering a fixed dose of 2.7 mg tetrahydrocannabinol (THC) and 2.5 mg cannabidiol (CBD), has been approved in Canada for multiple sclerosis-related central neuropathic pain.

Local anaesthetics

Lidocaine (lignocaine) and mexiletine are widely used local anaesthetics that are generally considered to be second-line agents for the management of localised neuropathic pain (Finnerup et al. 2015). This is because these agents not only block sodium channels on sensory nerves but also block sodium channels in cardiac tissue and the brain, potentially resulting in cardiac conduction block and neurotoxicity, respectively (Vadalouca et al. 2006).

Hence, to mitigate the systemic side effects of local anaesthetics, laidocaine patch 5% may be used for the relief of neuropathic pain in patients with postherpetic neuralgia and peripheral neuropathic pain (Khaliq et al. 2007; Meier et al. 2003). Randomised controlled trials show that the lidocaine patch 5% is well tolerated and systemic side effects are unusual (Heitz et al. 2009). However, a Cochrane review did not make firm conclusions due to the poor quality of the randomised trials (Derry et al. 2014).

Capsaicin patch

Capsaicin is a hydrophobic, colourless and odourless chemical irritant that is the pungent component of the red chilli pepper (Sawynok 2005). Capsaicin binds selectively to the transient receptor potential vanilloid (TRPV1) receptor on C fibres, resulting in initial excitation of neurons followed by a period of prolonged desensitisation and pain relief subsequent to depletion of substance P from presynaptic nerve terminals (Veronesi & Oortgiesen 2006). Topically applied capsaicin at a low concentration (0.075%) lacked efficacy for the alleviation of PDN, postherpetic neuralgia, human immunodeficiency virus (HIV) neuropathic pain or postsurgical neuropathic pain (Mason et al. 2004). However, when used at high concentration (8%), topically applied capsaicin produced long-lasting pain relief in HIV neuropathic pain (Simpson et al. 2008) and in postherpetic neuralgia (Backonja et al. 2008). Multiple systematic reviews of randomised clinical trials have shown the beneficial effects of capsaicin for relief of painful HIV neuropathy and diabetic neuropathy (Derry et al. 2017; Mou et al. 2013). Additionally, a network meta-analysis found the analgesic effects of capsaicin to be better than pregabalin and gabapentin (van Nooten et al. 2017).

α_2-adrenergic receptor agonists

After intrathecal administration, clonidine, an α_2-adrenoceptor agonist, evokes analgesia and has opioid-sparing effects (Smith & Elliott 2001). Opioid-sparing effects of α_2-agonists such as clonidine and dexmedetomidine were also evident after systemic dosing routes in the postoperative setting (Arain et al. 2004; Jalonen et al. 1997; Park et al. 1996).

Glucocorticoids

Glucocorticoids have potent antiinflammatory effects involving suppression of immune responses as well as the production of prostaglandins and leukotrienes (Goppelt-Struebe et al. 1989). In the postoperative setting, several randomised controlled trials have shown that addition of glucocorticoids to analgesic regimens improves postoperative pain relief while reducing analgesic consumption and reducing postoperative nausea, vomiting and fatigue (Kehlet 2007; Romundstad et al. 2006). However, they are generally considered to be of limited value in the management of chronic pain due to their severe adverse effect profile involving the CNS, musculoskeletal, endocrine, cardiovascular and gastrointestinal systems, with bone loss being one of the most serious side effects (Moghadam-Kia & Werth 2010). For short-term intraarticular use, corticosteroids such as triamcinolone, methylprednisolone and betamethasone show benefit for increasing joint mobility and for providing pain relief (Hepper et al. 2009; Habib et al. 2010).

Invasive procedures

Invasive procedures including reversible blockade with local anaesthetics, augmentation with spinal cord stimulation (SCS), ablation with neurolytic agents and intraspinal routes of delivery to improve an effective drug's therapeutic index are warranted for the treatment of chronic cancer and noncancer pain when conventional pharmacological therapies are unsuccessful due to either inadequate pain relief and/or intolerable side effects (Eisenberg et al. 2005; Markman & Philip 2007). Invasive interventions such as intrathecal opioids, neurolytic coeliac plexus blockade and SCS have been shown to be not only efficacious but also to reduce exposure to the side effects of systemically administered analgesic agents. These techniques need to be tailored to the individual patient, and they complement, rather than replace, pharmacological and nonpharmacological treatments for the management of chronic pain (Markman & Philip 2007).

Neurolytic celiac plexus blockade

Neurolytic coeliac plexus blockade using agents such as alcohol (50%–100%) or phenol is the most extensively utilised ablative procedure for the treatment of cancer pain, particularly intraabdominal cancer pain. This type of block has a duration of analgesia in the order of months (Markman & Philip 2007; Miguel 2000).

Implantable intrathecal drug delivery

Patients with noncancer pain experiencing inadequate pain relief and/or intolerable side effects with conventional pharmacotherapy may be considered for an implanted intrathecal drug delivery device (Markman & Philip 2007). Indications include failed back syndrome, neuropathic pain, axial spinal pain, complex regional pain syndrome, diffuse pain, brachial plexitis, central pain, failed SCS therapy, arachnoiditis, poststroke pain, spinal cord injury pain and peripheral neuropathy (Markman & Philip 2007).

Devices used to deliver analgesic agents into the epidural and intrathecal spaces include programmable implantable pumps, implanted accessible reservoir systems and tunnelled exteriorised catheters. A major benefit of intraspinal delivery systems is that they allow logarithmic scale reductions in the dosage requirements of analgesic agents relative to systemic routes of administration, but close monitoring of patients is essential, particularly during the initial dose titration phase (Markman & Philip 2007). Medications that have been given spinally include opioids, local anaesthetics, spasmolytics (e.g. baclofen), α_2-agonists (e.g. clonidine) and ziconotide (Markman & Philip 2007; Miguel 2000).

Following insertion of a small catheter into the cerebrospinal fluid in the intrathecal space, the catheter is attached to a small, subcutaneously implanted, battery-powered programmable pump, which is refilled at 1 to 3 monthly intervals (Markman & Philip 2007). This mode of delivery bypasses systemic metabolism and ensures that the administered medications are delivered in close proximity to target receptors. The net result is a longer duration of action and a reduced rate of systemic side effects relative to more conventional dosing routes. Before definitive pump implantation, selected patients undergo psychological profiling, and the potential therapeutic benefit of intrathecal drug delivery is tested via an external pump (Markman & Philip 2007).

Catheter-related problems that commonly occur in up to 25% of patients include kinking, disconnection, blockage and granuloma formation at the catheter tip as a result of prolonged high-rate infusion (Markman & Philip 2007).

Spinal cord stimulation

For the treatment of chronic radicular pain after lumbar and cervical spine surgery, SCS is commonly used as a late-stage therapy supported by the outcomes of randomised controlled trials showing superior outcomes relative to lumbar reoperation (Markman & Philip 2007). For SCS, cylindrical catheter-like leads or flat, paddle-shaped leads are positioned in the dorsal epidural space and an electrical field is generated via connection of the stimulating metal contacts with a programmable pulse generator (Markman & Philip 2007). The resulting electrical field stimulates the axons of the dorsal root and dorsal column fibres, resulting in activation of descending inhibition and blockade of activity in the lateral spinothalamic tract (Markman & Philip 2007). The battery, similar in size to a cardiac pacemaker, is implanted subcutaneously and connected to the leads via a subcutaneous tunnel (Markman & Philip 2007).

Conclusion

Considerable research over the last three decades has shown that the neurobiology of pain is highly complex, with multiple concurrent changes in expression levels of a broad array of receptors, ion channels and enzymes that represent potential novel targets for the development of the next generation of pain therapeutics. Although several potential new pain therapeutics are in preclinical or clinical development, these are yet to reach the market. Hence, the currently available analgesic and adjuvant medications will continue to be utilised for the foreseeable future to manage clinical pain, according to the principles succinctly summarised by the WHO three-step analgesic ladder (WHO 1986). Briefly, this involves use of nonopioid analgesics for the relief of mild pain, with adjuvants added when pain has a neuropathic component. When mild pain progresses to moderate pain, weak opioid analgesics are added to nonopioids and/or adjuvants as required. For moderate-to-severe pain, strong opioid analgesics are prescribed, often in combination with nonopioids and/or adjuvants as required. More invasive interventions are recommended for the 10%–30% of patients whose pain is not relieved by conventional pharmacotherapy.

Given the complexity of the pathobiology underpinning chronic pain revealed by research to date, it is difficult to conceive how there could ever be a single 'gold standard' drug treatment for the optimal management of all types of pain. Development of methods to enable mechanism-based pharmacotherapy of pain is required to improve our ability to individualise the pharmacological management of pain within a multidisciplinary approach that includes nonpharmacological and psychosocial interventions.

References

Abeyaratne, C., Lalic, S., Bell, J.S., Ilomaki, J., 2018. Spontaneously reported adverse drug events related to tapentadol and oxycodone/naloxone in Australia. Ther. Adv. Drug. Saf 9, 197–205.

AHRQ, 2009. Choosing nonopioid analgesics for osteoarthritis: clinician summary guide. J. Pain Palliat. Care Pharmacother. 23, 433–457.

Aiyer, R., Mehta, N., Gungor, S., Gulati, A., 2018. A systematic review of NMDA receptor antagonists for treatment of neuropathic pain in clinical practice. Clin. J. Pain 34, 450–467.

Alcantara Montero, A., Sanchez Carnerero, C.I., 2021. Voltage-gated sodium channel blockers: new perspectives in the treatment of neuropathic pain. Neurologia 36, 169–171.

Altman, R.D., Dreiser, R.L., Fisher, C.L., Chase, W.F., Dreher, D.S., Zacher, J., 2009. Diclofenac sodium gel in patients with primary hand osteoarthritis: a randomized, double-blind, placebo-controlled trial. J. Rheumatol. 36, 1991–1999.

Alviar, M.J., Hale, T., Dungca, M., 2016. Pharmacologic interventions for treating phantom limb pain. Cochrane Database Syst. Rev. 10, CD006380.

American College of Medical Toxicology, 2016. ACMT position statement: the use of methadone as an analgesic. J. Med. Toxicol. 12, 213–215.

Apkarian, A.V., 2008. Pain perception in relation to emotional learning. Curr. Opin. Neurobiol. 18, 464–468.

Arain, S.R., Ruehlow, R.M., Uhrich, T.D., Ebert, T.J., 2004. The efficacy of dexmedetomidine versus morphine for postoperative analgesia after major inpatient surgery. Anesth Analg. 98, 153–158 table of contents.

Argoff, C.E., Silvershein, D.I., 2009. A comparison of long- and short-acting opioids for the treatment of chronic noncancer pain: tailoring therapy to meet patient needs. Mayo. Clin. Proc 84, 602–612.

Attal, N., Cruccu, G., Haanpaa, M., Hansson, P., Jensen, T.S., Nurmikko, T., et al., 2006. EFNS guidelines on pharmacological treatment of neuropathic pain. Eur. J. Neurol 13, 1153–1169.

Baaklini, L.G., Arruda, G.V., Sakata, R.K., 2017. Assessment of the analgesic effect of magnesium and morphine in combination in patients with cancer pain: a comparative randomized double-blind study. Am. J. Hosp. Palliat. Care 34, 353–357.

Backonja, M., Wallace, M.S., Blonsky, E.R., Cutler, B.J., Malan Jr., P., Rauck, R., et al., 2008. NGX-4010, a high-concentration capsaicin patch, for the treatment of postherpetic neuralgia: a randomised, double-blind study. Lancet. Neurol 7, 1106–1112.

Bao, Y.J., Hou, W., Kong, X.Y., Yang, L., Xia, J., Hua, B.J., et al., 2016. Hydromorphone for cancer pain. Cochrane. Database. Syst. Rev 10, CD011108.

Baron, R., 2009. Neuropathic pain: a clinical perspective. Handb. Exp. Pharmacol 3–30.

Barthel, H.R., Haselwood, D., Longley 3rd, S., Gold, M.S., Altman, R.D., 2009. Randomized controlled trial of diclofenac sodium gel in knee osteoarthritis. Semin. Arthritis. Rheum 39, 203–212.

Basbaum, A.I., Bautista, D.M., Scherrer, G., Julius, D., 2009. Cellular and molecular mechanisms of pain. Cell 139, 267–284.

Battershill, A.J., Keating, G.M., 2006. Remifentanil : a review of its analgesic and sedative use in the intensive care unit. Drugs 66, 365–385.

Bell, R.F., Dahl, J.B., Moore, R.A., Kalso, E., 2006. Perioperative ketamine for acute postoperative pain. Cochrane. Database. Syst. Rev CD004603.

Benner, K.W., Durham, S.H., 2011. Meperidine restriction in a pediatric hospital. J. Pediatr. Pharmacol. Ther 16, 185–190.

Bhave, G., Hu, H.J., Glauner, K.S., Zhu, W., Wang, H., Brasier, D.J., et al., 2003. Protein kinase C phosphorylation sensitizes but does not activate the capsaicin receptor transient receptor potential vanilloid 1 (TRPV1). Proc. Natl. Acad. Sci. U. S. A 100, 12480–12485.

Bhave, G., Zhu, W., Wang, H., Brasier, D.J., Oxford, G.S., Gereau, R.W.T., 2002. cAMP-dependent protein kinase regulates desensitization of the capsaicin receptor (VR1) by direct phosphorylation. Neuron 35, 721–731.

Blieden, M., Paramore, L.C., Shah, D., Ben-Joseph, R., 2014. A perspective on the epidemiology of acetaminophen exposure and toxicity in the United States. Expert. Rev. Clin. Pharmacol 7, 341–348.

Boerner, U., 1975. The metabolism of morphine and heroin in man. Drug. Metab. Rev 4, 39–73.

Bovill, J.G., 1987. Which potent opioid? Important criteria for selection. Drugs 33, 520–530.

Bravo, L., Mico, J.A., Berrocoso, E., 2017. Discovery and development of tramadol for the treatment of pain. Expert. Opin. Drug. Discov 12, 1281–1291.

Bredlau, A.L., Thakur, R., Korones, D.N., Dworkin, R.H., 2013. Ketamine for pain in adults and children with cancer: a systematic review and synthesis of the literature. Pain. Med 14, 1505–1517.

Broad, L.M., Mogg, A.J., Beattie, R.E., Ogden, A.M., Blanco, M.J., Bleakman, D., 2009. TRP channels as emerging targets for pain therapeutics. Expert. Opin. Ther. Targets 13, 69–81.

Brown, A.J., 2007. Novel cannabinoid receptors. Br. J. Pharmacol 152 567-75.

Bruera, E., Belzile, M., Pituskin, E., Fainsinger, R., Darke, A., Harsanyi, Z., et al., 1998. Randomized, double-blind, cross-over trial comparing safety and efficacy of oral controlled-release oxycodone with controlled-release morphine in patients with cancer pain. J. Clin. Oncol 16, 3222–3229.

Burke, A., S., E., Fitzgerald, G.A., 2006. Analgesic-Antipyretic Agents. McGraw-Hill, New York.

Busserolles, J., Tsantoulas, C., Eschalier, A., Lopez Garcia, J.A., 2016. Potassium channels in neuropathic pain: advances, challenges, and emerging ideas. Pain 157 (suppl. 1), S7–S14.

Caparrotta, T.M., Antoine, D.J., Dear, J.W., 2018. Are some people at increased risk of paracetamol-induced liver injury? A critical review of the literature. Eur. J. Clin. Pharmacol 74, 147–160.

Capone, M.L., Tacconelli, S., Patrignani, P., 2005. Clinical pharmacology of etoricoxib. Expert. Opin. Drug. Metab. Toxicol 1, 269–282.

Cheer, S.M., Goa, K.L., 2001. Parecoxib (parecoxib sodium). Drugs 61, 1133–1141 discussion 1142-3.

Childers Jr., W.E., Baudy, R.B., 2007. N-methyl-D-aspartate antagonists and neuropathic pain: the search for relief. J. Med. Chem 50, 2557–2562.

Chizh, B.A., Headley, P.M., 2005. NMDA antagonists and neuropathic pain--multiple drug targets and multiple uses. Curr. Pharm. Des 11, 2977–2994.

Chung, J.W., Zeng, Y., Wong, T.K., 2013. Drug therapy for the treatment of chronic nonspecific low back pain: systematic review and meta-analysis. Pain. Phy 16, E685–E704.

Codd, E.E., Shank, R.P., Schupsky, J.J., Raffa, R.B., 1995. Serotonin and norepinephrine uptake inhibiting activity of centrally acting analgesics: structural determinants and role in antinociception. J. Pharmacol. Exp. Ther 274, 1263–1270.

Colucci, S.V., Perrino, P.J., Shram, M., Bartlett, C., Wang, Y., Harris, S.C., 2014. Abuse potential of intravenous oxycodone/naloxone solution in nondependent recreational drug users. Clin. Drug. Investig 34, 421–429.

Costigan, M., Scholz, J., Woolf, C.J., 2009. Neuropathic pain: a maladaptive response of the nervous system to damage. Annu. Rev. Neurosci 32, 1–32.

Cousins, M.J., 2007. Persistent pain: a disease entity. J. Pain. Symptom. Manag 33, S4–S10.

Crown, E.D., Gwak, Y.S., Ye, Z., Johnson, K.M., Hulsebosch, C.E., 2008. Activation of p38 MAP kinase is involved in central neuropathic pain following spinal cord injury. Exp. Neurol 213, 257–267.

Cuomo, A., Bimonte, S., Forte, C.A., Botti, G., Cascella, M., 2019. Multimodal approaches and tailored therapies for pain management: the trolley analgesic model. J. Pain. Res 12, 711–714.

D'mello, R., Dickenson, A.H., 2008. Spinal cord mechanisms of pain. Br. J. Anaesth 101, 8–16.

Damaj, M.I., Flood, P., Ho, K.K., May, E.L., Martin, B.R., 2005. Effect of dextrometorphan and dextrorphan on nicotine and neuronal nicotinic receptors: in vitro and in vivo selectivity. J. Pharmacol. Exp. Ther 312, 780–785.

Davis, M.P., 2005. Buprenorphine in cancer pain. Support. Care Cancer 13, 878–887.

Davis, M.P., 2006. Management of cancer pain: focus on new opioid analgesic formulations. Am. J. Cancer 5, 171–182.

Davison, S.N., Mayo, P.R., 2008. Pain management in chronic kidney disease: the pharmacokinetics and pharmacodynamics of hydromorphone and hydromorphone-3-glucuronide in hemodialysis patients. J. Opioid. Manag 4, 339–344 335-6.

Derry, S., Rice, A.S., Cole, P., Tan, T., Moore, R.A., 2017. Topical capsaicin (high concentration) for chronic neuropathic pain in adults. Cochrane. Database. Syst. Rev 1, CD007393.

Derry, S., Stannard, C., Cole, P., Wiffen, P.J., Knaggs, R., Aldington, D., et al., 2016. Fentanyl for neuropathic pain in adults. Cochrane. Database. Syst. Rev 10, CD011605.

Derry, S., Wiffen, P.J., Moore, R.A., Quinlan, J., 2014. Topical lidocaine for neuropathic pain in adults. Cochrane. Database. Syst. Rev CD010958.

Diatchenko, L., Nackley, A.G., Slade, G.D., Fillingim, R.B., Maixner, W., 2006. Idiopathic pain disorders--pathways of vulnerability. Pain 123, 226–230.

Dick, I.E., Brochu, R.M., Purohit, Y., Kaczorowski, G.J., Martin, W.J., Priest, B.T., 2007. Sodium channel blockade may contribute to the analgesic efficacy of antidepressants. J. Pain 8, 315–324.

Dickenson, A.H., Ghandehari, J., 2007. Anti-convulsants and anti-depressants. Handb. Exp. Pharmacol 145–177.

Doubell, T.P., Mannion, R.H., Woolf, C.J., 1999. The dorsal horn: state-dependent sensory processing, plasticity and the generation of pain. In: Wall, P.D., Melzack, R. (Eds.), Textbook of Pain, fourth ed. Churchill Livingstone, London.

Dowell, D., Haegerich, T.M., Chou, R., 2016. CDC guideline for prescribing opioids for chronic pain - United States, 2016. MMWR. Recomm. Rep. (Morb. Mortal. Wkly. Rep.) 65, 1–49.

Dray, A., 1997. Kinins and their receptors in hyperalgesia. Can. J. Physiol. Pharmacol 75, 704–712.

Dugowson, C.E., Gnanashanmugam, P., 2006. Nonsteroidal anti-inflammatory drugs. Phys. Med. Rehabil. Clin. N. Am 17, 347–354 vi.

Dworkin, R.H., O'Connor, A.B., Backonja, M., Farrar, J.T., Finnerup, N.B., Jensen, T.S., et al., 2007. Pharmacologic management of neuropathic pain: evidence-based recommendations. Pain 132, 237–251.

Ehret, G.B., Desmeules, J.A., Broers, B., 2007. Methadone-associated long QT syndrome: improving pharmacotherapy for dependence on illegal opioids and lessons learned for pharmacology. Expert. Opin. Drug. Saf 6, 289–303.

Eisenberg, E., Marinangeli, F., Birkhahn, J., Paladini, A., Varrassi, G., 2005. Time to modify the WHO analgesic ladder, vol. XIII. Clinical Updates, Pain.

Evans, H.C., Easthope, S.E., 2003. Transdermal buprenorphine. Drugs 63, 1999–2010 discussion 2011-2.

Fenton, C., Keating, G.M., Wagstaff, A.J., 2004. Valdecoxib: a review of its use in the management of osteoarthritis, rheumatoid arthritis, dysmenorrhoea and acute pain. Drugs 64, 1231–1261.

Fernandes, V., Sharma, D., Vaidya, S., Shantanu, P., A. Guan, Y., Kalia, K., et al., 2018. Cellular and molecular mechanisms driving neuropathic pain: recent advancements and challenges. Expert. Opin. Ther. Targets 22, 131–142.

Finnerup, N.B., Attal, N., Haroutounian, S., McNicol, E., Baron, R., Dworkin, R.H., et al., 2015. Pharmacotherapy for neuropathic pain in adults: a systematic review and meta-analysis. Lancet. Neurol 14, 162–173.

Finnerup, N.B., Otto, M., McQuay, H.J., Jensen, T.S., Sindrup, S.H., 2005. Algorithm for neuropathic pain treatment: an evidence based proposal. Pain 118, 289–305.

Frampton, J.E., 2010. Tapentadol immediate release: a review of its use in the treatment of moderate to severe acute pain. Drugs 70, 1719–1743.

Gidal, B.E., 2006. New and emerging treatment options for neuropathic pain. Am. J. Manag. Care 12, S269–S278.

Gilman, A.G., Goodman, L.S., Gilman, A., 1980. Opioid Analgesics and Antagonists. Macmillan, New York.

Gilron, I., Watson, C.P., Cahill, C.M., Moulin, D.E., 2006. Neuropathic pain: a practical guide for the clinician. CMAJ. (Can. Med. Assoc. J.) 175, 265–275.

Goppelt-Struebe, M., Wolter, D., Resch, K., 1989. Glucocorticoids inhibit prostaglandin synthesis not only at the level of phospholipase A2 but also at the level of cyclo-oxygenase/PGE isomerase. Br. J. Pharmacol 98, 1287–1295.

Gorman, A.L., Elliott, K.J., Inturrisi, C.E., 1997. The d- and l-isomers of methadone bind to the non-competitive site on the N-methyl-D-aspartate (NMDA) receptor in rat forebrain and spinal cord. Neurosci. Lett 223, 5–8.

Goudet, C., Magnaghi, V., Landry, M., Nagy, F., Gereau, R.W.T., Pin, J.P., 2009. Metabotropic receptors for glutamate and GABA in pain. Brain. Res. Rev 60, 43–56.

Green, J.L., Heard, K.J., Reynolds, K.M., Albert, D., 2013. Oral and intravenous acetylcysteine for treatment of acetaminophen toxicity: a systematic review and meta-analysis. West. J. Emerg. Med 14, 218–226.

Habib, G.S., Saliba, W., Nashashibi, M., 2010. Local effects of intra-articular corticosteroids. Clin. Rheumatol 29, 347–356.

Hagen, N., Thirlwell, M.P., Dhaliwal, H.S., Babul, N., Harsanyi, Z., Darke, A.C., 1995. Steady-state pharmacokinetics of hydromorphone and hydromorphone-3-glucuronide in cancer patients after immediate and controlled-release hydromorphone. J. Clin. Pharmacol 35, 37–44.

Hair, P.I., Keating, G.M., McKeage, K., 2008. Transdermal matrix fentanyl membrane patch (matrifen): in severe cancer-related chronic pain. Drugs 68, 2001–2009.

Hanani, M., 2005. Satellite glial cells in sensory ganglia: from form to function. Brain. Res. Rev 48, 457–476.

Harris, D.S., Mendelson, J.E., Lin, E.T., Upton, R.A., Jones, R.T., 2004. Pharmacokinetics and subjective effects of sublingual buprenorphine, alone or in combination with naloxone: lack of dose proportionality. Clin. Pharmacokinet 43, 329–340.

Hartrick, C.T., 2010. Tapentadol immediate-release for acute pain. Expert Rev. Neurother 10, 861–869.

Harvey, V.L., Dickenson, A.H., 2008. Mechanisms of pain in nonmalignant disease. Curr. Opin. Support. Palliat. Care 2, 133–139.

Hays, H., Hagen, N., Thirlwell, M., Dhaliwal, H., Babul, N., Harsanyi, Z., et al., 1994. Comparative clinical efficacy and safety of immediate release and controlled release hydromorphone for chronic severe cancer pain. Cancer 74, 1808–1816.

Heitz, J.W., Witkowski, T.A., Viscusi, E.R., 2009. New and emerging analgesics and analgesic technologies for acute pain management. Curr. Opin. Anaesthesiol 22, 608–617.

Hepper, C.T., Halvorson, J.J., Duncan, S.T., Gregory, A.J., Dunn, W.R., Spindler, K.P., 2009. The efficacy and duration of intra-articular corticosteroid injection for knee osteoarthritis: a systematic review of level I studies. J. Am. Acad. Orthop. Surg 17, 638–646.

Herndon, C.M., 2007. Iontophoretic drug delivery system: focus on fentanyl. Pharmacotherapy 27, 745–754.

Horn, E., Nesbit, S.A., 2004. Pharmacology and pharmacokinetics of sedatives and analgesics. Gastrointest. Endosc. Clin. N. Am 14, 247–268.

Hoy, S.M., Keating, G.M., 2008. Fentanyl transdermal matrix patch (Durotep MT patch; Durogesic DTrans; Durogesic SMAT): in adults with cancer-related pain. Drugs 68, 1711–1721.

Jalonen, J., Hynynen, M., Kuitunen, A., Heikkila, H., Perttila, J., Salmenpera, M., et al., 1997. Dexmedetomidine as an anesthetic adjunct in coronary artery bypass grafting. Anesthesiology 86, 331–345.

Jann, M.W., Slade, J.H., 2007. Antidepressant agents for the treatment of chronic pain and depression. Pharmacotherapy 27, 1571–1587.

Jensen, T.S., 2002. Anticonvulsants in neuropathic pain: rationale and clinical evidence. Eur. J. Pain 6 (Suppl. A), 61–68.

Ji, R.R., 2004. Peripheral and central mechanisms of inflammatory pain, with emphasis on MAP kinases. Curr. Drug Targets - Inflamm. Allergy 3, 299–303.

Jiang, B.C., Liu, T., Gao, Y.J., 2020. Chemokines in chronic pain: cellular and molecular mechanisms and therapeutic potential. Pharmacol. Ther 212, 107581.

Johnson, R.E., Fudala, P.J., Payne, R., 2005. Buprenorphine: considerations for pain management. J. Pain. Symptom. Manage 29, 297–326.

Kalso, E., 2005. Oxycodone. J. Pain. Symptom. Manage 29, S47–S56.

Kehlet, H., 2007. Glucocorticoids for peri-operative analgesia: how far are we from general recommendations? Acta Anaesthesiol. Scand 51, 1133–1135.

Khaliq, W., Alam, S., Puri, N., 2007. Topical lidocaine for the treatment of postherpetic neuralgia. Cochrane. Database. Syst. Rev CD004846.

King, M.R., Ladha, K.S., Gelineau, A.M., Anderson, T.A., 2016. Perioperative dextromethorphan as an adjunct for postoperative pain: a meta-analysis of randomized controlled trials. Anesthesiology 124, 696–705.

Klimas, R., Mikus, G., 2014. Morphine-6-glucuronide is responsible for the analgesic effect after morphine administration: a quantitative review of morphine, morphine-6-glucuronide, and morphine-3-glucuronide. Br. J. Anaesth 113, 935–944.

Kneip, C., Terlinden, R., Beier, H., Chen, G., 2008. Investigations into the drug-drug interaction potential of tapentadol in human liver microsomes and fresh human hepatocytes. Drug. Metab. Lett 2, 67–75.

Krantz, M.J., Lewkowiez, L., Hays, H., Woodroffe, M.A., Robertson, A.D., Mehler, P.S., 2002. Torsade de pointes associated with very-high-dose methadone. Ann. Intern. Med 137, 501–504.

Krenzischek, D.A., Dunwoody, C.J., Polomano, R.C., Rathmell, J.P., 2008. Pharmacotherapy for acute pain: implications for practice. Pain. Manag. Nurs 9, S22–S32.

Kreutzwiser, D., Tawfic, Q.A., 2019. Expanding role of NMDA receptor antagonists in the management of pain. CNS. Drugs 33, 347–374.

Kronenberg, R.H., 2002. Ketamine as an analgesic: parenteral, oral, rectal, subcutaneous, transdermal and intranasal administration. J. Pain Palliat. Care. Pharmacother 16, 27–35.

Kucukemre, F., Kunt, N., Kaygusuz, K., Kiliccioglu, F., Gurelik, B., Cetin, A., 2005. Remifentanil compared with morphine for postoperative patient-controlled analgesia after major abdominal surgery: a randomized controlled trial. Eur. J. Anaesthesiol 22, 378–385.

Lai, J., Ossipov, M.H., Vanderah, T.W., Malan Jr., T.P., Porreca, F., 2001. Neuropathic pain: the paradox of dynorphin. Mol. Interv 1, 160–167.

Lalovic, B., Kharasch, E., Hoffer, C., Risler, L., Liu-Chen, L.Y., Shen, D.D., 2006. Pharmacokinetics and pharmacodynamics of oral oxycodone in healthy human subjects: role of circulating active metabolites. Clin. Pharmacol. Ther 79, 461–479.

Larson, A.M., Polson, J., Fontana, R.J., Davern, T.J., Lalani, E., Hynan, L.S., et al., 2005. Acetaminophen-induced acute liver failure: results of a United States multicenter, prospective study. Hepatology 42, 1364–1372.

Latremoliere, A., Woolf, C.J., 2009. Central sensitization: a generator of pain hypersensitivity by central neural plasticity. J. Pain 10, 895–926.

Latta, K.S., Ginsberg, B., Barkin, R.L., 2002. Meperidine: a critical review. Am. J. Ther 9, 53–68.

Lee, C., Straus, W.L., Balshaw, R., Barlas, S., Vogel, S., Schnitzer, T.J., 2004. A comparison of the efficacy and safety of nonsteroidal antiinflammatory agents versus acetaminophen in the treatment of osteoarthritis: a meta-analysis. Arthritis. Rheum 51, 746–754.

Lenz, H., Sandvik, L., Qvigstad, E., Bjerkelund, C.E., Raeder, J., 2009. A comparison of intravenous oxycodone and intravenous morphine in patient-controlled postoperative analgesia after laparoscopic hysterectomy. Anesth. Analg 109, 1279–1283.

Leow, K.P., Smith, M.T., Williams, B., Cramond, T., 1992. Single-dose and steady-state pharmacokinetics and pharmacodynamics of oxycodone in patients with cancer. Clin. Pharmacol. Ther 52, 487–495.

Leppert, W., 2009. The role of methadone in cancer pain treatment--a review. Int. J. Clin. Pract 63, 1095–1109.

Lugo, R.A., Satterfield, K.L., Kern, S.E., 2005. Pharmacokinetics of methadone. J. Pain. Palliat. Care. Pharmacother 19, 13–24.

Luongo, L., Malcangio, M., Salvemini, D., Starowicz, K., 2015. Chronic pain: new insights in molecular and cellular mechanisms. BioMed. Res. Int 2015, 676725.

Maher TJ, Chaiyakul P. Opioids (Bench). In: Smith HS, editor. Drugs for pain. Philadelphia: Hanley and Belfus; 2003. p. 83–96.

Manfredi, P.L., Foley, K.M., Payne, R., Houde, R., Inturrisi, C.E., 2003. Parenteral methadone: an essential medication for the treatment of pain. J. Pain. Symptom. Manage 26, 687–688.

Marier, J.F., Lor, M., Potvin, D., Dimarco, M., Morelli, G., Saedder, E.A., 2006. Pharmacokinetics, tolerability, and performance of a novel matrix transdermal delivery system of fentanyl relative to the commercially available reservoir formulation in healthy subjects. J. Clin. Pharmacol 46, 642–653.

Marinella, M.A., 1997. Meperidine-induced generalized seizures with normal renal function. South. Med. J 90, 556–558.

Markman, J.D., Philip, A., 2007. Interventional approaches to pain management. Med. Clin. North. Am 91, 271–286.

Marret, E., Kurdi, O., Zufferey, P., Bonnet, F., 2005. Effects of nonsteroidal antiinflammatory drugs on patient-controlled analgesia morphine side effects: meta-analysis of randomized controlled trials. Anesthesiology 102, 1249–1260.

Martinez, V., Beloeil, H., Marret, E., Fletcher, D., Ravaud, P., Trinquart, L., 2017. Non-opioid analgesics in adults after major surgery: systematic review with network meta-analysis of randomized trials. Br. J. Anaesth 118, 22–31.

Mason, L., Moore, R.A., Derry, S., Edwards, J.E., McQuay, H.J., 2004. Systematic review of topical capsaicin for the treatment of chronic pain. BMJ 328, 991.

Massey, T., Derry, S., Moore, R.A., McQuay, H.J., 2010. Topical NSAIDs for acute pain in adults. Cochrane. Database. Syst. Rev 6, CD007402.

McCleane, G., 2003. Pharmacological management of neuropathic pain. CNS. Drugs 17, 1031–1043.

McDonagh, M.S., Selph, S.S., Buckley, D.I., Holmes, R.S., Mauer, K., Ramirez, S., et al., 2020. Nonopioid Pharmacologic Treatments for Chronic Pain. Comparative Effectiveness Review No. 228. Agency for Healthcare Research and Quality (US), Rockville.

McKeown, A., Seppi, V., Hodgson, R., 2017. Intravenous magnesium sulphate for analgesia after caesarean section: a systematic review. Anesthesiol. Res. Pract 2017, 9186374.

Meacham, K., Shepherd, A., Mohapatra, D.P., Haroutounian, S., 2017. Neuropathic pain: central vs. peripheral mechanisms. Curr. Pain. Headache. Rep 21, 28.

Meier, T., Wasner, G., Faust, M., Kuntzer, T., Ochsner, F., Hueppe, M., et al., 2003. Efficacy of lidocaine patch 5% in the treatment of focal peripheral neuropathic pain syndromes: a randomized, double-blind, placebo-controlled study. Pain 106, 151–158.

Mercadante, S., 2017. The role of tapentadol as a strong opioid in cancer pain management: a systematic and critical review. Curr. Med. Res. Opin 33, 1965–1969.

Merskey, H., Bogduk, N., 1994. Classification of Chronic Pain. IASP Press, Seattle, WA.

Michaud, K., Bombardier, C., Emery, P., 2007. Quality of life in patients with rheumatoid arthritis: does abatacept make a difference? Clin. Exp. Rheumatol 25, S35–S45.

Miguel, R., 2000. Interventional treatment of cancer pain: the fourth step in the World Health Organization analgesic ladder? Cancer. Control 7, 149–156.

Milne, R.W., Nation, R.L., Somogyi, A.A., 1996. The disposition of morphine and its 3- and 6-glucuronide metabolites in humans and animals, and the importance of the metabolites to the pharmacological effects of morphine. Drug. Metab. Rev 28, 345–472.

Mion, G., Villevieille, T., 2013. Ketamine pharmacology: an update (pharmacodynamics and molecular aspects, recent findings). CNS. Neurosci. Ther 19, 370–380.

Miotto, K., Cho, A.K., Khalil, M.A., Blanco, K., Sasaki, J.D., Rawson, R., 2017. Trends in tramadol: pharmacology, metabolism, and misuse. Anesth. Analg 124, 44–51.

Moghadam-Kia, S., Werth, V.P., 2010. Prevention and treatment of systemic glucocorticoid side effects. Int. J. Dermatol 49, 239–248.

Moore, R.A., Derry, S., Aldington, D., Wiffen, P.J., 2015. Single dose oral analgesics for acute postoperative pain in adults - an overview of cochrane reviews. Cochrane. Database. Syst. Rev CD008659.

Mou, J., Paillard, F., Turnbull, B., Trudeau, J., Stoker, M., Katz, N.P., 2013. Efficacy of Qutenza(R) (capsaicin) 8% patch for neuropathic pain: a meta-analysis of the Qutenza clinical trials database. Pain 154, 1632–1639.

Munir, M.A., Enany, N., Zhang, J.M., 2007. Nonopioid analgesics. Anesthesiol. Clin 25, 761–774 vi.

Murray, A., Hagen, N.A., 2005. Hydromorphone. J. Pain. Symptom. Manage 29, S57–S66.

Myers, S.H., Laporte, D.M., 2009. Acetaminophen: safe use and associated risks. J. Hand. Surg. Am 34, 1137–1139.

Nee, J., Zakari, M., Sugarman, M.A., Whelan, J., Hirsch, W., Sultan, S., et al., 2018. Efficacy of treatments for opioid-induced constipation: systematic review and meta-analysis. Clin. Gastroenterol. Hepatol 16, 1569–1584 e2.

Nelson, E.M., Philbrick, A.M., 2012. Avoiding serotonin syndrome: the nature of the interaction between tramadol and selective serotonin reuptake inhibitors. Ann. Pharmacother 46, 1712–1716.

Niesters, M., Proto, P.L., Aarts, L., Sarton, E.Y., Drewes, A.M., Dahan, A., 2014. Tapentadol potentiates descending pain inhibition in chronic pain patients with diabetic polyneuropathy. Br. J. Anaesth 113, 148–156.

O'Connor, A.B., Dworkin, R.H., 2009. Treatment of neuropathic pain: an overview of recent guidelines. Am. J. Med 122, S22–S32.

Ohara, P.T., Vit, J.P., Bhargava, A., Romero, M., Sundberg, C., Charles, A.C., et al., 2009. Gliopathic pain: when satellite glial cells go bad. Neuroscientist 15, 450–463.

Otto, M., Bach, F.W., Jensen, T.S., Brosen, K., Sindrup, S.H., 2008. Escitalopram in painful polyneuropathy: a randomized, placebo-controlled, cross-over trial. Pain 139, 275–283.

Park, J., Forrest, J., Kolesar, R., Bhola, D., Beattie, S., Chu, C., 1996. Oral clonidine reduces postoperative PCA morphine requirements. Can. J. Anaesth 43, 900–906.

Pasero, C., 2005. Fentanyl for acute pain management. J. Perianesth. Nurs 20, 279–284.

Patrono, C., Patrignani, P., Garcia Rodriguez, L.A., 2001. Cyclooxygenase-selective inhibition of prostanoid formation: transducing biochemical selectivity into clinical read-outs. J. Clin. Invest 108, 7–13.

Peng, P.W., Sandler, A.N., 1999. A review of the use of fentanyl analgesia in the management of acute pain in adults. Anesthesiology 90, 576–599.

Peng, Y.N., Sung, F.C., Huang, M.L., Lin, C.L., Kao, C.H., 2018. The use of intravenous magnesium sulfate on postoperative analgesia in orthopedic surgery: a systematic review of randomized controlled trials. Medicine (Baltim.) 97, e13583.

Perea, G., Araque, A., 2005. Properties of synaptically evoked astrocyte calcium signal reveal synaptic information processing by astrocytes. J. Neurosci 25, 2192–2203.

Picard, N., Cresteil, T., Djebli, N., Marquet, P., 2005. In vitro metabolism study of buprenorphine: evidence for new metabolic pathways. Drug. Metab. Dispos 33, 689–695.

Pick, C.G., Peter, Y., Schreiber, S., Weizman, R., 1997. Pharmacological characterization of buprenorphine, a mixed agonist-antagonist with kappa 3 analgesia. Brain. Res 744, 41–46.

Pickering, G., Loriot, M.A., Libert, F., Eschalier, A., Beaune, P., Dubray, C., 2006. Analgesic effect of acetaminophen in humans: first evidence of a central serotonergic mechanism. Clin. Pharmacol. Ther 79, 371–378.

Pickering, G., Morel, V., Simen, E., Cardot, J.M., Moustafa, F., Delage, N., et al., 2011. Oral magnesium treatment in patients with neuropathic pain: a randomized clinical trial. Magnes. Res 24, 28–35.

Portenoy, R.K., Lesage, P., 1999. Management of cancer pain. Lancet 353, 1695–1700.

Poyhia, R., Olkkola, K.T., Seppala, T., Kalso, E., 1991. The pharmacokinetics of oxycodone after intravenous injection in adults. Br. J. Clin. Pharmacol 32, 516–518.

Poyhia, R., Seppala, T., Olkkola, K.T., Kalso, E., 1992. The pharmacokinetics and metabolism of oxycodone after intramuscular and oral administration to healthy subjects. Br. J. Clin. Pharmacol 33, 617–621.

Przybyla, G.W., Szychowski, K.A., Gminski, J., 2020. Paracetamol - an old drug with new mechanisms of action. Clin. Exp. Pharmacol. Physiol.

Quigley, C., 2002. Hydromorphone for acute and chronic pain. Cochrane. Database. Syst. Rev CD003447.

Rainville, P., Duncan, G.H., Price, D.D., Carrier, B., Bushnell, M.C., 1997. Pain affect encoded in human anterior cingulate but not somatosensory cortex. Science 277, 968–971.

Raivich, G., 2005. Like cops on the beat: the active role of resting microglia. Trends. Neurosci 28, 571–573.

Raja, S.N., Carr, D.B., Cohen, M., Finnerup, N.B., Flor, H., Gibson, S., et al., 2020. The revised International Association for the Study of Pain definition of pain: concepts, challenges, and compromises. Pain 161, 1976–1982.

Rao, S.S., Go, J.T., 2010. Update on the management of constipation in the elderly: new treatment options. Clin. Interv. Aging 5.

Reichling, D.B., Levine, J.D., 2009. Critical role of nociceptor plasticity in chronic pain. Trends. Neurosci 32, 611–618.

Remy, C., Marret, E., Bonnet, F., 2006. State of the art of paracetamol in acute pain therapy. Curr. Opin. Anaesthesiol 19, 562–565.

Riley, J., Ross, J.R., Gretton, S.K., A'hern, R., Du Bois, R., Welsh, K., et al., 2007. Proposed 5-step World Health Organization analgesic and side effect ladder. Eur. J. Pain. Suppl 1, 23–30.

Robinson, S.E., 2002. Buprenorphine: an analgesic with an expanding role in the treatment of opioid addiction. CNS. Drug. Rev 8, 377–390.

Romundstad, L., Breivik, H., Roald, H., Skolleborg, K., Haugen, T., Narum, J., et al., 2006. Methylprednisolone reduces pain, emesis, and fatigue after breast augmentation surgery: a single-dose, randomized, parallel-group study with methylprednisolone 125 mg, parecoxib 40 mg, and placebo. Anesth. Analg 102, 418–425.

Rostom, A., Dube, C., Wells, G., Tugwell, P., Welch, V., Jolicoeur, E., et al., 2002. Prevention of NSAID-induced gastroduodenal ulcers. Cochrane. Database. Syst. Rev CD002296.

Rumack, B., Heard, K., Green, J., Albert, D., Bucher-Bartelson, B., Bodmer, M., et al., 2012. Effect of therapeutic doses of acetaminophen (up to 4 g/day) on serum alanine aminotransferase levels in subjects consuming ethanol: systematic review and meta-analysis of randomized controlled trials. Pharmacotherapy 32, 784–791.

Saarto, T., Wiffen, P.J., 2005. Antidepressants for neuropathic pain. Cochrane. Database. Syst. Rev CD005454.

Saliba, S.W., Marcotegui, A.R., Fortwangler, E., Ditrich, J., Perazzo, J.C., Munoz, E., et al., 2017. AM404, paracetamol metabolite, prevents prostaglandin synthesis in activated microglia by inhibiting COX activity. J. Neuroinflammation 14, 246.

Sawynok, J., 2005. Topical analgesics in neuropathic pain. Curr. Pharm. Des 11, 2995–3004.

Scholz, J., Broom, D.C., Youn, D.H., Mills, C.D., Kohno, T., Suter, M.R., et al., 2005. Blocking caspase activity prevents transsynaptic neuronal apoptosis and the loss of inhibition in lamina II of the dorsal horn after peripheral nerve injury. J. Neurosci 25, 7317–7323.

Serlin, R.C., Mendoza, T.R., Nakamura, Y., Edwards, K.R., Cleeland, C.S., 1995. When is cancer pain mild, moderate or severe? Grading pain severity by its interference with function. Pain 61, 277–284.

Seybold, V.S., 2009. The role of peptides in central sensitization. Handb. Exp. Pharmacol 451–491.

Shadnia, S., Brent, J., Mousavi-Fatemi, K., Hafezi, P., Soltaninejad, K., 2012. Recurrent seizures in tramadol intoxication: implications for therapy based on 100 patients. Basic. Clin. Pharmacol. Toxicol 111, 133–136.

Sherrington, C.S., 1906. The Integrative Action of the Nervous System. Scribner, New York.

Sheth, R.N., Dorsi, M.J., Li, Y., Murinson, B.B., Belzberg, A.J., Griffin, J.W., Meyer, R.A., 2002. Mechanical hyperalgesia after an L5 ventral rhizotomy or an L5 ganglionectomy in the rat. Pain 96, 63–72.

Simon, L.S., Grierson, L.M., Naseer, Z., Bookman, A.A., Zev Shainhouse, J., 2009. Efficacy and safety of topical diclofenac containing dimethyl sulfoxide (DMSO) compared with those of topical placebo, DMSO vehicle and oral diclofenac for knee osteoarthritis. Pain 143, 238–245.

Simpson, D.M., Brown, S., Tobias, J., 2008. Controlled trial of high-concentration capsaicin patch for treatment of painful HIV neuropathy. Neurology 70, 2305–2313.

Sindrup, S.H., Otto, M., Finnerup, N.B., Jensen, T.S., 2005. Antidepressants in the treatment of neuropathic pain. Basic. Clin. Pharmacol. Toxicol 96, 399–409.

Smith, H., Elliott, J., 2001. Alpha(2) receptors and agonists in pain management. Curr. Opin. Anaesthesiol 14, 513–518.

Smith, M.T., 2000. Neuroexcitatory effects of morphine and hydromorphone: evidence implicating the 3-glucuronide metabolites. Clin. Exp. Pharmacol. Physiol 27, 524–528.

Smith, S.R., Deshpande, B.R., Collins, J.E., Katz, J.N., Losina, E., 2016. Comparative pain reduction of oral non-steroidal anti-inflammatory drugs and opioids for knee osteoarthritis: systematic analytic review. Osteoarthritis. Cartilage 24, 962–972.

Srebro, D., Vuckovic, S., Milovanovic, A., Kosutic, J., Vujovic, K.S., Prostran, M., 2017. Magnesium in pain research: state of the art. Curr. Med. Chem 24, 424–434.

Sridharan, K., Sivaramakrishnan, G., 2018. Drugs for treating opioid-induced constipation: a mixed treatment comparison network meta-analysis of randomized controlled clinical trials. J. Pain. Symptom. Manage 55, 468–479 e1.

Stanley, T.H., 2005. Fentanyl. J. Pain. Symptom. Manage 29, S67–S71.

Stannard, C., Gaskell, H., Derry, S., Aldington, D., Cole, P., Cooper, T.E., et al., 2016. Hydromorphone for neuropathic pain in adults. Cochrane. Database. Syst. Rev CD011604.

Stevens, A.J., Higgins, M.D., 2017. A systematic review of the analgesic efficacy of cannabinoid medications in the management of acute pain. Acta. Anaesthesiol. Scand 61, 268–280.

Stockings, E., Campbell, G., Hall, W.D., Nielsen, S., Zagic, D., Rahman, R., et al., 2018. Cannabis and cannabinoids for the treatment of people with chronic noncancer pain conditions: a systematic review and meta-analysis of controlled and observational studies. Pain 159, 1932–1954.

Stone, L.S., Molliver, D.C., 2009. In search of analgesia: emerging roles of GPCRs in pain. Mol. Interv 9, 234–251.

Sultan, A., Gaskell, H., Derry, S., Moore, R.A., 2008. Duloxetine for painful diabetic neuropathy and fibromyalgia pain: systematic review of randomised trials. BMC. Neurol 8, 29.

Takeda, M., Takahashi, M., Matsumoto, S., 2009. Contribution of the activation of satellite glia in sensory ganglia to pathological pain. Neurosci. Biobehav. Rev 33, 784–792.

Tassone, D.M., Boyce, E., Guyer, J., Nuzum, D., 2007. Pregabalin: a novel gamma-aminobutyric acid analogue in the treatment of neuropathic pain, partial-onset seizures, and anxiety disorders. Clin. Ther 29, 26–48.

Teixeira, J.M., Oliveira, M.C., Parada, C.A., Tambeli, C.H., 2010. Peripheral mechanisms underlying the essential role of P2X7 receptors in the development of inflammatory hyperalgesia. Eur. J. Pharmacol 644, 55–60.

Thacker, M.A., Clark, A.K., Marchand, F., McMahon, S.B., 2007. Pathophysiology of peripheral neuropathic pain: immune cells and molecules. Anesth. Analg 105, 838–847.

The Australian and New Zealand College of Anaesthetists, 2021. Opioid Dose Equivalence Calculation Table. Available from: https://www.anzca.edu.au/getattachment/6892fb13-47fc-446b-a7a2-11cdfe1c9902/PS01(PM)-(Appendix)-Opioid-Dose-Equivalence-Calculation-Table.

Toms, L., McQuay, H.J., Derry, S., Moore, R.A., 2008. Single dose oral paracetamol (acetaminophen) for postoperative pain in adults. Cochrane. Database. Syst. Rev CD004602.

Traynelis, S.F., Wollmuth, L.P., McBain, C.J., Menniti, F.S., Vance, K.M., Ogden, K.K., et al., 2010. Glutamate receptor ion channels: structure, regulation, and function. Pharmacol. Rev 62, 405–496.

Trescot, A.M., Datta, S., Lee, M., Hansen, H., 2008. Opioid pharmacology. Pain. Physician 11, S133–S153.

Tzschentke, T.M., Christoph, T., Kogel, B.Y., 2014. The mu-opioid receptor agonist/noradrenaline reuptake inhibition (MOR-NRI) concept in analgesia: the case of tapentadol. CNS Drugs 28, 319–329.

Tzschentke, T.M., De Vry, J., Terlinden, R., Hennies, H.H., Lange, C., Strassburger, W., et al., 2006. Tapentadol HCl. Drugs. Future 31, 1053–1061.

Uceyler, N., Schafers, M., Sommer, C., 2009. Mode of action of cytokines on nociceptive neurons. Exp. Brain. Res 196, 67–78.

Vadalouca, A., Siafaka, I., Argyra, E., Vrachnou, E., Moka, E., 2006. Therapeutic management of chronic neuropathic pain: an examination of pharmacologic treatment. Ann. N. Y. Acad. Sci 1088, 164–186.

Vallejo, R., Tilley, D.M., Vogel, L., Benyamin, R., 2010. The role of glia and the immune system in the development and maintenance of neuropathic pain. Pain. Pract 10, 167–184.

Van Nooten, F., Treur, M., Pantiri, K., Stoker, M., Charokopou, M., 2017. Capsaicin 8% patch versus oral neuropathic pain medications for the treatment of painful diabetic peripheral neuropathy: a systematic literature review and network meta-analysis. Clin. Ther 39, 787–803 e18.

Vane, J.R., 1971. Inhibition of prostaglandin synthesis as a mechanism of action for aspirin-like drugs. Nat. New. Biol 231, 232–235.

Vanegas, H., Schaible, H.G., 2004. Descending control of persistent pain: inhibitory or facilitatory? Brain. Res. Brain. Res. Rev 46, 295–309.

Vergnolle, N., Ferazzini, M., D'Andrea, M.R., Buddenkotte, J., Steinhoff, M., 2003. Proteinase-activated receptors: novel signals for peripheral nerves. Trends. Neurosci 26, 496–500.

Veronesi, B., Oortgiesen, M., 2006. The TRPV1 receptor: target of toxicants and therapeutics. Toxicol. Sci 89, 1–3.

Vinik, A.I., Shapiro, D.Y., Rauschkolb, C., Lange, B., Karcher, K., Pennett, D., et al., 2014. A randomized withdrawal, placebo-controlled study evaluating the efficacy and tolerability of tapentadol extended release in patients with chronic painful diabetic peripheral neuropathy. Diabetes. Care 37, 2302–2309.

Viscusi, E.R., Martin, G., Hartrick, C.T., Singla, N., Manvelian, G., 2005. Forty-eight hours of postoperative pain relief after total hip arthroplasty with a novel, extended-release epidural morphine formulation. Anesthesiology 102, 1014–1022.

Walsh, D., 2005. Advances in opioid therapy and formulations. Support. Care. Cancer 13, 138–144.

Wang, S., 2019. Historical review: opiate addiction and opioid receptors. Cell. Transplant 28, 233–238.

Wang, Z., Ma, W., Chabot, J.G., Quirion, R., 2010. Morphological evidence for the involvement of microglial p38 activation in CGRP-associated development of morphine antinociceptive tolerance. Peptides 31, 2179–2184.

Watkins, L.R., Hutchinson, M.R., Ledeboer, A., Wieseler-Frank, J., Milligan, E.D., Maier, S.F., 2007. Norman Cousins Lecture. Glia as the "bad guys": implications for improving clinical pain control and the clinical utility of opioids. Brain. Behav. Immun 21, 131–146.

Wemmie, J.A., Taugher, R.J., Kreple, C.J., 2013. Acid-sensing ion channels in pain and disease. Nat. Rev. Neurosci 14, 461–471.

Whitcomb, D.C., Block, G.D., 1994. Association of acetaminophen hepatotoxicity with fasting and ethanol use. JAMA 272, 1845–1850.

WHO, 1986. Cancer Pain Relief. WHO, Geneva.

Wiffen, P., Collins, S., McQuay, H., Carroll, D., Jadad, A., Moore, A., 2005. Anticonvulsant drugs for acute and chronic pain. Cochrane. Database. Syst. Rev CD001133.

Wiffen, P.J., Derry, S., Moore, R.A., 2013. Lamotrigine for chronic neuropathic pain and fibromyalgia in adults. Cochrane. Database. Syst. Rev CD006044.

Wittenberg, R.H., Schell, E., Krehan, G., Maeumbaed, R., Runge, H., Schluter, P., et al., 2006. First-dose analgesic effect of the cyclo-oxygenase-2 selective inhibitor lumiracoxib in osteoarthritis of the knee: a randomized, double-blind, placebo-controlled comparison with celecoxib [NCT00267215]. Arthritis. Res. Ther 8, R35.

Woolf, C.J., Ma, Q., 2007. Nociceptors--noxious stimulus detectors. Neuron 55, 353–364.

Wyeth Pharmaceuticals, 2009. RELISTOR (Methylnaltrexone Bromide) Prescribing Information. Wyeth Pharmaceuticals Inc.

Xiao, J.P., Li, A.L., Feng, B.M., Ye, Y., Wang, G.J., 2017. Efficacy and safety of tapentadol immediate release assessment in treatment of moderate to severe pain: a systematic review and meta-analysis. Pain. Med 18, 14–24.

Yaksh, T.L., 2006. Calcium channels as therapeutic targets in neuropathic pain. J. Pain 7, S13–S30.

Zeilhofer, H.U., 2007. Prostanoids in nociception and pain. Biochem. Pharmacol 73, 165–174.

Zhang, J.M., Strong, J.A., 2008. Recent evidence for activity-dependent initiation of sympathetic sprouting and neuropathic pain. Sheng. Li. Xue. Bao 60, 617–627.

Zhang, M., Wang, Y., Geng, J., Zhou, S., Xiao, B., 2019. Mechanically activated piezo channels mediate touch and suppress acute mechanical pain response in mice. Cell. Rep 26, 1419–1431 e4.

Zhuo, M., 2007. Neuronal mechanism for neur'opathic pain. Mol. Pain 3, 14.

Zollner, C., Stein, C., 2007. Opioids. Handb. Exp. Pharmacol 31–63.

Chapter 16

Transcutaneous electrical nerve stimulation and acupuncture

Mark I. Johnson and Mike Cummings

CHAPTER CONTENTS

LEARNING OBJECTIVES

At the end of this chapter, readers will be able to:
1. Overview the use of TENS and acupuncture for pain management, including indications, contraindications and risks. To outline the principles that underpinning various techniques of TENS and acupuncture.
2. Describe the research supporting the analgesic mechanisms of action of TENS and acupuncture.
3. Summarise research evidence on clinical effectiveness for TENS and acupuncture.
4. Discuss why clinical experience of outcome when using TENS and acupuncture sometimes differs from some of the clinical research findings.

Part 1: Transcutaneous electrical nerve stimulation (TENS)

Context

TENS is a noninvasive technique for symptomatic relief of pain (Table 16.1). A portable battery-powered device passes electrical currents across the intact surface of the skin (transcutaneous) via adhesive electrode pads in order to stimulate low-threshold non-nociceptive peripheral afferents (Fig. 16.1). TENS is also used for nonpainful conditions such as postoperative nausea and vomiting, wound and bone healing, incontinence, constipation and dementia (for review see Johnson 2014d). TENS is popular and devices can be purchased without prescription in many countries. Approximately 50% of chronic pain patients who try TENS benefit in the short term.

When used to relieve pain, TENS is either a standalone treatment or can be combined with other treatments. Gladwell et al. (2015, 2016, 2020) suggest that TENS is a complex intervention because patients individualise usage patterns to achieve direct benefits such as reducing pain, distressing sensations associated with muscle tension and medication intake, with indirect benefits such as improving rest, function and well-being. Patient evaluation and education is critical for success, and an initial 30-minute treatment has been shown to help predict TENS responders (Vance et al. 2021). Generally, TENS effects are maximal when the sensation is strong but comfortable. Effects are immediate, which is particularly useful to manage severe breakthrough or incident pain. TENS does not produce side effects associated with drugs, such as sedation, dizziness, nausea and disorientation. Applying TENS for long periods of time does not produce toxicity, alleviating fears of overdose. Interactions with drugs are few, so TENS is often used in combination with analgesic medication to reduce drug dosage, side effects and

TABLE 16.1 Painful conditions commonly treated using TENS

Acute pain	Chronic pain
• Postoperative pain, e.g. thoracotomy • Painful minor surgical procedures • Physical trauma, e.g. sprains, strains and bone fractures • Labour pain • Dysmenorrhoea • Angina pectoris • Orofacial pain	• Chronic primary pain, e.g. chronic widespread pain, fibromyalgia, nonspecific back pain, irritable bowel syndrome and complex regional pain syndrome • Chronic secondary musculoskeletal pain, e.g. osteoarthritis and rheumatoid arthritis • Chronic secondary headache or orofacial pain, e.g. temporomandibular disorders • Chronic postsurgical or posttraumatic pain • Chronic secondary visceral pain arising from ischaemia, thrombosis, obstruction, distension and compression • Chronic neuropathic pain, e.g. poststroke, nerve trauma, or diabetic neuropathy, postamputation pain, postherpetic and trigeminal neuralgia • Chronic cancer-related pain associated with the disease and/or its treatment

costs (Bjordal et al. 2003; Kerai et al. 2014). TENS is most effective when patients administer it as required, following appropriate instruction by a healthcare professional.

Definition

Any technique that delivers electricity across the surface of the skin with the purpose of activating underlying nerves is TENS, although in healthcare, the term 'TENS' is used to describe stimulation using a standard TENS device.

Standard TENS

The features of standard TENS are shown in Table 16.2 and Fig. 16.2. Output specifications differ between manufacturers, with limited impact on physiological effects.

TENS-like devices

A variety of TENS-like devices are available (for review see Johnson 2014c). Some deliver microampere (μA) currents, much lower than a standard TENS device, some use pen-like electrodes and some deliver currents transcranially or transspinally. Critical reviews conclude that manufacturers' claims about TENS-like devices are overambitious and practitioners should use a standard TENS device in the first instance (Johnson 2001, 2014c). The remainder of this chapter will focus on standard TENS and will use the term 'TENS' to refer to a standard TENS device.

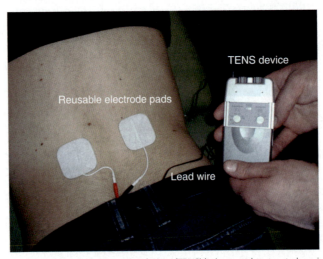

Fig. 16.1 Transcutaneous electrical nerve stimulation *(TENS)* being used to treat chronic low back pain.

TABLE 16.2 The technical specifications of a standard TENS device (pulsed current generator) and accessories

Pulsed current generator (device)	
Dimensions	Small device = 6 × 5 × 2 cm Large device = 12 × 9 × 4 cm (50–250 g)
Cost	£15–150 GBP
Pulse waveform	• Biphasic—symmetrical or asymmetrical • Monophasic
Pulse amplitude	Most devices deliver constant current output which is adjustable between 1 and 50 mA into a 1 kΩ load
Pulse duration	Adjustable between 50 and 500 µs
Pulse frequency (adjustable)	Adjustable between 1 and 250 pps
Pulse pattern	Options include continuous (normal), burst (intermittent trains of pulses), random pulse frequency, alternating pulse frequency, modulated amplitude, modulated frequency and modulated pulse duration
Channels	1 or 2
Additional features on device	Timer Some devices provide a range of preprogrammed settings
Accessories	
Batteries	PP3 (9 V), AA, USB rechargeable
Electrodes	Traditional electrodes—self-adhesive hypoalgesic in various shapes and sizes (e.g. square 5 cm × 5 cm) Wearable electrodes—electrodes woven into garments
Electrode lead wires	Connect device to electrodes Some modern devices use Bluetooth or WiFi interfaces between device and electrodes

Principles underpinning TENS

Electricity has been used to relieve pain since 2500 BC, when electrogenic fish were used to treat painful conditions. The use of medical electricity entered mainstream medical practice in the 18th century, but fell out of favour by the 20th century because of variable clinical results and the development of pharmacological treatments. In 1965, Melzack and Wall provided a physiological rationale for electroanalgesia, followed by clinical observations that chronic pain could be relieved by

electrical stimulation of neurons in skin, spinal cord dorsal columns and periaqueductal grey (Melzack & Wall 1965).

The purpose of TENS is to selectively activate different populations of neurons to initiate physiological responses that lead to pain relief. As the current amplitude is increased, low-threshold non-nociceptive Aβ axons are activated first (Fig. 16.3). The sensation beneath the electrodes is often described as 'tingling' or 'pins and needles' (electrical paraesthesia) with a nonpainful intensity. If current amplitude is increased further, smaller diameter Aδ- and C-fibre afferents (see Chapters 6 and 7) become active and the user experiences a painful sensation, which is undesirable. Activation of Aβ axons without concurrent activation of Aδ and C-fibre afferents is achieved using currents with low amplitude (intensity) and pulse durations of 50 to 500 µs. The rate of action potentials is determined by the pulse frequency. At higher frequencies, nerve impulse generation is limited by the absolute and relative refractory periods for the axon. In theory, TENS frequencies below 250 pps should be optimal.

Most TENS devices produce biphasic electrical pulse waveforms, resulting in zero net current flow between the electrodes, thus preventing skin irritation. Some devices produce monophasic waveforms, whereby the cathode (normally the black lead) is placed proximal to the anode because the cathode activates the axonal membrane and generates the nerve impulse. Currents delivered using TENS tend to remain superficial due to the high impedance of the skin and stimulate cutaneous rather than deep-seated tissue. It is possible to generate muscle contractions by placing electrodes over muscles or muscle efferents.

Clinical technique

The effects produced by TENS depend on location, number and type of electrodes, and electrical characteristics of currents. Protocols in manufacturers' materials may be used as guidance rather than an inflexible regimen. Pulse amplitude is the critical factor for selective recruitment of different neurons. Increasing pulse amplitude results in activation of neurons with higher thresholds of activation and stronger sensations. Two commonly used TENS techniques are *conventional TENS* and *acupuncture-like TENS* (*AL-TENS*) (Table 16.3).

TENS techniques

Conventional TENS (low intensity, high frequency)

The purpose of conventional TENS is to selectively activate peripheral Aβ afferents, leading to reduced onward transmission of nociceptive information in the central nervous system (see 'Mechanism of action'). TENS amplitude is increased to achieve a strong, comfortable, nonpainful

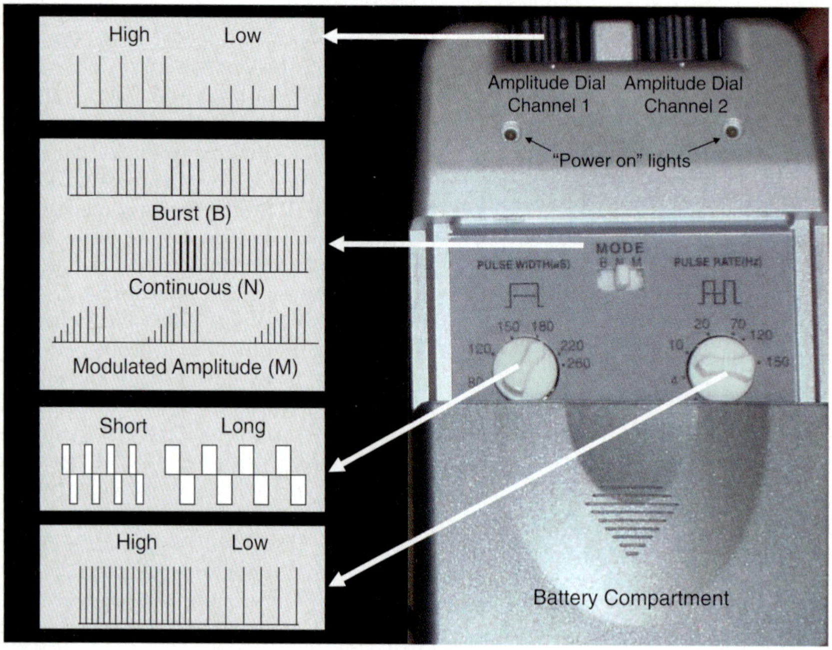

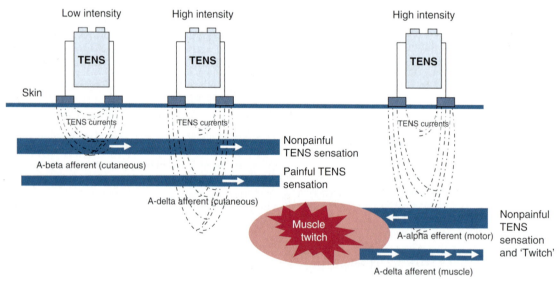

Fig. 16.2 Electrical characteristics of a standard transcutaneous electrical nerve stimulation device.

Fig. 16.3 Fibre recruitment by increasing the amplitude of electrical currents administered during conventional transcutaneous electrical nerve stimulation *(TENS)*.

electrical paraesthesia beneath the electrodes or in the relevant body part. The International Association for the Study of Pain (IASP) previously defined conventional TENS as high frequency (50–100 Hz), low intensity (paraesthesia, not painful), small pulse width (50–200 μs), although in clinical practice, frequencies of approximately 10 to 250 pps are used.

Acupuncture-like TENS

Acupuncture-like TENS (AL-TENS) was first described in the 1970s as a means to harness the mechanisms of action of TENS and acupuncture (Eriksson & Sjölund 1976). IASP defines AL-TENS as 'hyperstimulation' using currents

TABLE 16.3 The characteristics of different TENS techniques

Characteristic	Conventional TENS	AL-TENS
Peripheral action	Generally, stimulates cutaneous non-noxious afferents	Generally, stimulates small diameter cutaneous afferents and/or large diameter motor nerves leading to a muscle twitch and activity in small-diameter muscle afferents
Sensory experience	Nonpainful TENS paraesthesiae (minimal muscle activity)	Strong pulsating TENS sensation with simultaneous muscle twitching
Electrode location	Straddle site of pain (dermatomal) but if not successful main nerve bundles, across the spinal cord or contralateral positions are used	Over muscle belly or motor nerves (myotomal) at site of pain. If not successful contralateral positions, trigger points or acupuncture points are used
Pulse amplitude (intensity)	Low-current amplitude (nonpainful without muscle contraction)	High-current amplitude (nonpainful with mild muscle twitching)
Pulse frequency	High (>5–250 pulses per second) determined by patient preference	Low-frequency pulses (≤5 pulses per second) or low-frequency bursts (trains) of high-frequency pulses (≤5 bursts per second)
Pulse duration	Usually 50–200 μs determined by patient preference	Usually 100–200 μs. Lower pulse width will generate a weaker TENS sensation yet still create muscle twitching
Pulse pattern	Continuous in first instance but determined by patient preference	Burst in first instance, if not successful or uncomfortable amplitude modulated is used
Dose	Generally, used as much and as often as needed with a short break every hour or so	Generally, used for no more than 30 minutes at a time a few times each day as muscle fatigue may develop resulting in delayed onset muscle soreness the following day
Time course of pain relief	Rapid onset and offset of effects. Pain relief tends to be mediated via segmental mechanisms	Rapid onset and delayed offset of effects. Pain relief tends to be mediated via a combination of segmental and extrasegmental mechanisms

TENS, Transcutaneous electrical nerve stimulation.

that are of low frequency (2–4 Hz), higher intensity (to tolerance threshold) and longer pulse width (100–400 μs). In practice, AL-TENS is used to generate strong but nonpainful pulsating sensations and/or muscle twitching, generating impulses in small-diameter afferents from cutaneous and musculoskeletal structures, thus activating descending inhibitory pathways and the release of endogenous opioids in the central nervous system (Johnson 1998, 2014b).

AL-TENS uses single pulses at frequencies below 10 pps (usually 1–4 pps), or intermittent trains or bursts (2–4 Hz) of high-frequency pulses (~100 pps) administered close to the painful site, or over muscles, motor points, acupuncture points (APs) and trigger points. It is claimed that AL-TENS produces prolonged poststimulation effects and is useful for neuropathic pain, pain from deep structures, pain associated with altered skin sensitivity and/or patients resistant to conventional TENS (for review see Francis & Johnson 2011).

Other TENS techniques

TENS terminology is confusing, with a variety of overlapping techniques described in the literature. *Intense TENS* delivers currents at painful intensities for short periods and is used as a counterirritant for brief painful procedures such as wound-dressing changes, suture removal and venepuncture. The terms *acu-TENS* and *transcutaneous electric acupoint stimulation (TEAS)* have been used to describe the application of a variety of types of TENS devices to APs as a noninvasive alternative to acupuncture.

Principles of electrode placement

TENS electrodes are made of knitted stainless-steel fibres with adhesive gel. Sizes vary but 5 × 5 cm^2 is most common (see Fig. 16.1). Some evidence suggests that small electrodes (0.8 × 0.8 cm^2) are more comfortable for thin fat layers (0.25 cm) and stimulating superficial nerves, while larger electrodes (4.1 × 4.1 cm²) are more comfortable for thicker fat layers (2 cm) and stimulating deeper nerves (1.1 cm) (Alon et al. 1994). Glove, sock and belt electrodes are also available, and recently, array electrodes have been developed to target stimulation more precisely.

It is necessary to site electrodes on healthy skin with functioning nerves and normal sensation, so a sharp-blunt skin test should be conducted before use. Electrodes can be placed up to ~15 cm apart and a dual-channel device with four electrodes used for large areas of pain or simultaneous treatment of two body sites. During conventional TENS, electrodes are positioned so that TENS paraesthesiae cover the pain (Fig. 16.4). When this is not possible, TENS can be positioned at alternative sites, including:

- over main nerves proximal to the site of pain (especially useful to project TENS sensations distally)
- on skin from an ipsilateral or contralateral dermatome
- paravertebrally at the spinal segment related to the pain location.

Electrodes should not be placed over:

- skin with tactile allodynia or dysaesthesia, for example, because it may aggravate the pain, although paradoxically this is not always the case
- an open wound

- frail skin due to eczema, radiotherapy or reconstructive surgery
- the abdomen of a pregnant woman
- the anterior neck, because stimulation of baroreceptors at the carotid sinus may cause a hypotensive response and stimulation of laryngeal nerves may cause laryngeal spasm
- the eyes, because it may increase intraocular pressure
- internally except in specific circumstances and with a specially designed device for dental analgesia or incontinence
- through the chest using electrodes placed on the anterior and posterior thorax as this interferes with intercostal muscle activity, leading to severely compromised breathing.

As neuropathic pain conditions often present with hypersensitivity, electrodes should initially be placed over peripheral nerves proximal to the pain. Likewise, electrodes may be placed along the main nerves proximal to the site of pain, if TENS sensation cannot be produced at the site of pain because of diminished skin sensitivity resulting from nerve damage (e.g. numbness following peripheral neuropathy). For postoperative pain, 'strip-like' electrodes can be placed either side of the incision scar, provided there is no hypersensitivity. In phantom limb pain, it is possible to place electrodes along the main nerve trunk in the residual limb to project TENS sensation

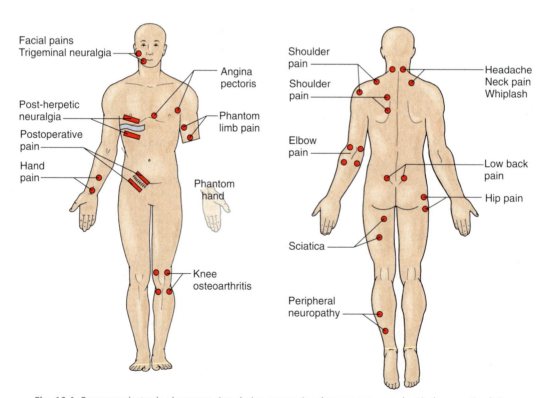

Fig. 16.4 Common electrode placement sites during conventional transcutaneous electrical nerve stimulation.

peripherally. Paravertebral electrode positions at spinal segments related to the pain can also be used. For example, during childbirth, electrodes are positioned on the back at spinal segments with afferents from cervix and lower uterine segment for the first stage of labour, and afferents from pelvis and perineum for the second stage.

Principles of choosing electrical characteristics

Much has been written about optimal settings for different conditions, but evidence of a relationship between pulse frequency or pattern and analgesia or diagnosis is sparse and inconsistent. The critical determinant of outcome is pulse amplitude (intensity). Studies using healthy pain-free human volunteers show that strong nonpainful TENS is superior to barely perceptible TENS (Lazarou et al. 2009; Moran et al. 2011). Electrophysiological research suggests that different TENS frequencies activate different neurophysiological mechanisms at submotor thresholds (for review see Johnson 2014b; Sluka & Walsh 2016), but this may not translate into differential outcomes in humans. Systematic reviews of studies using pain-free volunteers exposed to experimentally induced pain suggest that pulse frequency does not influence hypoalgesia per se during strong nonpainful TENS (Chen et al. 2008; Claydon et al. 2011). Patients appear to have individual preferences for electrical characteristics of TENS based on comfort rather than the amount of pain relief. Encouraging patients to experiment with TENS settings may produce the most effective outcome.

Clinical practice and dosage

Pain relief with conventional TENS is rapid in onset and offset. Long-term users report maximal benefit during stimulation and administer TENS for many hours each day. Electrodes may be left in situ and the device attached to a trouser belt to administer TENS intermittently throughout the day on an as-needed basis.

The intensity of TENS fades due to habituation, so users increase amplitude to maintain a strong nonpainful sensation. Some patients report that TENS effects wear off with repeated use (i.e. tolerance to TENS), and repeated use generates opioid tolerance in animals, with cholecystokinin and N-methyl-D-aspartate (NMDA) receptors being involved (DeSantana et al. 2010; Hingne & Sluka 2008). Patterns of pulsed currents using modulated and random modes have been shown to reduce habituation and tolerance (Avendano-Coy et al. 2019; Chen & Johnson 2009; Liebano et al. 2011; Lima et al. 2015). Changing electrode placement or temporarily withdrawing TENS may also help. *Sequential TENS*, i.e. strong nonpainful TENS punctuated with more intense TENS using muscle twitching, may be clinically useful to manage background pain with incidents of breakthrough pain.

Ideally, new TENS patients are given a supervised trial, to ensure TENS does not aggravate pain and to teach safe technique (Box 16.1). A 30-minute in-clinic trial of TENS treatment predicts longer-term outcome in women with fibromyalgia and may be generalisable to other conditions (Vance et al. 2021). Patients should be competent operating the device on leaving the clinic and have a point of contact if they encounter problems. Patients are advised to administer TENS as a 30-minute treatment the first few times and use it as much as they like thereafter. They are advised to experiment with all settings to achieve the most comfortable stimulation each time. Children as young as 4 years old are able to understand TENS, and short-duration treatments have been useful for dental pain and minor procedures such as wound dressing and venepuncture.

BOX 16.1 **Safe TENS technique**

1. Check contraindications and test skin for normal sensation.
2. Adjust initial transcutaneous electrical nerve stimulation (TENS) settings when device is switched off as follows:
   - Pulse pattern (mode) = continuous (normal)
   - Pulse frequency (rate) = mid-range (80–100 pps)
   - Pulse duration (width) = mid-range (100–200 μs)
   - Timer (if available) = continuous
3. Connect electrode lead wires to electrodes.
4. Position electrodes on skin at site of pain or over main nerve bundle.
5. Connect electrode lead wires to TENS device.
6. Switch TENS device on and slowly increase intensity until patient reports first TENS 'tingling' sensation.
7. Ask patient whether the sensation is acceptable.
8. Slowly increase intensity until patient reports a strong but nonpainful TENS sensation.
9. Check that the sensation is acceptable and monitor patient for any signs of an autonomic response.
10. Allow patient to experiment with device settings by:
    - reducing amplitude so TENS is barely perceptible, then
    - change the device setting and then increase pulse amplitude to a strong nonpainful level.
11. Instruct patient to adjust duration of stimulation according to need.

Contraindications, precautions and adverse events

Safety guidelines for TENS are available in Australia, the United Kingdom and the United States. An excellent web-based resource is http://www.electrotherapy.org. Active implants such as pacemakers and ventricular assist devices (*artificial hearts*) are absolute contraindications, although TENS has been used in these situations following approval from the medical specialist. TENS interferes with internal cardiac defibrillators, producing inadvertent shocks, and generates artefacts on foetal monitoring equipment (Carlson et al. 2009). Patients are advised not to administer TENS over the abdomen during pregnancy; on the neck or head if they have epilepsy; or close to bleeding tissue, malignancy (except in palliative care) or active epiphysis. TENS should be used with care over metal implants, as there is a case report of skin burn after interferential therapy (Ford et al. 2005). TENS appears to be safe when used with stents, percutaneous central catheters or drainage systems, although consideration is given to mechanical stresses resulting from TENS-induced muscle contractions. TENS is used with caution for patients on an anticoagulant treatment and not delivered close to transdermal drug delivery systems because they may iontophoretically drive the drug through the skin, leading to drug toxicity. TENS must not be used while operating hazardous equipment, including motor vehicles.

Serious adverse events from TENS are rare. There is a single case report of respiratory compromise due to electrodes positioned on the anterior and posterior chest, a single case report of repetitive epileptic seizures in an individual with coexisting psychomotor disturbances and a few cases of minor electrical burns due to inappropriate technique (for review see Johnson 2014a). Minor skin irritation is more common and necessary to monitor in all patients. TENS worsens pain in some individuals and may produce a vasovagal response, leading to nausea, dizziness and even syncope.

Mechanism of action

TENS generates impulses in low-threshold peripheral afferents that are conducted to brainstem nuclei (e.g. nucleus gracilis and nucleus cuneatus), thalamus and somatosensory cortex. The resultant paraesthesic sensation is due to ectopic impulses generated by TENS. Pain relief from TENS is due to peripheral, spinal and supraspinal actions.

Peripheral mechanisms

Electrodes deliver currents through the skin that generate impulses travelling along axons in both directions (Fig. 16.5). Impulses travelling towards the periphery extinguish impulses arising from sensory receptors activated by natural stimuli (e.g. arising from nociceptors, mechanoreceptors and thermoreceptors) via a 'busy line' effect (Walsh et al. 1998).

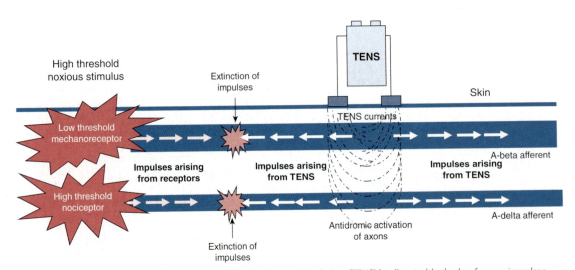

Fig. 16.5 Axonal activation during transcutaneous electrical nerve stimulation *(TENS)* leading to blockade of nerve impulses travelling in peripheral afferents.

Spinal mechanisms

Conventional TENS is used to activate non-noxious afferents, which branch as they enter the central nervous system. They synapse with interneurons, which release inhibitory neurotransmitters (e.g. γ-amino butyric acid (GABA) and met-enkephalin), inhibiting central transmission of nociceptive information and reducing central sensitisation (Ma & Sluka 2001) (Fig. 16.6). This mechanism is rapid in onset and offset, and maximal when delivered to somatic receptive fields of the central nociceptive transmission cells (i.e. segmental). At higher intensities, longer duration poststimulation inhibition of central nociceptor cells occurs for up to 2 hours (Sandkühler et al. 1997).

Supraspinal mechanisms

Stronger stimulation using low-frequency single pulses (i.e. AL-TENS) produces a pulsate sensation in the skin and may generate muscle twitching. Bursts of high-frequency pulses can produce a similar effect and are more comfortable for the patient. In both instances, phasic muscle twitching generates impulses in muscle afferents (e.g. proprioceptors) resulting in activity in descending inhibitory pathways (e.g. periaqueductal grey and ventromedial medulla), which inhibit central nociceptive transmission in the spinal cord (for review see Johnson 2014b; Fig. 16.7; Chapter 7). Stronger and longer lasting inhibition of central nociceptive transmission occurs when muscle rather than skin afferents are activated (Radhakrishnan & Sluka 2005). Evidence suggests that low-frequency TENS involves μ-opioid receptors, and high-frequency TENS involves δ-opioid receptors (Kalra et al. 2001). GABA is a key neurotransmitter for conventional TENS, although cholinergic, adrenergic and serotonergic systems may also be involved (for review see Johnson 2014b).

TENS delivered at intensities at or above the pain threshold (i.e. intense TENS) activates Aδ afferents, leading to pain relief through counterirritation in a process referred to as conditioned pain modulation (CPM) via diffuse noxious inhibitory pathways (Chapters 6 and 7; Morton et al. 1988). TENS also activates peripheral parasympathetic and sympathetic efferents, leading to the release of acetylcholine and noradrenaline at autonomic effectors, respectively. There has been surprisingly little research into the effects of TENS on the autonomic nervous system and studies are conflicting (for review see Johnson 2014d).

Clinical research: benefits and harms

There is a long-standing debate whether public health systems (e.g. the National Health Service, UK) or private healthcare insurance (e.g. Center for Medicare Services, USA) should offer TENS because clinical guidelines appear contradictory (for review see Johnson 2021). For example, the National Institute of Health and Care Excellence (NICE, UK) advises against TENS for chronic primary pain (NICE 2021) or nonspecific chronic low back pain (NICE 2016) but does recommend TENS for osteoarthritis (NICE 2014) and rheumatoid arthritis (NICE 2018). Guidelines are generated according to traditional pathology-based classifications of pain which restricts the quantity of randomised controlled trials (RCTs) included for evaluation, resulting in concern about the validity of some 'expert panel' evaluations. For example, the Therapeutics and Technology Assessment Subcommittee of the American Academy of Neurology concluded that TENS should not be recommended for the treatment of chronic low back pain based on 'Level A evidence' (Dubinsky & Miyasaki 2010). However, this Level A evidence consisted of 114 participants receiving TENS and 87 receiving sham TENS. A rebuttal stated 'It seems unreasonable that the effectiveness of TENS, and subsequent clinical recommendations, can be established from studies with so few participants' (Johnson & Walsh 2010).

Ongoing uncertainty about offering TENS is scandalous considering there are over 350 published RCTs and over 100 systematic reviews, including Cochrane reviews (Johnson et al. 2022b). The majority of systematic reviews are inconclusive resulting in an 'efficacy-impasse' due to a variety of factors, including methodological challenges associated with delivering robust RCTs (for in-depth reviews see Bennett et al. 2011; Johnson 2021). A summary of the current status of clinical research on TENS is provided below.

TENS for any type of pain

It has been argued that RCTs from specific pain conditions could be pooled for meta-analysis because of commonalities in the way that pain presents and because TENS acts via nonspecific therapeutic neuromodulation irrespective of pathology (Johnson et al. 2019). The largest meta-analysis on TENS undertaken to date found moderate-certainty evidence of lower pain intensity of clinical importance during or immediately after TENS compared with placebo, irrespective of the type of pain (i.e. acute or chronic) and was part of a systematic review of 381 RCTs and 24,532 participants (Johnson et al. 2022a). The Meta-TENS study found low or very low-certainty evidence for other outcomes and comparisons including adverse events.

TENS for acute pain

The most recent Cochrane review found tentative evidence that TENS given as a sole treatment reduced the intensity of a variety of acute pain conditions compared with placebo (Johnson et al. 2015). A subgroup analysis within the

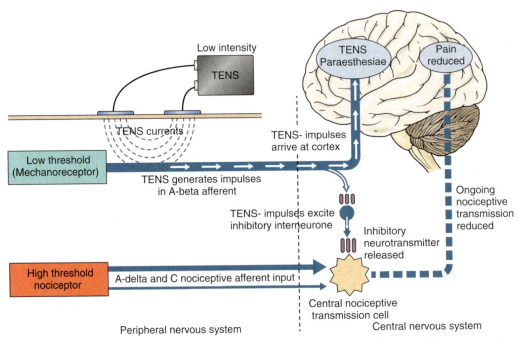

Fig. 16.6 The mechanism of action of conventional transcutaneous electrical nerve stimulation *(TENS)* ▮▮▮-neurotransmitters.

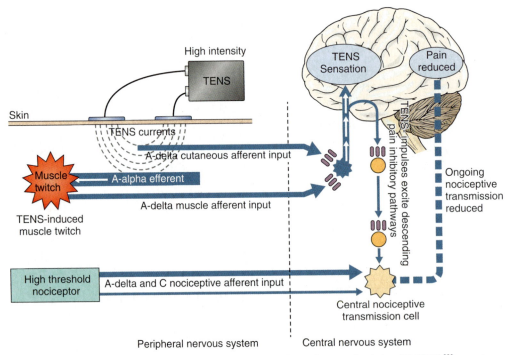

Fig. 16.7 The mechanism of action of acupuncture-like transcutaneous electrical nerve stimulation *(AL-TENS)* ▮▮▮-neurotransmitters.

Meta-TENS study provided moderate-certainty evidence of lower acute pain intensity during TENS compared with placebo (Johnson et al. 2022a).

TENS for postoperative pain

Systematic reviews in the 1990s concluded that TENS was not effective in postoperative pain (Carroll et al. 1996). In 2003, Bjordal et al.'s meta-analysis of 21 RCTs (1350 patients) with a subgroup analysis of 11 trials (964 patients) found larger reductions in analgesic consumption in RCTs using adequate TENS technique (i.e. strong stimulation at the pain site) (Bjordal et al. 2003). Recently, a systematic review and meta-analysis suggested that TENS is beneficial as an adjunct to alleviate pain following pulmonary and cardiothoracic surgery (Zhou et al. 2020). A critical review of TENS for postoperative pain concluded that TENS reduces analgesic consumption and improves pain, pulmonary function, and nausea and vomiting when used as an adjunct to core treatment (Johnson 2017).

TENS for labour pain

Systematic reviews in the 1990s concluded that TENS was not effective for labour pain (Carroll et al. 1997). The most recent Cochrane review published in 2009 was inconclusive, although the use of TENS at home in early labour was not assessed (Bedwell et al. 2011; Dowswell et al. 2009). Recently, a systematic review of 26 RCTs (3348 parturients) included a meta-analysis that found small but significant reductions in pain intensity during TENS (Thuvarakan et al. 2020). NICE guidelines recommend that TENS should not be offered to women in established labour, although it may be beneficial in the early stages of labour (NICE 2007).

TENS for other types of acute pain

TENS may be beneficial for a wide range of conditions associated with acute pain, including orofacial pain, fractured ribs, acute musculoskeletal pain, painful surgical procedures (e.g. dental pain), angina pectoris and dysmenorrhoea. There is a paucity of evidence for efficacy.

A systematic review of three RCTs evaluating TENS for acute low back pain was inconclusive (Binny et al. 2019), although a network meta-analysis to compare conservative care strategies provided moderate-quality evidence that TENS improved physical function for women with pregnancy-related low back pain compared with placebo (Chen et al. 2019).

The most recent Cochrane review evaluating TENS for dysmenorrhoea was published in 2002 and concluded that high-frequency but not low-frequency TENS was superior to placebo, although this was based on an analysis that pooled too few participants (7 RCTs, 213 patients) (Proctor et al. 2002). Recently, the authors of a meta-analysis of four RCTs (260 patients) claimed that pain intensity during TENS was lower than sham TENS for women with primary dysmenorrhoea, but again there were too few participants to have any degree of certainty (Arik et al. 2020).

NICE guidelines recommend that TENS should not be offered to patients for the management of stable angina (NICE 2011).

TENS for chronic pain

In 2019, an overview of eight Cochrane reviews (51 RCTs, 2895 participants) was inconclusive (Gibson et al. 2019). Reviewers were reluctant to meta-analyse data due to concerns about methodological and clinical heterogeneity. However, a subgroup analysis within the Meta-TENS study provided moderate-certainty evidence of lower pain intensity during TENS compared with placebo for chronic pain (Johnson et al. 2022a).

TENS for chronic musculoskeletal pain

A systematic review of 32 RCTs on TENS and 6 studies on percutaneous electrical nerve stimulation (PENS) for chronic musculoskeletal pain included a meta-analysis that pooled data from 29 RCTs (1227 participants) and concluded that both TENS and PENS were effective for chronic musculoskeletal pain (Johnson & Martinson 2007).

TENS for chronic nonspecific back and neck pain

The most recent Cochrane review evaluating TENS for chronic nonspecific low back pain was inconclusive (4 RCTs, 585 patients) (Khadilkar et al. 2008). Recent systematic reviews have been contradictory (Jauregui et al. 2016; Wu et al. 2018).

The most recent Cochrane review on TENS for neck pain was inconclusive, because it was not possible to pool data, although immediate posttreatment pain relief favouring TENS compared with placebo was reported by the authors of four of the included RCTs (Kroeling et al. 2013). Recently, a systematic review of seven RCTs (651 participants) found insufficient data for meta-analysis and concluded that there was very low-certainty evidence of a difference between TENS and sham TENS (Martimbianco et al. 2019).

TENS for osteoarthritis

The most recent Cochrane review on osteoarthritic knee pain (18 RCTs, 813 patients) was inconclusive (Rutjes et al. 2009). However, a meta-analysis of 7 RCTs administering TENS at optimal doses found that TENS produced short-term reductions in pain of 22.2 mm (95% confidence interval (CI): 18.1–26.3) on a 100-mm visual analogue scale (VAS) (Bjordal et al. 2007), and this magnitude of effect was confirmed in 2015 in a meta-analysis of 14 RCTs comparing TENS with control groups (Chen et al. 2015).

TENS for rheumatoid arthritis

The most recent Cochrane review of TENS for rheumatoid arthritis of the hand (3 RCTs, 78 people) was published in 2003 and was inconclusive (Brosseau et al. 2003). There have been no recent systematic reviews. Clinical practice guidelines recommended the use of TENS for short-term pain relief (NICE 2018; Ottawa Panel 2004).

TENS for fibromyalgia

A Cochrane review of eight RCTs in 2017 found insufficient evidence efficacy for fibromyalgia (Johnson et al. 2017), although the authors of a systematic review of eight RCTs published 2 years later concluded that TENS was effective (Megia Garcia et al. 2019). Since then, a high-quality RCT of approximately 100 participants in each trial arm found that TENS was superior to placebo TENS for alleviating movement-evoked pain and fatigue in fibromyalgia (Dailey et al. 2019)

TENS for neuropathic pain

A Cochrane review of 15 studies (724 participants) and pooled data from 5 studies (six comparisons, 207 participants with various neuropathic conditions) found a mean postintervention difference in effect size favouring TENS of −1.58 (95% CI −2.08 to −1.09, six comparisons from five studies), although this was judged to be very low-quality evidence (Gibson et al. 2017).

TENS for cancer pain

A Cochrane review of two studies on cancer-related pain was inconclusive (Hurlow et al. 2012), although a feasibility study provided preliminary evidence that TENS may be of benefit for cancer-induced bone pain (Bennett et al. 2010).

TENS for other chronic pains

Generally, there is a paucity of RCTs to determine efficacy for sickle cell pain (Pal et al. 2020), spinal cord injury (Harvey et al. 2016), multiple sclerosis (Amatya et al., 2018), spasticity (Fernandez-Tenorio et al. 2019) or chronic recurrent headache (i.e. migraine and tension-type headache) (Bronfort et al. 2004), although a recent meta-analysis suggested that TENS may be effective for the management of migraine (Tao et al. 2018).

Conclusion

TENS has been used to provide immediate and short-term relief of any type of acute and chronic pain since the 1970s. Strong physiological evidence supports that TENS reduces activity and excitability of nociceptive transmission neurons (i.e. physiological plausibility). Clinical literature supports the view that TENS is beneficial and safe for some individuals (i.e. clinical experience). There has been a long-standing debate about clinical efficacy due to systematic reviews that are generally inconclusive resulting in some expert panels recommending that TENS should not be paid for by public (government) funds (Johnson 2021). Nevertheless, some large meta-analyses demonstrate superiority of TENS over placebo, so TENS should be considered as an adjunct to core treatment.

Part 2: Acupuncture

Context

Therapeutic needling techniques may date back more than 5000 years. Ötzi, the Tyrolean iceman, is the most well persevered human mummy ever found in Europe (Dorfer 1998; Dorfer et al. 1999). He has 61 tattoos that may have been applied for acupuncture-like therapeutic purposes, possibly pain relief, 3 millennia before the first recorded use in China. They were produced by superficial piercing of the skin with a needle made from bone followed by the application of charcoal. Several locations of these tattoos were in areas where Ötzi may have suffered pain from degenerative joint disease.

Such high-threshold stimulation techniques have developed independently in human communities across the globe. In the case of a more persistent discomfort, many cultures use local and regional massage applied deeply and vigorously, even though doing so may temporarily exacerbate the discomfort. This is likely to be conditioned behaviour resulting from the analgesic effect of somatic sensory stimulation. It is easy to hypothesise a progression of therapeutic techniques, ultimately resulting in piercing the skin, fascia and muscle at a site of persistent pain. It may be that treatment of pain through pressure and piercing at the location of symptoms became recognised and accepted as a method of treating pain associated with myofascial tissues. Over time these locations were given names such as acupressure points, APs, myofascial trigger points (MTrPs), tender points and muscle knots. In some parts of the world, people developed superficial techniques of scratching or cauterising the skin, whereas in the Far and Middle East, the technique of acupuncture developed (Cummings 2004).

Definitions

Traditional Chinese acupuncture (TCA)

Acupuncture techniques became part of the medical system in China around 2000 years ago when they were adopted and documented together with the techniques and remedies handed down within families and communities for many generations (Buck 2015; Unschuld 2016).

Acupuncture using metal needles does not seem to have developed in China before 168 BCE, according to silk scrolls found in the Han Tomb No. 3 at Mawangdui, Changsha, in the early 1970s (Bai & Baron 2001). These scrolls described meridians and the use of moxibustion, but there was no mention of APs or needling. However, within a span of less than 200 years, a comprehensive system of needle therapy had been documented and interwoven into the cultural and philosophical backdrop of ancient China (Unschuld 2016).

The *bian shi*, or sharpened stones claimed by some to represent the earliest forms of acupuncture, may have been used therapeutically to prick the body (Ma 1992). However, it seems unlikely that the sophisticated acupuncture system that developed in the Han dynasty grew out of these primitive roots (P.U. Unschuld, 2018, personal communication).

A system of lines running from the chest to the hand, the hand to the face, the face to the foot and the foot back to the chest were developed. It has been argued that these meridians, or channels, were based on early anatomical studies of blood vessels (Shaw 2014; Shaw & McLennan 2016). An influential Chinese physician in the early 20th century, Cheng Dan'an, rejected the point positions based on blood vessels in favour of nerves (Andrews 2014). Whether the lines were based on blood vessels, nerves or another system, the locations (points) where needles were inserted occurred along these meridians.

Dry needling

Dry needling (DN) was developed as a therapeutic technique that focused on the importance of the needle effect rather than the effect of an injected substance. Lewit was the first to write about the needle effect in myofascial pain (Lewit 1979). Prior to this, the accepted treatments for myofascial pain consisted of manual therapy or injection (Lewit & Simons 1984; Steindler 1940; Travell & Rinzler 1952). With the advent of the systematic review of evidence, it became clear that the injected substance might not affect the outcome of treatment, so the use of a needle may have been the key component of either DN or injection (Cummings & White 2001). While DN initially utilised hypodermic needles (Hong 1994), the much less traumatic filiform acupuncture

needles are currently used. The principal targets for DN are MTrPs, although more contemporary practice has seen an expansion of the targets for DN and an increasing overlap between DN and acupuncture techniques.

Western medical acupuncture

The term Western medical acupuncture (WMA) was first introduced over 20 years ago to differentiate a developing system of needle therapy with a basis in Western medical science (Filshie & Cummings 1999). WMA is defined as: 'a therapeutic modality involving the insertion of fine needles; it is an adaptation of Chinese acupuncture using current knowledge of anatomy, physiology and pathology, and the principles of evidence-based medicine' (White & Editorial Board of Acupuncture in Medicine 2009). WMA principally focusses on trigger point needling or DN of local tissues, together with segmental or regional acupuncture (Macdonald et al. 1983), and takes into account the central and systemic effects of acupuncture needling (Cummings 2016; White et al. 2018).

Theoretical overlaps between these approaches

DN is a practice that appears to have developed independently from the popularity and acceptance of TCA in the West. WMA developed out of a scientific evaluation of TCA and then adopted MTrPs as a target for needling (Lapeer & Monga 1986; Macdonald et al. 1983; Melzack 1981; Travell & Simons 1983). There is some overlap between MTrPs and APs (Travell & Simons 1983) and a strong similarity between meridian paths and pain referral patterns from MTrPs (Dorsher 2009), but it is difficult to equate TCA and DN. Indeed, DN techniques distinct from TCA have been adopted in China (Jin et al. 2020), where some intriguing and novel research on MTrPs is currently being published. WMA spans the conceptual divide between TCA and DN by combining both MTrPs and APs as sites for therapeutic needling.

Principles underpinning acupuncture

Point selection

The two main approaches to point selection in WMA are DN of trigger points and segmental acupuncture (Cummings 2016). The latter is defined as the technique of needling an area of the tissue innervated by the same spinal segment as the structure under treatment (Filshie & Cummings 1999). Nerve signals created by needling travel into the same segments of the spinal cord as the nociceptive signals from the area of the body being treated, thus maximising the potential for sensory modulation.

Based on neurophysiological and clinical evidence (Bowsher 1998; Ceccherelli et al. 1998; Chapman et al. 1977; Lundeberg et al. 1987, 1989; Sato et al. 1993; White 1999), the principle in point selection is to stimulate the tissue as close as is practical to the seat of the pathology, or at least within the same innervated-related segment. Trigger points, tender points or APs can be chosen for treatment according to the needling approach.

If the key element of the somatic pathology is an MTrP, this is arguably the only point that it is necessary to treat. In most other cases, the analgesia afforded by local needling may be enhanced by using additional points at a distance from the pathology. Distant points may be chosen because they stimulate the appropriate related segment, or because they are conveniently located and are likely to generate the desired needling sensation. In individual cases, point selection may be modified by the need to avoid local conditions, e.g. skin infection, ulceration, moles, tumours and varicosities; or to avoid regional conditions such as hydrostatic oedema, lymphoedema, anaesthetic or hyperaesthetic areas, or ischaemic tissues. As a general rule, therapeutic needling should be performed in healthy tissue.

Clinical technique

Needle technique

Sterile, single-use, disposable needles should always be used. In most cases, acupuncture needling involves stimulation of muscle tissue and possibly fascial planes between muscle tissue, which produces a characteristic sensation often described as a dull, diffuse ache, pressure, swelling or numbness, which can be referred some distance from the point of stimulation. Needling of other tissues of the soma, such as skin, ligament, tendon, periosteum and the fascial covering of muscle, produces relatively localised and often sharp sensations, although there appear to be differences with age, particularly with periosteal needling. Rapid insertion through the skin and superficial layers minimises discomfort for the patient. Practitioners who are learning the technique find that the use of an introducer facilitates a rapid, often painless insertion through skin. If an introducer is not used, the practitioner stretches the skin over the point during insertion. Once through the skin, the needle should be carefully advanced to the desired position and depth and is then stimulated by rotation back and forth combined with a varying degree of 'lift and thrust' (slight withdrawal and reinsertion) until the desired sensation is achieved. If constant stimulation of the needle is required, a specifically designed electroacupuncture device can be used to deliver electrical impulses. Pulse frequency is most commonly applied at low (2 Hz) or intermediate (10–15 Hz)

frequencies and intensities of 1–6 mA, provided the pulse width is approximately 100 to 200 μs.

DN of MTrPs involves a very similar procedure, although the practitioner will often lift and thrust the needle (fast-in and fast-out technique) to a greater degree and with a variation in needle direction, aiming to hit the MTrP precisely. When the needle directly impinges on an MTrP, a local twitch response is often seen or felt in the associated taut band of muscle, and the symptoms derived from that point are usually reproduced.

In clinical practice, a wide variety of needling techniques and depth have been described. Superficial needling of APs is common in Japanese forms of acupuncture and Baldry described a superficial needling technique exclusively over MTrPs (Baldry 2005). Periosteal needling was first described by Mann (1992, 1998), although he, as most Western practitioners after him, used a variety of techniques. As suggested above, muscle is the most common site of stimulation. Depth and strength of needling in this tissue range from brief, superficial stimulation of the muscle surface to deep, repetitive intramuscular stimulation. The latter is not uncommon in Chinese acupuncture, but is also promoted by some practitioners in the West, in particular Gunn, who favoured targeting motor points and paraspinal muscles (Gunn 1989, 1996).

Clinical aspects

There is a range of responses to WMA or DN treatment, from no effect in 5% or 10% of the population, to profound analgesia and improved well-being, in a similar proportion (Brockhaus & Elger 1990). Patient selection will influence success, and a healthy patient with a short-lived myofascial pain syndrome is much more likely to have a beneficial outcome than a debilitated patient with a chronic, ill-defined and complex chronic pain problem.

It is difficult to define a 'dose' for needling (White et al. 2008), because a judicious single needle insertion may have the same effect as 10 or more needles left in place for 20 minutes, and similar strength, sequential treatments often have increasing potency in early stages of a course of treatment. Experimental work appears to support a dose–response relationship for sensory stimulation (Lundeberg & Lund 2016), but it is unlikely to be linear and recent meta-analysis has not been able to identify exceptional acupuncture responders within a very large dataset drawn from clinical trials (Foster et al. 2020). There is probably a stepwise increase in potency from 1 to 5 in the following list:

1. superficial, heterosegmental needling with minimal sensation
2. superficial, segmental needling with minimal sensation
3. deep, heterosegmental needling with strong sensation
4. deep, segmental needling with strong sensation
5. deep, segmental needling with electrical stimulation sufficient to cause muscle contraction.

While needling is likely to do more than simply offer pain relief, the effect from treatment is most easily appreciated in terms of analgesia. There may be little or no effect after the first session, as the practitioner will usually start with a limited treatment to avoid aggravation of symptoms in people sensitive to needling. The initial response is seen within the first 72 hours after treatment, and its onset is often not perceived until the day after needling. Repeat treatments are performed either bi-weekly or weekly, and the interval can be lengthened with the response. Typically, there is a progressive increase in the quality and duration of the effect following repeated sessions. In chronic pain states, symptoms control can be maintained for some patients with relatively infrequent treatments, perhaps every 4 to 6 weeks.

Contraindications, precautions and adverse events

Safety aspects of therapeutic needling with filiform needles have been studied extensively (Lin et al. 2019; White 2004; Witt et al. 2009). The principles apply equally to DN (Boyce et al. 2020; Brady et al. 2014). Most adverse events from DN and acupuncture are minor and serious adverse events are rare.

The most important adverse event to consider when needling in the region of the neck, back or chest is pneumothorax. This is particularly relevant when needling points in the shoulder girdle muscles overlying the thorax such as trapezius, rhomboid major and minor, levator scapulae, latissimus dorsi, pectoralis major and minor. The estimated incidence of clinically apparent pneumothorax after needling in these areas is 1.75 per million treatments (Lin et al. 2019).

Other main categories of adverse events are infection and trauma. In the past, the most prevalent infection related to needling was hepatitis B, but with widespread use of disposable needles, avoidance of needlestick injuries and implementation of contaminated sharps disposal, hepatitis B cases related to therapeutic needling have almost disappeared in modern medical environments (Walsh 2001).

Inoculation of bacteria from the skin surface is very rare cause of infection because of the size and shape of the fine filiform needle tip (Hoffman 2001). The risk is likely to be greatest where there are surgical implants close to the skin surface. There is one known case report of glenohumeral joint infection following acupuncture (Kirschenbaum & Rizzo 1997).

Safety is often used as a reason for employing imaging techniques during needling; however, this may give a false sense of security since fine needles cannot be visualised all the time. One report of cardiac tamponade following ultrasound guided trigger point injection of pectoralis major may illustrate this (Jung et al. 2014).

Many practitioners worry about using acupuncture techniques in patients with coagulopathies, but serious bleeding-related adverse events are extremely rare. For example, there is only one reported case of compartment syndrome in the literature in a patient taking warfarin (Smith et al. 1986).

Mechanism of action

Mechanisms of needling

The acute analgesic effects of acupuncture are mediated principally through stimulation of the peripheral nervous system and can thus be abolished by local anaesthetic blockade (Chiang et al. 1973). In particular, stimulation of Aδ or type III afferents has been implicated as the key component in producing acupuncture-related analgesia (Chung et al. 1984). The therapeutic effects of needling interventions are divided into three categories based on the area influenced: local (peripheral), segmental (spinal cord) and general (brainstem) (Fig. 16.8).

Local (peripheral) effects

Local effects are mediated through antidromic stimulation of high-threshold afferent nerves, in the same way as the 'triple response' (Lewis 1927). Release of trophic and vasoactive neuropeptides, including neuropeptide Y (NPY), calcitonin gene-related peptide (CGRP) and vasoactive intestinal peptide (VIP), has been found following acupuncture in patients with xerostomia (Dawidson et al. 1998a, b). It is likely that the release of CGRP and VIP from peripheral nerves results in enhanced circulation and wound healing in rats (Jansen et al. 1989a, b). Equivalent sensory stimulation has proved effective in humans (Lundeberg et al. 1988).

Increased circulation resulting from nerve stimulation is an important local effect of acupuncture. In rats, it appears to be principally mediated by the release of CGRP (Sato et al. 2000). However, the effect of acupuncture on muscle blood flow may not rely solely on nerve stimulation (Shinbara et al. 2008). Under normal circumstances, in healthy subjects, blood flow in muscle and skin is increased by needling muscle points and less affected by needling skin (Sandberg et al. 2003). However, this situation may be reversed if the subject is very sensitive, for example, in patients with fibromyalgia (Sandberg et al.

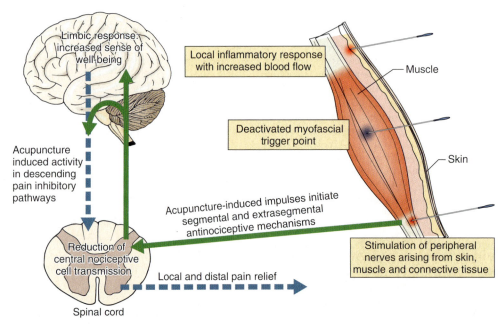

Fig. 16.8 An overview of the mechanism of action of manual acupuncture.

2004). The increase in muscle and skin blood flow following local needling of muscles in patients with work-related trapezius myalgia appears to be lower than in healthy individuals, which may reflect the degree of sympathetic activation and hypersensitivity in these patients (Sandberg et al. 2005). Since hypoxia is thought to be one of the key components in chronic myalgia and hypothetically plays a role in the pathophysiology of myofascial pain (Donnelly et al. 2019), any increase in blood flow caused by needling muscle may contribute to therapeutic responses.

Goldman et al. (2010) demonstrated a unilateral distal antinociceptive effect of acupuncture needling with manual stimulation via release of adenosine, including data from multiple experiments in animal (rodent) models of inflammatory and neuropathic pain. Moré et al. (2013) showed that a similar antinociceptive effect could be abolished by high levels of caffeine consumption in rodents. The release of adenosine by acupuncture needling has also been demonstrated in humans using microdialysis (Takano et al. 2012).

Segmental (spinal cord) effects

Through stimulation of high-threshold ergoreceptors in muscle tissue, needling can have an influence on sensory modulation within the dorsal horn at the relevant segmental level. C-fibre nociceptive transmission is inhibited via enkephalinergic interneurons in lamina II (Bowsher 1998; White 1999). Segmental stimulation appears to have a more powerful effect than equivalent stimulation from a distant segment on pain modulation (Chapman et al. 1977; Lundeberg et al. 1989; Zhao 2008), local autonomic activity (Sato et al. 1993) and itch (Lundeberg et al. 1987). Aδ or type III afferent neurons can be stimulated by superficial needling as well as by needling deeper tissues, but it seems that segmental stimuli from the latter (usually muscle) have a more powerful effect (Ceccherelli et al. 1998; Lundeberg et al. 1987, 1989; Zhao 2008).

General (brainstem) effects: heterosegmental

While segmental stimulation appears to be the more powerful effect, needling anywhere in the body can influence afferent processing throughout the spinal cord. Heterosegmental needle stimulation affects descending inhibitory pathways and the diffuse noxious inhibitory system (DNIC) (see Chapters 6 and 7). It exerts influence through the different pain inhibitory mechanisms to varying degrees (Bowsher 1998; White 1999).

Recent evidence showed that strong electroacupuncture (EA) (>2.0 mA) applied daily to patients (n = 301) with knee osteoarthritis is able to significantly increase descending inhibition as measured by CPM, compared with a milder form of EA (<0.5 mA) (Lv et al. 2019).

Clinically relevant changes in pain and functional outcomes were apparent at 1 week, after five treatment sessions, but significant changes in CPM were only apparent after 2 weeks (10 treatment sessions).

General (brainstem) effects: systemic

These are more difficult to define and there is clearly some overlap with heterosegmental effects. The latter term is used here to denote effects mediated at every segment of the spinal cord, as opposed to effects on higher centres in the central nervous system or those mediated by humeral means. Acupuncture needling has proven efficacy in the treatment of nausea and vomiting (Lee et al. 2015; Lee & Done 2004; Lee & Fan 2009; Vickers 1996), and this effect is likely to be mediated centrally. A substantial body of work indicates the importance of beta-endorphin and other endogenous opioids in acupuncture-related analgesia (Han 2004, 2011; Han & Terenius 1982; Zhao 2008), and correlations have been identified between the endorphin releasing effect of acupuncture and that of prolonged exercise (Thoren et al. 1990). Further correlations in terms of neuropeptide release have also been noted (Bucinskaite et al. 1996). It has been suggested that activation of opioid systems, by exercise and potentially acupuncture, may mediate enhanced immunity (Jonsdottir 1999).

Functional magnetic resonance imaging (fMRI) studies indicate general effects on limbic structures (Hui et al. 2000) and the importance of the nature of the needle stimulus in achieving this effect (Hui et al. 2007, 2009, 2010). A meta-analysis by Chae et al. (2013) concluded that acupuncture is not only able to activate several areas located in the sensorimotor cortical network, including the insula, thalamus, anterior cingulate cortex and primary and secondary somatosensory cortices, but it also is able to deactivate the limbic–paralimbic neocortical network, including the medial prefrontal cortex, caudate, amygdala, posterior cingulate cortex, and parahippocampus. This is compatible with a reduction in the affective component of pain experienced by patients treated with acupuncture.

While target-directed expectation may theoretically play a role in the mechanism of acupuncture under some circumstances (Benedetti et al., 1999), the effects of acupuncture may not be explained entirely by expectation (Kong et al. 2009a, b). In clinical practice, context-driven effects are considered important in acupuncture analgesia (Finniss et al. 2010), and areas of affective and cognitive processing are consistently activated by acupuncture (Huang et al. 2012), so it is challenging to disentangle the direct effects of acupuncture needling on central nervous system structures from the indirect effects related to the context of treatment (Cummings 2016).

Mechanisms of trigger point dry needling

The mechanisms by which DN exerts its analgesic effects share aspects with acupuncture, but additional aspects related to a direct effect of DN on the MTrP are considered (Cagnie et al. 2013; Chou et al. 2012). In addition to the neurophysiological mechanisms explaining DN-related analgesia, it is possible that the more vigorous and fast insertion of the needle has a mechanical effect on endplates, muscle spindles or fibres themselves. Simons et al. suggested that the therapeutic factor of needling interventions was the mechanical effect of the needle consisting of disruption of dysfunctional endplates, an increase of sarcomere length and a reduction of the overlapping between actin and myosin filaments (Donnelly et al. 2019). These potential mechanical effects are supported by studies showing that DN decreased spontaneous electrical activity and acetylcholine levels of the MTrP area (Liu et al. 2017). A more extensive discussion of possible mechanisms of trigger point DN can be found in Dommerholt & Fernández-de-las-Peñas 2018 and Fernández-de-Las-Peñas & Nijs 2019.

Clinical research: benefits and harms

As stated previously, harmful outcomes related to acupuncture are rare, but short-lived exacerbation of pain is more common and may dissuade some patients from continuing treatment.

The biggest and most reliable dataset derived from RCTs of acupuncture in pain conditions is the individual patient data meta-analysis by Vickers et al. (2012, 2018). It includes trials on headache, osteoarthritis and musculoskeletal pain, and the latest update includes a total of 20,827 patients from 39 trials. The results clearly indicate small but statistically significant effects (~0.2 standardised mean difference) over sham acupuncture and moderate effects (~0.5 standardised mean difference) over no acupuncture controls (Vickers et al. 2018).

The main methodological challenge in efficacy trials of acupuncture is finding a sham control that is not an active treatment itself and adequately blinds patient and outcome assessor. In the large GERAC (German Acupuncture Trials) trials, which were part of a major research initiative funded by health insurance providers Modellvorhaben Akupunktur (Cummings 2009), sham acupuncture was either similar in effect or markedly superior to guideline-based conventional care (Diener et al. 2006; Haake et al. 2007; Scharf et al. 2006).

TABLE 16.4 A comparison of the characteristics of TENS and acupuncture

	TENS	Electroacupuncture
Applied via	Pads on skin	Needles inserted through skin, usually into muscle
Nerves mediating principal effects	Aβ fibre in skin	Aδ and C fibres in deep somatic tissues
Region of influence (neurophysiological)	Segmental	Local Segmental Systemic/general
Onset of effects	Immediate	Delayed
Duration of effects	Short	24–48 hours
Frequencies (Hz)	Conventional TENS: 5–250 pulses per second (often between 20 and 100 pulses per second) AL-TENS: low-frequency single pulses (<5 pulses per second) or bursts of high-frequency pulses (<5 bursts per second)	2–100 Typically, 2/15 or 4/100
Pulse width (μs)	Typically, 50–200	Typically, 100–200
Current (mA)	Typically, 10–60	Typically, 0.5–20
Cost of device (typical)	£20–£70	£200–£700

TENS, Transcutaneous electrical nerve stimulation.

Conclusion

Acupuncture is a useful technique with a long and interesting history. The scientific evaluation is extensive and modern versions have sprung up in a variety of professional settings. As yet it is underutilised in the West but is gradually finding its way into clinical guidelines as the methodological difficulties associated with rigorous evaluation of such techniques are more fairly appreciated.

A comparison of the characteristics of TENS and acupuncture is provided in Table 16.4.

Competing interests

MIJ has received royalties from Oxford University for his book *TENS: Research to Support Clinical Practice*. MIJ's employer has received support from Glaxo-SmithKline plc and TENSCare Ltd for expert consultancy services. MC is employed full time as Medical Director by the British Medical Acupuncture Society, which is a charity. In addition to his salary, he receives a small income from an educational partnership teaching Western Veterinary Acupuncture and some modest royalties from textbooks.

Accessing materials

Materials related to our paper (e.g. data, samples or models) can be accessed by contacting Professor Mark I. Johnson.

Review questions   Q

1. List the contraindications and relative contraindications for TENS and acupuncture.
2. Identify and prioritise the risks that patients face when using TENS and provide simple patient advice to manage these risks.
3. Outline to a patient with nonspecific low back pain how to administer TENS at home and what they should expect in terms of pain relief.
4. List three major differences between traditional Chinese and Western style acupuncture.
5. Describe, briefly, the main physiological mechanisms by which TENS and acupuncture relieve pain.
6. List reasons why clinical research on TENS and acupuncture is still not conclusive.

References

Alon, G., Kantor, G., Ho, H.S., 1994. Effects of electrode size on basic excitatory responses and on selected stimulus parameters. J. Orthop. Sports. Phys. Ther. 20, 29–35.

Amatya, B., Young, J., Khan, F., 2018. Non–pharmacological interventions for chronic pain in multiple sclerosis. Cochrane Database Syst. Rev. 12. https://doi.org/10.1002/14651858.CD012622.pub2.

Andrews, B., 2014. The Making of Modern Chinese Medicine, 1850–1960, first ed. University of British Columbia Press, Vancouver.

Arik, M.I., Kiloatar, H., Aslan, B., Icelli, M., 2020. The Effect of Tens for Pain Relief in Women with Primary Dysmenorrhea: A Systematic Review and Meta-Analysis, p. 2541 Explore (NY).

Avendano-Coy, J., Bravo-Esteban, E., Ferri-Morales, A., Martinez-de la Cruz, R., Gomez-Soriano, J., 2019. Does frequency modulation of transcutaneous electrical nerve stimulation affect habituation and mechanical hypoalgesia? A randomized, double-blind, sham-controlled crossover trial. Phys. Ther. 99 (7), 924–932.

Bai, X., Baron, R.B., 2001. Acupuncture: Visible Holism. Butterworth-Heinemann, Oxford.

Baldry, P.E., 2005. Acupuncture, Trigger Points & Musculoskeletal Pain, third ed. Churchill Livingstone, Edinburgh.

Bedwell, C., Dowswell, T., Neilson, J.P., Lavender, T., 2011. The use of transcutaneous electrical nerve stimulation (TENS) for pain relief in labour: a review of the evidence. Midwifery 27 (5), e141–e148.

Benedetti, F., Arduino, C., Amanzio, M., 1999. Somatotopic activation of opioid systems by target-directed expectations of analgesia. J. Neurosci. 19 (9), 3639–3648.

Bennett, M.I., Hughes, N., Johnson, M.I., 2011. Methodological quality in randomised controlled trials of transcutaneous electric nerve stimulation for pain: low fidelity may explain negative findings. Pain 152 (6), 1226–1232.

Bennett, M.I., Johnson, M.I., Brown, S.R., Radford, H., Brown, J.M., Searle, R.D., 2010. Feasibility study of transcutaneous electrical nerve stimulation (TENS) for cancer bone pain. J. Pain 11 (4), 351–359.

Binny, J., Joshua Wong, N.L., Garga, S., Lin, C.W.C., Maher, C.G., McLachlan, A.J., et al., 2019. Transcutaneous electric nerve stimulation (TENS) for acute low back pain: systematic review. Scand. J. Pain 19 (2), 225–233.

Bjordal, J.M., Johnson, M.I., Ljunggreen, A.E., 2003. Transcutaneous electrical nerve stimulation (TENS) can reduce postoperative analgesic consumption. A meta-analysis with assessment of optimal treatment parameters for postoperative pain. Eur. J. Pain 7 (2), 181–188.

Bjordal, J.M., Johnson, M.I., Lopes-Martins, R.A., Bogen, B., Chow, R., Ljunggren, A.E., 2007. Short-term efficacy of physical interventions in osteoarthritic knee pain. A systematic review and meta-analysis of randomised placebo-controlled trials. BMC Musculoskelet. Disord. 8, 51. https://doi.org/10.1186/1471-2474-8-51. PMID: 17587446; PMCID: PMC1931596.

Bowsher, D., 1998. Mechanisms of acupuncture. In: Filshie, J., White, A. (Eds.), Medical Acupuncture - A Western Scientific Approach, first ed. Churchill Livingstone, Edinburgh, pp. 69–82.

Boyce, D., Wempe, H., Campbell, C., Fuehne, S., Zylstra, E., Smith, G., et al., 2020. Adverse events associated with therapeutic dry needling. Int. J. Sports. Phys. Ther. 15 (1), 103–113.

Brady, S., McEvoy, J., Dommerholt, J., Doody, C., 2014. Adverse events following trigger point dry needling: a prospective survey of chartered physiotherapists. J. Man. Manip. Ther. 22 (3), 134–140.

Brockhaus, A., Elger, C.E., 1990. Hypalgesic efficacy of acupuncture on experimental pain in man. Comparison of laser acupuncture and needle acupuncture. Pain. 43 (2), 181–185.

Bronfort, G., Nilsson, N., Haas, M., Evans, R., Goldsmith, C.H., Assendelft, W.J., et al., 2004. Non-invasive physical treatments for chronic/recurrent headache. Cochrane Database Syst. Rev. 3, CD001878.

Brosseau, L., Yonge, K.A., Robinson, V., Marchand, S., Judd, M., Wells, G., et al., 2003. Transcutaneous electrical nerve stimulation (TENS) for the treatment of rheumatoid arthritis in the hand. Cochrane Database Syst. Rev. 3, CD004287.

Bucinskaite, V., Theodorsson, E., Crumpton, K., Stenfors, C., Ekblom, A., Lundeberg, T., 1996. Effects of repeated sensory stimulation (electro-acupuncture) and physical exercise (running) on open-field behaviour and concentrations of neuropeptides in the hippocampus in WKY and SHR rats. Eur. J. Neurosci. 8 (2), 382–387.

Buck, C., 2015. Acupuncture and Chinese Medicine - Roots of Modern Practice, first ed. Singing Dragon, London and Philadelphia.

Cagnie, B., Dewitte, V., Barbe, T., Timmermans, F., Delrue, N., Meeus, M., 2013. Physiologic effects of dry needling. Curr. Pain. Headache. Rep. 17 (8), 348.

Carlson, T., Andrell, P., Ekre, O., Edvardsson, N., Holmgren, C., Jacobsson, F., et al., 2009. Interference of transcutaneous electrical nerve stimulation with permanent ventricular stimulation: a new clinical problem? Europace. 11 (3), 364–369.

Carroll, D., Moore, R.A., Tramer, M.R., McQuay, H.J., 1997. Transcutaneous electrical nerve stimulation does not relieve labor pain: updated systematic review. Contemp. Rev. Obstet. Gynaecol. 9 (3), 195–205.

Carroll, D., Trame, M., McQuay, R.H., Nye, B., Moore, A., 1996. Randomization is important in studies with pain outcomes: systematic review of transcutaneous electrical nerve stimulation in acute postoperative pain. Br. J. Anaesth. 77 (6), 798–803.

Ceccherelli, F., Gagliardi, G., Visentin, R., Giron, G., 1998. Effects of deep vs. superficial stimulation of acupuncture on capsaicin-induced edema. A blind controlled study in rats. Acupunct. Electro-Ther. Res. 23 (2), 125–134.

Chae, Y., Chang, D.S., Lee, S.H., Jung, W.M., Lee, I.S., Jackson, S., et al., 2013. Inserting needles into the body: a meta-analysis of brain activity associated with acupuncture needle stimulation. J. Pain. 14 (3), 215–222.

Chapman, C.R., Chen, A.C., Bonica, J.J., 1977. Effects of intrasegmental electrical acupuncture on dental pain: evaluation by threshold estimation and sensory decision theory. Pain. 3 (3), 213–227.

Chen, C.-C., Tabasam, G., Johnson, M.I., 2008. Does the pulse frequency of transcutaneous electrical nerve stimulation (TENS) influence hypoalgesia? A systematic review of studies using experimental pain and healthy human participants. Physiotherapy. 94 (1), 11–20.

Chen, C.C., Johnson, M.I., 2009. An investigation into the effects of frequency-modulated transcutaneous electrical nerve stimulation (TENS) on experimentally-induced pressure pain in healthy human participants. J. Pain. 10 (10), 1029–1037.

Chen, L., Ferreira, M., Beckenkamp, P., Caputo, E., Ferreira, P., 2019. Comparative efficacy and safety of conservative care for pregnancy-related low back pain: a systematic review and network meta-analysis. Osteoarthritis. Cartilage. 27, S456–S457.

Chen, L.X., Zhou, Z.R., Li, Y.L., Ning, G.Z., Li, Y., Wang, X.B., et al., 2015. Transcutaneous electrical nerve stimulation in patients with knee osteoarthritis: evidence from randomized controlled trials. Clin. J. Pain. 32 (2), 146–154 2016.

Chiang, C., Chang, C., Chu, H., Yang, L., 1973. Peripheral afferent pathway for acupuncture analgesia. Sci. Sin. 16 (2), 210–217.

Chou, L.-W., Kao, M.-J., Lin, J.-G., 2012. Probable mechanisms of needling therapies for myofascial pain control. Evid. Based Complement. Alternat. Med. 2012, 1–11.

Chung, J.M., Fang, Z.R., Hori, Y., Lee, K.H., Willis, W.D., 1984. Prolonged inhibition of primate spinothalamic tract cells by peripheral nerve stimulation. Pain. 19 (3), 259–275.

Claydon, L.S., Chesterton, L.S., Barlas, P., Sim, J., 2011. Dose-specific effects of transcutaneous electrical nerve stimulation (TENS) on experimental pain: a systematic review. Clin. J. Pain. 27 (7), 635–647.

Cummings, M., 2004. Acupuncture and trigger point needling. In: Hazelman, B., Riley, G., Speed, C. (Eds.), Soft Tissue Rheumatology. Oxford University Press, Oxford, pp. 275–282.

Cummings, M., 2009. Modellvorhaben Akupunktur–a summary of the ART, ARC and GERAC trials. Acupunct. Med. 27 (1), 26–30.

Cummings, M., 2016. Western medical acupuncture – the approach to treatment. In: Filshie, J., White, A., Cummings, M. (Eds.), Medical Acupuncture – A Western Scientific Approach, second ed. Edinburgh; Elsevier, pp. 100–124.

Cummings, T.M., White, A.R., 2001. Needling therapies in the management of myofascial trigger point pain: a systematic review. Arch. Phys. Med. Rehabil. 82 (7), 986–992.

Dailey, D.L., Vance, C.G., Rakel, B.A., Zimmerman, M.B., Embree, J., Merriwether, E.N., et al., 2019. A randomized controlled trial of TENS for movement-evoked pain in women with fibromyalgia. Arthritis. Rheumatol. 72 (5), 824–836.

Dawidson, I., Angmar-Mansson, B., Blom, M., Theodorsson, E., Lundeberg, T., 1998a. The influence of sensory stimulation (acupuncture) on the release of neuropeptides in the saliva of healthy subjects. Life. Sci. 63 (8), 659–674.

Dawidson, I., Angmar-Mansson, B., Blom, M., Theodorsson, E., Lundeberg, T., 1998b. Sensory stimulation (acupuncture) increases the release of vasoactive intestinal polypeptide in the saliva of xerostomia sufferers. Neuropeptides. 32 (6), 543–548.

DeSantana, J.M., da Silva, L.F., Sluka, K.A., 2010. Cholecystokinin receptors mediate tolerance to the analgesic effect of TENS in arthritic rats. Pain. 148 (1), 84–93.

Diener, H.C., Kronfeld, K., Boewing, G., Lungenhausen, M., Maier, C., Molsberger, A., et al., 2006. Efficacy of acupuncture for the prophylaxis of migraine: a multicentre randomised controlled clinical trial. Lancet. Neurol. 5 (4), 310–316.

Direct and Indirect Benefits Reported by Users of Transcutaneous Electrical Nerve Stimulation for Chronic Musculoskeletal Pain: Qualitative Exploration Using Patient Interviews. Gladwell PW, Badlan K, Cramp F, Palmer S. Physical Therapy, 2015, 95(11):1518–1528.

Dommerholt, J., Fernández-de-las-Peñas, C., 2018. Proposed mechanisms and effects of trigger point dry needling. In: Dommerholt, J., Fernández-de-las-Peñas, C. (Eds.), Trigger Point Dry Needling, second ed. Elsevier, pp. 21–30.

Donnelly, J., Fernández-de-las-Peñas, C., Finnegan, M., Freeman, J., 2019. Travell, Simons & Simons' myofascial pain & dysfunction. The Trigger Point Manual, third ed. Wolters Kluwer.

Dorfer, L., 1998. 5200-year-old acupuncture in central Europe? Science. 282 (5387), 242–243.

Dorfer, L., Moser, M., Bahr, F., Spindler, K., Egarter-Vigl, E., Giullen, S., et al., 1999. A medical report from the stone age? Lancet. 354 (9183), 1023–1025.

Dorsher, P.T., 2009. Myofascial referred-pain data provide physiologic evidence of acupuncture meridians. J. Pain. 10 (7), 723–731.

Dowswell, T., Bedwell, C., Lavender, T., Neilson, J.P., 2009. Transcutaneous electrical nerve stimulation (TENS) for pain relief in labour. Cochrane Database Syst. Rev. 2, CD007214.

Dubinsky, R.M., Miyasaki, J., 2010. Assessment: efficacy of transcutaneous electric nerve stimulation in the treatment of pain in neurologic disorders (an evidence-based review): report of the Therapeutics and Technology Assessment Subcommittee of the American Academy of Neurology. Neurology. 74 (2), 173–176.

Eriksson, M., Sjölund, B., 1976. Acupuncture-like electroanalgesia in TNS resistant chronic pain. In: Zotterman, Y. (Ed.), Sensory Functions of the Skin. Pergamon Press, Oxford, pp. 575–581.

Fernández-de-Las-Peñas, C., Nijs, J., 2019. Trigger point dry needling for the treatment of myofascial pain syndrome: current perspectives within a pain neuroscience paradigm. J. Pain. Res. 12, 1899–1911.

Fernandez-Tenorio, E., Serrano-Munoz, D., Avendano-Coy, J., Gomez-Soriano, J., 2019. Transcutaneous electrical nerve stimulation for spasticity: a systematic review. Neurologia. 34 (7), 451–460.

Filshie, J., Cummings, M., 1999. Western medical acupuncture. In: Ernst, E., White, A. (Eds.), Acupuncture - A Scientific Appraisal, first ed. Butterworth Heinemann, pp. 31–59.

Finniss, D.G., Kaptchuk, T.J., Miller, F., Benedetti, F., 2010. Biological, clinical, and ethical advances of placebo effects. Lancet. 375 (9715), 686–695.

Ford, K.S., Shrader, M.W., Smith, J., McLean, T.J., Dahm, D.L., 2005. Full-thickness burn formation after the use of electrical stimulation for rehabilitation of unicompartmental knee arthroplasty. J. Arthroplasty. 20 (7), 950–953.

Foster, N.E., Vertosick, E.A., Lewith, G., Linde, K., MacPherson, H., Sherman, K.J., et al., 2020. Identifying patients with chronic pain who respond to acupuncture: results from an individual patient data meta-analysis. Acupunct. Med. 39 (2), 83–90.

Francis, R.P., Johnson, M.I., 2011. The characteristics of acupuncture-like transcutaneous electrical nerve stimulation (acupuncture-like TENS): a literature review. Acupunct. Electro-Therapeutics. Res. 36 (3–4), 231–258.

Gibson, W., Wand, B.M., Meads, C., Catley, M.J., O'Connell, N.E., 2019. Transcutaneous electrical nerve stimulation (TENS) for chronic pain - an overview of Cochrane Reviews. Cochrane Database Syst. Rev. 2, CD011890. https://doi.org/10.1002/1465 1858.CD011890.pub2.

Gibson, W., Wand, B.M., O'Connell, N.E., 2017. Transcutaneous electrical nerve stimulation (TENS) for neuropathic pain in adults. Cochrane Database Syst. Rev. 9, CD011976. https://doi.org/10.1002/14651858.CD011976.pub2.

Gladwell, P.W., Badlan, K., Cramp, F., Palmer, S., 2016. Problems, solutions, and strategies reported by users of transcutaneous electrical nerve stimulation for chronic musculoskeletal pain: qualitative exploration using patient interviews. Phys. Ther. 96 (7), 1039–1048.

Gladwell, P.W., Cramp, F., Palmer, S., 2020. Matching the perceived benefits of Transcutaneous Electrical Nerve Stimulation (TENS) for chronic musculoskeletal pain against patient reported outcome measures using the International Classification of Functioning, disability and health (ICF). Physiotherapy. 106, 128–135.

Goldman, N., Chen, M., Fujita, T., Xu, Q., Peng, W., Liu, W., et al., 2010. Adenosine A1 receptors mediate local anti-nociceptive effects of acupuncture. Nat. Neurosci. 13 (7), 883–888. https://doi.org/10.1038/nn.2562.

Gunn, C.C., 1989. Treating Myofascial Pain, Intramuscular Stimulation (IMS) for Myofascial Pain Syndromes of Neuropathic Origin. University of Washington.

Gunn, C.C., 1996. Treating myofascial pain. Acupunct. Med. 14 (1), 20–21.

Haake, M., Müller, H.-H., Schade-Brittinger, C., Basler, H.D., Schäfer, H., Maier, C., et al., 2007. German Acupuncture Trials (GERAC) for chronic low back pain: randomized, multicenter, blinded, parallel-group trial with 3 groups. Arch. Intern. Med. 167 (17), 1892–1898.

Han, J.-S., 2004. Acupuncture and endorphins. Neurosci. Lett. 361 (1–3), 258–261.

Han, J.S., 2011. Acupuncture analgesia: areas of consensus and controversy. Pain. 152 (Suppl 3), S41–S48.

Han, J.S., Terenius, L., 1982. Neurochemical basis of acupuncture analgesia. Annu. Rev. Pharmacol. Toxicol. 22, 193–220.

Harvey, L.A., Glinsky, J.V., Bowden, J.L., 2016. The effectiveness of 22 commonly administered physiotherapy interventions for people with spinal cord injury: a systematic review. Spinal. Cord. 54 (11), 914–923.

Hingne, P.M., Sluka, K.A., 2008. Blockade of NMDA receptors prevents analgesic tolerance to repeated transcutaneous electrical nerve stimulation (TENS) in rats. J. Pain. 9 (3), 217–225.

Hoffman, P., 2001. Skin disinfection and acupuncture. Acupunct. Med. 19 (2), 112–116. https://doi.org/10.1136/aim.19.2.112.

Hong, C.-Z., 1994. Lidocaine injection versus dry needling to myofascial trigger point. The importance of the local twitch response. Am. J. Phys. Med. Rehabil. 73 (4), 256–263.

Huang, W., Pach, D., Napadow, V., Park, K., Long, X., Neumann, J., et al., 2012. Characterizing acupuncture stimuli using brain imaging with FMRI--a systematic review and meta-analysis of the literature. PLoS. One. 7 (4), e32960.

Hui, K.K., Liu, J., Makris, N., Gollub, R.L., Chen, A.J., Moore, C.I., et al., 2000. Acupuncture modulates the limbic system and subcortical gray structures of the human brain: evidence from fMRI studies in normal subjects. Hum. Brain. Mapp. 9 (1), 13–25.

Hui, K.K., Marina, O., Claunch, J.D., Nixon, E.E., Fang, J., Liu, J., et al., 2009. Acupuncture mobilizes the brain's default mode and its anti-correlated network in healthy subjects. Brain. Res. 1287, 84–103.

Hui, K.K., Marina, O., Liu, J., Rosen, B.R., Kwong, K.K., 2010. Acupuncture, the limbic system, and the anticorrelated networks of the brain. Auton. Neurosci. 157 (1–2), 81–90.

Hui, K.K., Nixon, E.E., Vangel, M.G., Liu, J., Marina, O., Napadow, V., et al., 2007. Characterization of the "deqi" response in acupuncture. BMC. Complement. Altern. Med. 7, 33.

Hurlow, A., Bennett, M.I., Robb, K.A., Johnson, M.I., Simpson, K.H., Oxberry, S.G., 2012. Transcutaneous electric nerve stimulation (TENS) for cancer pain in adults. Cochrane Database Syst. Rev. 3, CD006276. https://doi.org/10.1002/14651858.CD006276.pub3.

Jansen, G., Lundeberg, T., Kjartansson, J., Samuelson, U.E., 1989a. Acupuncture and sensory neuropeptides increase cutaneous blood flow in rats. Neurosci. Lett. 97 (3), 305–309.

Jansen, G., Lundeberg, T., Samuelson, U.E., Thomas, M., 1989b. Increased survival of ischaemic musculocutaneous flaps in rats after acupuncture. Acta. Physiol. Scand. 135 (4), 555–558.

Jauregui, J.J., Cherian, J.J., Gwam, C.U., Chughtai, M., Mistry, J.B., Elmallah, R.K., et al., 2016. A meta-analysis of transcutaneous electrical nerve stimulation for chronic low back pain. Surg. Technol. Int. 296–302. http://www.ncbi.nlm.nih.gov/pubmed/27042787.

Jin, F., Guo, Y., Wang, Z., Badughaish, A., Pan, X., Zhang, L., et al., 2020. The pathophysiological nature of sarcomeres in trigger points in patients with myofascial pain syndrome: a preliminary study. Eur. J. Pain. ejp.1647.

Johnson, M.I., Paley, C., Jones, G., Mulvey, M.R., Wittkopf, P.G., 2022a. Efficacy and safety of transcutaneous electrical nerve stimulation (TENS) for acute and chronic pain in adults: a systematic review and meta-analysis of 381 studies (the meta-TENS study). BMJ Open 12 (2), e051073. https://doi.org/10.1136/bmjopen-2021-051073. https://bmjopen.bmj.com/content/12/2/e051073.

Johnson, M.I., Paley, C.A., Wittkopf, P.G., Mulvey, M.R., Jones, G., 2022b. Characterising the features of 381 clinical studies evaluating transcutaneous electrical nerve stimulation (TENS) for pain relief: a secondary analysis of the meta-TENS study to improve future research. Medicina 58 (6), 803. 2022. https://doi.org/10.3390/medicina58060803.

Johnson, M., 1998. Acupuncture-like transcutaneous electrical nerve stimulation (AL-TENS) in the management of pain. Phys. Ther. Rev. 3, 73–93.

Johnson, M.I., 2014a. Contraindications, precautions, and adverse events. In: Johnson, M. (Ed.), Transcutaneous Electrical Nerve Stimulation (TENS). Research to Support Clinical Practice. Oxford University Press, pp. 93–115.

Johnson, M.I., 2014b. Mechanism of action. In: Johnson, M. (Ed.), Transcutaneous Electrical Nerve Stimulation (TENS). Research to Support Clinical Practice. Oxford University Press, pp. 172–192.

Johnson, M.I., 2014c. TENS-like devices. In: Johnson, M. (Ed.), Transcutaneous Electrical Nerve Stimulation (TENS). Research to Support Clinical Practice. Oxford University Press, pp. 203–212.

Johnson, M.I., 2014d. The use of TENS for non-painful conditions. In: Johnson, M. (Ed.), Transcutaneous Electrical Nerve Stimulation (TENS). Research to Support Clinical Practice. Oxford University Press, pp. 193–202.

Johnson, M., Martinson, M., 2007. Efficacy of electrical nerve stimulation for chronic musculoskeletal pain: a meta-analysis of randomized controlled trials. Pain. 130 (1–2), 157–165.

Johnson, M.I., 2001. A critical review of the analgesic effects of TENS-like devices. Phys. Ther. Rev. 6, 153–173.

Johnson, M.I., 2017. Transcutaneous electrical nerve stimulation (TENS) as an adjunct for pain management in perioperative settings: a critical review. Expert. Rev. Neurother. 17 (10), 1013–1027.

Johnson, M.I., 2021. Resolving long-standing uncertainty about the clinical efficacy of transcutaneous electrical nerve stimulation (TENS) to relieve pain: a comprehensive review of factors influencing outcome. Medicina (Kaunas) 57 (4).

Johnson, M.I., Claydon, L.S., Herbison, G.P., Jones, G., Paley, C.A., 2017. Transcutaneous electrical nerve stimulation (TENS) for fibromyalgia in adults. Cochrane Database Syst. Rev. 10, CD012172. https://doi.org/10.1002/14651858.CD012172.pub2.

Johnson, M.I., Jones, G., Paley, C.A., Wittkopf, P.G., 2019. The clinical efficacy of transcutaneous electrical nerve stimulation (TENS) for acute and chronic pain: a protocol for a meta-analysis of randomised controlled trials (RCTs). BMJ. Open. 9 (10), e029999.

Johnson, M.I., Paley, C.A., Howe, T.E., Sluka, K.A., 2015. Transcutaneous electrical nerve stimulation for acute pain (Cochrane review) [with consumer summary]. Cochrane Database Syst. Rev. 2015, 6.

Johnson, M.I., Walsh, D.M., 2010. Pain: continued uncertainty of TENS' effectiveness for pain relief. Nat. Rev. Rheumatol. 6 (6), 314–316.

Jonsdottir, I., 1999. Physical exercise, acupuncture and immune function. Acupunct. Med. 17 (1), 50–53.

Jung, J.-W., Kim, S.R., Jeon, S.Y., Bang, S.R., Kim, Y.H., Lee, S.E., 2014. Cardiac tamponade following ultrasonography-guided trigger point injection. J. Muscoskel. Pain. 22 (4), 389–391.

Kalra, A., Urban, M.O., Sluka, K.A., 2001. Blockade of opioid receptors in rostral ventral medulla prevents antihyperalgesia produced by transcutaneous electrical nerve stimulation (TENS). J. Pharmacol. Exp. Ther. 298 (1), 257–263.

Kerai, S., Saxena, K.N., Taneja, B., Sehrawat, L., 2014. Role of transcutaneous electrical nerve stimulation in post-operative analgesia. Indian. J. Anaesth. 58 (4), 388–393. https://doi.org/10.4103/0019-5049.138966.

Khadilkar, A., Odebiyi, D.O., Brosseau, L., Wells, G.A., 2008. Transcutaneous electrical nerve stimulation (TENS) versus placebo for chronic low-back pain. Cochrane Database Syst. Rev. 4, CD003008.

Kirschenbaum, A.E., Rizzo, C., 1997. Glenohumeral pyarthrosis following acupuncture treatment. Orthopedics. 20 (12), 1184–1186.

Kong, J., Kaptchuk, T., Polich, G., Kirsch, I.V., Angel, M., Zyloney, C., et al., 2009a. An fMRI study on the interaction and dissociation between expectation of pain relief and acupuncture treatment. Neuroimage. 45 (3), 940–949.

Kong, J., Kaptchuk, T.J., Polich, G., Kirsch, I., Vangel, M., Zyloney, C., et al., 2009b. Expectancy and treatment interactions: a dissociation between acupuncture analgesia and expectancy evoked placebo analgesia. Neuroimage. 45 (3), 940–949.

Kroeling, P., Gross, A., Goldsmith, C.H., Burnie, S.J., Haines, T., Graham, N., et al., 2013. Electrotherapy for neck pain. Cochrane Database Syst. Rev. (8), N.PAG-N.PAG. https://doi.org/10.1002/14651858.CD004251.pub3.

Lapeer, G.L., Monga, T.N., 1986. Myofascial trigger-point acupuncture in relieving chronic pain after endarterectomy. Can. Fam. Physician. 32, 1955–1958.

Lazarou, L., Kitsios, A., Lazarou, I., Sikaras, E., Trampas, A., 2009. Effects of intensity of transcutaneous electrical nerve stimulation (TENS) on pressure pain threshold and blood pressure in healthy humans: a randomized, double-blind, placebo-controlled trial. Clin. J. Pain. 25 (9), 773–780.

Lee, A., Chan, S.K.C., Fan, L.T.Y., 2015. Stimulation of the wrist acupuncture point PC6 for preventing postoperative nausea and vomiting. Cochrane Database Syst. Rev. 11, CD003281.

Lee, A., Done, M.L., 2004. Stimulation of the wrist acupuncture point P6 for preventing postoperative nausea and vomiting. Cochrane Database Syst. Rev. 3, CD003281.

Lee, A., Fan, L.T., 2009. Stimulation of the wrist acupuncture point P6 for preventing postoperative nausea and vomiting. Cochrane Database Syst. Rev. 2, CD003281.

Lewis, T., 1927. The Blood Vessels of the Human Skin and Their Responses. Shaw, London.

Lewit, K., 1979. The needle effect in the relief of myofascial pain. Pain. 6 (1), 83–90.

Lewit, K., Simons, D.G., 1984. Myofascial pain: relief by post-isometric relaxation. Arch. Phys. Med. Rehabil. 65 (8), 452–456.

Liebano, R.E., Rakel, B., Vance, C.G., Walsh, D.M., Sluka, K.A., 2011. An investigation of the development of analgesic tolerance to TENS in humans. Pain. 211, 335–342.

Lima, L.V., Cruz, K.M., Abner, T.S., Mota, C.M., Agripino, M.E., Santana-Filho, V.J., et al., 2015. Associating high intensity and modulated frequency of TENS delays analgesic tolerance in rats. Eur. J. Pain. 19 (3), 369–376.

Lin, S.-K., Liu, J.-M., Hsu, R.-J., Chuang, H.-C., Wang, Y.-X., Lin, P.-H., 2019. Incidence of iatrogenic pneumothorax following acupuncture treatments in Taiwan. Acupunct. Med. 37 (6), 332–339.

Liu, Q.-G., Liu, L., Huang, Q.-M., Nguyen, T.-T., Ma, Y.-T., Zhao, J.-M., 2017. Decreased spontaneous electrical activity and acetylcholine at myofascial trigger spots after dry needling treatment: a pilot study. Evid. Based. Complement. Alternat. Med. 2017, 1–7.

Lundeberg, T., Bondesson, L., Thomas, M., 1987. Effect of acupuncture on experimentally induced itch. Br. J. Dermatol. 117 (6), 771–777.

Lundeberg, T., Eriksson, S., Lundeberg, S., Thomas, M., 1989. Acupuncture and sensory thresholds. Am. J. Chin. Med. 17 (3–4), 99–110.

Lundeberg, T., Kjartansson, J., Samuelsson, U., 1988. Effect of electrical nerve stimulation on healing of ischaemic skin flaps. Lancet. (London, England) 2 (8613), 712–714.

Lundeberg, T., Lund, I., 2016. Peripheral components of acupuncture stimulation – their contribution to the specific clinical effects of acupuncture. In: Filshie, J., White, A., Cummings, M. (Eds.), Medical Acupuncture – A Western Scientific Approach, second ed. Elsevier, pp. 22–58.

Lv, Z.-T., Shen, L.-L., Zhu, B., Zhang, Z.-Q., Ma, C.-Y., Huang, G.-F., et al., 2019. Effects of intensity of electroacupuncture on chronic pain in patients with knee osteoarthritis: a randomized controlled trial. Arthritis. Res. Ther. 21 (1), 120.

Ma, K., 1992. The roots and development of Chinese Acupuncture: from prehistory to early 20th century. Acupunct. Med. 10 (Suppl. ment), 92–99.

Ma, Y.T., Sluka, K.A., 2001. Reduction in inflammation-induced sensitization of dorsal horn neurons by transcutaneous electrical nerve stimulation in anesthetized rats. Exp. Brain. Res. 137 (1), 94–102.

Macdonald, A.J., Macrae, K.D., Master, B.R., Rubin, A.P., 1983. Superficial acupuncture in the relief of chronic low back pain. Ann. R. Coll. Surg. Engl. 65 (1), 44–46.

Macdonald, A.J.R., 1983. Segmental acupuncture therapy. Acupunct. Electro-Ther. Res. 8 (3), 267–282.

Mann, F., 1992. Reinventing Acupuncture: A New Concept of Ancient Medicine. Butterworth-Heinemann, Oxford.

Mann, F., 1998. A new system of acupuncture. In: Filshie, J., White, A. (Eds.), Medical Acupuncture - A Western Scientific Approach, first ed. Churchill Livingstone London. pp. 61–66.

Martimbianco, A.L.C., Porfirio, G.J., Pacheco, R.L., Torloni, M.R., Riera, R., 2019. Transcutaneous electrical nerve stimulation (TENS) for chronic neck pain. Cochrane Database Syst. Rev. 12, CD011927. https://doi.org/10.1002/14651858.

Megia Garcia, A., Serrano-Munoz, D., Bravo-Esteban, E., Ando Lafuente, S., Avendano-Coy, J., Gomez-Soriano, J., 2019. Analgesic effects of transcutaneous electrical nerve stimulation (TENS) in patients with fibromyalgia: a systematic review. Aten. Primaria. 51 (7), 406–415. https://doi.org/10.1016/j.aprim.2018.03.010.

Melzack, R., 1981. Myofascial trigger points: relation to acupuncture and mechanisms of pain. Arch. Phys. Med. Rehabil. 62 (3), 114–117.

Melzack, R., Wall, P.D., 1965. Pain mechanisms: a new theory. Science. 150 (3699), 971–979.

Moran, F., Leonard, T., Hawthorne, S., Hughes, C.M., McCrum-Gardner, E., Johnson, M.I., et al., 2011. Hypoalgesia in response to transcutaneous electrical nerve stimulation (TENS) depends on stimulation intensity. J. Pain. 12 (8), 929–935.

Moré, A.O., Cidral-Filho, F.J., Mazzardo-Martins, L., Martins, D.F., Nascimento, F.P., Li, S.M., et al., 2013. Caffeine at moderate doses can inhibit acupuncture-induced analgesia in a mouse model of postoperative pain. J. Caffeine. Res. 3 (3), 143–148.

Morton, C., Du, H., Xiao, H., Maisch, B., Zimmermann, M., 1988. Inhibition of nociceptive responses of lumbar dorsal horn neurones by remote noxious afferent stimulation in the cat. Pain. 34 (1), 75–83.

NICE: National Institute for Health and Care Excellence, 2007. NICE Clinical Guideline 55 Intrapartum Care: Care of Healthy Women and Their Babies during Childbirth.

NICE: National Institute for Health and Care Excellence, 2011. NICE Clinical Guideline 126. Management of Stable Angina.

NICE: National Institute for Health and Care Excellence, 2014. Osteoarthritis: Care and Management. Available from http://nice.org.uk/guidance/cg177.

NICE: National Institute for Health and Care Excellence, 2016. Low Back Pain and Sciatica in over 16s: Assessment and Management. National Institute for Health and Care Excellence (NICE), London, pp. 1–18. Clinical guideline [NG59].

NICE: National Institute for Health and Care Excellence, 2018. Rheumatoid Arthritis in Adults. Available from www.nice.org.uk/NG100.

NICE: National Institute for Health and Care Excellence, 2021. Chronic Pain (Primary and Secondary) in over 16s: Assessment of All Chronic Pain and Management of Chronic Primary Pain (NG193). National Institute for Health and Care Excellence (NICE), London, UK.

Ottawa Panel, 2004. Ottawa Panel evidence-based clinical practice guidelines for therapeutic exercises in the management of rheumatoid arthritis in adults. Phys. Ther. 84 (10), 934–972.

Pal, S., Dixit, R., Moe, S., Godinho, M.A., Abas, A.B., Ballas, S.K., et al., 2020. Transcutaneous electrical nerve stimulation (TENS) for pain management in sickle cell disease. Cochrane Database Syst. Rev. 3, CD012762. https://doi.org/10.1002/14651858.CD012762.pub2.

Proctor, M., Farquhar, C., Stones, W., He, L., Zhu, X., Brown, J., 2002. Transcutaneous Electrical Nerve Stimulation and Acupuncture for Primary Dysmenorrhoea. Cochrane Database Syst. Rev. N.PAG-N.PAG.

Radhakrishnan, R., Sluka, K.A., 2005. Deep tissue afferents, but not cutaneous afferents, mediate transcutaneous electrical nerve stimulation-Induced antihyperalgesia. J. Pain. 6 (10), 673–680.

Rutjes, A.W., Nuesch, E., Sterchi, R., Kalichman, L., Hendriks, E., Osiri, M., et al., 2009. Transcutaneous electrostimulation for osteoarthritis of the knee. Cochrane Database Syst. Rev. 4, CD002823.

Sandberg, M., Larsson, B., Lindberg, L.G., Gerdle, B., 2005. Different patterns of blood flow response in the trapezius muscle following needle stimulation (acupuncture) between healthy subjects and patients with fibromyalgia and work-related trapezius myalgia. Eur. J. Pain. 9 (5), 497–510.

Sandberg, M., Lindberg, L.-G., Gerdle, B., 2004. Peripheral effects of needle stimulation (acupuncture) on skin and muscle blood flow in fibromyalgia. Eur. J. Pain. 8 (2), 163–171.

Sandberg, M., Lundeberg, T., Lindberg, L.G., Gerdle, B., 2003. Effects of acupuncture on skin and muscle blood flow in healthy subjects. Eur. J. Appl. Physiol. 90 (1–2), 114–119.

Sandkühler, J., Chen, J.G., Cheng, G., 1997. Low-frequency stimulation of afferent adelta-fibers induces long-term depression at primary afferent synapses with substantia gelatinosa neurons in the rat. J. Neurosci. 17 (16), 6483–6491.

Sato, A., Sato, Y., Shimura, M., Uchida, S., 2000. Calcitonin gene-related peptide produces skeletal muscle vasodilation following antidromic stimulation of unmyelinated afferents in the dorsal root in rats. Neurosci. Lett. 283 (2), 137–140.

Sato, A., Sato, Y., Suzuki, A., Uchida, S., 1993. Neural mechanisms of the reflex inhibition and excitation of gastric motility elicited by acupuncture-like stimulation in anesthetized rats. Neurosci. Res. 18 (1), 53–62.

Scharf, H.P., Mansmann, U., Streitberger, K., Witte, S., Kramer, J., Maier, C., et al., 2006. Acupuncture and knee osteoarthritis: a three-armed randomized trial. Ann. Intern. Med. 145 (1), 12–20.

Shaw, V., 2014. Chōng meridian an ancient Chinese description of the vascular system? Acupunct. Med. 32 (3), 279–285.

Shaw, V., McLennan, A.K., 2016. Was acupuncture developed by Han Dynasty Chinese anatomists? Anat. Rec. 299 (5), 643–659.

Shinbara, H., Okubo, M., Sumiya, E., Fukuda, F., Yano, T., Kitade, T., 2008. Effects of manual acupuncture with sparrow pecking on muscle blood flow of normal and denervated hindlimb in rats. Acupunct. Med. 26 (3), 149–159.

Sluka, K., Walsh, D., 2016. Chapter 8: transcutaneous electrical nerve stimulation and interferential therapy. In: KA, S. (Ed.), Mechanisms and Management of Pain for the Physical Therapist, second ed. IASP Press, pp. 203–224.

Smith, D.L., Walczyk, M.H., Campbell, S., 1986. Acupuncture needle induced compartment syndrome. West. J. Med. 144 (4), 478–479.

Steindler, A., 1940. The interpretation of sciatic radiation and the syndrome of low-back pain. J. Bone. Joint. Surg. Am. 22 (1), 28–34.

Takano, T., Chen, X., Luo, F., Fujita, T., Ren, Z., Goldman, N., et al., 2012. Traditional acupuncture triggers a local increase in adenosine in human subjects. J. Pain. 13 (12), 1215–1223. https://doi.org/10.1016/j.jpain.2012.09.012.

Tao, H., Wang, T., Dong, X., Guo, Q., Xu, H., Wan, Q., 2018. Effectiveness of transcutaneous electrical nerve stimulation for the treatment of migraine: a meta-analysis of randomized controlled trials. J. Headache Pain. 19 (1), 42.

Thoren, P., Floras, J.S., Hoffmann, P., Seals, D.R., 1990. Endorphins and exercise: physiological mechanisms and clinical implications. Med. Sci. Sports. Exerc. 22, 417–428 (0195-9131 SB - M).

Thuvarakan, K., Zimmermann, H., Mikkelsen, M.K., Gazerani, P., 2020. Transcutaneous electrical nerve stimulation as a pain-relieving approach in labor pain: a systematic review and meta-analysis of randomized controlled trials. Neuromodulation. 23 (6), 732–746.

Travell, J., Rinzler, S.H., 1952. The myofascial genesis of pain. PGM (Postgrad. Med.) 11 (5), 425–434.

Travell, J.G., Simons, D.G., 1983. Myofascial Pain & Dysfunction. The Trigger Point Manual. Volume 1. The Upper Extremities, first ed. Williams & Wilkins, Philadelphia.

Unschuld, P.U., 2016. Huang Di Nei Jing Ling Shu - the Ancient Classic on Needle Therapy, first ed. University of California Press.

Vance, C.G.T., Zimmerman, M.B., Dailey, D.L., Rakel, B.A., Geasland, K.M., Chimenti, R.L., et al., 2021. Reduction in movement-evoked pain and fatigue during initial 30-minute transcutaneous electrical nerve stimulation treatment predicts transcutaneous electrical nerve stimulation responders in women with fibromyalgia. Pain. 162 (5), 1545–1555.

Vickers, A.J., 1996. Can acupuncture have specific effects on health? A systematic review of acupuncture antiemesis trials. J. R. Soc. Med. 89 (6), 303–311.

Vickers, A.J., Cronin, A.M., Maschino, A.C., Lewith, G., MacPherson, H., Foster, N.E., et al., 2012. Acupuncture for chronic pain: individual patient data meta-analysis. Arch. Intern. Med. 172 (19), 1444–1453.

Vickers, A.J., Vertosick, E.A., Lewith, G., MacPherson, H., Foster, N.E., Sherman, K.J., et al., 2018. Acupuncture for chronic pain: update of an individual patient data meta-analysis. J. Pain. 19 (5), 455–474.

Walsh, B., 2001. Control of infection in acupuncture. Acupunct. Med. 19 (2), 109–111.

Walsh, D.M., Lowe, A.S., McCormack, K., Willer, J.C., Baxter, G.D., Allen, J.M., 1998. Transcutaneous electrical nerve stimulation: effect on peripheral nerve conduction, mechanical pain threshold, and tactile threshold in humans. Arch. Phys. Med. Rehabil. 79 (9), 1051–1058.

White, A., 1999. Neurophysiology of acupuncture analgesia. In: Ernst, E., White, A. (Eds.), Acupuncture: A Scientific Appraisal. Butterworth-Heinemann, Oxford.

White, A., 2004. A cumulative review of the range and incidence of significant adverse events associated with acupuncture. Acupunct. Med. 22 (3), 122–133.

White, A., Cummings, M., Barlas, P., Cardini, F., Filshie, J., Foster, N.E., et al., 2008. Defining an adequate dose of acupuncture using a neurophysiological approach--a narrative review of the literature. Acupunct. Med. 26 (2), 111–120.

White, A., Cummings, M., Filshie, J., 2018. An Introduction to Western Medical Acupuncture, second ed. Elsevier.

White, A., & Editorial Board of Acupuncture in Medicine, 2009. Western medical acupuncture: a definition. Acupunct. Med. 27 (1), 33–35.

Witt, C.M., Pach, D., Brinkhaus, B., Wruck, K., Tag, B., Mank, S., et al., 2009. Safety of acupuncture: results of a prospective observational study with 229,230 patients and introduction of a medical information and consent form. Forsch. Komplementmed. 16 (2), 91–97.

Wu, L.C., Weng, P.W., Chen, C.H., Huang, Y.Y., Tsuang, Y.H., Chiang, C.J., 2018. Literature review and meta-analysis of transcutaneous electrical nerve stimulation in treating chronic back pain. Reg. Anesth. Pain. Med. 43 (4), 425–433.

Zhao, Z.Q., 2008. Neural mechanism underlying acupuncture analgesia. Prog. Neurobiol. 85 (4), 355–375.

Zhou, J., Dan, Y., Yixian, Y., Lyu, M., Zhong, J., Wang, Z., et al., 2020. Efficacy of transcutaneous electronic nerve stimulation in postoperative analgesia after pulmonary surgery: a systematic review and meta-analysis. Am. J. Phys. Med. Rehabil. 99 (3), 241–249.

Chapter | 17 |

Workplace rehabilitation

Susan E. Peters

LEARNING OBJECTIVES

At the end of this chapter, readers will understand the:
1. Role of healthcare professionals in facilitating the RTW process for a worker with an injury/pain.
2. Different conceptual models that can be applied to facilitating the RTW process.
3. Roles of key stakeholders in the RTW process.
4. Multidimensional factors that influence RTW.
5. Overcoming barriers and identifying facilitators for RTW.
6. Types of interventions (and components of programmes) that facilitate early and safe RTW.
7. Steps involved in a work rehabilitation programme for the injured worker.

Introduction

Work is central to our identity and social roles (Waddell & Burton 2006) and is a social determinant of health and well-being (Lovejoy et al. 2021). Being unemployed has been related to increased mortality rates, hospitalisation rates and poorer physical and mental health (Mathers & Schofield 1998). Work rehabilitation is an important part of healthcare professionals' role and the treatments they provide. Work rehabilitation consists of any intervention that is geared towards the prevention of work disability, facilitating participation in work and satisfactory fulfilment of the worker role (AOTA 2017). It is 'a managed process involving timely intervention with appropriate and adequate services based on assessed need, and which is aimed at maintaining injured or ill employees in, or returning them to, suitable employment' (Heads of Workers' Compensation Authorities 2019, p. 17). Work disability can be operationally defined as 'time off work, reduced productivity or working with functional limitations as a result (outcome), or either traumatic or non-traumatic clinical conditions' (Schultz et al. 2007, p. 329).

Therefore the goals of work rehabilitation are wide-ranging, and can include primary, secondary and tertiary interventions (Box 17.1). The return-to-work (RTW) process and the type of intervention implemented also depend on whether the worker with pain is able to:
- Stay at work: worker can remain at work, possibly with work accommodations, and self-manage their pain and other symptoms. This also involves preventing an injury or illness from occurring.
- Early RTW: worker returns as early as reasonably and safely possible after the pain inciting event with an RTW programme including modified, meaningful and suitable work duties.
- Prolonged RTW: worker may have a failed RTW attempt or require longer work absence due to the extreme severity of the injury.
- Unemployed but seeking work (jobseeker): worker has a disability or health condition with work limitations and is not currently in the workforce but is seeking competitive employment.

Aetiology of pain in the workplace

Musculoskeletal disorders (MSDs) and injuries are the most common reasons for pain in the workplace: they are inflammatory and degenerative conditions that impact muscles, nerves, tendons and joints (Punnett & Wegman 2004). Substantial evidence exists to support the multifactorial nature of work-related pain, and associated conditions and disorders (Oakman et al. 2019). Work-related musculoskeletal problems are generally acknowledged as those that: (1) the work environment, job tasks and/or demands contributed significantly to the condition, or (2) the condition was made worse or persisted for longer due to work. Hazardous and ill-designed working conditions are the main cause of MSDs and work-related pain including physical work environment, job demands (e.g. high physical demands and fast work pace), psychosocial factors (e.g. supervisor and co-worker support) and the way work is designed (e.g. shifts, and longer work hours) can all contribute to MSDs (Oakman et al. 2019). High work demands and/or low control over one's job have been found to contribute significantly to symptoms (Karasek & Theorell 1991) and early mortality (Gonzalez-Mule & Cockburn 2016).

For acute MSDs, the relationship with work can usually be easily established. However, for chronic pain conditions (such as neck and back pain), the aetiology is often cumulative and a result of multiple work hazards, and establishing the connection to work can be challenging. In countries where workers' compensation systems exist, there is often a requirement to identify the work-related hazard or event that triggered the injury or condition (e.g. Safe Work Australia 2019). Healthcare providers, generally

medical doctors and occupational physicians, are responsible for making the work-related designation for an injury or disease. In the situation of complex or chronic conditions, the multiple hazards that may have been contributed to the injury or condition may not be fully appreciated, and subsequent controls may be overlooked (Oakman et al. 2019).

Other conditions causing pain include arthritis, acute musculoskeletal injuries (such as fractures and amputations), neck pain, work-related cancers, migraines and other systematic illnesses. The ageing workforce also poses a significant challenge. Older workers are more vulnerable to injury and may have other painful health conditions (Peng & Chan 2019; Steenstra et al. 2017). They are also needing to work longer before retirement and remain productive at work (Steenstra et al. 2017). Research suggests that older workers find returning to work after an injury more challenging (Durand et al. 2021a, b). They are less likely to RTW after an injury due to other health conditions, no financial need to work or having spouse or child still at home who can support them (Fan et al. 2020).

Incidence of pain in the workplace

MSDs are the leading contributor to disability globally: approximately 1.7 billion people experience MSDs globally, with low back pain being the leading cause affecting nearly 600 million people (Cieza et al. 2020; Hartvigsen et al. 2018). These conditions, typically characterised by pain, can result in considerable time off work, work disability and even early retirement from work. They are also the largest contributor to years lived with a disability (YLD) worldwide, resulting in lower quality of life and well-being (Vos et al. 2016).

Persistent MSDs have been associated with opioid misuse (Dale et al. 2021). In some countries, such as the United States, opioid use has been found to be higher in some occupational groups that also experience high incidence of pain-related conditions, such as construction (Hawkins et al. 2019; Morano et al. 2018). This is significant, as opioid misuse is common and can lead to overdose and long-term (work-) disability (Hawkins et al. 2020; Webster et al. 2007).

Cost of pain

Disability and costs associated with MSDs and pain-related conditions are projected to increase in future decades. Economic impacts occur at the individual, employer, insurer and societal levels. The societal cost of workers' pain is high, estimated in some countries, like the United States, to be around $560 to $635 billion annually (Gaskin & Richard 2012). In Australia, MSDs contribute to 12% of the country's burden of disease and injury, and 23% of nonfatal burden, ranking second only to mental health and substance use (Australian Institute of Health and Welfare 2017); lost productivity due to days missed from work, lost work hours and lower wages due to time missed are estimated to account for about 50% of this amount. In addition, a small proportion of cases that experience higher disability and time off work contribute to a high proportion of these costs (Chou et al. 2007; Maetzel & Li 2002). The burden of these types of injuries will likely increase in low- and medium-income countries where health and workers' compensation systems are weak or limited (Hartvigsen et al. 2018). Therefore there is increasing consensus that countries around the world need to implement strategies to reduce the costs of pain in the workforce; improve RTW processes; and facilitate early, safe and meaningful RTW or stay at work (SAW) for workers with injuries and pain (Waddell & Burton 2006).

Contextual considerations

While there is international recognition of the importance of keeping workers with pain at work, the social, political and economic contexts of different countries drive how health and work disability policies and programmes are implemented (Sorensen et al. 2021). Prevailing legislation and the different arrangement of systems within each country (and state or provincial jurisdictions) influence how policies, programmes and practices impact workers' RTW and healthcare journeys. In general, policies, standard guidelines and programmes are geared towards fostering and maintaining engagement in the labour force. However, differences exist across the globe in how workers' compensation, social security, unemployment benefits, employment services, healthcare systems and insurance, as well as programmes to facilitate work participation, are implemented and directed towards injured workers (MacEachen 2018). This, in turn, also impacts the role that a healthcare professional has in assisting the worker with pain to SAW, or RTW. Because of the differences in systems that exist globally, workers' experiences of the process can vary significantly, and their experiences can also impact their work-related outcomes (Collie et al. 2016; Kilgour et al. 2015).

Given the varied roles that healthcare professionals can play and the significant number of different systems around the world that influence these roles, this chapter will focus on broad principles for work rehabilitation.

Conceptual frameworks

Work disability prevention and work rehabilitation has been studied from various disciplinary and epistemological perspectives, resulting in differing conceptual models and definitions.

Conceptual models can be very useful in helping to understand (1) various factors that can influence the RTW process and work disability, and (2) the different levels at which interventions can be implemented. While a comprehensive review of all the models (see examples of other useful models in Costa-Black et al. 2013; Knauf et al. 2014; Kristman et al. 2020) that are available is out of the scope of this chapter, four examples of models are described below, and are useful for the healthcare provider to understand the complex nature and the various systems involved in work rehabilitation.

Biopsychosocial model

The biopsychosocial model recognises that work disability not only has biological and physical determinants, but may also be influenced by psychological, behavioural (e.g. lifestyle, health behaviours), cognitive and social conditions (e.g. cultural, family, social supports) (Knauf & Schultz 2016). For work rehabilitation, this means that healthcare professionals should broaden their perspective on injury and pain to understand the complex interplay of factors impacting recovery and RTW, and to better address these factors through the treatments they recommend and provide. The model also accepts that there is an interaction between the individual and systems level, and focuses on motivations, perceptions, beliefs and expectations of recovery and disability, self-efficacy and coping (Knauf & Schultz 2016). The World Health Organization's International Classification of Functioning, Disability and Health (WHO 2018) reinforces this model and focuses our attention on work functioning rather than limitations.

Work disability prevention arena model

This model, depicted in Fig. 17.1, is an example of an ecological case management model focused on secondary prevention that considers the key stakeholders involved in work rehabilitation (Loisel et al. 2005). This interdisciplinary model depicts the complexity and interaction of the multiple systems across healthcare, insurance/compensation, employer, and the individual worker within the broader socio-political-economic system (including relevant disability and work rehabilitation legislation and standards). This model highlights the different perspectives, motivations for RTW, and paradigms of the key stakeholders, and the critical roles that they play in facilitating the RTW process. All have a common goal to return the worker back to work in a safe and timely manner. Often this goal is financially motivated, but to the worker it is also related to their quality of life and sense of self-worth. Within this model, stakeholder collaboration is instrumental in facilitating RTW and preventing

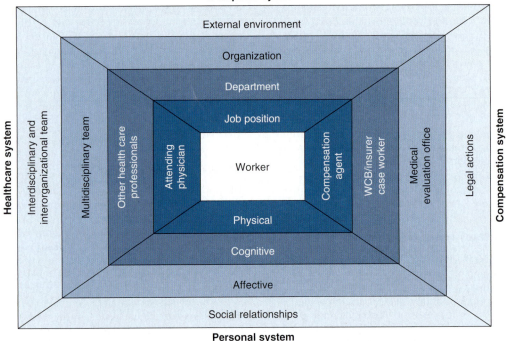

Fig. 17.1 Work disability arena model. *WCB*, Workers' Compensation Board. (From Loisel et al. 2005.)

work disability. Decision-making can be influenced by the actions, behaviours, interactions, and motivations of each stakeholder within the system.

Readiness to RTW model

This model acknowledges the temporal nature of the RTW process, and the recurrent nature of work-related pain and injury (Franche & Krause 2002). RTW is viewed as a process – from the time the injury occurs to the time a person returns to work and remains at work long-term. Based on the Readiness for Change Model (Prochaska & DiClemente 1983), the Readiness to RTW Model postulates that an individual worker's readiness to RTW is based on five progressive phases: pre-contemplation, contemplation, preparation for action, action, and maintenance (Franche & Krause 2002). Each phase recognises that worker decisional balance, self-efficacy, change processes and motivation play a role at each stage of the RTW process.

Harvard Center for work, health and well-being's safety, health and well-being model

This transdisciplinary model (Fig. 17.2) provides a systems-level framework which focuses on the role of

working conditions—physical work environment, psychosocial work environment, job design—and how they shape worker and enterprise outcomes, such as RTW outcomes, both related to the worker (e.g. work ability, individual productivity, lost wages) and the enterprise (e.g. absenteeism rates, productivity, and lost costs) (Sorensen et al. 2021). For example, a healthcare provider who has a primary job task of transferring a patient might need to consider how various working conditions impact on the successful and safe completion of that task, and the various hospital policies that might impact those conditions (Box 17.2).

Evidence consistently indicates that with good working conditions, workers with injuries and illness are able to remain at work or RTW with accommodations before they reach full recovery to produce a safe and sustainable transition to regular full duties (Cancelliere et al. 2016; Cullen et al. 2018; Franche et al. 2005; Gouin et al. 2019; Palmer et al. 2012). Moreover, working conditions are changing as technology advances, different and flexible work arrangements are made possible, such as through telecommuting, which may act as novel work hazards but may also provide expanded opportunities for work accommodations (Peters et al., 2022).

This model also emphasises the importance of organisational and public policy on influencing working

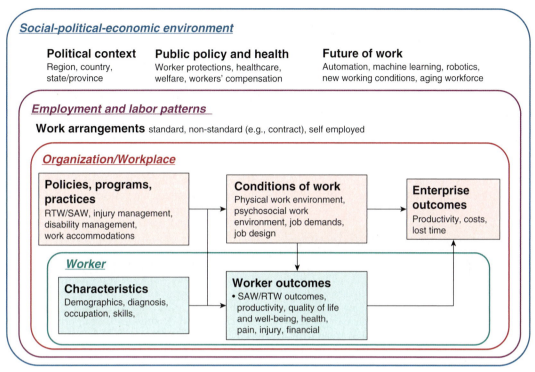

Fig. 17.2 Harvard Center model. *RTW*, Return-to-work; *SAW*, stay-at-work. (Modified from Sorensen et al. 2021.)

BOX 17.2 Example of different working conditions impacting the health and safety of a healthcare worker during a patient transfer

Physical work environment:	Psychosocial work environment:	Job demands:	Job design:
Is there equipment to transfer the patient available? Is the equipment in good working order? Does the hospital have policies for maintenance and availability of the equipment?	What is the hospital culture for using equipment to transfer patients? Are supervisors and co-workers supportive of appropriate equipment use, or is there a tendency to select the easiest method of transfer? How much decision-making ability does the worker have in their role? e.g. Nursing assistants may feel like they need to follow the orders of nurses.	Is there sufficient time to use the equipment safely? If something goes wrong during the transfer, what is the policy for protecting the safety of the patient?	Is the patient's mobility status and type of transfer needed always accurately documented in the patient's care plan? Does the worker receive adequate rest breaks if their main role involves physical demands?

---

conditions and can be used as a framework for work rehabilitation for primary, secondary or tertiary interventions. It considers how different policies, programmes, and practices can influence the working conditions, either hindering or supporting RTW.

The employer and workplace are considered within the broader context of the socio-political-economic environment and employment and labour patterns, which can have implications for RTW process and stakeholder engagement, motivations, and decisions. This model also recognises that the trends in the broader context, such as increasing technological innovation, changes in work arrangements, globalisation, and demographic workforce changes (e.g. increasing ageing workforce) impact jobs and workers' experiences (Sorensen et al. 2021). The focus on thinking about the different working conditions that a worker is exposed to in their job can aid the healthcare professional in thinking about which conditions are supportive or hindering the worker's RTW, or ability to SAW. Often the focus is placed on physical work environment and job demands, but psychosocial factors (e.g. supervisor and co-worker support), or job design (e.g. shifts, schedules), can also play an important role for RTW.

Stakeholders in work rehabilitation

The injured worker and employer are the central actors in work rehabilitation. In addition, there are a range of external stakeholders involved, depending on whether the focus is primary, secondary or tertiary intervention; the circumstances and severity of the injury or condition; and the complexity of the work situation and RTW. The employer is responsible for providing a safe work environment and, in many contexts, is required to have policies, programmes and practices geared towards supporting injured workers either SAW or RTW. In some countries, the insurer also plays a key role, often providing income replacement to workers, rehabilitation and managing a worker's compensation claim. Healthcare providers are nearly always involved, especially if the injury or condition is work-related in origin or in jurisdictions that have workers' compensation systems. These can include medical doctors, occupational physicians, physiotherapists, occupational therapists and other allied health professionals. Additionally, return-to work coordinators (RTW coordinators) may be in place to facilitate and coordinate the RTW process. Achieving a positive work outcome relies on the commitment and collaborative participation of the stakeholders involved.

In this chapter, we focus mainly on the role of allied health professionals in work rehabilitation.

Worker

Workers have differing work and RTW experiences based on their own unique personal circumstances, their work and employer, as well as the jurisdiction and associated legislation, insurance, and RTW procedures. Workers also have rights and responsibilities in the work rehabilitation process: they need to report their injury to their employer, and to make reasonable efforts to participate in the design

and implementation of their rehabilitation and RTW plans. A worker may be receiving workers' compensation or welfare payments, and these systems may be funding their treatment and work rehabilitation.

Most workers manage to continue working despite their injury and symptoms, and for many that require time off work, their RTW is relatively straightforward. However, for some workers, their pain and work situation may require more attention. Approximately one in five workers require additional time off after their first return after their injury or pain onset, and about 15% experience ongoing limitations with work tasks when they return (Social Research Centre 2018). Workers' RTW experiences also vary depending on their occupation and the working conditions to which they are exposed: workers with high job demands and limited control over their work have poorer RTW outcomes (Haveraaen et al. 2017).

A safe and supportive workplace culture, free of stigma associated with workers' compensation and modified RTW programmes—that focus on meaningful and good work—are necessary to support the worker in pain in the workplace. The most effective approaches are tailored to the worker; however, supportive injury and disability management policies and other upstream approaches provide benefits to all workers. Workers can find navigating the RTW and insurance or workers' compensation systems challenging (Kilgour et al. 2015). For example, a systematic review found that stigma hinders a sustainable work outcome and negatively impacts worker well-being (van Beukering et al. 2021). Another qualitative study of the effect of the workers' compensation process on workers in Quebec found that the stigma and prejudice due to their injured worker status and stereotypes about them 'playing the system', as well as experiences of power imbalance in the workers' compensation system (with the worker having the least amount of power of all stakeholders) contributed to higher mental health issues (Lippel 2007). However, participants also identified the positive health effects of being in the process, such as more expedient access to healthcare and a valuable, supportive relationship with someone in power, such as a health professional or RTW coordinator, who knew the system and the process. Healthcare professionals can have a role in educating the worker about the RTW process and legislation, as well as building the worker's health literacy to empower them to take a more active role in their recovery and RTW.

Worker factors, workplace factors and the RTW process itself can have impacts on the worker and work-related outcomes, which can vary by pain duration. Table 17.1 summarises the best evidence synthesis of 56 systematic reviews of factors affecting RTW outcomes after injury or illness (Cancelliere et al. 2016). This review of reviews found that positive RTW outcomes were influenced by: higher education and socio-economic status, higher

TABLE 17.1 Summary of factors influencing RTW outcomes for workers with MSDs

	Positive RTW outcomes	Negative RTW outcomes
Demographic factors	Higher education and socio-economic status	Older age
Worker psychosocial	Higher self-efficacy and recovery/RTW expectations	
Biological and body structure	Lower severity of injury	Higher pain and disability
Workplace	Pre-injury employment Work modification/accommodation	Higher physical job demands Previous sickness absence
Intervention-related	Multidisciplinary interventions Early intervention Stakeholder participation in RTW process RTW coordination Educational interventions Psychological interventions	

MSDs, Musculoskeletal disorders; *RTW,* Return-to-work.
From Cancelliere et al. (2016).

self-efficacy and optimistic recovery and RTW expectations, lower severity of injury and pain, effective RTW coordination and multidisciplinary interventions that include the employer and other key stakeholders. They also found that negative RTW outcomes were impacted by being older, higher pain or disability, occupations with higher physical work demands, previous sick leave and unemployment.

Up to 27% of workers who experience a musculoskeletal injury also experience significant psychological impacts and mental health symptoms (Collie et al. 2020). A review of the literature examined factors influencing RTW for workers who have a psychological response to their injury and found that the following worker psychological and physical factors influenced RTW outcomes (Safe Work Australia 2019): (1) workers who have high levels of pain catastrophising and fear avoidance, (2) workers' concerns about making a claim for workers' compensation, (3) workers' own recovery expectations', (4) workers' self-efficacy to achieve their recovery or RTW goals and (5) perceived work ability.

Many factors, including many that are not listed in this chapter, can play a role in either facilitating or limiting a workers' RTW (Peters et al. 2017). Each worker's experience is unique, and some factors may not have been fully examined empirically. However, it does illustrate the multidimensional nature of factors influencing work-related outcomes. Interventions need to address the multidimensional factors of the worker and workplace impacting RTW.

In another review of 41 qualitative studies focused on workers with chronic pain and employer experiences of challenges for RTW (Grant et al. 2020), a mismatch of expectations between the worker and employer resulted in tension and the worker feeling judged or having difficulty asking for assistance. When a worker can navigate obstacles and participate in the RTW planning, this will likely result in a successful RTW outcome despite the pain.

Healthcare professionals may need to support and provide advice to the injured worker to help them navigate the healthcare and RTW systems and processes. This could include knowledge of the insurer claims management processes, coordinated approaches to recovery and RTW, assistance with navigating employer processes and practices and providing workplace support, interventions to support the workers' psychological response to the injury and tailored treatments and support based on the worker circumstances (Safe Work Australia 2019). Healthcare professionals should also acknowledge that workers are dealing with multiple stakeholders throughout their recovery, and navigating these relationships (on top of all their other concerns) may be challenging. Workers may need additional support outside the role of the healthcare professional, such as formal advocates who may be union representations, lawyers and other community organisations. Informal advocates such as family, friends or religious leaders may also play a key role in the recovery and support of the injured worker (Snippen et al. 2019).

Employer

The employer has a responsibility to provide a safe work environment with good working conditions. They also need to reasonably accommodate workers who have pain, injury or disability. The organisational culture and climate of the employer, the availability of suitable, meaningful and modified work, the need for flexibility as the worker recovers, all need to be balanced with organisational productivity, financial impacts and avoiding placing undue burden on co-workers or supervisors (Jansen et al. 2021; Main et al. 2021).

Supervisors are integral to facilitating the RTW process and can have a great influence on the worker's work-related outcomes (MacEachen et al. 2006; Van Oostrom et al. 2009). However, supervisors can find disability management and their role in the RTW process challenging. A study of supervisors in Australia identified the following difficulties when supporting the injured worker including: juggling the RTW process with their current workload, identifying and problem solving suitable duties and work accommodations, interpreting the doctor's capacity for work certificate, ensuring the worker is performing safe duties to their capacity, understanding the RTW process and their responsibilities, balancing the needs of the worker and organisation, managing conflict as a result of the worker's RTW and being honest with the worker especially if it is news the worker will not want to hear (Johnston et al. 2015).

Lower levels of co-worker support have also been associated with prolonged work absences (Campbell et al. 2013; Steenstra et al. 2005), and have been found to be as important as supervisor support or return to meaningful duties (Mielenz et al. 2008).

There can be many challenges when working with employers to implement organisational change (Amick et al. 2000; Whysall et al. 2006). When consulting to employers, allied health professionals may need to provide transformative safety leadership strategies and training (Clarke 2013), as well as providing practical tools and techniques to enable supervisors to facilitate a smooth RTW. Employers should provide budgetary control and time for supervisors to deal with health and safety issues; however, this is not always the case. Small and medium businesses may face unique challenges due to limited resources, limited experiences dealing with workers experiences of pain and work ability, limited capacity to provide suitable duties and higher proportionate financial costs related to accommodating a worker with chronic pain (Australian Small Business and Family Enterprise Ombudsman 2016).

RTW coordinators

An RTW coordinator is someone with expert training, knowledge and skills to support workers to return or remain at work after being ill or injured (Safe Work Australia 2019). They are often employed by an employer or are contracted to perform the role. RTW coordinators have been found to facilitate an earlier RTW (Dol et al. 2021). Within the bounds of the legislation of a jurisdiction,

an RTW coordinator's main role is to support workers as they recover, facilitate return to good and safe work and provide a link between the various stakeholders involved. This professional title may also be called other names in different countries, such as case manager, rehabilitation counsellor or disability prevention specialist, and may not be mandated. Sometimes healthcare professionals act in these roles; however, they may also be other safety or insurance personnel who have received additional training. Studies have examined the required competencies for RTW coordinators (Pransky et al. 2010; Shaw et al. 2008) which range from knowledge of the legal, insurance aspects and RTW process, assessment (e.g. workplace assessment and interviewing), identifying barriers and facilitators for RTW, planning for modified duty, implementing the RTW plan, communication, problem solving and conflict management and workplace mediation.

Role of healthcare professionals

Around the world, the role of the healthcare professional can be greatly influenced by the healthcare and labour systems in place. They may only have a role in medical treatment and intervention and have little involvement with the workplace. They may be involved only if the worker claims workers' compensation, and collaborate with the claimant and the insurer to develop a suitable or modified duties programme to get the worker back to functional employment.

Medical practitioners, often acting as the treating specialist, provide and recommend treatments for the injured worker. They are also often required to provide a diagnosis, work-related determination, establish capacity for work, communicate with other stakeholders and complete certification (such as, medical certificates, fit for work certificates, and approving suitable duties plans) (Denne et al. 2015). In some cases, an occupational physician may be involved. The role of occupational physicians varies greatly across jurisdictions. For example, in some European countries, the occupational physician provides all primary care for work-related injuries (Horppu et al. 2016). Whereas, in other countries, such as Australia, New Zealand or the United States, the occupational physician may only be involved depending on the employer, workers' compensation insurer and complexity of the workers' injury and case (ACOEM 2008; Australasian Faculty of Occupational and Environmental Medicine 2022).

Role of allied health providers

Allied health professionals are involved in either providing clinical treatments, or as a workplace rehabilitation provider (WRP). Allied health professionals can also have different roles depending on the worker's current work status. Allied health professionals who are providing clinical care, such as physical therapy or psychological services, have an important role in facilitating early RTW, as well as improving function and symptoms. A substantial body of evidence suggests that pain-relieving treatments alone do not guarantee RTW, and therefore clinical interventions also need to have work-focused goals (Cullen et al. 2018; Hutting et al. 2020). Accordingly, therapists should include work-focused conversations in their rehabilitation (Hutting et al. 2020).

Some allied health providers, such as physiotherapists and occupational therapists, may also provide integrated rehabilitation at the workplace, either as a contractor or as an employee of the organisation. Onsite therapy can provide benefits to the organisation and the worker by reducing the incidence of prolonged work injuries, providing early symptom management and facilitating early recovery to enable workers to remain at work (Donovan et al. 2021). An Australian study examining the benefits of an onsite physiotherapist reported cost savings to the insurer and employer, fewer injuries, shorter work absences and fewer workers' compensation claims (Donovan et al. 2021).

A WRP is generally a healthcare professional who is specialised in work rehabilitation. In this role, they may be engaged to provide recommendations and advice on RTW and other interventions to enable a workers' recovery and safe and meaningful participation at work. They frequently coordinate with other stakeholders, such as medical doctors, insurer and employer, to facilitate the RTW process.

The WRP can provide primary, secondary or tertiary intervention—largely dependent on whether the worker has a job to which they are aiming to return, or the worker is returning to the workforce in a different job or occupation. The WRP provides advice on primary prevention, such as ergonomics; improving working conditions; and even advice on policies, programmes and practices. They may provide 'occupational rehabilitation' services and be heavily involved in the RTW process, liaising with workers and managers to provide workplace-based early intervention and ensure the worker can safely remain at work beyond the first return. They may also work with people with persistent pain who cannot return to their usual occupation and are considering returning to the workforce in a new occupation; this is commonly called 'vocational rehabilitation'.

The role of the WRP in some countries also encompasses absenteeism management for workers with any injury or illness—regardless of whether it is work-related or not—where early intervention is provided no matter what the reason for days off work and whether the cause is work-related or not, and to manage presenteeism, for workers who do not take time off work but are not at full productivity due to injury, illness or disability (Calkins et al. 2000).

Knowledge and skills required by allied health providers for workplace rehabilitation practice

In some jurisdictions, allied health professionals may require specific qualifications and additional work rehabilitation training to become a work rehabilitation provider (Heads of Workers' Compensation Authorities 2019). Most commonly, they are occupational therapists, physiotherapists, psychologists, nurses, social workers, and less commonly, medical practitioners.

They require a range of knowledge and skills to practice in the work rehabilitation field. This includes knowledge of the prevailing legislation, such as workers' compensation, occupational health and safety, injury and disability management, disability discrimination and welfare legislation. They also require knowledge of the specific disability management and RTW processes, as well as other jurisdiction-specific procedures, to communicate to and assist the worker in navigating the systems and processes in place, such as workers' compensation regulations and processes (Jetha et al. 2021). There is also a need for a strong grounding in the nature, prognosis and functional impact of the pain-related injury, including the implications of treatments for RTW issues, e.g. the effect of pain medications on driving. In addition, they need to be able to address the workers' and employers' concerns and attitudes towards returning to work and provide strategies to overcome any barriers (Jetha et al. 2021). Importantly, providers need an understanding of the evidence for their practice and any treatments they recommend (Heads of Workers' Compensation Authorities 2019).

Effective communication skills are instrumental for the healthcare professional involved in work rehabilitation. These include communicating support and encouragement for the injured worker (and also the employer) throughout the RTW process; providing the information early or at the optimal time and throughout the process; considering word choice that is inclusive, supportive and easily understood; framing messages to highlight the benefits of being at work; and tailoring the communication to the specific worker and stakeholder(s) involved (Jetha et al. 2021).

Moving beyond a biomedical paradigm

Healthcare professionals can positively or negatively impact recovery and RTW outcomes (Spink et al. 2021). For a healthcare professional to focus on work in their treatment plans, or to provide specific work rehabilitation services, it assumes health professionals develop specific work-focused care is not in their scope of practice (Bartys et al. 2019). This has been addressed in various countries by the development of standards, and policies, directing healthcare professionals to have work-focused conversations with their patients, setting work-related treatment goals and addressing obstacles for RTW (Bartys et al. 2019). However, allied health professionals have also reported that they lack time and sufficient funding and resources to be able to achieve work-focused care in their practice (Johnston et al. 2012). Thus there is also a need for systems to adequately reimburse providers time for any increased engagement with the workplace and case management. Lastly, work-focused care needs to be included in healthcare professionals training and university curricula to facilitate this approach.

Evidence-based principles

Healthcare professionals practising in the work rehabilitation field can be involved in primary, secondary and tertiary interventions to promote good work. Evidence indicates that pain and function improve more rapidly for workers with an immediate or early (1–7 days) RTW after an acute inciting event (Shaw et al. 2018). However, it is important for this work to be 'good work'. 'Good work' defined by the Australasian Faculty of Occupational and Environmental Medicine (2022) means 'good work is engaging, fair, respectful and balances job demands, autonomy and job security. It is characterised by safe and healthy work practices, and it strikes a balance between the interests of individuals, employers and society. It requires effective change management, clear and realistic performance indicators, matches the work to the individual and uses transparent productivity metrics. Good work accepts the importance of culture and traditional beliefs. Healthcare professionals should strive to ensure that in their role, workers are exposed to good work conditions'. The next section provides a summary and examples of the types of interventions that healthcare professionals might implement in their role to support the injured worker to return to 'good work'.

work-focused goals as well as consider the multidimensional factors that may impact recovery and achieving a successful work outcome—that is, moving beyond a biomedical framework towards a multidimensional systems-level, biopsychosocial one. However, historically this has not been the case for healthcare professionals. For example, a study of Canadian physiotherapists found that only about 20% of physiotherapists focused on improving function and capacity for work in their practice, and this resulted in less than 50% of workers returning to work at the end of therapy (Poitras et al. 2005). Recent approaches have found that when providers move beyond the biomedical paradigm, with treatment being tailored to the worker including work-focused rehabilitation, both functional and work outcomes improved (Hutting et al. 2020; Xie et al. 2021). As healthcare professionals provide treatments soon after the injury or pain onset, they play an essential role in facilitating an early transition back to work. This can include having structured work-focused conversations (Box 17.3) and conducting work-related assessments, such as functional capacity evaluations (FCEs), work hardening, workplace-based self-management strategies and graded activity programmes.

Other challenges faced by the healthcare professionals

There have been concerns that treating healthcare professionals can compound the issues for workers returning to work, for example by certifying workers as unfit for all duties (when they are able to perform some meaningful role), lack of identification of suitable duties (when they are available), or by providing inaccurate education about timely resumption of activity and work (Waddell & Burton 2006). Some healthcare professionals feel that

Primary prevention

Primary prevention are interventions that are implemented before the injury or pain occurs. This is often achieved by preventing exposure to hazardous working conditions, providing working conditions that promote health and well-being and altering unsafe or unhealthy worker behaviours (IWH 2015). Employers have a duty to eliminate risks and where this is not practically possible, they need to reduce risks. They should also work towards

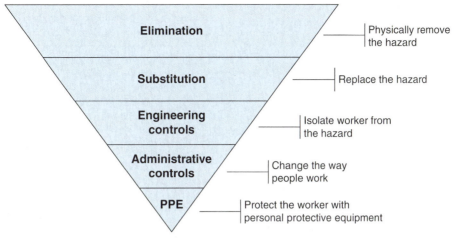

Fig. 17.3 Hierarchy of controls.

conditions that enable workers to thrive both at work and in their lives outside of work (Peters et al. 2021). Healthcare professionals can play a key role in primary prevention. For example, healthcare professionals often provide recommendations (such as ergonomic improvements, or injury reporting and prevention policies) to an organisation to control hazardous exposures to working conditions to protect workers from pain and injury.

Policies are another example of primary prevention. Policy changes occur at the system level: (1) public policy and legislation changes such as employer compliance, welfare supports, healthcare delivery, insurance regulation or workers' compensation claim processes and disability management and (2) organisational level, such as workplace policies surrounding reporting and addressing workplace hazards, safe and good working conditions, and standardised RTW and disability management practices. As the overlying public and organisation policy landscape can be complex and dynamic, healthcare professionals need to be well versed on how these policies might impact their practice, and the RTW, for specific workers.

A 'hierarchy of controls' framework is a useful tool for healthcare professionals who are focused on providing advice to employers for minimising risk of pain and injury in the workplace (Fig. 17.3) (CDC 2015). Although often used in primary prevention, it can also be used when making changes in the workplace when a worker is returning to work following an injury (that is, secondary intervention). Starting at the top of the hierarchy, eliminating the working condition/ risk is the most effective. If this cannot be achieved, reducing the risk should be undertaken by (1) substituting the risk with a lesser risk, (2) isolating workers from the hazard (e.g. providing guards or barriers), (3) or providing engineering controls to change the way work is complemented, e.g. providing a trolley to

move heavy items. In cases where this cannot be achieved, implementing administrative controls to minimise exposure reduces the level of risk or harm (e.g. procedures for safe use of equipment or manual handling, or limiting the amount of time someone is exposed). Lastly, personal protective equipment should be provided, and appropriate training provided, to protect workers in cases where no other more effective strategies can be implemented.

Secondary interventions

Secondary interventions target individual workers or groups of workers that demonstrate pain or early musculoskeletal injury and attempts to prevent the development of long-term (work-) disability through the reduction of symptoms and improvements in function (IWH 2015). These can be through symptom-reduction treatments that healthcare professionals implement and recommend in their clinical practice. However, as mentioned earlier, these should include a focus on both function- and work-related goal setting. These may also include RTW interventions designed to facilitate RTW after an injury, illness or disease, or to help the worker SAW while they recover or have ongoing symptoms. In a Cochrane systematic review, workplace-based interventions have been found to be effective in reducing work absences and time to RTW (van Vilsteren et al. 2015).

Workplace-based self-management programmes

Workplace-based *self-management programmes* are designed to improve workplace functioning and engagement for workers with work limitations. In a randomised controlled trial of US-based workers, mainly with pain conditions,

283

such as chronic MSDs and headaches, a self-management psychoeducation programme based on concepts of facilitated health self-management, self-efficacy, ergonomics and communication, was found to improve work engagement and reduce turnover intention (Shaw et al. 2022).

Principles for RTW interventions

Principles for successful RTW, based on a comprehensive review of the most effective workplace-based intervention conducted by the Institute for Work and Health, and Safe Work Australia, can guide RTW planning and interventions (Box 17.4) (Cullen et al. 2018; IWH 2014; Safe Work Australia 2019). These principles inform the role of the healthcare professional in supporting RTW and their engagement with other key RTW stakeholders. These principles provide important directions for healthcare professionals in their roles with workers who have work-related pain. These implications include the need for healthcare professionals to communicate with employers (with the worker's consent) about workplace demands and the potential impact on the worker's condition. For health professionals directly involved in the RTW planning process, there is a need to ensure the modified duties are safe, suitable to the worker's abilities and enacted as soon as is safely possible without disadvantaging co-workers and supervisors. They also have implications for a potential role, working with employers to help them improve their commitment to health and safety, to educate management and line supervisors about work disability prevention and RTW planning and to assist them to develop processes for early communication and effective in-house RTW coordination processes.

Stepped care and stratified care model

Increasing evidence supports a multidisciplinary multidimensional intervention model due to the complex nature of recovery and RTW (Cancelliere et al. 2016; Cullen et al. 2018). Various multidimensional secondary intervention models have been proposed and tested in various settings. Most of these work-focused models focus on providing different treatments to workers based on their recovery (Kongsted et al. 2020):

Stepped care: where treatment is guided by the chronicity of their condition, recovery and RTW stage, with more comprehensive care being provided to those at later stages.

Stratified care: treatment is delivered based on the early identification of workers with higher predicted risk for a poor RTW outcome, and their risk profiles.

These types of interventions incorporate healthcare provision, RTW coordination and communication, and

---

BOX 17.4 **Principles for successful RTW interventions**

1. The employer has a strong commitment to worker health, safety and well-being, which is demonstrated by positive and proactive behaviours and actions of the employer and workplace stakeholders.
2. The employer provides meaningful suitable and/or modified *good work* tailored to the injured workers' capabilities so they can return-to-work (RTW) as early and safely as feasibly possible. The RTW process should neither exacerbate the existing condition(s) or pain, not create new ones. It should support optimal recovery and engagement in work that is productive for both worker and employer. Workplaces should be physically and psychologically safe.
3. Work rehabilitation healthcare professionals and other stakeholders involved in the RTW planning ensure the RTW plan supports the early return of workers without disadvantaging the worker, or the workers' supervisors or co-workers, and are worker-centred.
4. Supervisors who are trained in providing work disability prevention and supportive RTW are included in the RTW planning.
5. The employer makes early, appropriate and considerate contact with the injured worker.
6. An appropriate person is identified as being responsible for coordinating and facilitating the RTW.
7. Employer, health professionals and other key stakeholders communicate openly, honestly and collaboratively with each other in a coordinated fashion to facilitate the RTW plan, with the workers' involvement and consent.
8. Evidence and data should drive all underlying processes, recommendations, strategies and treatments.

Institute for Work and Health (2014), Cullen et al. (2018) and Safe Work Australia (2019).

---

suitable duties and work accommodation components (Cullen et al. 2018). Often these programmes are tailored to address individual worker (e.g. worker expectations, capacity, psychological state), as well as workplace needs (e.g. employer expectations, job design and work accommodations), and coordinate approaches between all stakeholders. They are often called *occupational rehabilitation*. These models dictate which treatments are delivered and when. They frequently contain the steps and components for work rehabilitation programmes that are described later in this chapter. Context, differing healthcare and insurance systems, among other factors, influence how each model might be implemented.

In a *stepped care* model, different types of clinical treatments can be recommended depending on the stage of the recovery process, with more work-focused multidisciplinary treatments starting at a later timepoint, often at 6 to 8 weeks, if RTW has not been achieved. In a study of workers with soft tissue injuries, physical therapy was provided early within the first 4 weeks (Stephens & Gross 2007). Workers who had not returned to work within 4 to 6 weeks were referred for work conditioning physiotherapy, and at 6 to 8 weeks, multidisciplinary assessment and rehabilitation. This study found that workers returned to work faster with significant economic benefits, and workers also reported being more satisfied with their care.

In another *stepped care* approach, different treatments are also applied at different stages, but it includes an RTW plan in which stakeholders, led by a health provider, work together using participatory methods to identify suitable duties and work modifications when workers do not RTW. The integrated models include workplace-based strategies such as development of an RTW plan, identifying barriers to RTW, conducting workplace visits to identify work accommodations, resolving any concerns identified, and case management. This model has been found to result in higher functional levels in workers, earlier resumption of work, no increase in symptoms and economic savings (Lambeek et al. 2010a, b; Loisel et al. 1997, 2002).

In a *stratified care* model, screening instruments, such as worker questionnaires, are generally used to stratify workers into different risk profiles. Then, different treatments are provided for workers based on their risk level and/or profile, with more intensive treatments provided for those who are higher risk. An example of a stratified care model is the STarT Back intervention, using the STarT back screening tool, which places workers into subgroups based on their risk of persistent disability. When compared to usual nonstratified care, this stratified approach resulted in less disability, higher quality of life and cost savings (Foster et al. 2014; Hill et al. 2011). In an Australian study that implemented a stratified care approach, using the Orebro Musculoskeletal Pain Questionnaire, high-risk workers were referred to psychological intervention and a comprehensive RTW plan to overcome obstacles (Nicholas et al. 2020). Workers who were at low risk received standard (stepped) care. This study found that workers reported higher health benefits, and there were more cost savings for the workers' compensation insurer.

Some have proposed combining stratified and stepped care models—due to their overlapping practical applications (Kongsted et al. 2020)—to move towards a common model for intervention. Different countries practice guidelines currently recommend one, or the other, or either approach. Also, neither model of care has been found to be more effective than the other (Kongsted et al. 2020; Linton et al. 2018). A combined approach would allow interventions to be directed to those who are most in need, be guided by those who are responding (or not) to treatment and also be based on prognostic factors for RTW outcomes. However, the evidence for these models is still emerging, and more testing in different settings is required to determine their effectiveness (Linton et al. 2018).

Other types of secondary interventions

Other promising strategies that might be useful—as adjuncts to standard care or any of the aforementioned models—are emerging as practitioners and researchers try to tackle the complex nature of work-related pain/injury. One approach is *motivational interviewing*, an interviewing technique that can be employed in a health professionals' practice to identify and focus on RTW. Motivational interviewing is a worker-centred goal-oriented counselling approach used in work rehabilitation that focuses on behaviour change by strengthening the worker's motivation and commitment to RTW based on their readiness to RTW. In a randomised controlled trial of workers with chronic musculoskeletal conditions, motivational interviewing used in conjunction with a functional restoration programme was found to increase RTW rates as well as improve sustained work outcomes, compared to a group of workers who only received the functional restoration approach (focused on RTW planning, improving work capacity through graded activity and exercise, group education sessions and multistakeholder involvement in RTW process) (Gross et al. 2017). However, some healthcare providers have reported that the skills for this technique take time to be proficient (Foldal et al. 2021).

New interventions and decision-making tools based on technological advancements, such as machine learning are now being trialled and evaluated (Gross et al. 2020a). An example of this is the Workplace Assessment Triage Tool—a novel clinical decision support tool that uses machine learning to identify appropriate interventions for workers by categorising workers based on their characteristics and associated with the highest probability of a positive work outcome, but is still in its infancy (Gross et al. 2020b). Other researchers are attempting to develop robotic FCE solutions incorporating machine learning to overcome the limitations of traditional FCE (Fong et al. 2020). Researchers are still refining methods to improve accuracy above that of human clinical recommendations (Gross et al. 2020a). While still in the early stages, these types of models are frequently being sought to identify which workers need specific interventions to support their RTW. As technologies continue to advance, we expect that more novel and innovative solutions will be developed; however, WRPs will need to ensure that the tools they use are valid and reliable.

Tertiary interventions

Tertiary intervention focuses on minimising the impact on chronic or complex pain and injury (IWH 2015). This includes *vocational rehabilitation* programmes that aim to retrain workers or find new jobs that are suitable for the workers' chronic pain condition. It also includes strategies to ensure that workers with ongoing persistent or fluctuating pain problems can remain at work long term beyond their first return. Workers may be returning to a job in their current occupational field, or alternatively they may need to change occupations due to the nature of their pain-related condition.

The aim of vocational rehabilitation is to optimise work participation for workers who have health-related impairments. Vocational rehabilitation can be implemented for workers with chronic pain who are unemployed or are in temporary work arrangements (such as contract workers, app-based workers, self-employed workers). As the nature of work continues to evolve, work arrangements also change. People in nonstandard work arrangements represent a substantial proportion of workers in our workforces and are more vulnerable to job loss and unemployment. For example, in Europe, workers in nonstandard work arrangements represent about 40% of the workforce (OECD 2020). For unemployed workers or those in nonstandard work arrangements, their RTW process may look quite different from those who are employed and can return to their original employer, and may receive supports through a workers' compensation insurer.

Similar barriers and facilitators for RTW have been found for workers in vocational rehabilitation programmes as injured workers in occupational rehabilitation settings. Facilitators include individualised and tailored support with a focus on the workers' capacity, stakeholder cooperation and communication (Larsson et al. 2021). Barriers include differences in stakeholders' goals and motivations, limitations in resources including limited time in a vocational rehabilitation programme and labour market limitations and worker's financial situations.

Principles for vocational rehabilitation are similar to occupational rehabilitation strategies and have been described in the work rehabilitation section in this chapter. Effective vocational rehabilitation interventions are also worker-centred and tailored to the individual, evidence-based, have a biopsychosocial multidimensional approach and are multidisciplinary, involve contact with the employer, and a RTW and symptom self-management plan (Escorpizo et al. 2011; Pinto et al. 2018; Reneman 2015). In a randomised control trial, a multicomponent comprehensive vocational rehabilitation programme with these characteristics was associated with positive work outcomes (Beemster et al. 2021) and cost savings (Reneman et al. 2021).

An example of another tailored and multidimensional vocational rehabilitation intervention is the Individual Placement and Support (IPS) model. This model is a promising integrated employment- and health-focused intervention with the goal to support workers to obtain competitive employment. Originally developed for workers with mental health diagnoses, it is currently being used as an intervention to support workers with chronic MSDs in the United States and Norway (Bond et al. 2019), but no large trials have yet been conducted.

The work rehabilitation process

The basic steps of a multidisciplinary workplace rehabilitation process include (1) referral for a work rehabilitation service; (2) work rehabilitation needs assessment; (3) planning; (4) implementation, review and evaluation and (5) repeat the process if required due to either improvement or a failed RTW attempt. Regardless of the names and numbers of steps, these basic steps tend to be completed across jurisdictions, especially those that are receiving benefits from an insurer, such as workers' compensation. Work rehabilitation in this sense is the same as occupational rehabilitation. Depending on the context, the terms are often used interchangeably.

The steps in the work rehabilitation process are generally conducted face to face, in person. However, the COVID-19 pandemic has accelerated the adoption of videoconferencing in rehabilitation to limit the spread of transmission (Prvu & Resnik 2020). During this period, many in-person services were stopped or limited, including occupational and vocational rehabilitation services. In a Canadian evaluation, occupational rehabilitation services were able to successfully transition to a fully remote model during the COVID-19 pandemic using videoconferencing or telerehabilitation (Gross et al. 2021). Because of the increasing acceptance of these digital methods, we expect to see them being used more frequently in the future.

The following section explains each of the steps in the process. These steps draw on the conceptual models and types of interventions already described in this chapter.

Referral

Referral for work rehabilitation may come from several sources depending on the prevailing system in any one country, state or province. These sources include the insurer or workers' compensation insurer, the person's treating medical practitioner, the employer, other health or welfare professionals, solicitors/attorneys, union representative, the injured worker or jobseeker with a disability and their family. In some countries, such as Australia, this referral can happen early in the recovery trajectory, whereas in other countries, such as the Netherlands, it may only be commenced when the duration of work absence exceeds a certain time threshold (Kristman et al. 2020).

Work rehabilitation needs assessment

The objectives of the needs assessment are to assess the capabilities and intervention needs of the injured worker to enable RTW planning. When the person is a worker who has a job available, the assessment focuses on the current work duties, working conditions, work environment, worker's current work ability, medical contraindications and social supports. The focus needs to be on the workers' capabilities rather than their limitations to identify what the worker can do at work, rather than what their work limitations are. Information about performance in daily living and leisure activities may also be sought, not necessarily to consider what interventions can be provided to improve these, as workplace rehabilitation may not cover such interventions, but to establish a sense of the functional effects of the pain-related injury or disability, especially when the person is not currently working. When the person is a jobseeker and cannot RTW, detailed information about aspects such as their work and education history may also be needed.

Screening of biopsychosocial factors may be indicated, particularly if there has been prolonged RTW or unsuccessful prior attempts at RTW. A plethora of multidimensional tools are available for early measurement of different prognostic factors for RTW and poor recovery outcomes (Karran et al. 2017; Veirman et al. 2019). Several instruments have shown promising ability to identify and stratify workers. The Orebro Musculoskeletal Pain Screening Questionnaire (Linton & Boersma 2003; Nicholas 2010) has been able to predict workers' RTW outcome in a sample of recently injured workers (Nicholas et al. 2019). Shaw and colleagues developed the PRICE screening tool which identifies those workers at elevated risk of long-term back pain disability and places workers in one of four groups: (1) minimal risk, (2) workplace concerns, (3) activity limitations and (4) emotional distress (Reme et al. 2012). Based on this categorisation, workers can then be recommended appropriate interventions. STarT back tool is another screening tool designed to identify high-risk workers for a stratified care intervention model, as already described (Hill et al. 2011). A promising newer instrument, the Work Disability Diagnosis Interview (WoDDI) is a semi-structured interview designed to guide healthcare professionals in identifying factors contributing to work disability and based on this identify other rehabilitation needs that will facilitate recovery and RTW (Durand et al. 2021a, b; Marois & Durand 2009).

For the jobseeker with pain, there are also some tools that may be useful to the WRP in this early stage of rehabilitation needs assessment. One is the job-seeking self-efficacy scale (Strauser & Berven 2006), which asks the jobseeker about their confidence in a range of areas, including self-presentation, handling disability and barriers in the job-seeking process and in executing the job search.

It is at this stage that, if not already provided by the referrer, consent is obtained from the worker to contact other important stakeholders in the rehabilitation process, such as the treating medical practitioner and other treatment providers (physiotherapists, chiropractors, etc.), the employer, RTW coordinator, union representative, etc. For workers returning to a specific employer, the WRP may contact the employer to explore work accommodation options, and to set up a time for a workplace assessment to be conducted so that a modified RTW plan can begin as early as reasonably possible.

Functional capacity evaluations

If requested, the FCE may form part of the needs assessment. FCEs are used to determine capacity to RTW, identify functional capability and guide rehabilitation decision-making. Many different methods of FCEs exist (De Baets et al. 2018). There are also vast differences in how FCEs are conducted around the world (Edelaar et al. 2020). The value of FCEs has more recently been debated (Pransky & Dempsey 2004), and their psychometric validity questioned (De Baets et al. 2018). A Canadian study found that FCEs were able to expedite RTW, but were not associated with lower recurrence of injury, pain intensity or disability (Gross & Battie 2005). Further, in a study of workers with upper extremity conditions, FCEs did not predict quicker or sustained recovery (Gross & Battie 2006). A randomised trial also found that an FCE integrated with occupational rehabilitation did not increase work ability at follow-up or increase RTW rates compared to a semi-structured interview (Gross et al. 2014). Biopsychosocial factors have been found to influence FCE results (Ansuategui Encheita et al. 2019), and therefore should be considered in conjunction with the FCE findings. Gross et al. (2007) also advocated that a short-form FCE protocol was just as effective as a more intensive FCE fitness for work assessment. Recently, there have been calls for more research to develop standardised and evidence-based methods to improve the components, delivery and implementation of FCEs (Ansuategui Encheita et al. 2019; Edelaar et al. 2020).

Planning

Developing the RTW goal and plan

An important part of managing the overall RTW process is developing the RTW goal and plan in conjunction with the worker, employer, treating medical provider and other key parties. The WRP needs to be able to select and consult appropriate members of the multidisciplinary team, including the person's medical practitioners, in order to propose and then monitor and review the RTW programme (Gibson 2009). In some cases, the WRP may also be working closely with an RTW coordinator.

RTW plans (often called RTW programmes) are key tools for facilitating a successful RTW outcome (Durand et al. 2014). RTW plans can also be used for workers who do not need a leave of absence but have work limitations, for workers returning to their employer after a work absence and for jobseekers with pain-related limitations who are commencing employment. In some jurisdictions, a written RTW plan is compulsory for insured employers, whereas, in other jurisdictions, they may be optional. The plan provides a reference document that relevant stakeholders can use throughout the RTW process, and is the cornerstone for a successful RTW programme (Kristman et al. 2020). The format for RTW plans varies in different jurisdictions. However, it usually contains one or more of these components: the RTW goal, services to achieve the goal, any medical contraindications (e.g. unable to drive due to pain medication), the suitable duties plan and work accommodations, recommendations for treatment and stakeholder roles and responsibilities. In developing the plan, the WRP can consider the strengths, facilitators or positive factors for the person's RTW, as well as the associated barriers, risks or negative factors, and available evidence supporting any recommendations. For the jobseeker with an injury, programmes offer early, intensive job-seeking support, which may include worksite evaluations, and in some cases, skills training if the worker cannot return to their previous occupation.

In the past, there has been a strong focus on assessing the compatibility between the demands of the job and the functional capacity of the worker. This approach could potentially lead to unnecessary sickness certification delaying RTW. The complexity of the nature of work, including the impact of psychosocial factors, can make accurate matching of functional capacities to job demands difficult (Pransky et al. 2004). This is not to say that workers should return to duties that are not deemed safe and suitable for their capacities. But rather functional capacity is just one piece to the puzzle. Safety of the injured worker and co-workers is always paramount in designing the RTW programme. Thus early and effective communication between stakeholders, centred on the worker, is critical (Pransky et al. 2004).

Evidence indicates that when an RTW plan is in place, workers have a greater likelihood of returning to work. Having a RTW plan or programme in place doubled the odds of workers' sustained RTW in Australia (Lane et al. 2017) and enabled workers to RTW 1.4 times more quickly than those without a RTW programme in a cohort of US-based workers whose employers were self-insured (McLaren et al. 2017). A national review of workers' compensation claims in Australia also found that when plans are put in place within 30 days of the injury or pain onset, it increases the worker's odds of returning to work by 1.7, and when a written plan was still in place after 30 days, the odds of remaining at work increased by 3.4 times (Sheehan et al. 2018).

Workplace assessment

A workplace assessment is an evaluation of the worker's job. It is usually conducted in a specific workplace but may also be conducted elsewhere depending on the worker's work arrangement. For example, nonstandard workers may work across various worksites, some workers may work remotely or from home, some workers duties may involve mainly driving in a vehicle, and a construction worker may work on different worksites every day. Regardless of where the assessment occurs, this assessment informs the modified work or suitable duties programme. Workplace assessment usually involves a review or observation of the work activities, interviews with the worker and supervisor and, in some cases, co-workers.

A cornerstone of this approach is the analysis of the physical, psychosocial, cognitive and emotional job demands and the working conditions to which the worker is exposed. Anema et al. (2003) described a promising approach to workplace assessment for the development of modified work programmes based on the participatory ergonomics approach successfully used in injury prevention. In this approach, the worker and supervisor are interviewed separately about the job and then the worker is observed in the workplace performing work tasks. A joint meeting to develop solutions for RTW then follows. In the separate interviews, the tasks and their resultant problems for the injured worker are noted, and the frequency and severity of each problem is rated then prioritised. In the observations, checklists are used to note the different working conditions and demands of the job. In the joint meeting, the possible solutions are brainstormed separately, then prioritised jointly based on their existence, feasibility and problem-solving capability. The collaborative nature of the process -with the focus on the worker and supervisor co-developing the solution -is pivotal to obtain buy-in from all parties involved; the WRP facilitates the development of solutions.

Work accommodations and suitable duties planning

A key activity and deliverable in the RTW plan is the identification of work accommodations and development of a suitable duties plan. Accommodations can be made for those who are able to remain at work after the injury or diagnosis, for those returning after a work absence and for those with chronic pain and disability. Tailored and individualised work accommodations should focus on including meaningful, suitable and modified duties that are graduated as the worker recovers to ensure workers return early and safely. Evidence has consistently found that modified work and suitable duties plans are effective in facilitating early and safe work outcomes (Cancelliere et al. 2016; Cullen et al. 2018; Krause et al. 1998).

The development of a suitable duties plan (SDP) is based on the needs assessment and workplace assessment, and common principles include (Innes 1997):

1. Based on the hierarchy of control model (see Fig. 17.1), first eliminate any problematic working conditions. If this cannot be achieved, move to next level within the model.
2. Duties need to be *compatible with the person's functional abilities*, or the person has the potential to perform them in a modified way to allow them to be safely accomplished.
3. The duties can be conducted *safely.*
4. The duties are *meaningful* and allow the worker to be productive. The duties have a purpose and contribute to the role of the worker, and the process or business of the workplace.
5. The duties need to be *compatible* with the worker's education, skills and experience: When workers are from high-level physically demanding jobs in physically demanding industries, such as labouring jobs in construction, and may have little education, it may be inappropriate for workers on suitable duties plans to be placed in what are considered 'lighter' office jobs that require higher level literacy.
6. A plan needs to be developed with the *input of all key stakeholders.* The worker and the supervisor will be involved. It is important that the worker's treating medical practitioner be consulted for potential medical contraindications or precautions. Some jurisdictions require the signed approval of the treating medical practitioner or occupational physician on the SDP plan. The person's co-workers and/or the union or labour representative may also need to be consulted if the duties impact on other workers.
7. The SDP will be *graduated* to align with the workers' recovery. It is important to start the worker at a level appropriate to their capacities without the likelihood for

> ### BOX 17.5 **Examples of work accommodations and suitable duties**
>
> - Modifying workplace policy (e.g. work from home policies or remote work, flexible leave, extended health benefits, disability management)
> - Modifying the physical environment and architecture (e.g. ramps, modified furniture)
> - Modification of job responsibilities (e.g. job redesign, reassigning duties, modifying duties, controlling work pace and order, job sharing)
> - Supportive personal provision (e.g. co-worker supports, paid additional supports)
> - Flexible scheduling (e.g. modifying work hours, break schedules, work schedules, adjusting arrival and departure times)
> - Providing assistive technologies and equipment
>
> Wong et al. (2021).

aggravation of the injury, but also productive enough to contribute to the work process without being disruptive. When deciding on the starting point and subsequent grading of the worker's duties, the WRP can consider choosing and grading specific duties, specific tasks within the duties and hours and days of work. Duties and tasks can be graded from light to heavy and/or occasional to frequent. The WRP may reduce the number of hours and shifts, or work on alternate days. In increasing hours, shifts or duties, it is important to try to change in small increments so that, if aggravation of the pain occurs, the likely cause of the aggravation can be identified.

8. WRP *checks in regularly* with the worker and employer. However, the WRP should not contact the worker so frequently that they feel like they are being monitored or policed. The WRP may ask the worker to provide a regular check-in through an email, phone call or completion of a check-list with the worker and supervisor. Sometimes the WRP may need to revisit the workplace to revise or update an SDP.

Examples of the types of work accommodations that may be needed are detailed in Box 17.5.

One challenge in implementing work accommodations and suitable duties is aligning the expectations of the worker, supervisor, co-workers and the employer. Employees who feel able to articulate what job accommodations might be needed and advocate for themselves are likely to transition back to work more smoothly. Workers are also more likely to accept job accommodations when they understand their own work capacity, know what accommodations they might need, have higher self-efficacy and recovery expectations, have good relationships and communication with their supervisors, have access to supportive resources and experience less stress when asking for accommodations. Also, studies have found that workers who have more job control tend to be able to implement work accommodations more easily (Wong et al. 2021). Often employers have limited knowledge with respect to what job accommodations might be needed or are possible. If job accommodations might impact co-workers, they should be engaged in the RTW process to ensure that they are not overly burdened by the new situation.

Employers' attitudes towards the types of work accommodations proposed can pose as a challenge or an enabler in the RTW process. For example, they might be concerned about the costs of some modifications or how the accommodation might impact workplace productivity. These need to be discussed and addressed to ensure all parties are comfortable with the proposed accommodations. In some cases, there may be external support to help the worker and employer fund needed modifications or purchase of equipment, such as through their health insurance, workers' compensation insurance, government-funded programmes, or community organisations.

Implementation, review and evaluation

The WRP needs to conduct regular reviews to ensure that services are implemented in a timely and cost-effective manner, streamlining with any concurrent treatment services, and avoiding duplication of services (Heads of Workers' Compensation Authorities 2019). In this phase, collaboration with the RTW coordinator, if one is involved, is important. This phase is where dialogue between key parties can be critical to prevent possible breakdowns in communication and ensure prevention of reinjury. Effective and timely communication is critical to ensure the RTW goal is sustained. The objective here is to provide guidance and further recommendations by reviewing the RTW plan. For workers with chronic pain and permanent impairments, this step is even more important to prevent exacerbation of symptoms and secondary work disability. In a cohort of Canadian workers with permanent impairment, at 1 year post workers' compensation claim closure, 66% reported moderate-to-severe pain, 40% reported ongoing work limitations and 47% reported difficulty keeping their job because of their impairment (Sears et al. 2021). These workers may be more vulnerable to job loss and economic impacts if they need to work fewer hours (Sears et al. 2021).

If the identified RTW goal is not achieved, a worker has a recurrence of symptoms or another work absence, the preceding stages are repeated and should include a revised RTW plan and potentially new interventions; thus the process can be iterative and cyclical. Attention should be focused on any contextual factors or working conditions that might have contributed to the failed RTW. Importantly, continued communication and collaboration between stakeholders is integral in these cases. On case closure, the WRP needs to consider and advise on any ongoing or potential future needs of the worker to be able to remain at work long term (Heads of Workers' Compensation Authorities 2019). This may include recommendations for ongoing health services or equipment maintenance or replacement.

It is also important for the WRP to develop criteria and methods for evaluation of the interventions and RTW plan. This is where objective measures are used to determine the efficiency and/or effectiveness of interventions (Clifton 2005). Efficiency usually relates to administrative aspects (Clifton 2005), such as cost and length of the RTW programme. Effectiveness can include outcomes such as durable RTW and satisfaction with the service. Different schemes may have different outcome evaluation requirements, for example a person sustains a return to employment for 13 weeks before the case can be closed or payment forwarded by the funder to the rehabilitation provider. Some workers' compensation authorities, such as in Australia, conduct a regular survey of workers (Safe Work Australia 2021).

Other work rehabilitation services

On-the-job training

On-the-job training—also called work training schemes or host employment placements (WorkCover Queensland 2021)—can be a powerful tool for getting jobseekers with a disability into new jobs, or for those workers who cannot return to their original job. These schemes vary in different systems and countries, but the principles are much the same. The schemes allow employers the opportunity to give the worker a trial on the job without having to pay them (the jobseeker remains on welfare, workers' compensation or insurance payments) and without risk of exposure to workers' compensation claims for any aggravation of the injury, as the schemes cover the jobseeker for workers' compensation, sometimes for all claims, but at least for aggravation of pre-existing injuries. This can be an excellent way for (1) a jobseeker with a disability to trial employment and to demonstrate to employers that they can perform the duties of the job and (2) to build work tolerance if the workers cannot return to their original job.

The principles for developing and monitoring SDPs outlined earlier in this chapter should also be applied to the development and monitoring of work training.

Vocational assessment

Sometimes, jobseekers with persistent pain who cannot return to their previous occupation have no existing or suitable transferable skills that they can draw on to gain employment. In these cases, a more comprehensive vocational assessment may be required to help ascertain potential new occupations for the jobseeker and the need for training. Such assessment can include exploration of work interests, values and transferable skills. It may be carried out as a formal assessment of intelligence and aptitudes (Power 2000) through use of standardised tests, such as questionnaires and profiles, or it may take a naturalistic form, using interviews and on-the-job assessments (Hagner 2010). Specific questionnaires and tools to assess work-related function for jobseekers have also been developed and psychometrically evaluated for reliability and validity, such as the Work Rehabilitation Questionnaire (Roels et al. 2021). One 'silver lining' of the COVID-19 pandemic is that remote working options and telecommuting are becoming more accessible and employers are becoming more accepting of this work arrangement (Schur et al. 2020). For workers in certain occupations with disabilities and persistent pain problems that may have caused them to exit the workforce, they may be more easily able to accommodate their work limitations if they are able to work from home (Sears et al. 2021).

Conclusion

Work rehabilitation for workers with pain problems can be complex and multifactorial. Understanding the various factors at different systems levels can provide a framework for interventions. They require a holistic and multi-layered approach aimed at preventing injury and pain and assist both employed and unemployed workers to have meaningful and safe work roles and be productive members of the workforce. Healthcare professionals play an important and integral role from primary prevention of injury and pain to tertiary prevention of long-term (work-) disability.

Review questions   Q

1. What are some physical/emotional/social/financial problems an injured worker might face when returning to work, and how can the WRP help to overcome these?
2. What types of interventions might be effective in facilitating RTW for a worker who is currently off work after a painful injury?
3. What are some problems supervisors and/or co-workers might face in relation to an injured worker returning to work, and how can the WRP help to address these?
4. Which assessments might the WRP perform to establish the needs and preferences of the injured worker or jobseeker?
5. Which assessments might the WRP perform to establish the suitability of a workplace/workload for the injured worker or jobseeker?
6. What steps are involved in achieving a successful RTW for an injured worker?
7. How might these steps differ for a worker who is currently unemployed and seeking to re-enter the workforce?

References

ACOEM Special Committee on Competencies, 2008. American College of Occupational and Environmental Medicine competencies—2008. J. Occup. Environ. Med. 50 (6), 712–724.

American Occupational Therapy Association (AOTA), 2017. Occupational therapy services in facilitating work participation and performance. Am. J. Occup. Ther. 71 (Suppl. 2).

Amick, B.C., Habeck, R.V., Hunt, A., Fossel, A.H., Chapin, A., Keller, R.B., et al., 2000. Measuring the impact of organizational behaviors on work disability prevention and management. J. Occup. Rehabil. 10 (1), 21–38.

Anema, J.R., Steenstra, I.A., Urlings, I.J.M., Bongers, P.M., De Vroome, E.M.M., Van Mechelen, W., 2003. Participatory ergonomics as a return–to–work intervention: a future challenge? Am. J. Ind. Med. 44 (3), 273–281.

Ansuategui Echeita, J., Bethge, M., van Holland, B.J., Gross, D.P., Kool, J., Oesch, P., et al., 2019. Functional capacity evaluation in different societal contexts: results of a multicountry study. J. Occup. Rehabil. 29 (1), 222–236.

Australian Faculty of Occupational and Environmental Medicine. 2022. Consensus Statement on the Health Benefits for Good work. Available at: https://www.racp.edu.au/advocacy/division-faculty-and-chapter-priorities/faculty-of-occupational-environmental-medicine/health-benefits-of-good-work.

Australian Small Business and Family Enterprise Ombudsman, 2016. Small Business Counts: Small Business in the Australian Economy. Available from https://www.asbfeo.gov.au/sites/default/files/Small_Business_Statistical_Report-Final.pdf.

Australian Institute of Health and Welfare, 2017. The burden of Musculoskeletal Conditions in Australia: A Detailed Analysis of the Australian Burden of Disease Study 2011. Australian Burden of Disease Study series no. 13. BOD 14. Canberra: AIHW. ISSN 2204-4108 (PDF).

Bartys, S., Edmondson, A., Burton, K., Parker, C., Martin, R., 2019. Work Conversations in Healthcare: How, where, when and by Whom: A Review to Understand Conversations about Work in Healthcare and Identify Opportunities to Make Work Conversations a Part of Everyday Health Interactions. Public Health England, London.

Beemster, T.T., van Bennekom, C.A., van Velzen, J.M., Frings-Dresen, M.H., Reneman, M.F., 2021. Vocational rehabilitation with or without work Module for Patients with chronic musculoskeletal pain and sick leave from work: Longitudinal impact on work Participation. J. Occup. Rehabil. 31 (1), 72–83.

Bond, G.R., Drake, R.E., Pogue, J.A., 2019. Expanding individual placement and support to populations with conditions and disorders other than serious mental illness. Psychiatr. Serv. 70 (6), 488–498.

Calkins, J., Lui, J.W., Wood, C., 2000. Recent developments in integrated disability management: implications for professional and organisational development. J. Vocat. Rehabil. 15 (1), 31–37.

Campbell, P., Wynne-Jones, G., Muller, S., Dunn, K.M., 2013. The influence of employment social support for risk and prognosis in nonspecific back pain: a systematic review and critical synthesis. Int. Arch. Occup. Environ. Health 86 (2), 119–137. https://doi.org/10.1007/s00420-012-0804-2. Epub 2012/08/10. PubMed PMID: 22875173; PubMed Central PMCID: PMC3555241.(1).

Cancelliere, C., Donovan, J., Stochkendahl, M.J., Biscardi, M., Ammendolia, C., Myburgh, C., et al., 2016. Factors affecting return to work after injury or illness: best evidence synthesis of systematic reviews. Chiropr. Man. Ther. 24 (1), 1–23.

Centers for Disease Control (CDC), National Institute for Occupational Safety and Health, 2015. Hierarchy of controls. Available from https://www.cdc.gov/niosh/topics/hierarchy/default.html.

Chou, R., Qaseem, A., Snow, V., Casey, D., Cross Jr., J.T., Shekelle, P., et al., 2007. Diagnosis and treatment of low back pain: a joint clinical practice guideline from the American College of Physicians and the American Pain Society. Ann. Intern. Med. 147 (7), 478–491.

Cieza, A., Causey, K., Kamenov, K., Hanson, S.W., Chatterji, S., Vos, T., 2020. Global estimates of the need for rehabilitation based on the global burden of disease study 2019: a systematic analysis for the global burden of disease study 2019. Lancet 396 (10267), 2006–2017.

Clarke, S., 2013. Safety leadership: a meta–analytic review of transformational and transactional leadership styles as antecedents of safety behaviours. J. Occup. Organ. Psychol. 86 (1), 22–49.

Clifton, D.W., 2005. Outcomes management. In: Clifton, D.W. (Ed.), Physical Rehabilitation's Role in Disability Management: Unique Perspectives for Success. Elsevier Saunders, St Louis, MO.

Collie, A., Lane, T.J., Hassani-Mahmooei, B., Thompson, J., McLeod, C., 2016. Does time off work after injury vary by jurisdiction? A comparative study of eight Australian workers' compensation systems. BMJ Open 6 (5), e010910.

Collie, A., Sheehan, L., Lane, T.J., Iles, R., 2020. Psychological distress in workers' compensation claimants: prevalence, predictors and mental health service use. J. Occup. Rehabil. 30 (2), 194–202.

Costa-Black, K.M., Feuerstein, M., Loisel, P., 2013. Work disability models: past and present. In: Loisel, P., Anema, J.R., Feuerstein, M., MacEachen, E., Pransky, G., Costa-Black, K. (Eds.), Handbook of Work Disability. Springer, New York, NY, pp. 71–93.

Cullen, K.L., Irvin, E., Collie, A., et al., 2018. Effectiveness of workplace interventions in return-to-work for musculoskeletal, pain-related and mental health conditions: an update of the evidence and messages for practitioners. J. Occup. Rehabil. 28, 1–15.

Dale, A.M., Buckner–Petty, S., Evanoff, B.A., Gage, B.F., 2021. Predictors of long–term opioid use and opioid use disorder among construction workers: analysis of claims data. Am. J. Ind. Med. 64 (1), 48–57.

De Baets, S., Calders, P., Schalley, N., Vermeulen, K., Vertriest, S., Van Peteghem, L., et al., 2018. Updating the evidence on functional capacity evaluation methods: a systematic review. J. Occup. Rehabil. 28 (3), 418–428.

Denne, J., Kettner, G., Ben-Shalom, Y., 2015. The Role of the Physician in the Return-To-Work Process Following Disability Onset. Mathematica Center for Studying Disability Policy. Available from https://www.dol.gov/sites/dolgov/files/odep/topics/pdf/rtw_role%20of%20physician_2015-03.pdf.

Donovan, M., Khan, A., Johnston, V., 2021. The contribution of onsite physiotherapy to an integrated model for managing work injuries: a follow up study. J. Occup. Rehabil. 31, 207–218.

Durand, M.J., Corbiere, M., Coutu, M.F., Reinharz, D., Albert, V., 2014. A review of best work-absence management and return-to-work practices for workers with musculoskeletal or common mental disorders. Work 48 (4), 579–589.

Durand, M.J., Coutu, M.F., Tremblay, D., et al., 2021a. Insights into the sustainable return to work of aging workers with a work disability: an interpretative description study. J. Occup. Rehabil. 31, 92–106.

Durand, M.J., Coutu, M.F., Berbiche, D., 2021b. Validation of the work disability diagnosis interview for musculoskeletal and mental disorders. J. Occup. Rehabil. 31, 232–242.

Dol, M., Varatharajan, S., Neiterman, E., McKnight, E., Crouch, M., McDonald, E., Malachowski, C., et al., 2021. Systematic review of the impact on return to work of return-to-work coordinators. J. Occup. Rehabil. 31 (4), 675–698.

Edelaar, M.J.A., Oesch, P.R., Gross, D.P., James, C.L., Reneman, M.F., 2020. Functional capacity evaluation research: report from the fourth international functional capacity evaluation research meeting. J. Occup. Rehabil. 30 (3), 475–479.

Escorpizo, R., Reneman, M.F., Ekholm, J., Fritz, J., Krupa, T., Marnetoft, S.U., et al., 2011. A conceptual definition of vocational rehabilitation based on the ICF: building a shared global model. J. Occup. Rehabil. 21 (2), 126–133.

Fan, J.K., Gignac, M.A., Harris, M.A., Smith, P.M., 2020. Age differences in return-to-work following injury. J. Occup. Environ. Med. 62 (12), e680–e687.

Foldal, V.S., Solbjør, M., Standal, M.I., Fors, E.A., Hagen, R., Bagøien, G., et al., 2021. Barriers and facilitators for implementing motivational interviewing as a return to work intervention in a Norwegian social insurance setting: a mixed methods process evaluation. J. Occup. Rehabil. 31 (4), 785–795.

Fong, J., Ocampo, R., Gross, D.P., Tavakoli, M., 2020. Intelligent robotics incorporating machine learning algorithms for improving functional capacity evaluation and occupational rehabilitation. J. Occup. Rehabil. 30 (3), 362–370.

Foreman, P., Murphy, G., Swerissen, H., 2006. Barriers and Facilitators to Return to Work: A Literature Review. Australian Institute for Primary Care, La Trobe University, Melbourne.

Foster, N.E., Mullis, R., Hill, J.C., Lewis, M., Whitehurst, D.G., Doyle, C., et al., 2014. Effect of stratified care for low back pain in family practice (IMPaCT Back): a prospective population-based sequential comparison. Ann. Fam. Med. 12 (2), 102–111.

Franche, R.L., Krause, N., 2002. Readiness for return to work following injury or illness: conceptualizing the interpersonal impact of health care, workplace, and insurance factors. J. Occup. Rehabil. 12 (4), 233–256.

Franche, R.L., Cullen, K., Clarke, J., Irvin, E., Sinclair, S., Frank, J., 2005. Workplace-based return-to-work interventions: a systematic review of the quantitative literature. J. Occup. Rehabil. 15 (4), 607–631.

Gaskin, D.J., Richard, P., 2012. The economic costs of pain in the United States. J. Pain 13 (8), 715–724.

Gibson, L., 2009. Functional capacity evaluation: an integrated approach to assessing work activity limitations. In: Söderback, I. (Ed.), International Handbook of Occupational Therapy Interventions. Springer Science+Business Media, Inc, Dordrecht, pp. 497–505.

Gonzalez-Mulé, E., Cockburn, B., 2016. Worked to death: the relationships of job demands and job control with mortality. Person. Psychol. 70, 73–112.

Gouin, M., Coutu, M., Durand, M., 2019. Return-to-work success despite conflicts: an exploration of decision-making during a work rehabilitation program. Disabil. Rehabil. 41 (5), 523–533.

Grant, M., O-Beirne-Elliman, J., Froud, R., Underwood, M., Seers, K., 2019. The work of return to work. Challenges of returning to work when you have chronic pain: a meta-ethnography. BMJ Open 9 (6), e025743. https://doi.org/10.1136/bmjopen-2018-025743. PMID: 31227529; PMCID: PMC6596973.

Gross, D.P., Battié, M.C., 2005. Functional capacity evaluation performance does not predict sustained return to work in claimants with chronic back pain. J. Occup. Rehabil. 15, 285–294.

Gross, D.P., Battié, M.C., 2006. Does functional capacity evaluation predict recovery in workers' compensation claimants with upper extremity disorders? Occup. Environ. Med. 63, 404–410.

Gross, D.P., Battié, M.C., Asante, A.K., 2007. Evaluation of a short-form functional capacity evaluation: less may be best. J. Occup. Rehabil. 17, 422–435.

Gross, D.P., Asante, A.K., Miciak, M., Battié, M.C., Carroll, L.J., Sun, A., et al., 2014. A cluster randomized clinical trial comparing functional capacity evaluation and functional interviewing as components of occupational rehabilitation programs. J. Occup. Rehabil. 24 (4), 617–630.

Gross, D.P., Park, J., Rayani, F., Norris, C.M., Esmail, S., 2017. Motivational interviewing improves sustainable return to work in injured workers after rehabilitation: a cluster randomized controlled trial. Arch. Phys. Med. Rehabil. 98 (12), 2355–2363.

Gross, D.P., Steenstra, I.A., Shaw, W., Yousefi, P., Bellinger, C., Zaïane, O., 2020a. Validity of the Work Assessment Triage Tool for selecting rehabilitation interventions for workers' compensation claimants with musculoskeletal conditions. J. Occup. Rehabil. 30 (3), 318–330.

Gross, D.P., Steenstra, I.A., Harrell, F.E., Bellinger, C., Zaïane, O., 2020. Machine learning for work disability prevention: introduction to the special series. J. Occup. Rehabil. 30 (3), 303–307.

Gross, D.P., Asante, A., Pawluk, J., Niemeläinen, R., 2021. A descriptive study of the implementation of remote occupational rehabilitation services due to the COVID-19 pandemic within a workers' compensation context. J. Occup. Rehabil. 31 (2), 444–453.

Hagner, D., 2010. The role of naturalistic assessment in vocational rehabilitation. J. Rehabil. 76 (1), 28–34.

Hartvigsen, J., Hancock, M.J., Kongsted, A., Louw, Q., Ferreira, M.L., Genevay, S., et al., 2018. What low back pain is and why we need to pay attention. Lancet 391 (10137), 2356–2367.

Haveraaen, L.A., Skarpaas, L.S., Aas, R.W., 2017. Job demands and decision control predicted return to work: the rapid-RTW cohort study. BMC Publ. Health 17, 154.

Hawkins, D., Roelofs, C., Laing, J., Davis, L., 2019. Opioid–related overdose deaths by industry and occupation—Massachusetts, 2011–2015. Am. J. Ind. Med. 62 (10), 815–825.

Hawkins, D., Davis, L., Punnett, L., Kriebel, D., 2020. Disparities in the deaths of despair by occupation, Massachusetts, 2000 to 2015. J. Occup. Environ. Med. 62 (7), 484–492.

Heads of Workers' Compensation Authorities, 2019. Principles of Practice for Workplace Rehabilitation Providers. Available from https://www.hwca.org.au/wp-content/uploads/2019/11/HWCA-Principles-of-Practice-for-Workplace-Rehabilitation-Providers-2019_.pdf.

Hill, J.C., Whitehurst, D.G., Lewis, M., Bryan, S., Dunn, K.M., Foster, N.E., et al., 2011. Comparison of stratified primary care management for low back pain with current best practice (STarT Back): a randomised controlled trial. Lancet 378 (9802), 1560–1571.

Horppu, R., Martimo, K.P., Viikari-Juntura, E., Lallukka, T., MacEachen, E., 2016. Occupational physicians' reasoning about recommending early return to work with work modifications. PLoS One 11 (7), e0158588.

Hutting, N., Oswald, W., Staal, J.B., Heerkens, Y.F., 2020. Self-management support for people with non-specific low back pain: a qualitative survey among physiotherapists and exercise therapists. Musculoskelet. Sci. Pract. 50, 102269.

Innes, E., 1997. Work assessment options and the selection of suitable duties: an Australian perspective. N. Z. J. Occup. Ther. 48 (1), 14–20.

Institute for Work and Health (IWH), 2014. Seven 'principles' for Successful Return to Work. Available from https://www.iwh.on.ca/sites/iwh/files/iwh/tools/seven_principles_rtw_2014.pdf.

Institute for Work and Health, 2015. Primary, Secondary and Tertiary Prevention. Available from https://www.iwh.on.ca/what-researchers-mean-by/primary-secondary-and-tertiary-prevention.

Jansen, J., van Ooijen, R., Koning, P.W.C., Boot, C.R., Brouwer, S., 2021. The role of the employer in supporting work participation of workers with disabilities: a systematic literature review using an interdisciplinary approach. J. Occup. Rehabil. 31 (4), 916–949.

Jetha, A., Le Pouésard, M., Mustard, C., Backman, C., Gignac, M.A., 2021. Getting the message right: evidence-based insights to improve organizational return-to-work communication practices. J. Occup. Rehabil. 1–12.

Johnston, V., Nielsen, M., Corbiere, M., Franche, R.L., 2012. Experiences and perspectives of physical therapists managing patients covered by workers' compensation in Queensland, Australia. Phys. Ther. 92 (10), 1306–1315.

Johnston, V., Way, K., Long, M.H., Wyatt, M., Gibson, L., Shaw, W.S., 2015. Supervisor competencies for supporting return to work: a mixed-methods study. J. Occup. Rehabil. 25 (1), 3–17.

Karasek, R., Theorell, T., 1991. Healthy Work: Stress, Productivity, and the Reconstruction of Working Life. Basic Books, New York, NY.

Karran, E.L., McAuley, J.H., Traeger, A.C., Hillier, S.L., Grabherr, L., Russek, L.N., et al., 2017. Can screening instruments accurately determine poor outcome risk in adults with recent onset low back pain? A systematic review and meta-analysis. BMC Med. 15 (1), 1–15.

Kilgour, E., Kosny, A., McKenzie, D., Collie, A., 2015. Interactions between injured workers and insurers in workers' compensation systems: a systematic review of qualitative research literature. J. Occup. Rehabil. 25 (1), 160–181.

Knauf, M. T., Schultz, I. Z., Stewart, A. M., & Gatchel, R. J. (2014). Models of return to work for musculoskeletal disorders: advances in conceptualization and research. In *Handbook of musculoskeletal pain and disability disorders in the workplace* (pp. 431-452). Springer, New York, NY.

Knauf, M.T., Schultz, I.Z., 2016. Current conceptual models of return to work. In: Schultz, I.Z., Gatchel, R.J. (Eds.), Handbook of Return to Work. Springer, Boston, MA, pp. 27–51.

Kongsted, A., Kent, P., Quicke, J.G., Skou, S.T., Hill, J.C., 2020. Risk-stratified and stepped models of care for back pain and osteoarthritis: are we heading towards a common model? Pain. Rep. 5 (5), e843.

Krause, N., Dasinger, L.K., Neuhauser, F., 1998. Modified work and return to work: a review of the literature. J. Occup. Rehabil. 8 (2), 113–139.

Kristman, V.L., Boot, C.R., Sanderson, K., Sinden, K.E., Williams-Whitt, K., 2020. Implementing best practice models of return to work. In: Bültmann, U., Siegrist, J. (Eds.), Handbook of Disability, Work and Health. Springer, Cham, pp. 589–613.

Lambeek, L.C., Bosmans, J.E., Van Royen, B.J., Van Tulder, M.W., Van Mechelen, W., Anema, J.R., 2010a. Effect of integrated care for sick listed patients with chronic low back pain: economic evaluation alongside a randomised controlled trial. BMJ 341, c6414.

Lambeek, L.C., van Mechelen, W., Knol, D.L., Loisel, P., Anema, J.R., 2010b. Randomised controlled trial of integrated care to reduce disability from chronic low back pain in working and private life. BMJ 340, c1035.

Lane, T.J., Lilley, R., Hogg-Johnson, S., LaMontagne, A.D., Sim, M.R., Smith, P.M., 2017. A prospective cohort study of the impact of return-to-work coordinators in getting injured workers back on the job. J. Occup. Rehabil. 28, 298–306.

Larsson, K., Hurtig, A.L., Andersén, Å.M., Anderzén, I., 2021. Vocational rehabilitation professionals' perceptions of facilitators and barriers to return to work: a qualitative descriptive study. Rehabil. Counsel. Bull. p.00343552211060013.

Linton, S., Nicholas, M., Shaw, W., 2018. Why wait to address high-risk cases of acute low back pain? A comparison of stepped, stratified, and matched care. Pain 159 (12), 2437–2441.

Linton, S.J., Nicholas, M., MacDonald, S., 2011. Development of a short form of the Örebro musculoskeletal pain screening questionnaire. Spine 36 (22), 1891–1895.

Linton, S.J., Boersma, K., 2003. Early identification of patients at risk of developing a persistent back problem: the predictive validity of the Örebro Musculoskeletal Pain Questionnaire. Clin. J. Pain 19 (2), 80–86.

Lippel, K., 2007. Workers describe the effect of the workers' compensation process on their health: a Quebec study. Int. J. Law Psychiatr. 30 (4–5), 427–443.

Loisel, P., Abenhaim, L., Durand, P., Esdaile, J.M., Suissa, S., Gosselin, L., et al., 1997. A population-based, randomized clinical trial on back pain management. Spine 22 (24), 2911–2918.

Loisel, P., Lemaire, J., Poitras, S., Durand, M.J., Champagne, F., Stock, S., et al., 2002. Cost-benefit and cost-effectiveness analysis of a disability prevention model for back pain management: a six year follow up study. Occup. Environ. Med. 59 (12), 807–815.

Loisel, P., Buchbinder, R., Hazard, R., Keller, R., Scheel, I., Van Tulder, M., et al., 2005. Prevention of work disability due to musculoskeletal disorders: the challenge of implementing evidence. J. Occup. Rehabil. 15 (4), 507–524.

Lovejoy, M., Kelly, E.L., Kubzansky, L.D., Berkman, L.F., 2021. Work redesign for the 21st century: promising strategies for enhancing worker well-being. Am. J. Public. Health 111 (10), 1787–1795.

MacEachen, E. (Ed.), 2018. The Science and Politics of Work Disability Prevention. Routledge, New York.

MacEachen, E., Clarke, J., Franche, R.L., Irvin, E., 2006. Workplace-based Return to Work Literature Review G. Systematic review of the qualitative literature on return to work after injury. Scand. J. Work. Environ. Health 32 (4), 257–269 Epub 2006/08/26. PubMed PMID: 16932823.

Maetzel, A., Li, L., 2002. The economic burden of low back pain: a review of studies published between 1996 and 2001. Best Pract. Res. Clin. Rheumatol. 16 (1), 23–30.

Main, L., Chris, J.a, Shaw, W.S.b,*, Nicholas, M.K.c, Linton, S.J.d, 2022. System-level efforts to address pain-related workplace challenges. Pain 163 (8), 1425–1431. https://doi.org/10.1097/j.pain.0000000000002548.

Marois, E., Durand, M.J., 2009. Does participation in interdisciplinary work rehabilitation programme influence return to work obstacles and predictive factors? Disabil. Rehabil. 31 (12), 994–1007.

Mathers, C.D., Schofield, D.J., 1998. The health consequences of unemployment: the evidence. Med. J. Aust. 168 (4), 178–182.

McLaren, C.F., Reville, R.T., Seabury, S.A., 2017. How effective are employer return to work programs? Int. Rev. Law Econ. 52 (Suppl. C), 58–73.

Mielenz, T.J., Garrett, J.M., Carey, T.S., 2008. Association of psychosocial work characteristics with low back pain outcomes. Spine 33 (11), 1270–1275.

Morano, L.H., Steege, A.L., Luckhaupt, S.E., 2018. Occupational patterns in unintentional and undetermined drug-involved and opioid-involved overdose deaths—United States, 2007–2012. MMWR (Morb. Mortal. Wkly. Rep.) 67 (33), 925.

Nicholas, M.K., Costa, D.S.J., Linton, S.J., Main, C.J., Shaw, W.S., Pearce, R., et al., 2019. Predicting return to work in a heterogeneous sample of recently injured workers using the brief ÖMPSQ-SF. J. Occup. Rehabil. 29 (2), 295–302.

Nicholas, M.K., Costa, D.S.J., Linton, S.J., Main, C.J., Shaw, W.S., Pearce, G., et al., 2020. Implementation of early intervention protocol in Australia for 'high risk' injured workers is associated with fewer lost work days over 2 years than usual (stepped) care. J. Occup. Rehabil. 30 (1), 93–104.

Oakman, J., Clune, S., Stuckey, R., 2019. Work-Related Musculoskeletal Disorders in Australia, 2019. Safe Work Australia, Canberra.

OECD, 2020. Distributional Risks Associated with Non-standard Work: Stylised Facts and Policy Considerations. Available from https://www.oecd.org/coronavirus/policy-responses/distributional-risks-associated-with-non-standard-work-stylised-facts-and-policy-considerations-68fa7d61/.

Palmer, K.T., Harris, E.C., Linaker, C., Barker, M., Lawrence, W., Cooper, C., et al., 2012. Effectiveness of community-and workplace-based interventions to manage musculoskeletal-related sickness absence and job loss: a systematic review. Rheumatology 51 (2), 230–242.

Peng, L., Chan, A.H., 2019. A meta-analysis of the relationship between ageing and occupational safety and health. Saf. Sci. 112, 162–172.

Peters, S.E., Dennerlein, J.T., Wagner, G.R., Sorensen, G., 2022. Work and worker health in the post-pandemic world: a public health perspective. Lancet Public Health 7 (2), e188–e194.

Peters, S.E., Coppieters, M.W., Ross, M., Johnston, V., 2017. Perspectives from employers, insurers, lawyers and healthcare providers on factors that influence workers' return-to-work following surgery for non-traumatic upper extremity conditions. J. Occup. Rehabil. 27 (3), 343–358.

Peters, S.E., Sorensen, G., Katz, J.N., Gundersen, D.A., Wagner, G.R., 2021. Thriving from work: conceptualization and measurement. Int. J. Environ. Res. Publ. Health 18 (13), 7196.

Pinto, A.D., Hassen, N., Craig-Neil, A., 2018. Employment interventions in health settings: a systematic review and synthesis. Ann. Fam. Med. 16 (5), 447–460.

Poitras, S., Blais, R., Swaine, B., Rossignol, M., 2005. Management of work-related low back pain: a population-based survey of physical therapists. Phys. Ther. 85 (11), 1168–1181.

Power, P.W., 2000. A Guide to Vocational Assessment, third ed. Pro-Ed, Austin, TX.

Pransky, G.S., Dempsey, P.G., 2004. Practical aspects of functional capacity evaluations. J. Occup. Rehabil. 14, 217–229. https://doi.org/10.1023/B:JOOR.0000022763.61656.b1.

Pransky, G., Shaw, W.S., Loisel, P., Hong, Q.N., Désorcy, B., 2010. Development and validation of competencies for return to work coordinators. J. Occup. Rehabil. 20 (1), 41–48.

Prochaska, J.O., DiClemente, C.C., 1983. Stages and processes of self-change of smoking: toward an integrative model of change. J. Consult. Clin. Psychol. 51 (3), 390.

Prvu Bettger, J., Resnik, L.J., 2020. Telerehabilitation in the age of COVID-19: an opportunity for learning health system research. Phys. Ther. 100 (11), 1913–1916.

Punnett, L., Wegman, D.H., 2004. Work-related musculoskeletal disorders: the epidemiologic evidence and the debate. J. Electromyogr. Kinesiol. 14 (1), 13–23.

Reme, S.E., Shaw, W.S., Steenstra, I.A., Woiszwillo, M.J., Pransky, G., Linton, S.J., 2012. Distressed, immobilized, or lacking employer support? A sub-classification of acute work-related low back pain. J. Occup. Rehabil.

Reneman, M.F., 2015. State of vocational rehabilitation and disability evaluation in chronic musculoskeletal pain conditions. In: Escorpizo, R., Brage, S., Homa, D., Stucki, G. (Eds.), Handbook of Vocational Rehabilitation and Disability Evaluation. Handbooks in Health, Work, and Disability. Springer, Cham. https://doi-org.ezp-prod1.hul.harvard.edu/10.1007/978-3-319-08825-9_9.

Reneman, M.F., Beemster, T.T., Welling, S.J., et al., 2021. Vocational rehabilitation for patients with chronic musculoskeletal pain with or without a work module: an economic evaluation. J. Occup. Rehabil. 31, 84–91. https://doi.org/10.1007/s10926-020-09921-y.

Roels, E.H., Reneman, M.F., Post, M.W., 2021. Measurement properties of the full and brief version of the work rehabilitation questionnaire in persons with physical disabilities. J. Occup. Rehabil. 1–9.

Safe Work Australia, 2019. National Return to Work Strategy 2020-2030. Available from https://www.safeworkaustralia.gov.au/system/files/documents/1909/national_return_to_work_strategy_2020-2030.pdf.

Safe Work Australia, 2021. 2021 National Return to Work Survey. Available from https://www.safeworkaustralia.gov.au/doc/2021-national-return-work-survey-headline-measures-report.

Schultz, I.Z., Stowell, A.W., Feuerstein, M., Gatchel, R.J., 2007. Models of return to work for musculoskeletal disorders. J. Occup. Rehabil. 17 (2), 327–352.

Schur, L.A., Ameri, M., Kruse, D., 2020. Telework after COVID: a "silver lining" for workers with disabilities? J. Occup. Rehabil. 30 (4), 521–536.

Sears, J.M., Schulman, B.A., Fulton-Kehoe, D., Hogg-Johnson, S., 2021. Workforce reintegration after work-related permanent impairment: a look at the first year after workers' compensation claim closure. J. Occup. Rehabil. 31 (1), 219–231.

Shaw, W., Hong, Q.N., Pransky, G., Loisel, P., 2008. A literature review describing the role of return-to-work coordinators in trial programs and interventions designed to prevent workplace disability. J. Occup. Rehabil. 18 (1), 2–15.

Shaw, W.S., Nelson, C.C., Woiszwillo, M.J., Gaines, B., Peters, S.E., 2018. Early return to work has benefits for relief of back pain and functional recovery after controlling for multiple confounds. J. Occup. Environ. Med. 60 (10), 901–910.

Shaw, W. S., McLellan, R. K., Besen, E., Namazi, S., Nicholas, M. K., Dugan, A. G., & Tveito, T. H. (2022). A Worksite Self-management Program for Workers with Chronic Health Conditions Improves Worker Engagement and Retention, but not Workplace Function. Journal of Occupational Rehabilitation, 32(1), 77–86.

Sheehan, L.R., Lane, T.J., Gray, S.E., Beck, D., Collie, A., 2018. Return to Work Plans for Injured Australian Workers: Overview and Association with Return to Work. Insurance Work and Health Group. Monash University, Melbourne.

Snippen, N.C., de Vries, H.J., van der Burg-Vermeulen, S.J., Hagedoorn, M., Brouwer, S., 2019. Influence of significant others on work participation of individuals with chronic diseases: a systematic review. BMJ Open 9 (1), e021742.

Social Research Centre, 2018. National Return to Work Survey 2018. Available from https://www.safeworkaustralia.gov.au/system/files/documents/1811/national-rtw-survey-2018-summary-report.pdf.

Sorensen, G., Dennerlein, J.T., Peters, S.E., Sabbath, E.L., Kelly, E.L., Wagner, G.R., 2021. The future of research on work, safety, health and wellbeing: a guiding conceptual framework. Soc. Sci. Med. 269, 113593.

Spink, A., Wagner, I., Orrock, P., 2021. Common reported barriers and facilitators for self-management in adults with chronic musculoskeletal pain: a systematic review of qualitative studies. Musculoskelet. Sci. Pract. 102433.

Steenstra, I., Cullen, K., Irvin, E., Van Eerd, D., Alavinia, M., Beaton, D., et al., 2017. A systematic review of interventions to promote work participation in older workers. J. Saf. Res. 60, 93–102.

Steenstra, I.A., Verbeek, J.H., Heymans, M.W., Bongers, P.M., 2005. Prognostic factors for duration of sick leave in patients sick listed with acute low back pain: a systematic review of the literature. Occup. Environ. Med. 62 (12), 851–860. https://doi.org/10.1136/oem.2004.015842. Epub 2005/11/22. PubMed PMID: 16299094; PubMed Central PMCID: PMC1740930.

Stephens, B., Gross, D.P., 2007. The influence of a continuum of care model on the rehabilitation of compensation claimants with soft tissue disorders. Spine 32 (25), 2898–2904.

Strauser, D., Berven, N.L., 2006. Construction and field testing of the job seeking self-efficacy scale. Rehabil. Counsel. Bull. 49 (4), 207–218.

Van Beukering, I.E., Smits, S.J.C., Janssens, K.M.E., Bogaers, R.I., Joosen, M.C.W., Bakker, M., et al., 2021. In what ways does health related stigma affect sustainable employment and well-being at work? A systematic review. J. Occup. Rehabil. 1–15.

van Vilsteren, M., van Oostrom, S.H., de Vet, H.C., Franche, R.L., Boot, C.R., Anema, J.R., 2015. Workplace interventions to prevent work disability in workers on sick leave. Cochrane Database Syst. Rev. (10).

Veirman, E., Van Ryckeghem, D.M.L., De Paepe, A., Kirtley, O.J., Crombez, G., 2019. Multidimensional screening for predicting pain problems in adults: a systematic review of screening tools and validation studies. Pain. Rep. 4 (5), e775.

Vos, T., Allen, C., Arora, M., Barber, R.M., Bhutta, Z.A., Brown, A., et al., 2016. Global, regional, and national incidence, prevalence, and years lived with disability for 310 diseases and injuries, 1990–2015: a systematic analysis for the Global Burden of Disease Study 2015. lancet 388 (10053), 1545–1602.

van Oostrom, S.H., Driessen, M.T., de Vet, H.C., Franche, R.L., Schonstein, E., Loisel, P., et al., 2009. Workplace interventions for preventing work disability. Cochrane Database Syst. Rev. 2 (2), CD006955. https://doi.org/10.1002/14651858.CD006955.pub2. Epub 2009/04/17. PubMed PMID: 19370664.

Waddell, G., Burton, A.K., 2006. Is Work Good for Your Health and Well-Being? TSO, London.

Webster, B.S., Verma, S.K., Gatchel, R.J., 2007. Relationship between early opioid prescribing for acute occupational low back pain and disability duration, medical costs, subsequent surgery and late opioid use. Spine 32 (19), 2127–2132.

Whysall, Z., Haslam, C., Haslam, R., 2006. Implementing health and safety interventions in the workplace: an exploratory study. Int. J. Ind. Ergon. 36 (9), 809–818.

Wong, J., Kallish, N., Crown, D., Capraro, P., Trierweiler, R., Wafford, Q.E., et al., 2021. Job accommodations, return to work and job retention of people with physical disabilities: a systematic review. J. Occup. Rehabil. 31 (3), 474–490.

WorkCover Queensland, 2021. Host Employment Placement Guideline. Available from https://www.health.qld.gov.au/__data/assets/pdf_file/0023/632147/qh-gdl-401-5-1.pdf.

World Health Organization (WHO), 2018. International Classification of Functioning, Disability and Health. ICF, Geneva.

Xie, Y., Hutting, N., Bartys, S., Johnston, V., 2021. Interventions to promote work–focused care by healthcare providers for individuals with musculoskeletal conditions a scoping review. J. Occup. Rehabil. 31 (4), 840–865.

Section | 3 |

Special issues

Chapter 18

Multidisciplinary and interprofessional working

Bronwyn Lennox Thompson

CHAPTER CONTENTS

LEARNING OBJECTIVES

At the end of this chapter, readers will understand the:
1. Value of teamwork in pain management and rehabilitation.
2. Different models of teamwork.
3. Clinical skills for collaborative teamwork.
4. Processes and skills used by effective teams.

Overview

Pain is always a multidimensional experience, so treatments must address multiple aspects of the pain experience. No single profession holds the breadth of knowledge needed to help a person who has been living with pain for months or years, with difficulties spanning physical, emotional, social and economic domains. Pharmacological and procedural approaches may reduce pain intensity, but will fail to address physical capabilities, participation in life roles and distress (Lin et al. 2020). A team of clinicians from a range of professional backgrounds working together is best placed to ensure comprehensive assessment, treatment planning and delivery (Chou et al. 2009). Although team-based treatments are common in persistent pain management, persistent pain is influenced by factors that either precede pain onset or develop rapidly after pain begins. Many of these factors are amenable to change, e.g. beliefs and attitudes towards pain (Smith et al. 2021). Attention should be given to them early in the recovery process, with this approach requiring a team of clinicians with skills to intervene in a person's areas of need (Katz et al. 2019).

A combination of clinical expertise and skills for collaborative work are needed for effective pain management teamwork. This chapter will introduce readers to terminology, the value of teamwork, skills for collaborative teamwork and practices to enhance team working (Box 18.1).

Box 18.1 **Reflective practice**

The reader has probably been a member of many teams. There may have been group assignments for school or university, a sports team, a choir or a team of co-workers. Take a moment to reflect on the best team and the 'worst' team you have been part of.

Write three key points associated with the experience of each of those two teams.
How can you use these observations to shed light on working in a pain management team?

Working in a team

Teams are 'a distinguishable set of two or more people who interact dynamically, interdependently, and adaptively towards a common and valued goal/objective/mission' (Salas et al. 1992, p. 4). While the term is often applied only to the *clinicians* working with a person experiencing pain, the core team must also include *the person with pain*.

Three types of teams in healthcare are multidisciplinary, interdisciplinary and interprofessional

(Chamberlain-Salaun et al. 2013). Additional terms include transdisciplinary, transprofessional and multiprofessional. Although each term has a particular meaning, they are often used interchangeably. Different team types are illustrated in Fig. 18.1.

A note about terminology: Throughout this chapter, the term *professional* is used in preference to *disciplinary*, recognising that disciplines are a branch of learning or field of study, while professions not only hold learning unique to that profession but also adhere to unique values, beliefs and regulatory requirements in which they apply their knowledge (Smith & Clouder 2010).

Multidisciplinary/multiprofessional teams involve people from different health professions working alongside one another, while using their profession's clinical models (Körner 2010). The team members recognise the contributions of the other professions, but there is limited role overlap. Clinicians usually have high professional autonomy, generating their own treatment goals and plans for the patient. Treatments proceed in parallel, although one clinician may take the lead in coordinating and communicating with the whole team (Ruan & Kaye 2016). For example, in postoperative pain management, different professionals may independently contribute their skills, with a nurse practitioner as coordinator. The International Association for the Study of Pain specifically points to multidisciplinary pain management centres as the most effective way to meet the needs of people with pain (Sluka et al. 2009).

Interdisciplinary/interprofessional teams also involve different health professionals working alongside one another using their areas of expertise, but where all use a common overarching model such as a biopsychosocial approach. Teams meet regularly to collaborate on treatment goals and priorities (Ruan & Kaye 2016). There is limited hierarchy and extensive communication, cooperation and overlap between team members (Körner 2010). The patient may be included in team discussions and decision-making. Some multiprofessional teams may evolve into interprofessional teams, particularly over time as clinicians work together, and when using a biopsychosocial framework (Katz et al. 2019). Comprehensive interprofessional pain management has demonstrated long-term effectiveness for patients with complex presentations (Oslund et al. 2009; Phillips et al. 2014).

Transprofessional teams are a recent phenomenon and can be described as a process of collaboration between two or more professionals *across and beyond* professional and disciplinary boundaries, such that boundaries blur and new synergies flourish (Chiocchio & Richer 2015). Gordon et al. (2014) described a transdisciplinary team in which all clinicians used the same pain management strategies (e.g. meditation, guided imagery and a structured medication schedule) to support a woman with ovarian cancer. They suggested that the unique features of a transdisciplinary team are: integrated goal-setting shared across the team; co-treatment can occur; several disciplines may conduct assessments together; learning occurs across

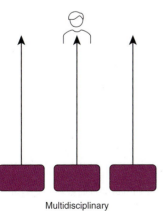

Work in parallel/independently
Separate goals and treatment priorities
Hierarchical
Meet infrequently

Multidisciplinary

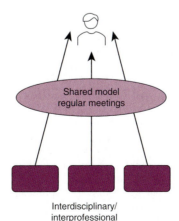

Work collaboratively
Shared goals and treatment priorities
Non-hierarchical
Meet frequently, often informally as well as formally

Shared model regular meetings

Interdisciplinary/
interprofessional

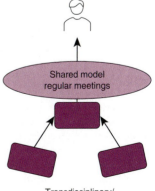

Work collaboratively
Clinician with most to contribute at any time steps forward, with support from others
"Key" clinician may change over time
Shared goals and treatment priorities
Non-hierarchical
Meet frequently, often informally as well as formally

Shared model regular meetings

Transdisciplinary/
transprofessional

Fig. 18.1 Types of teamwork.

disciplinary lines; and communication is consistent to people with pain and their families (Gordon et al. 2014).

Patients' perspective on teams

Pain patients receiving multi- or interprofessional pain management have described feeling validated (Mathias et al. 2014) and supported as they learned how to manage their pain (Bryl et al. 2021). They have reported enhanced confidence in treatments because of the application of a consistent treatment model (Nordin et al. 2013) and have indicated that coordinated and comprehensive treatment is a more efficient use of time and resources for them and their family (Joypaul et al. 2019). A participant in one study said: 'Leaving a team-conference meeting sensing having been respected, listened to and grasping that they (the health professionals) want to help me, gave me a boost to continue [the rehabilitation] … I felt happier, strengthened and felt less pain' (Nordin et al. 2013, p. 583). Unfortunately, there may also be mixed messages from different members of a team causing confusion for the person (Stewart 2018; see Chapter 3), but when teams collaborate closely, patients report benefits (Phillips et al. 2014).

Clinicians' perspectives on teams

Qualitative enquiry has shown that clinicians find treating people with persistent pain highly challenging, unrewarding and may feel underprepared to address these patients' needs (Gardner et al. 2017; Synnott et al. 2015). However, there is minimal research that has explored clinicians' experiences of teamwork in pain treatment.

Stenberg et al. (2017) found that team members thought teamwork was enriching, and that good teamwork was a strength. They reported that working in the team supported and strengthened their clinical skills. In another team, clinicians emphasised that, despite professional differences, the motivators for team collaboration were being there for the patient and reaching a higher level together that 'we are here for the patient' (Pype et al. 2018, Emergent pattern 1, first bullet point).

Nevertheless, navigating professional interactions is not always straightforward, because each decision made by a clinician may have an impact on the approach taken by others. Teamwork may be problematic if each clinician retains their own professional and personal perspective without incorporating the team stance. Team members in an interprofessional pain management team in Norway, for example, identified clinicians with discrepant beliefs about pain, describing them as 'villains' of the story (Battin et al. 2021). Gergerich and colleagues (2019) identified that even during pre-licensure training, tensions between team members arose from perceptions of hierarchy, marginalisation and failure to resolve these issues. Active steps are needed to develop a team that can work closely together.

Despite the challenges of close collaboration with different professionals, the value of interprofessional teamwork for people with pain, as well as the clinicians working together, appears evident especially when working with patients with complex presentations. For decades there have been strong recommendations calling for interprofessional team treatment to become the norm in pain management and rehabilitation (Loeser 2005). Research from both within healthcare teams, and more broadly from organisational psychology, has identified features of effective teamwork, and the remainder of this chapter discusses these processes.

Skills for collaborative teamwork

Effective teams do not develop without time and support. Achieving quality coordination and cohesion in a team requires team members to have both taskwork and teamwork skills. *Taskwork skills* are clinical skills from each clinician's professional background, relevant to pain management. *Teamwork skills* relate to team processes such as communication, interpersonal relationships, decision-making processes and shared mental models (Zajac et al. 2021).

Taskwork/clinical skills

Proffering a list of the various professionals within an interprofessional team does not guarantee successful team functioning. Gaps and duplications can occur when clinicians believe that a certain area of practice belongs to theirs or another profession, or when there are conflicting approaches to practice. The range of skills within a team are listed in Table 18.1, recognising that contributions to a team overlap as members work together, while the titles and scopes of professions may differ depending on jurisdiction.

Team members must be skilled in their own professional domains of concern and well versed in a modern understanding of pain as a multifactorial experience (Sluka et al. 2009). Treatment or care should be person-centred, based on evidence and focused on:

- reducing or managing pain where possible
- optimising physical, psychological and social role functioning
- optimising healthcare resource and medication use
- improving quality of life
- enhancing self-efficacy for preventing or managing future pain episodes (Wilkinson & Whiteman 2017).

TABLE 18.1 Clinical skills and competencies for pain rehabilitation teams

Foundational skills

- Skilled in own professional domains of concern
- Comprehensive understanding of a modern view of pain as a multifactorial experience
- Person-centred care
- Based on evidence
- Focused on reducing or managing pain intensity, optimising physical psychological and social role functioning, optimising medication and healthcare use, improving quality of life, enhancing self-efficacy for preventing or managing future episodes

Assessment and planning

Assessment and synthesis	• Pain diagnosis where established causal mechanisms and clear-cut responses to treatments are available • Case formulation to answer why this person is presenting in this way at this time, and what might be maintaining their predicament • Identifies treatment targets and valued outcomes
Diagnosis	• Pain diagnosis where established causal mechanisms and clear-cut responses to treatment are available • Predominant pain mechanistic descriptor • Biological contributors to pain • Exclude possible diagnoses • Establishes a 'label' for the person's pain problem
Understanding the impact of pain on performance	• Physical performance assessment • Recognising the effect of environmental contexts and personal values on performance • Help to establish what a person is willing to do • Collaborate with the person to identify functional status
Identifying psychosocial factors relevant to pain and disability	• Pain-specific attitudes, beliefs and emotions • Factors that influence behaviour/disability • Interaction between person, important others and disability
Collecting and interpreting intake and outcome data	• Understand, interpret and use data for treatment planning and outcome measurement (all team members) • Value the data for what it offers to all stakeholders, including people with pain • Analyse and present information in meaningful ways (specialised clinicians and support staff) • Collecting, storing and managing data long term
Establishing treatment/ management order and priorities	• Integrate goals, values and preferences of the person with pain • Recognise constraints of team capabilities, funding and evidence • Open discussion about expectations, pain reduction and/or self-management • Progress review and treatment adjustment

Treatment and rehabilitation

Medical treatments	• Used for pain reduction, where possible • Integrated with, and supporting rehabilitation treatment
Pain mechanism explanations	• Used to encourage active participation in rehabilitation, reduce fear of harm • Must be consistent within the team
Movement-based approaches	• Personally valued activities that can be incorporated into a person's daily life routines • Used to reduce fear and avoidance, enhance self-efficacy • To counter the effects of reduced activity levels • To support consistent performance in daily life

Continued

TABLE 18.1 Clinical skills and competencies for pain rehabilitation teams—cont'd	
Skills for working with thoughts and feelings	• Understanding and managing the relationship between thoughts, emotions and actions • Self-management skills to help clinicians manage their own responses to seeing people in pain
Behaviour change expertise	• Skills to encourage long-term adoption and generalisation of strategies developed in a clinic setting
Generalising pain rehabilitation	• Identifying obstacles to knowledge transfer outside the clinic • Establishing set-back plans • Needed to support long-term behaviour change
Couple, family and group facilitation skills	• Where couples, families and groups are included in the rehabilitation programme

Clinicians should recognise that their patients are individuals with strengths, vulnerabilities and a preexisting life trajectory into which pain has intruded. People also bring their cultural perspectives, values and priorities when they seek treatment for their pain. They are part of families, workplaces and communities. For people with pain to collaborate as equal partners, clinicians must develop expertise in individualised communication, negotiation and integration of evidence-based approaches (Santana et al. 2018), while supporting the person with pain to express what matters to them (Howarth et al. 2014). Using these skills ensures personalised treatment rather than a standardised treatment algorithm. While clinicians working without the support of a team also need these skills, the strength of an interprofessional team lies in its ability to offer coordinated interventions in combinations that can accommodate the unique needs of their patients.

Gordon et al. (2018) detailed core competencies for interprofessional pain management in a model which has the needs of the person in pain at its centre. This model has four overlapping knowledge domains: (1) pain as a multidimensional experience, (2) assessing and measuring pain, (3) managing pain and (4) pain in specific clinical conditions. The core values and principles of the model are advocacy, empathy, collaboration, ethical treatment, communication, evidence-based practice, compassion, health disparities reduction, comprehensive care, interprofessional teamwork, cultural inclusiveness and patient-centred care (Gordon et al. 2018).

Clinical skills for an interprofessional pain management and rehabilitation team may superficially appear to be no different from skills required when working individually or in other clinical areas. Where interprofessional teamwork in pain differs from other team contexts is that professionals may hold different models of pain from one another and the patient, while responses to treatments vary widely. Psychosocial factors contribute greatly to a person's presentation, so the conventional biomedical model used in much healthcare is less relevant. Treating the disease may have little impact on a person's participation in what matters to them. There is much that is unknown about pain and its management, and both clinicians and people with pain may hold different views on the desired outcomes; achieving agreement between all those involved requires a sophisticated level of teamwork. Conversely, interprofessional teamwork offers both clinicians and people with pain opportunities for individually tailored treatment delivered in a consistent and comprehensive way.

Assessment, diagnosis and synthesis

Chapter 9 provided guidance about pain assessment and measurement tools that can help the clinician. Pain as an experience, its impact on an individual and contributing factors are usually part of assessment, but how teams *synthesise* this information to generate an explanatory model is seldom discussed.

There are two broad approaches to synthesising assessment information. Where there are established causal mechanisms and clear-cut responses to specific treatments, a *pain diagnosis* may be useful, and it will guide treatment. When causal mechanisms are uncertain, diagnosis is unclear, there are many treatment options or multiple aspects of the person's presentation to address, a *case formulation* approach may be more useful (Nicholas & George 2011). Please refer to Chapters 5 and 13 for further understanding of the value of case formulation.

Case formulations aim to explain why *this* person is presenting in *this* way at *this* time, and what might be *maintaining* their predicament (Lennox Thompson 2021). Case formulations are used to integrate information gathered from biological, psychological and social/environmental perspectives. A set of hypotheses about the relationships between contributing factors and a person's presentation can be generated (Nicholas & George 2011; Vertue & Haig 2008). Case formulations can incorporate pain diagnoses along with predisposing and contributing factors to identify why and how a person is distressed or disabled. Doing so provides an idiographic approach to

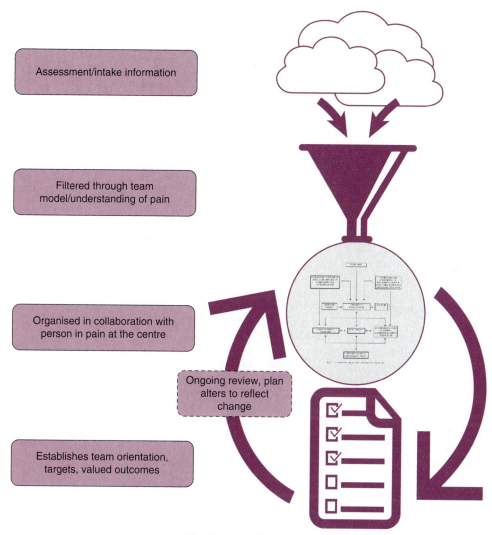

Fig. 18.2 Case formulation.

treatment, establishing an understanding of the person's situation, and identifying treatment targets and outcomes that are valued by the person in pain (Fig. 18.2).

There is no standardised framework for case formulation, but a formulation should include the following at a minimum:

1. Diagnosis, or biological contributions to the pain problem. This may also include comorbid health problems.
2. The impact of pain on performance in the person's life context.
3. Relevant psychosocial factors influencing pain and disability.

More detailed information about formulation is to be found elsewhere in this textbook (Chapters 5 and 13).

The interdependencies between pain reduction, self-efficacy, social reinforcement, physical fitness and contextual factors need to be incorporated into the formulation. Each clinician will bring their area of expertise to the team when contributing to clinical reasoning, when considering what may be offered to the person and when negotiating the timing and intensity of treatment components.

A formulation allows all team members to know the goals of treatment, maintaining a consistent approach that supports therapeutic change. This means that while movement-based therapy may be the major contribution from a physical therapist, a nurse may also ask a patient about the progress they are making in exercise class, while the physical therapist may report on specific fears held about medications to the nurse. Because of the need to recognise and contribute to goals in common, clinicians need to be somewhat conversant with one another's treatment approaches. This ensures consistency for patients, and in turn, this offers them greater certainty that they are following a coherent treatment plan (Nordin et al. 2013).

Treatment planning

After assessing and formulating, teams need to identify how they will approach treatment or management. The person with pain's goals, values and preferences must be central in this process, within the constraints of the team, funding and current evidence base. There is little research detailing how pain management teams undertake this process and the effectiveness of such deliberations. Actively involving the person with pain in clinical decision-making and teamwork may only be given lip service (Stewart 2018). Teamwork skills will have an impact on how effectively the treatment plan will be developed and implemented.

Whether treatment strategies focused on pain reduction can be combined with self-management approaches and which should be prioritised can be complex issues for interprofessional teams. For example, a biomedical approach focusing on identifying and treating peripheral contributors to pain may delay the person's readiness to engage with treatments targeting 'top-down' approaches such as cognitive therapy. Mismatched expectations may exist between people with pain and professionals, and differing emphases between clinicians may be present (Schultz et al. 2021). This will impact on team deliberations and treatment planning, requiring careful negotiations and leadership.

Treatment planning in pain management and rehabilitation is an iterative process. Regular reviews involving the entire team, including the person with pain, are crucial. They allow clinicians to titrate the intensity of any treatment (e.g. exercise frequency, medication dose) and monitor carryover into the person's daily life. Important factors influencing progress may be highlighted at team meetings. For example, a person may respond well to a medication but fail to report unhelpful side-effects to the prescribing clinician but may discuss this within an exercise class; a person may show improvement in exercise classes but be unable to transfer gains to household or work tasks. Team meetings enable collaboration to develop creative solutions as different perspectives are brought to the discussion.

Integrating psychosocial and physical treatments

The definition of pain explicitly includes qualities of unpleasantness and that it is both a sensory and emotional experience, so it is unsurprising that negative emotions are common when a person experiences pain. Human emotion is bidirectionally communicated both verbally and nonverbally. Pain clinicians' burnout is high (Ashton-James et al. 2021) and they need skills to manage their own responses to witnessing people in distress, while also helping people with pain to manage their emotions. Support from within the team has been identified as one strength of interprofessional teamwork (Körner et al. 2015), while staff turnover is associated with poorer outcomes for patients attending the service (Williams & Potts 2010).

Clinicians will also need skills to assist people with pain appreciate the relationship between thoughts and their emotional responses and pain intensity. While cognitive behavioural therapy and acceptance and commitment therapy (ACT) are formal therapies used in pain rehabilitation (Williams et al. 2020), it is useful to consider that all clinicians offer explanations to engage patients and influence beliefs, and dealing with emotional responses is common in many clinical settings. A cognitive behavioural approach to managing pain has been employed by interprofessional teams since the 1980s (Turk & Flor 1984).

While all clinicians should have some competence in this area, those with specialised training and expertise in working with thoughts and emotions may need to be willing to share strategies with less specialised clinicians. This ensures the person with pain is offered appropriate support at the time they need it. For example, if a person becomes distressed while returning to functional activities or exercise, the clinician present at the time should have sufficient skills to address unhelpful beliefs or help reduce distress rather than suggest the person waits to see the dedicated clinician.

Teams need to develop strategies to enable the three clinical skill areas unique to interprofessional teamwork (assessment and synthesis, treatment planning and integrating psychosocial and physical treatments) to be undertaken successfully. The processes underpinning success in these activities are effective teamwork and team processes.

Skills for effective teamwork and team processes

Most teamwork research in pain management and rehabilitation has investigated team *effectiveness*, with relatively few studies examining the *processes* used by teams to undertake their work in this setting. Team effectiveness can be characterised as (1) achieving goals by drawing on current resources and cues for action, (2) establishing consistent processes that are flexible and responsive, (3) selecting actions that fit the current situation even if these actions differ slightly from usual practice and (4)

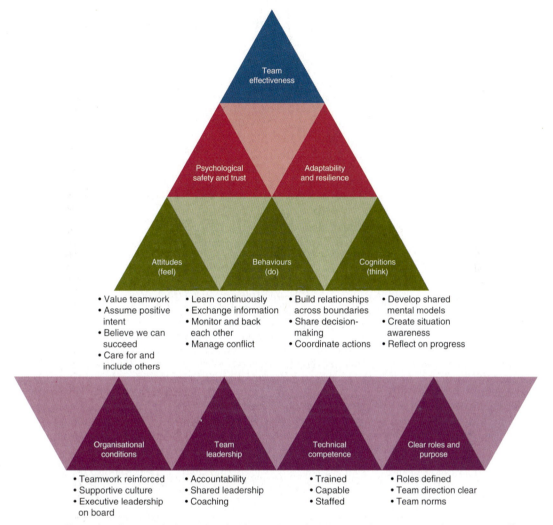

Fig. 18.3 Team effectiveness framework. (Reproduced with permission from Zajac et al. 2021. Comprehensive Team Effectiveness Framework. From Overcoming challenges to teamwork in healthcare: A team effectiveness framework and evidence-based guidance. S. Zajac, et al. (2021), Frontiers in Communication, 6(6), doi: 10.3389/fcomm.2021.606445. Copyright 2021 by Stephanie Zajac. Reprinted with permission.)

being able to innovate in response to novel challenges (Gorman et al. 2018). In other words, an effective team should influence patient outcomes, be cost effective, maintain consistency even when patients or team composition changes and respond to unexpected demands. Zajac and colleagues (2021) have suggested that team effectiveness is the product of team performance (results), team functioning and team viability (Fig. 18.3).

Team performance outcomes and cost effectiveness are extensively examined in pain literature (e.g. Cheung et al. 2019; Fullen et al. 2014; Gagnon et al. 2018; Hampel et al. 2019). Team functioning refers to how a team performs day to day and includes both clinical skills as well as teamwork. Team viability relates to predictions of how a team will perform over time (Zajac et al. 2021). These processes have received less attention in research, and there is less to guide their development specific to pain management teams.

Drawing from what is known about teamwork in other contexts, there are three main factors for effective team functioning in pain management (Cannon-Bowers & Salas 2014). *Attitudes* are what team members feel or believe, and include mutual trust, team cohesion and collective efficacy. These influence interactions between team members. *Behaviours* are what team members do, and include processes associated with exchanging information, supporting team members and problem-detection. *Cognitions* are what team members think or know and refer to knowledge distributed among team members that is used to enable treatment planning and implementation. Cognitions include contextual awareness of factors potentially impacting on team performance, as well as collective critical thinking. Collective critical thinking describes team information acquisition, deliberations and eventual decisions about the adopted approach (Fiore et al. 2010). All three of these factors are emergent team-level processes developed as clinicians work together.

In the sections below, aspects of teamwork are discussed first, followed by research-based strategies that teams have used to support their development. It is important to recognise the interconnectivity and emergent nature of these factors. How a team works is different from how each member functions individually.

Team attitudes

Cooperation, team efficacy and team orientation (the belief and preference for teamwork) are important team attitudes and are associated with psychological trust and safety and positive team behaviours (actions) (Salas et al. 2015). Trust and safety in this context do not necessitate that team members are friends or that there are no disagreements. It describes a team atmosphere where discussions are directed towards issues, not people, with a foundational expectation that team members have the best interests of both patients and team in mind. The distinction between trust and safety has been defined by Vaida & Ardelean (2019): 'When talking about psychological safety, it is others [who]will give you the benefit of a doubt when taking a risk, while with trust, it is you that will give others the benefit of a doubt when taking a risk'.

A key benefit of having an interprofessional team is the contribution of differing perspectives. When team members believe it is safe for them to take interpersonal risks, they are more likely to express an opinion that differs from another member of the team (Edmondson & Lei 2014; Grossman & Feitosa 2018). Expressing different opinions allows for a comprehensive understanding of what is going on for the person in pain, and the rehabilitation options that might be most suitable for them. Team members, however, may share already common knowledge yet fail to share their unique perspectives, particularly during detailed discussion, requiring team leadership to use strategies to ensure all voices are heard (Zijl et al. 2021). Detailed discussion enables the team to exchange and synthesise disparate views. For example, a person's progress in an exercise class may be discussed, but if the team member who is aware of the difficulties that person

> ### Box 18.2 **Team attitude activities**
>
> **Team attitude activities**
> A well-established pain service has used these approaches to develop positive team attitudes.
> *Recruitment:* Potential new team members can spend time with the existing team to establish "team fit"
> *Induction:* New team members follow clinicians from other professions for one day a week for the first month.
> *Continuing professional development:* All team members are included in monthly journal club meetings over lunch with shared responsibility for providing a paper to discuss; opportunities for ongoing learning are open to all clinicians irrespective of profession
> *Centre day:* this is a full day set aside each year to review data collected on patient characteristics, referral sources, episode of care durations, and outcomes. The day is also used for appreciative inquiry and a social event.

has in generalising their progress to daily life contexts feels uncomfortable about sharing their observation, it may not be discussed in sufficient detail for the team to establish an appropriate intervention.

Elevating the opinions of some team members over others can influence what information is valued and therefore discussed (Fox & Comeau-Vallée 2020). High-trust teams demonstrate inclusiveness (all team members can express their views), trust in the team's collective responsibility (decisions are made by the team, rather than individuals) and use open communication (Thorgren & Caiman 2019).

Team efficacy refers to the confidence that a team can successfully perform and is influenced by the team's previous performance (Goncalo et al. 2010). Team cohesion (the strength and extent of interpersonal connection) influences how people with dissenting views are included. Team efficacy and team cohesion influence how willing teams are to review their performance and make changes (Salas et al. 2015). Limited opportunities to obtain feedback on performance, and lack of coaching from leadership to meet performance objectives can reduce team efficacy, as can unclear objectives (Zajac et al. 2021). Supporting a shared responsibility for outcomes and routine reviews of outcomes and processes may offer openings for teams to reflect on their performance, while social teambuilding occasions can enhance team cohesion. Box 18.2 illustrates some ways teams have supported positive team attitudes.

Team behaviours

Open information exchange supports effective team performance. Griffin & Hay-Smith (2019) found that communication enhanced team decision-making and information sharing, mutual support for difficult situations, consistent messages to patients and feedback and support for clinicians. Communicating about emerging aspects of the patient's pain experience, in turn, enhanced confidence in expertise within the team, and supported clinicians to question team decisions (Griffin & Hay-Smith 2019).

Skills in managing conflict, communication and providing mutual support are critical for successful team functioning. Conflict may arise in pain teams because clinicians have interprofessional differences in their training, values, priorities and approaches to team decision-making (Kane & Perry 2016), as well as interpersonal conflict arising from personal characteristics, conflict management and communication styles and burnout (Kim et al. 2017). Managing conflict well is crucial for developing trust and safety. *Task-related* conflict during decision-making can be positive because it generates multiple solutions, whereas *interpersonal* conflict is detrimental (O'Neill et al. 2013). Interpersonal conflict reduces psychological trust and safety, and can lead to restricted information flow, reduced risk-taking and apportioning blame (Zajac et al. 2021). Fostering conflicting and divergent perspectives in clinical reasoning, however, offers the potential for creative problem solving (Farh et al. 2010). Achieving open discussion without risking interpersonal conflict requires establishing ground rules for the discussion: address the ideas, not the person.

There are always areas of risk in communication. Lack of clarity during handover from clinician-to-clinician risks duplicating or omitting information (Griffin & Hay-Smith 2019). Having limited time may mean clinicians fail to share what is assumed to be common knowledge when new clinicians join the team, hampering collaboration and the shared mental model (Grand et al. 2016; Hellman et al. 2016). Each profession uses its own jargon: ensuring that a common understanding exists between clinicians may involve translating profession-specific terms into language used by all the team members (Schot et al. 2020). In-depth conversations are particularly important when new clinicians join the team, and with the introduction of new treatments or technology as they are integrated within the team's mental model. New clinicians bring with them new ideas and habits, while new treatments or technology may affect the timing of other aspects of the treatment plan. If teams fail to have opportunities for deep conversations and reflection, issues may remain unresolved, eroding trust and safety.

Mutual support enhances trust and safety while building team efficacy. It is aligned with open communication and reflexivity (discussed later). Mutual support involves reciprocated recognition and responses to emotional and practical needs of team members (Cooke 2016). It

---

Box 18.3 Team behaviours activities

Actions to support effective team behaviours: Case formulation process

Each assessing clinician provides their information in turn without discussion, entering this into a structured formulation diagram. Treatment recommendations are not shared until all the assessment information is integrated into the formulation. Once the formulation is developed, each clinician in turn makes their recommendation.

This approach allows each clinician an opportunity to share their assessment information in its entirety. All the information is assembled before reducing the risk of prematurely making decisions. Treatment priorities are identified on the basis of the patient's goals, and clinical reasoning. The formulation diagram and treatment plan is shared with the patient.

---

may include informal conversations about difficult situations, temporarily stepping in to replace a clinician who is overloaded, offering back-up help to team members to ensure the team continues to perform despite changes in circumstances. Blurring or overlapping of roles forms part of mutual support but fails to capture 'emotional labour' aspects of this emergent team behaviour (Schot et al. 2020).

Mutual support has mainly positive effects but there are some risks. Clinicians may not disclose role overload and inadequate resourcing to managers, because their immediate needs are met. New team members may initially find it difficult to become part of the team where strong mutual support has led to in-group formation.

Efforts to enhance positive team behaviours such as TeamSTEPPS, a programme developed by the U.S. Department of Defense and the Agency for Healthcare Research and Quality (2008), have shown positive effects on team attitudes and behaviours (Cooke 2016).

See Box 18.3 for some ways teams have introduced and supported positive team behaviours.

Team cognition

Team cognition refers to how teams process information (encode, store and retrieve information) as well as the product of that process (Fiore et al. 2010). It includes the mental models that the team develop about themselves and their modus operandi and their reflexivity. In pain management teams, a shared model of pain is important, while how information from each patient is synthesised depends on team members forming a deep understanding of the relevance of this information to the case formulation and to other members of the team.

As teams work together, a mutual understanding forms about what others bring to the team (role definitions), how the team prioritises information and develops case formulations (mental models) and how the team acquires and generates information relevant to their work (DeChurch & Mesmer-Magnus 2010). Grand et al. (2016) identified that learning and sharing are integral to team-level knowledge emergence. Learning at the team level is the process of recognising and acquiring team-relevant information; sharing is how team members communicate, interact and disseminate knowledge within the team (Grand et al 2016). Sharing depends on levels of trust, safety and communication. Therefore for teams to develop effective team cognitions, the team's attitudes and behaviours are crucial. Formal team orientation training (induction) and shared continuing education about pain may help to ensure the team mental model integrates information within a biopsychosocial framework.

Aligning mental models of pain within the team is particularly relevant for pain management and rehabilitation because conflicting models may undermine the consistent messages needed by the person with pain. For example, teams with a dominant biomechanical model may struggle to appreciate the importance of family or behavioural reinforcement factors and consequently ignore family member responses that can increase pain catastrophising (Martire et al. 2019). Team members may fail to acquire an understanding of these factors and their influence on outcomes (team learning) if they are not valued when they are shared (team sharing). Information about factors that could be relevant to the person seeking help may not be shared within the team (team sharing). Lack of shared knowledge also makes it more difficult to establish team trust and psychological safety and in turn can foster unhelpful team behaviours such as limited mutual support (Grand et al. 2016). Active steps to form a biopsychosocial model of pain and disability with common language may enhance sharing and learning.

Structured case formulations are an explicit form of mental modelling. Teams also hold mental models of available treatment options and contextual factors such as patient demographics, location, travel times, funding and relationships with other teams and clinicians. Together, case formulations and mental models form a pool of shared knowledge that influences what is offered to the person seeking help.

Team reflexivity describes how the team selects and adds relevant information to the shared mental model, deliberates on it during problem solving and then coordinates action (Schmutz & Eppich 2017). It is a form of collective critical thinking and involves setting aside time to focus on the team's purpose and processes now and for the future (Zajac et al. 2021).

Anticipating and recognising when rehabilitation strategies should change in response to progress is part of team

---

Box 18.4 Team reviews: case conference

Team reviews

One tertiary pain management centre has held a weekly case conference for all clinical staff since 1987. The case conference is in two parts:
1. Clinical cases submitted by team members for review because the person's response to treatment is not as expected.
2. Case presentation made by a clinician to illustrate something the clinician learned.

At the conclusion, the clinicians bringing cases to the meeting are not obligated to follow recommendations from the team but have more information with which to make their clinical decisions.

The case conference has a rotating chair so every team member can facilitate discussion. All team members can contribute to the discussion, irrespective of scope of practice.

---

reflexivity. The shared mental model informs all clinicians, even those who may not be directly responsible for that aspect of treatment. For example, a person with pain may choose to talk with an occupational therapist with whom they feel comfortable about having stopped a medication. The therapist needs to retain this knowledge, recognise possible effects of medication cessation and share the discussion with the other professionals. Knowing what is relevant for whom and how to best share that knowledge is therefore a combination of both taskwork (clinical skills) and teamwork.

Teamwork is carried out in a dynamic environment where the team must remain responsive to the person experiencing pain, changes within the team and external factors influencing service delivery. Actively reviewing team processes and outcomes (including routine practices) relies on effective communication and high levels of trust between team members (McHugh et al. 2020). Reflexive reviews enable teams to detail 'taken-as-given' processes so they can examine assumptions, review outcomes and generate creative alternatives. This in turn promotes learning from experience and adaptation to contextual factors.

Box 18.4 offers two ways teams have developed and maintained a shared mental model.

Additional practices to enhance teamwork

Most processes described in the previous sections are emergent, i.e. they arise from time spent as a team and interactions that occur between team members. Organisational conditions, team leadership, technical competence and purpose contribute to teams developing the attitudes, behaviours and cognitions described previously (Zajac et al. 2021).

Organisational conditions: Rydenfalt and colleagues (2017) identified three organisational design principles that influence characteristics of effective teams. (1) Team stability supports trust, and in turn is associated with open communication, conflict resolution, mutual support and team reflexivity. They suggest reducing staff rotation through different areas of practice and keeping teams small so each team member can relate to fewer people. (2) Occasions for communication include formal team meetings as well as informal coffee and lunch breaks and can also include the built environment that invites connection such as shared lunchrooms, comfortable couches and an open-door office policy. Co-location has been identified as a major facilitator of informal 'corridor conversations', and is as an important contributor to effective pain management teamwork (Griffin & Hay-Smith 2019). (3) A participative and adaptive approach to leadership is the third principle (Rydenfalt et al. 2017). This means that a person is acknowledged as the leader, especially in decision-making, but as Silva et al. (2021) have suggested, there is growing awareness that collective leadership has been found to improve patient experience, maintain quality improvement and support collective responsibility for outcomes. Coaching other members of the team to develop leadership capabilities will facilitate shared leadership.

Team leadership: Interprofessional leadership in healthcare emphasises slightly different skills and contributions from multiprofessional teams (Smith et al. 2018). The research literature highlights that leadership in interprofessional teamwork is often collective, with a transformational role that supports creativity and innovation. Leadership can therefore function as a catalyst. Zajac et al. (2021) also endorse accountability by all team members for commitments made to and by the team, and that coaching and teamwork development is shared by team members. This suggests that leadership training should be provided to all team members. Leadership training may include conflict resolution (negotiation skills), communication, facilitation skills, feedback and coaching skills. Training should be temporally spaced, i.e. delivered over weeks rather than a single day, employ an external trainer and be delivered on-site (Lacerenza et al. 2017). Leaders can use team coaching such as the GROUP (Goal-Reality-Options-Understand others-Perform) framework (Brown & Grant 2010) to help teams develop solutions.

Technical competence: This refers to clinical skills, which clinicians working in pain management teams must continue to develop. Clinical supervision or peer review helps support technical competence (Dysvik & Stephens 2010).

Purpose and clarity: Zajac et al. (2021) found that having defined roles, a clear team direction (with objectives, goals and priorities) and team norms (standards, or informal rules for behaviour) were also prerequisites for effective team functioning. Strategies to achieve these may include mission statements that articulate the vision of the team (Tingle 2017); action points with timeframes and responsibility established and documented in meetings; and written policies and procedures.

Conclusion

Interprofessional teamwork can be complex to establish and requires investment in time, training and ongoing support. Despite gaps in knowledge about teamwork processes, interprofessional teamwork in pain rehabilitation outperforms single discipline or multidisciplinary approaches. People seeking help, their family and friends, and clinicians benefit when a team with effective clinical and teamwork skills delivers pain rehabilitation.

Research is needed to further examine effective interprofessional team processes in pain management. There are differences between interprofessional teamwork in healthcare and in other areas of work (Griffin & Hay-Smith 2019), and it is likely that differences exist between pain management teams and teamwork in other areas of practice. Investigating how teams collaborate and developing strategies to optimise their working, including teams who work at a distance from one another (virtual teams), are all areas that need further attention.

Review questions   Q

1. What are the essential differences between a multiprofessional and an interprofessional team?
2. In addition to clinical skills usual for pain practitioners, what other skills should clinicians working in an interprofessional team work to develop?
3. What are the three team factors that influence team effectiveness?
4. How does a case formulation help interprofessional teamwork?
5. List the three organisational design principles that support effective interprofessional teamwork.

References

Agency for Healthcare Research and Quality, 2008. TeamSTEPPS: Team Strategies and Tools to Enhance Performance and Patient Safety. Available from https://www.ahrq.gov/teamstepps/index.html.

Ashton-James, C.E., McNeilage, A.G., Avery, N.S., Robson, L.H.E., Costa, D., 2021. Prevalence and predictors of burnout symptoms in multidisciplinary pain clinics: a mixed-methods study. Pain 162 (2), 503–513.

Battin, G.S., Romsland, G.I., Christiansen, B., 2021. The puzzle of therapeutic emplotment: creating a shared clinical plot through interprofessional interaction in biopsychosocial pain rehabilitation. Soc. Sci. Med. 277, 113904.

Brown, S.W., Grant, A.M., 2010. From GROW to GROUP: theoretical issues and a practical model for group coaching in organisations. Coaching 3 (1), 30–45.

Bryl, K., Wenger, S., Banz, D., Terry, G., Ballester, D., Bailey, C., et al., 2021. Power over pain - an interprofessional approach to chronic pain: program feedback from a medically underserved community. J. Eval. Clin. Pract. 27, 1223–1234.

Cannon-Bowers, J.A., Salas, E., 2014. Teamwork competencies: the interaction of team member knowledge, skills, and attitudes. In: O'Neil, H.F. (Ed.), Workforce Readiness: Competencies and Assessment. Lawrence Erlbaum Associates, New Jersey, Psychology Press: New York, pp. 151–174.

Chamberlain-Salaun, J., Mills, J., Usher, K., 2013. Terminology used to describe health care teams: an integrative review of the literature. J. Multidiscip. Healthc. 6, 65–74.

Cheung, K., Tse, M.M.Y., Wong, C.K., Mui, K.W., Lee, S.K., Ma, K.Y., et al., 2019. The effectiveness of a multidisciplinary exercise program in managing work-related musculoskeletal symptoms for low-skilled workers in the low-income community: a pre-post-follow-up study. Int. J. Environ. Res. Publ. Health. 16 (9).

Chiocchio, F., Richer, M.-C., 2015. From multi-professional to trans-professional healthcare teams: the critical role of innovation projects. In: Gurtner, S., Soyez, K. (Eds.), Challenges and Opportunities in Health Care Management. Springer, Berlin, pp. 161–169.

Chou, R., Loeser, J., Owens, D.K., Rosenquist, R.W., Atlas, S.J., Baisden, J., et al., 2009. Interventional therapies, surgery, and interdisciplinary rehabilitation for low back pain: an evidence-based clinical practice guideline from the American Pain Society. Spine 34 (10), 1066–1077.

Cooke, M., 2016. TeamSTEPPS for health care risk managers: improving teamwork and communication. J. Healthc. Risk Manag. 36 (1), 35–45.

DeChurch, L.A., Mesmer-Magnus, J.R., 2010. The cognitive underpinnings of effective teamwork: a meta-analysis. J. Appl. Psychol. 95 (1), 32–53.

Dysvik, E., Stephens, P., 2010. Conducting rehabilitation groups for people suffering from chronic pain. Int. J. Nurs. Pract. 16 (3), 233–240.

Edmondson, A.C., Lei, Z., 2014. Psychological safety: the history, renaissance, and future of an interpersonal construct. Annu. Rev. Organ. Psychol. Organ. Behav. 1 (1), 23–43.

Farh, J.L., Lee, C., Farh, C.I., 2010. Task conflict and team creativity: a question of how much and when. J. Appl. Psychol. 95 (6), 1173–1180.

Fiore, S.M., Elias, J., Salas, E., Warner, N.W., Letsky, M.P., 2010. From data, to information, to knowledge: measuring knowledge building in the context of collaborative cognition. In: Patterson, E.S., Miller, J.E. (Eds.), Macrocognition Metrics and Scenarios: Design and Evaluation for Real-World Teams. CRC Press, London, pp. 179–200.

Fox, S., Comeau-Vallée, M., 2020. The negotiation of sharing leadership in the context of professional hierarchy: interactions on interprofessional teams. Leadership 16 (5), 568–591.

Fullen, B.M., Blake, C., Horan, S., Kelley, V., Spencer, O., Power, C.K., 2014. Ulysses: the effectiveness of a multidisciplinary cognitive behavioural pain management programme-an 8-year review. Ir. J. Med. Sci. 183 (2), 265–275.

Gagnon, C.M., Scholten, P., Atchison, J., 2018. Multidimensional patient impression of change following interdisciplinary pain management. Pain. Pract. 18 (8), 997–1010.

Gardner, T., Refshauge, K., Smith, L., McAuley, J., Hubscher, M., Goodall, S., 2017. Physiotherapists' beliefs and attitudes influence clinical practice in chronic low back pain: a systematic review of quantitative and qualitative studies. J. Physiother. 63 (3), 132–143.

Gergerich, E., Boland, D., Scott, M.A., 2019. Hierarchies in interprofessional training. J. Interprof. Care. 33 (5), 528–535. https://doi.org/10.1080/13561820.2018.1538110.

Goncalo, J.A., Polman, E., Maslach, C., 2010. Can confidence come too soon? Collective efficacy, conflict and group performance over time. Organ. Behav. Hum. Decis. Process. 113 (1), 13–24.

Gordon, R.M., Corcoran, J.R., Bartley-Daniele, P., Sklenar, D., Sutton, P.R., Cartwright, F., 2014. A transdisciplinary team approach to pain management in inpatient health care settings. Pain Manag. Nurs. 15 (1), 426–435.

Gordon, D.B., Watt-Watson, J., Hogans, B.B., 2018. Interprofessional pain education-with, from, and about competent, collaborative practice teams to transform pain care. Pain Rep. 3 (3), e663.

Gorman, J. C., Grimm, D. A., & Dunbar, T. A. (2018). Defining and measuring team effectiveness in dynamic environments and implications for team ITS. In Building Intelligent Tutoring Systems for Teams (vol. 19, pp. 55-74). Emerald Publishing Limited, West Yorkshire, UK. https://doi.org/10.1108/S1534-085620180000019007.

Grand, J.A., Braun, M.T., Kuljanin, G., Kozlowski, S.W., Chao, G.T., 2016. The dynamics of team cognition: a process-oriented theory of knowledge emergence in teams. J. Appl. Psychol. 101 (10), 1353–1385.

Griffin, H., Hay-Smith, E.J.C., 2019. Characteristics of a well-functioning chronic pain team: a systematic review. N. Z. J. Physiother. 47 (1).

Grossman, R., Feitosa, J., 2018. Team trust over time: modeling reciprocal and contextual influences in action teams. Hum. Resour. Manag. Rev. 28 (4), 395–410.

Hampel, P., Kopnick, A., Roch, S., 2019. Psychological and work-related outcomes after inpatient multidisciplinary rehabilitation of chronic low back pain: a prospective randomized controlled trial. BMC. Psychol. 7 (1), 6.

Hellman, T., Jensen, I., Bergstrom, G., Bramberg, E.B., 2016. Essential features influencing collaboration in team-based non-specific back pain rehabilitation: findings from a mixed methods study. J. Interprof. Care. 30 (3), 309–315.

Howarth, M., Warne, T., Haigh, C., 2014. Pain from the inside: understanding the theoretical underpinning of person-centered care delivered by pain teams. Pain Manag. Nurs. 15 (1), 340–348.

Joypaul, S., Kelly, F.S., King, M.A., 2019. Turning pain into gain: evaluation of a multidisciplinary chronic pain management program in primary care. Pain. Med. 20 (5), 925–933.

Kane, A.T., Perry, D.J., 2016. What we're trying to solve: the back and forth of engaged interdisciplinary inquiry. Nurs. Inq. 23 (4), 327–337.

Katz, J., Weinrib, A.Z., Clarke, H., 2019. Chronic postsurgical pain: from risk factor identification to multidisciplinary management at the Toronto General Hospital Transitional Pain Service. Can. J. Pain. 3 (2), 49–58.

Kim, S., Bochatay, N., Relyea-Chew, A., Buttrick, E., Amdahl, C., Kim, L., et al., 2017. Individual, interpersonal, and organisational factors of healthcare conflict: a scoping review. J. Interprof. Care. 31 (3), 282–290.

Körner, M., 2010. Interprofessional teamwork in medical rehabilitation: a comparison of multidisciplinary and interdisciplinary team approach. Clin. Rehabil. 24 (8), 745–755.

Körner, M., Wirtz, M.A., Bengel, J., Goritz, A.S., 2015. Relationship of organizational culture, teamwork and job satisfaction in interprofessional teams. BMC. Health. Serv. Res. 15, 243.

Lacerenza, C.N., Reyes, D.L., Marlow, S.L., Joseph, D.L., Salas, E., 2017. Leadership training design, delivery, and implementation: a meta-analysis. J. Appl. Psychol. 102 (12), 1686–1718.

Lennox Thompson, B., 2021. Whole-person clinical reasoning. In: Erb, M., Schmid, A.A. (Eds.), Integrative Rehabilitation Practice. Singing Dragon, London, pp. 92–106.

Lin, I., Wiles, L., Waller, R., Goucke, R., Nagree, Y., Gibberd, M., et al., 2020. What does best practice care for musculoskeletal pain look like? Eleven consistent recommendations from high-quality clinical practice guidelines: systematic review. Br. J. Sports Med. 54 (2), 79–86.

Loeser, J.D., 2005. Quo vadis, poena. J. Muscoskel. Pain. 13 (3), 3–9.

Martire, L.M., Zhaoyang, R., Marini, C.M., Nah, S., Darnall, B.D., 2019. Daily and bidirectional linkages between pain catastrophizing and spouse responses. Pain. 160 (12), 2841–2847.

Mathias, B., Parry-Jones, B., Huws, J.C., 2014. Individual experiences of an acceptance-based pain management programme: an interpretative phenomenological analysis. Psychol. Health. 29 (3), 279–296.

McHugh, S.K., Lawton, R., O'Hara, J.K., Sheard, L., 2020. Does team reflexivity impact teamwork and communication in interprofessional hospital-based healthcare teams? A systematic review and narrative synthesis. BMJ. Qual. Saf. 29 (8), 672–683.

Nicholas, M.K., George, S.Z., 2011. Psychologically informed interventions for low back pain: an update for physical therapists. Phys. Ther. 91 (5), 765–776.

Nordin, C., Gard, G., Fjellman-Wiklund, A., 2013. Being in an exchange process: experiences of patient participation in multimodal pain rehabilitation. J. Rehabil. Med. 45 (6), 580–586.

O'Neill, T.A., Allen, N.J., Hastings, S.E., 2013. Examining the "pros" and "cons" of TeamConflict: a team-level meta-analysis

of task, relationship, and process conflict. Hum. Perform. 26 (3), 236–260.

Oslund, S., Robinson, R.C., Clark, T.C., Garofalo, J.P., Behnk, P., Walker, B., et al., 2009. Long-term effectiveness of a comprehensive pain management program: strengthening the case for interdisciplinary care. Proc. Bayl. Univ. Med. Cent. 22 (3), 211–214.

Phillips, R.L., Short, A., Kenning, A., Dugdale, P., Nugus, P., McGowan, R., et al., 2014. Achieving patient-centred care: the potential and challenge of the patient-as-professional role. Health. Expect. 18, 2616–2628.

Pype, P., Mertens, F., Helewaut, F., Krystallidou, D., 2018. Healthcare teams as complex adaptive systems: understanding team behaviour through team members' perception of interpersonal interaction. BMC. Health. Serv. Res. 18 (1), 570.

Ruan, X., Kaye, A.D., 2016. A call for saving interdisciplinary pain management. J. Orthop. Sports. Phys. Ther. 46 (12), 1021–1023.

Rydenfalt, C., Odenrick, P., Larsson, P.A., 2017. Organizing for teamwork in healthcare: an alternative to team training? J. Health. Organ. Manag. 31 (3), 347–362.

Salas, E., Dickinson, T.L., Converse, S.A., Tannenbaum, S.I., 1992. Toward an understanding of team performance and training. In: Teams: Their Training and Performance. Ablex Publishing, New York, Norwood, pp. 3–29.

Salas, E., Shuffler, M.L., Thayer, A.L., Bedwell, W.L., Lazzara, E.H., 2015. Understanding and improving teamwork in organizations: a scientifically based practical guide. Hum. Resour. Manag. 54 (4), 599–622.

Santana, M.J., Manalili, K., Jolley, R.J., Zelinsky, S., Quan, H., Lu, M., 2018. How to practice person-centred care: a conceptual framework. Health. Expect. 21 (2), 429–440.

Schmutz, J.B., Eppich, W.J., 2017. Promoting learning and patient care through shared reflection: a conceptual framework for team reflexivity in health care. Acad. Med. 92 (11), 1555–1563.

Schot, E., Tummers, L., Noordegraaf, M., 2020. Working on working together. A systematic review on how healthcare professionals contribute to interprofessional collaboration. J. Interprof. Care. 34 (3), 332–342.

Schultz, R., Brostrom Kousgaard, M., Davidsen, A.S., 2021. We have two different agendas": the views of general practitioners, social workers and hospital staff on interprofessional coordination for patients with chronic widespread pain. J. Interprof. Care. 35 (2), 284–292.

Silva, J. A. M., Fernandes Agreli, H., Harrison, R., Peduzzi, M., Mininel, V. A., & Xyrichis, A. (2021). Collective leadership to improve professional practice, healthcare outcomes, and staff well-being. Cochrane Database of Systematic Reviews. https://doi.org/10.1002/14651858.Cd013850.

Sluka, K., Turner, J., Collett, B., Miaskowski, C., Eccleston, C., Justins, D., et al., 2009. Pain Treatment Services. International Association for the Study of Pain. Available from: https://www.iasp-pain.org/resources/guidelines/pain-treatment-services/.

Smith, C.R., Baharloo, R., Nickerson, P., Wallace, M., Zou, B., Fillingim, R.B., et al., 2021. Predicting long-term postsurgical pain by examining the evolution of acute pain. Eur. J. Pain. 25 (3), 624–636.

Smith, S., Clouder, D.L., 2010. Interprofessional and interdisciplinary learning: an exploration of similarities and differences. In: Bromage, A., Clouder, L., Thistlethwaite,

J., Gordon, F. (Eds.), Interprofessional E-Learning and Collaborative Work: Practices and Technologies. IGI Global, Pennsylvania, pp. 1–13.

Smith, T., Fowler-Davis, S., Nancarrow, S., Ariss, S.M.B., Enderby, P., 2018. Leadership in interprofessional health and social care teams: a literature review. Leader. Health. Serv. 31 (4), 452–467. https://doi.org/10.1108/LHS-06-2016-0026.

Stenberg, G., Stalnacke, B.M., Enthoven, P., 2017. Implementing multimodal pain rehabilitation in primary care - a health care professional perspective. Disabil. Rehabil. 39 (21), 2173–2181.

Stewart, M.A., 2018. Stuck in the middle: the impact of collaborative interprofessional communication on patient expectations. Shoulder Elbow. 10 (1), 66–72.

Synnott, A., O'Keeffe, M., Bunzli, S., Dankaerts, W., O'Sullivan, P., O'Sullivan, K., 2015. Physiotherapists may stigmatise or feel unprepared to treat people with low back pain and psychosocial factors that influence recovery: a systematic review. J. Physiother. 61 (2), 68–76.

Thorgren, S., Caiman, E., 2019. The role of psychological safety in implementing agile methods across cultures. Res. Technol. Manag. 62 (2), 31–39.

Tingle, J., 2017. Improving patient safety and healthcare quality: examples of good practice. Br. J. Nurs. 26 (14), 828–829.

Turk, D.C., Flor, H., 1984. Etiological theories and treatments for chronic back pain. II. Psychological models and interventions. Pain. 19 (3), 209–233.

Vaida, S., Ardelean, I., 2019. Psychological safety and trust. A conceptual analysis. Studia. UBB. Psychol.Paed. 64 (1), 87–101.

Vertue, F.M., Haig, B.D., 2008. An abductive perspective on clinical reasoning and case formulation. J. Clin. Psychol. 64 (9), 1046–1068.

Wilkinson, P., Whiteman, R., 2017. Pain management programmes. BJA. Educ. 17 (1), 10–15.

Williams, A.C.C., Fisher, E., Hearn, L., Eccleston, C., 2020. Psychological therapies for the management of chronic pain (excluding headache) in adults. Cochrane Database Syst. Rev. 8, CD007407. https://doi.org/10.1002/14651858.CD007407.pub4.

Williams, A.C., Potts, H.W., 2010. Group membership and staff turnover affect outcomes in group CBT for persistent pain. Pain. 148 (3), 481–486.

Zajac, S., Woods, A., Tannenbaum, S., Salas, E., Holladay, C.L., 2021. Overcoming challenges to teamwork in healthcare: a team effectiveness framework and evidence-based guidance. Front. Commun. 6 (6). https://doi.org/10.3389/fcomm.2021.606445.

Zijl, A.L.V., Vermeeren, B., Koster, F., Steijn, B., 2021. Interprofessional teamwork in primary care: the effect of functional heterogeneity on performance and the role of leadership. J. Interprof. Care. 35 (1), 10–20.

Chapter | 19 |

Pain in childhood

Cate Sinclair and Adrienne Ruth Harvey

LEARNING OBJECTIVES

At the end of this chapter, readers will understand the:
1. Prevalence of pain in children and adolescents.
2. Guiding models for understanding children's pain.
3. Developmental and social processes related to pain in childhood and adolescence.
4. Assessment of pain in children and adolescents.
5. Management of pain in family, school and community contexts.

Overview

Pain is a frequent occurrence in childhood. It is experienced from infancy and due to a plethora of mechanisms, including medically required heel pricks and vaccinations, disease, injuries, social exclusion from peers and the loss of loved ones. Pain can be intense and overwhelming for children due to anatomical and functional aspects of the developing nervous system. And yet, unfortunately, pain in this age group is often not well managed.

Children initially express pain nonverbally and develop the capacity to identify and communicate pain verbally as they age. Overt expressions of pain are influenced by family and cultural norms, and it is dependent on parents and other carers to observe and decode the pain experienced. For younger children, and children who do not have the capacity to verbalise or communicate effectively, the absence of overt pain expression can result in an underestimation of pain intensity (Rajasagaram et al. 2009). The multiple factors influencing pain perception and expression can contribute to inadequate pain management which can increase suffering, potentiate long-term sensitivity of bodily tissue and lead to chronic pain and disability. Childhood pain needs to be managed more effectively, with the need to make pain matter, make pain understood, make pain visible and make pain better (Eccleston et al. 2021). In this chapter, we will articulate two guiding models for understanding children's pain and its management, provide tools to assist health professionals working in this area and highlight some useful management strategies.

Prevalence of pain in childhood and adolescence

Although pain is common in childhood, epidemiological studies are sparse and have focused on persistent pain (Table 19.1). Acute pain is most often caused by childhood disease, medical procedures and injury, with unintentional falls, burns, cuts and collisions at home, school and road traffic accidents contributing one third of admissions to emergency departments globally (Mickalide & Carr 2012). Medically, pain from multiple needles is reported to be the most aversive pain experience related to hospitalisation (Friedrichsdorf et al. 2015). Acute and persistent pain is also

TABLE 19.1 Prevalence of chronic pain in children and adolescents

Reference	Pain type	Frequency (%)
The epidemiology of chronic pain in children and adolescents revisited: a systematic review (King et al. 2011)	Back pain	18.0–24.0
	Headache	26.0–69.0
	Recurrent abdominal pain	3.8–41.2
	Musculoskeletal/limb pain	38.9
	Multiple pains	16.0
	Other/general body pain	60.0
Health Behaviour of School Children: WHO Collaborative Cross-Cultural Survey (HBSC) (Swain et al. 2014)	Headache	54.1
	Stomach pain	49.8
	Back pain	37

experienced by children with diseases such as juvenile idiopathic arthritis (Lalloo & Stinson 2014), cancer (Duran et al. 2020) and sickle cell disease (Brandow & DeBaun 2018).

The prevalence of persistent pain increases with age, with girls having a higher prevalence of pain than boys (King et al. 2011; Swain et al. 2014). Between 70% and 93% of adolescent girls are also affected by dysmenorrhea (Sachedina & Todd 2020). Increased levels of pain for adolescent girls may be related to different sex hormones and immune responses (Kozlowska et al. 2020). Pain in childhood is predictive of pain in adulthood. Prognostic factors which predict the presence of ongoing pain are older age, weekly day tiredness, weekly abdominal pain and waking during the night (Pate et al. 2020).

Pain is common yet often under-recognised in children with intellectual and developmental disabilities; there has been a lack of scientific attention given to pain in these individuals (Barney et al. 2020). Pain is the most prevalent comorbidity in children with cerebral palsy, the most common physical disability of childhood. Prevalence rates of pain vary from 14% to 76% of children and young people with cerebral palsy, due to the heterogeneity in this group (McKinnon et al. 2019). Pain is more prevalent with increasing age, severity of motor impairment, in females and in those with dyskinesia (McKinnon et al. 2019; Ostojic et al. 2019a). Persistent pain is experienced at a significantly higher rate for adolescents with physical disabilities in comparison with their able-bodied peers (de la Vega et al. 2018), and children with autism spectrum disorder have been found to have altered pain processing (Hauer & Houtrow 2017).

Guiding models for managing pain in children and adolescents

Two related models support the understanding, assessment and management of pain in childhood

The World Health Organization's (WHO) International Classification of Functioning, Disability and Health (ICF) (WHO 2001) provides a framework for describing health outcomes. It considers the potential influences on an individual's functioning and disability including body functions (physiology) and structures (anatomy), activity (ability to execute tasks and actions), participation (involvement in life situations), as well as contextual factors related to the environment (e.g. home, school and community settings) and personal factors (e.g. age, gender, preferences) (Fig. 19.1).

Biopsychosocial model of pain

The biopsychosocial model of pain (Gatchel et al. 2007) is important to consider when working with children, as children's development and growth is nested within parental, family, educational and community social systems. Biological processes influencing children's pain include genetics and bodily systems undergoing development and growth including the musculoskeletal systems, peripheral and central nervous systems, endocrine and inflammatory systems. Other biological processes include disease and disease-related processes, injury and medical treatments. Stress and trauma at key developmental stages influence the modulation of pain through neuroimmune,

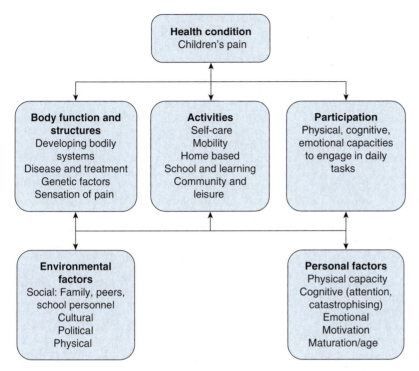

Health condition
Children's pain

Body function and structures
Developing bodily systems
Disease and treatment
Genetic factors
Sensation of pain

Activities
Self-care
Mobility
Home based
School and learning
Community and leisure

Participation
Physical, cognitive, emotional capacities to engage in daily tasks

Environmental factors
Social: Family, peers, school personnel
Cultural
Political
Physical

Personal factors
Physical capacity
Cognitive (attention, catastrophising)
Emotional
Motivation
Maturation/age

Fig. 19.1 Aspects of children's pain in accordance with the International Classification of Functioning, Disability, and Health.

neuroendocrine and nervous system changes (Fitzgerald & McKelvey 2016; Zouikr & Karshikoff 2017). Social systems found to influence pain include parent pain history and coping (Pavlova et al. 2020), family functioning (Birnie et al. 2017a, b), school, teacher and peer relationships (Jones et al. 2018), and generational and current histories of trauma (Nelson et al. 2017). From a psychological perspective, stress, mood, cognitions such as catastrophising, adaptive coping, self-efficacy and memories influence pain perception (Noel et al. 2015). An understanding of the interconnection between these factors and the contribution to pain perception and expression promotes health professionals' capacity to understand and manage pain.

Developmental perspective: body structure and function

As a child grows, the sensory, affective, motivational and cognitive components of their nervous systems, which modulate pain, develop according to genetic make-up and environmental conditions. Current understanding of pain and brain function is that pain arises from changes across regions of the brain, which are not specific to pain, creating a dynamic pain connectome (Verriotis et al. 2016). Pain is exacerbated or reduced as different brain regions

are recruited. Unlike primary sensory systems, which are dependent on activity and sensory input at key stages for effective development, the pain experienced by neonates reflects aspects of the pain connectome which are present from early life. Please refer to Verriotis et al. (2016) for a comprehensive review of the development of the anatomical and functional components of the pain connectome.

Pain in neonates, infants and young children can be of higher intensity and longer lasting due to developmental aspects of peripheral and central nervous systems. For neonates, neurotrophic factors enhance local sensory nerve sprouting when skin is wounded (Beggs et al. 2012), creating local and sustained pain sensitisation. Painful procedures, such as heel pricks or lances, have been found to elicit long-lasting reflex activity (Cornelissen et al. 2013), while repeated innocuous input reduces neural thresholds and causes a greater mechanical response for infants. At the dorsal horn of an infant's spinal cord, sensory input is facilitated, strengthening activity-dependent synapses but reducing sensory discrimination and localisation (Cornelissen 2013). Longitudinal studies show that children have lower pain thresholds than adolescents, with decreasing pain sensitivity with age for cold, pressure and mechanical pain (Hirschfeld et al. 2012).

Stressful early life experiences in a child's life impact the developing endocrine, immune and nervous systems, and in turn the developing pain system (Zouikr & Karshikoff 2017). In the early stages of life, the immune system is antiinflammatory, supressing excitation at the dorsal horn and preventing neuropathic pain (Fitzgerald & McKelvey 2016). Nerve damage resulting in neuropathic pain is rare in infants and uncommon in children under 6 years of age. The immune system becomes proinflammatory as children develop and latent responses to previous nerve injuries can emerge. This developmental process may explain why the median age of diagnosis for complex regional pain syndrome, phantom limb pain and neuropathic pain in adolescence is 13 years (Fitzgerald & McKelvey 2016), and why the prevalence of persistent pain increases with age (Perquin et al. 2000).

Inhibitory control and modulation of pain increases throughout childhood; therefore younger children are dependent on parents and carers to calm and inhibit pain through social and physical interactions. In earlier childhood, the developing sensory nervous system is facilitatory to optimise development within social and physical environments and descending inhibitory control of spinal reflexes develops during preadolescence (Hathway et al. 2012). Impaired development of inhibitory processes, through early exposure to stress (Ebner & Singewald 2017), potentially renders some children more vulnerable to developing persistent pain. Young adolescents with musculoskeletal pain related to acute injury are more likely to develop persistent pain if they have lower pain modulation through inhibition and are female (Holley et al. 2017); those who are depressed are more likely to have higher pain-related disability and lower quality of life. More vulnerable children and adolescents who have exposure to stress are likely to require targeted support to inhibit pain.

Personal and environmental factors and participation

Personal and environmental factors impact upon a child's pain intensity and the ability to function with pain. Stress, mood and cognitions directly impact acute pain. For example, children and adolescents with higher pain catastrophising experience higher pain intensity after surgery (Birnie et al. 2017a, b). From a social perspective, children and adolescents with persistent pain frequently have parents who also suffer persistent pain. It has been suggested that alterations may occur in parent and child brain circuits, which create a dyadic or contagious effect for pain (Simons et al. 2016). The experience of adverse childhood events increases the risk of developing persistent pain (Burke et al. 2017).

The capacity for children and adolescents with persistent pain to function in daily life is complex and impacted by multiple factors. Higher levels of disability are associated with child or adolescent depression, catastrophising, pain and anxiety, and parent protectiveness

and catastrophising (Sinclair et al. 2016). Persistent pain reduces children and adolescent's school attendance and cognitive performance (Dick & Riddell 2010), and school attendance and overall performance can also be predicted by parental catastrophising and protectiveness (Logan et al. 2012). Extreme sensory processing patterns, such as sensory sensitivity, and insecure attachment are also associated with reduced function and quality of life (Sinclair et al. 2020). Insecure attachment is indicative of stress within family relationships and poorer family functioning, which is more closely related to pain-related disability than pain intensity (Lewandowski et al. 2010). In a clinical setting, physical limitations related to pain are also observed to impact function in self-care, learning and leisure activities, and need to be addressed in treatment.

Assessment of pain in children and adolescents

'Pain should be made visible by doing developmentally appropriate valid pain assessment in every child' (Eccleston et al. 2021, p. 17). Infants, children and adolescents conceptualise and communicate pain differently, and their age indicates the developmentally appropriate measure to be used, except for children who have cognitive and communication deficits (Michaleff et al. 2017). Accurate assessment helps clinicians and adult carers to understand the child's pain experience, treat appropriately and monitor change. Pain is assessed by measuring physiological responses, observing behaviours, and child or adolescent self-report. It is important to recognise that physiological indictors, such as heart rate and blood pressure, are also associated with distress and anxiety and should not be used in isolation. Parents can be interviewed about the observed pain experience and context, and the child's normal pain expression. However, parent report is subject to bias related to their own pain memories and gender bias (Earp et al. 2019; Noel et al. 2015) and should not be the sole source of information. See Michaleff et al. (2017) for a full description of measurement tools.

Although children as young as 4 years are able to identify pain cause, location, meaning and quality (Pope et al. 2017), for children younger than 6 years, behavioural observation scales are recommended and should be coded by trained adults. For children with acute pain aged 6 years or more, the numerical rating scale with an 11-point scale from 0 (no pain) to 10 (worst hurt you could ever imagine) is strongly recommended for pain assessment (Birnie et al. 2019). Likewise, pain scales using faces, such as the Wong-Baker FACES Pain Rating Scale, are strongly recommended for children 7 years and

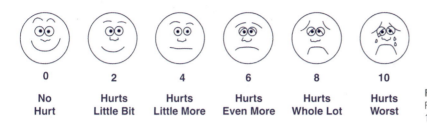

0	2	4	6	8	10
No Hurt	**Hurts Little Bit**	**Hurts Little More**	**Hurts Even More**	**Hurts Whole Lot**	**Hurts Worst**

Fig. 19.2 Wong-Baker FACES Pain Rating Scale. (From Wong & Baker 1988)

over (Wong & Baker 1988) (Fig. 19.2). The Colour Analogue Scale is another scale recommended for children 8 years and over.

Several multidimensional pain scales have been developed to assess the complexity of the persistent pain experience. These scales measure pain location, frequency, intensity, and duration and fluctuation over time, the impact of pain on daily life (such as school absenteeism, sport participation, interferences with activities of daily living), mood, pain catastrophising and quality of life, along with the use of medication and healthcare. Encouragingly, some of the scales also include parent factors, which measure the impact of parenting a child with persistent pain. For example, the Bath Pain Questionnaire measures parent stress, mood, catastrophising, parenting behaviour, marital adjustment and general functioning (Eccleston et al. 2007). In Australia, the Paediatric electronic Persistent Pain Outcome Collaboration (Paed ePPOC; see https://www.uow.edu.au/ahsri/eppoc/) has been effectively integrated into children's pain clinics to provide point-of-care information to clinicians and families to plan and measure treatment outcomes (Lord et al. 2019). Electronic methods using communication through smart phones and internet technology are also being developed to capture time stamped, accurate pain measurement for young people, such as the Pain-QuILT which is freely available (see https://painquilt.wordpress.com/.) (Lalloo & Stinson 2014).

Pain assessment in children with developmental disabilities is challenging due to varying intellectual capacity, communication types and functional ability (Kingsnorth et al. 2015). Self-report is often not possible and use of parent-report and observational assessment is often required. One important advance has been the creation of the 'Chronic pain assessment toolbox for children with disabilities' to guide clinicians and researchers (Kingsnorth et al. 2015; Orava et al. 2019). The toolbox includes 15 self-report or observational tools, able to measure pain interference and pain coping tools. However, not all tools are suitable across the spectrum of disability, and many have not yet been validated in the disability population. The case study of Alice (Case study 19.1) illustrates how

the assessment process can be tailored to meet the needs of the individual child and their family.

Managing pain in family, school and community contexts

The biopsychosocial complexity of acute and persistent pain in children has led to the development of guidelines to inform practice (Barney et al. 2020; Friedrichsdorf et al. 2018; Liossi et al. 2019). For children with acute pain, multimodal pharmacological interventions are used most, with evidence supporting adjunctive application of psychological management strategies: distraction, hypnosis, breathing exercises and combined cognitive behavioural therapies (CBT) (Birnie et al. 2018). Physical interventions such as cold and vibratory sensory input have also been found to reduce nociception (Bergomi et al. 2018), along with distraction through virtual reality (Gates et al. 2020). For infants and younger children, non-nutritive sucking and breastfeeding, swaddling and positioning to provide skin-to-skin contact reduce pain and distress (Pillai Riddell et al. 2015). Children's pain is reduced when parents and health professionals work together to create low-stress environments, incorporating low noise and lightning (Pancekauskaite & Jankauskaite 2018), and online parent education campaigns, such as 'It doesn't have to hurt', have improved access to information for parents (please see the link in the 'Resources for Health Professionals and Families') (Chambers et al. 2020).

Management of persistent pain has a different focus to the strategies recommended for conditions associated with acute pain, such as rest and distraction. Persistent pain requires active management and a shared understanding of emotional, behavioural and physical processes. Health professional provision of parent and family education begins this process which needs to be tailored for the age of the child or adolescent in pain (Robins et al. 2016). Psychological treatments are the most studied for children's persistent pain, with strong evidence to support cognitive behavioural therapies, including acceptance and commitment therapy (ACT), for persistent and episodic pain (Fisher et al. 2018). The aim of these treatment modalities is to reduce distress and to support children and adolescents to participate in age appropriate developmental activities, such as self-care, school and community tasks, and to prevent long-term disability.

For children and adolescents with complex persistent pain, evidence supports the provision of interdisciplinary team care (Liossi et al. 2019). Treating teams include pain specialists, psychologists, occupational therapists, physiotherapists and specialist nursing staff. Along with CBT or ACT provided by psychologists, occupational therapists and physiotherapists provide goal-directed therapy incorporating sensory-desensitising and graded functional return (Logan et al. 2012). The physiotherapy role includes physical conditioning and graded weight bearing. Occupational therapy focus incorporates daily activities in the provision of treatment, and optimisation of the child or adolescent's capacity to function in self-care, school, social and leisure activities. The case study of Naomi (Case study 19.2) illustrates the different roles of the team members. Systematic review and subset meta-analysis of these programs show minimal difference between inpatient and outpatient provision of care (Eccleston et al. 2021). However, studies often exclude children with complex comorbidities, and children from low-income communities who may not be able to access these programs. Pain management needs to address the specific needs of children in these populations. Online evidence-based therapies such as those provided by smart phones offer an alternative to direct care for children with persistent pain and pain associated with disease such as sickle cell disease (Fisher et al. 2019; Palermo et al. 2018) and have been found to have similar outcomes (Shaygan et al. 2021). These emerging therapies have the potential to reach a broader group of children and adolescents with pain.

Home and school environments create opportunities for the application of pain management strategies for children with persistent pain, and parents, teachers and peers can be integral to the treatment process. Parent factors directly impact persistent pain and disability for children and adolescents with persistent pain and are an essential component of pain treatment programs. Acceptance and commitment therapy provided to both children and their parents has resulted in improvements in pain interference on function, depression, reactivity and psychological flexibility for children, and higher levels of change in reactivity and psychological flexibility of parents (Kanstrup et al. 2016). School impairment can be extensive for children with persistent pain, whereby pain interrupts physical capacities, cognitive attention and working memory, peer relationships, and participation in academic, sporting and recreational activities. A recent review of school functioning of children with pain has recommended that health professionals work with teachers and peers to facilitate education programming through sufficient support and fairness to optimise school function (Jones et al. 2018).

Pain in children with developmental disabilities tends to be undertreated due to pain being under-recognised in this population. In addition, high-quality evidence for the effective management of pain in this group is limited. Medical management predominates, primarily analgesic use, as well as techniques such as heat, hydrotherapy, rest, massage, distraction and stretching (Ostojic et al. 2019a, b). There is limited evidence for nonpharmacological/nonsurgical options utilising a multidisciplinary approach for pain management in children with cerebral palsy (Ostojic et al. 2019b). A critical need exists for adopting evidence-based management principles based on the biopsychosocial model that is employed in the typically developing population and modifying where required for children with developmental disabilities.

Resources for health professionals and families

The Paediatric Listserv (https://pediatric-pain.ca/resources/pediatric-pain-mailing-list/) and the Paediatric Pain Letter (http://ppl.childpain.org/) offer resources and advice for health professionals about paediatric pain management. The International Symposium on Paediatric Pain is a biannual event organised by the Special Interest Group on Pain in Children of the International Association for the Study of Pain (http://childpain.org).

The following websites have been developed by hospitals and research groups for health professionals and families to access information on pain research and management:

It Doesn't have to Hurt https://itdoesnthavetohurt.ca
Support Kids in Pain SKiP website http://www.skip.org.au/
Holland Bloorview Kids Rehabilitation Hospital https://hollandbloorview.ca
Boston Children's Hospital Pain Treatment Centre https://www.childrenshospital.org/centers-and-services/programs/o-_-z/pain-treatment-center
Hospital for Sick Kids, Toronto, Canada https://www.sickkids.ca/en/care-services/centres/pain-centre/; https://www.sickkids.ca/en/learning/continuing-professional-development/pain-assessment-infants/
Pain Learning Hub https://www.aboutkidshealth.ca/pain
ACI NSW Pain Management Network, Pain Bytes Program for Youth http://www.aci.health.nsw.gov.au/chronic-pain/painbytes
Pain Education: Understanding Pain and What's to be done about it in 10 minutes https://www.youtube.com/watch?v=lVdulzi6oYw

Recently, Kozlowska and colleagues have published Functional Somatic Symptoms in Children and Adolescents: A Stress System Approach to Assessment and Treatment (Kozlowska et al. 2020) via open access which summarises a multisystem understanding of persistent pain and provides detailed information on assessment and treatment.

CASE STUDY 19.1

Alice, a 13-year-old with upper-limb cerebral palsy

Alice is a 13-year-old girl with dyskinetic CP who uses a wheelchair for mobility. Alice communicates effectively with those who know her through augmentative and alternative communication (AAC). However, effective communication can be impaired and take significantly longer with those unfamiliar with her. She has ongoing pain affecting her daily activities which impacts her quality of life. Alice's pain is managed primarily through medications including Baclofen, Gabapentin and Diazepam; however, this is not always effective. Alice and her parents would like to explore different options for her pain management including psychological support, massage, physical activity and relaxation as the medications leave her feeling drowsy and weak. To assess Alice's pain comprehensively and to monitor the effects of any future intervention, a combination of self-report and parent-report tools is necessary as is consideration of modifying existing pain tools to ensure that she can self-report using her AAC without it being overly burdensome for her.

CASE STUDY 19.2

Naomi, a 15-year-old with complex regional pain syndrome of the right upper limb

Naomi is a 15-year-old with complex regional pain syndrome of the right upper limb. She had fallen in her ballet class and had received a soft tissue injury to the right wrist. The pain in her wrist developed quickly following the fall and is radiating to her forearm. Her hand and arm can change colour, described to sometimes appear blotchy and red and at other times blue, and is cool to touch. Naomi describes that the pain feels like burning and electric shocks, and she has been holding her arm in a flexed position since the fall. She has been unable to shower because the pain is heightened with the touch and temperature of water. Naomi is right handed and has been unable to write at school. She has previously felt anxious socially in the school environment and has not attended since the fall 6 weeks ago. Naomi lives with her mother and younger sister and has regular contact with her father although the relationship between her parents is acrimonious.

Initially, Naomi's parents were both invited to attend a pain education session to assist them to develop a consistent management plan in the home. The psychologist then met with Naomi. She was taught mindfulness strategies and began to explore times when she felt her pain increase, recognising that this coincided with higher anxiety. Naomi began mobilisation and physical reconditioning exercises with the physiotherapist. The occupational therapist commenced sensory desensitising. Initially, Naomi was introduced to warm sensations which provided gentle pressure, such as draping warmed theraputty over the skin of her forearm which she tolerated with the assistance of mindfulness strategies. These sensations have a calming effect and reduce pain. Naomi progressed to tolerating light sensation which has an alerting effect, such as cotton wool, and was able to wear light clothing over her forearm. The occupational therapist liaised with the school and provided pain education to the teachers and Naomi's peers. Naomi then engaged in a graded return to school program and increased her capacity to handwrite and engage in sport while practicing pain management strategies such as mindfulness in the school environment.

Conclusion

The experience of pain in children is influenced by multiple factors, and health clinicians can be guided by the ICF and Biopsychosocial Model of Pain when assessing and managing both acute and persistent pain. In this chapter, evidence-based assessment and management have been provided. Along with internet-based assessment tools and treatment modalities, these strategies make pain management more effective and accessible for children and their families.

References

Barney, C.C., Andersen, R.D., Defrin, R., Genik, L.M., McGuire, B.E., et al., 2020. Challenges in pain assessment and management among individuals with intellectual and developmental disabilities. Pain Rep. 5 (4), e821.

Beggs, S., Alvares, D., Moss, A., Currie, G., Middleton, J., Salter, M.W., et al., 2012. A role for NT-3 in the hyperinnervation of neonatally wounded skin. Pain 153 (10), 2133–2139.

Bergomi, P., Scudeller, L., Pintaldi, S., Dal Molin, A., 2018. Efficacy of non-pharmacological methods of pain management in children undergoing venipuncture in a pediatric outpatient clinic: a randomized controlled trial of audiovisual distraction and external cold and vibration. J. Pediatr. Nurs. 42, e66–e72.

Birnie, K.A., Chambers, C.T., Chorney, J., Fernandez, C.V., McGrath, P.J., 2017a. A Multi-Informant multi-method investigation of family functioning and parent-child coping during children's acute pain. J. Pediatr. Psychol. 42 (1), 28–39.

Birnie, K.A., Chorney, J., El-Hawary, R., 2017b. Child and parent pain catastrophizing and pain from presurgery to 6 weeks postsurgery: examination of cross-sectional and longitudinal actor-partner effects. Pain 158 (10), 1886–1892.

Birnie, K.A., Noel, M., Chambers, C.T., Uman, L.S., Parker, J.A., 2018. Psychological interventions for needle-related procedural pain and distress in children and adolescents. Cochrane Database Syst. Rev. 10 (10):Cd005179.

Birnie, K.A., Hundert, A.S., Lalloo, C., Nguyen, C., Stinson, J.N., 2019. Recommendations for selection of self-report pain intensity measures in children and adolescents: a systematic review and quality assessment of measurement properties. Pain 160 (1), 5–18.

Brandow, A.M., DeBaun, M.R., 2018. Key components of pain management for children and adults with sickle cell disease. Hematol. Oncol. Clin. N. Am. 32 (3), 535–550.

Burke, N.N., Finn, D.P., McGuire, B.E., Roche, M., 2017. Psychological stress in early life as a predisposing factor for the development of chronic pain: clinical and preclinical evidence and neurobiological mechanisms. J. Neurosci. Res. 95 (6), 1257–1270.

Chambers, C.T., Dol, J., Parker, J.A., Caes, L., Birnie, K.A., Taddio, A., et al., 2020. Implementation effectiveness of a parent-directed YouTube video ("it doesn't have to hurt") on evidence-based strategies to manage needle pain: descriptive survey study. JMIR. Pediatr. Parent. 3 (1), e13552.

Cornelissen, L., Fabrizi, L., Patten, D., Worley, A., Meek, J., Boyd, S., et al., 2013. Postnatal temporal, spatial and modality tuning of nociceptive cutaneous flexion reflexes in human infants. PLoS One 8 (10), e76470.

de la Vega, R., Groenewald, C., Bromberg, M.H., Beals-Erickson, S.E., Palermo, T.M., 2018. Chronic pain prevalence and associated factors in adolescents with and without physical disabilities. Dev. Med. Child Neurol. 60 (6), 596–601. https://doi.org/10.1111/dmcn.13705.

Dick, B.R.R., Riddell, R.P., 2010. Cognitive and school functioning in children and adolescents with chronic pain: a critical review. Pain Res. Manag. 15 (4), 238–244.

Duran, J., Bravo, L., Torres, V., Craig, A., Heidari, J., Adlard, K., et al., 2020. Quality of life and pain experienced by children and adolescents with cancer at home following discharge from the hospital. J. Pediatr. Hematol. Oncol. 42 (1), 46–52.

Earp, B.D., Monrad, J.T., LaFrance, M., Bargh, J.A., Cohen, L.L., Richeson, J.A., 2019. Featured article: gender bias in pediatric pain assessment. J. Pediatr. Psychol. 44 (4), 403–414.

Ebner, K., Singewald, N., 2017. Individual differences in stress susceptibility and stress inhibitory mechanisms. Curr. Opin. Behav. Sci. 14, 54–64. https://doi.org/10.1016/j.cobeha.2016.11.016.

Eccleston, C., McCracken, L.M., Jordan, A., Sleed, M., 2007. Development and preliminary psychometric evaluation of the parent report version of the Bath Adolescent Pain Questionnaire (BAPQ-P): a multidimensional parent report instrument to assess the impact of chronic pain on adolescents. Pain 131 (1–2), 48–56.

Eccleston, C., Fisher, E., Howard, R., Slater, R., Forgeron, P., Palermo, T.M., et al., 2021. Delivering transformative action in paediatric pain: a Lancet Child & Adolescent Health Commission. Lancet. Child. Adolesc. Health. 5 (1), 47–87.

Fisher, E., Law, E., Dudeney, J., Palermo, T.M., Stewart, G., Eccleston, C., 2018. Psychological therapies for the management of chronic and recurrent pain in children and adolescents. Cochrane Database Syst. Rev. 9, CD003968. https://doi.org/10.1002/14651858.CD003968.pub5.

Fisher, E., Law, E., Dudeney, J., Eccleston, C., Palermo, T.M., 2019. Psychological therapies (remotely delivered) for the management of chronic and recurrent pain in children and adolescents. Cochrane Database Syst. Rev. 4 (4), Cd011118. https://doi.org/10.1002/14651858.CD011118.pub3.

Fitzgerald, M., McKelvey, R., 2016. Nerve injury and neuropathic pain - a question of age. Exp. Neurol. 275 (Pt 2), 296–302.

Friedrichsdorf, S.J., Postier, A., Eull, D., Weidner, C., Foster, L., Gilbert, M., et al., 2015. Pain outcomes in a US children's hospital: a prospective cross-sectional survey. Hosp. Pediatr. 5 (1), 18–26.

Friedrichsdorf, S.J., Eull, D., Weidner, C., Postier, A., 2018. A hospital-wide initiative to eliminate or reduce needle pain in children using lean methodology. Pain Rep. 3 (Suppl. 1), e671.

Gatchel, R.J., Peng, Y.B., Peters, M.L., Fuchs, P.N., Turk, D.C., 2007. The biopsychosocial approach to chronic pain: scientific advances and future directions. Psychol. Bull. 133 (4), 581–624.

Gates, M., Hartling, L., Shulhan-Kilroy, J., MacGregor, T., Guitard, S., Wingert, A., et al., 2020. Digital technology distraction for acute pain in children: a meta-analysis. Pediatrics 145 (2).

Hathway, G.J., Vega-Avelaira, D., Fitzgerald, M., 2012. A critical period in the supraspinal control of pain: opioid-dependent changes in brainstem rostroventral medulla function in preadolescence. Pain 153 (4), 775–783.

Hauer, J., Houtrow, A.J., 2017. Pain assessment and treatment in children with significant impairment of the central nervous system. Pediatrics 39 (6), e1–27.

Hirschfeld, G., Zernikow, B., Kraemer, N., Hechler, T., Aksu, F., Krumova, E., et al., 2012. Development of somatosensory perception in children: a longitudinal QST-study. Neuropediatrics 43 (1), 10–16.

Holley, A.L., Wilson, A.C., Palermo, T.M., 2017. Predictors of the transition from acute to persistent musculoskeletal pain in children and adolescents: a prospective study. Pain 158 (5), 794–801.

Jones, K., Nordstokke, D., Wilcox, G., Schroeder, M., Noel, M., 2018. The work of childhood understanding school functioning in youth with chronic pain. Pain Manag. 8 (2), 139–153.

Kanstrup, M., Wicksell, R.K., Kemani, M., Wiwe Lipsker, C., Lekander, M., Holmstrom, L., 2016. A clinical pilot study of individual and group treatment for adolescents with chronic pain and their parents: effects of acceptance and commitment therapy on functioning. Children (Basel) 3 (4).

King, S., Chambers, C.T., Huguet, A., MacNevin, R.C., McGrath, P.J., Parker, L., et al., 2011. The epidemiology of chronic pain in children and adolescents revisited: a systematic review. Pain 152 (12), 2729–2738.

Kingsnorth, S., Orava, T., Provvidenza, C., Adler, E., Ami, N., Gresley-Jones, T., et al., 2015. Chronic pain assessment tools for cerebral palsy: a systematic review. Pediatrics 136 (4), e947–960.

Kozlowska, K., Scher, S., Helgeland, H., 2020. Functional Somatic Symptoms in Children and Adolescents: A Stress System Approach to Assessment and Treatment. Palgrave Macmillan.

Lalloo, C., Stinson, J.N., 2014. Assessment and treatment of pain in children and adolescents. Best Pract. Res. Clin. Rheumatol. 28 (2), 315–330.

Lalloo, C., Kumbhare, D., Stinson, J.N., Henry, J.L., 2014. Pain-QuILT: clinical feasibility of a web-based visual pain assessment tool in adults with chronic pain. J. Med. Internet Res. 16 (5), e127.

Liossi, C., Johnstone, L., Lilley, S., Caes, L., Williams, G., Schoth, D.E., 2019. Effectiveness of interdisciplinary interventions in paediatric chronic pain management: a systematic review and subset meta-analysis. Br. J. Anaesth. 123 (2), e359–e371.

Lewandowski, A. S., Palermo, T. M., Stinson, J., Handley, S., & Chambers, C. T. (2010). Systematic review of family functioning in families of children and adolescents with chronic pain. The Journal of Pain, 11(11), 1027–1038.

Logan, D.E., Carpino, E.A., Chiang, G., Condon, M., 2012. A day-hospital approach to treatment of pediatric complex regional pain syndrome: initial functional outcomes. Clin. J. Pain 28 (9), 766–774.

Logan, D.E., Simons, L.E., Carpino, E.A., 2012. Too sick for school? Parent influences on school functioning among children with chronic pain. Pain 153 (2), 437–443.

Lord, S.M., Tardif, H.P., Kepreotes, E.A., Blanchard, M., Eagar, K., 2019. The Paediatric electronic Persistent Pain Outcomes Collaboration (PaedePPOC): establishment of a binational system for benchmarking children's persistent pain services. Pain 160 (7), 1572–1585.

McKinnon, C.T., Meehan, E.M., Harvey, A.R., Antolovich, G.C., Morgan, P.E., 2019. Prevalence and characteristics of pain in children and young adults with cerebral palsy: a systematic review. Dev. Med. Child Neurol. 61 (3), 305–314.

Michaleff, Z.A., Kamper, S.J., Stinson, J.N., Hestbaek, L., Williams, C.M., Campbell, P., et al., 2017. Measuring musculoskeletal pain in infants, children, and adolescents. J. Orthop. Sports Phys. Ther. 47 (10), 712–730.

Mickalide, A., Carr, K., 2012. Safe Kids Worldwide: preventing unintentional childhood injuries across the globe. Pediatr. Clin. 59 (6), 1367–1380.

Nelson, S.M., Cunningham, N.R., Kashikar-Zuck, S., 2017. A conceptual framework for understanding the role of adverse childhood experiences in pediatric chronic pain. Clin. J. Pain 33 (3), 264–270.

Noel, M., Rabbitts, J.A., Tai, G.G., Palermo, T.M., 2015. Remembering pain after surgery: a longitudinal examination of the role of pain catastrophizing in children's and parents' recall. Pain 156 (5), 800–808.

Orava, T., Provvidenza, C., Townley, A., Kingsnorth, S., 2019. Screening and assessment of chronic pain among children with cerebral palsy: a process evaluation of a pain toolbox. Disabil. Rehabil. 41 (22), 2695–2703.

Ostojic, K., Paget, S., Kyriagis, M., Morrow, A., 2019a. Acute and chronic pain in children and adolescents with cerebral palsy: prevalence, interference, and management. Arch. Phys. Med. Rehabil. 31060–31063.

Ostojic, K., Paget, S.P., Morrow, A.M., 2019b. Management of pain in children and adolescents with cerebral palsy: a systematic review. Dev. Med. Child Neurol. 61 (3), 315–321.

Palermo, T.M., Zempsky, W.T., Dampier, C.D., Lalloo, C., Hundert, A.S., Murphy, L.K., et al., 2018. iCanCope with Sickle Cell Pain: design of a randomized controlled trial of a smartphone and web-based pain self-management program for youth with sickle cell disease. Contemp. Clin. Trials 74, 88–96.

Pancekauskaite, G., Jankauskaite, L., 2018. Paediatric pain medicine: pain differences, recognition and coping acute procedural pain in paediatric emergency room. Medicina (Kaunas, Lithuania) 54 (6).

Pate, J.W., Hancock, M.J., Hush, J.M., Gray, K, Pounder, M,. Pacey, V., 2020. Prognostic factors for pain and functional disability in children and adolescents with persisting pain: A systematic review and meta-analysis. Eur. J. Pain. 24, 722–741. https://doi.org/10.1002/ejp.1539.

Pavlova, M., Orr, S.L., Noel, M., 2020. Parent-child reminiscing about past pain as a preparatory technique in the context of children's pain: a narrative review and call for future research. Children (Basel) 7 (9).

Pillai Riddell, R.R., Racine, N.M., Gennis, H.G., Turcotte, K., Uman, L.S., Horton, R.E., et al., 2015. Non-pharmacological management of infant and young child procedural pain. Cochrane Database Syst. Rev. 12, CD006275. https://doi.org/10.1002/14651858.CD006275.pub3.

Pope, N., Tallon, M., McConigley, R., Leslie, G., Wilson, S., 2017. Experiences of acute pain in children who present to a healthcare facility for treatment: a systematic review of qualitative evidence. JBI. Database. System. Rev. Implement. Rep. 15 (6), 1612–1644.

Perquin, C. W., Hazebroek-Kampschreur, A. A., Hunfeld, J. A., Bohnen, A. M., van Suijlekom-Smit, L. W., Passchier, J., & Van Der Wouden, J. C. (2000). Pain in children and adolescents: a common experience. Pain, 87(1), 51–58.

Rajasagaram, U., Taylor, D.M., Braitberg, G., Pearsell, J.P., Capp, B.A., 2009. Paediatric pain assessment: differences between triage nurse, child and parent. J. Paediatr. Child Health 45 (4), 199–203.

Robins, H., Perron, V., Heathcote, L.C., Simons, L.E., 2016. Pain neuroscience education: state of the art and application in pediatrics. Children (Basel) 3 (4).

Sachedina, A., Todd, N., 2020. Dysmenorrhea, endometriosis and chronic pelvic pain in adolescents. J. Clin. Res. Pediatr. Endocrinol. 12 (Suppl. 1), 7–17.

Shaygan, M., Jahandide, Z., Zarifsanaiey, N., 2021. An investigation of the effect of smartphone-based pain management application on pain intensity and the quality-of-life dimensions in adolescents with chronic pain: a cluster randomized parallel-controlled trial. Qual. Life Res. 30 (12), 3431–3442.

Sinclair, C., Meredith, P., Strong, J., Feeney, R., 2016. Personal and contextual factors affecting the functional ability of children and adolescents with chronic pain: a systematic review. J. Dev. Behav. Pediatr. 37 (4), 327–342.

Sinclair, C., Meredith, P., Strong, J., 2020. Pediatric persistent pain: associations among sensory modulation, attachment, functional disability, and quality of life. Am. J. Occup. Ther. 74 (2), 7402205040p7402205041–7402205040p7402205011.

Swain, M.S., Henschke, N., Kamper, S.J., Gobina, I., Ottová-Jordan, V., Maher, C.G., 2014. An international survey of pain in adolescents. BMC Publ. Health 14, 447.

Verriotis, M., Chang, P., Fitzgerald, M., Fabrizi, L., 2016. The development of the nociceptive brain. Neuroscience 338, 207–219.

Wong, D.L., Baker, C.M., 1988. Pain in children: comparison of assessment scales. Pediatr. Nurs. 14 (1), 9–17.

World Health Organisation, 2001. International Classification of Functioning, Disability and Health. World Health Organisation, Geneva.

Zouikr, I., Karshikoff, B., 2017. Lifetime modulation of the pain system via neuroimmune and neuroendocrine interactions. Front. Immunol. 8, 276.

Pain in older adults

Maria O'Reilly

LEARNING OBJECTIVES

At the end of this chapter, readers will understand:
1. How the pain experience differs with age.
2. The particular conditions that commonly cause pain among middle-aged and older people.
3. The differences in pain report and coping strategies among people of different age groups.
4. How age-related changes in neurophysiology may alter the pain experience.
5. How the pain experience is unique for older people in special populations, such as those with dementia.
6. How to approach the assessment of pain in older adults.
7. Some key points about pain management in older people.

Overview

Throughout the world, there has been an increase in the number of people living into old age. The number of people aged over 60 years is anticipated to double by 2050, and the number over 80 years of age is expected to increase by more than three-fold (United Nations 2017, 2019). This is relevant for many nations, including Australia, Japan, South Korea and the United States. For example, South Korea has experienced a rapid escalation of the number of older persons in recent decades, with older adults expected to increase from 15.7% of its total population in 2020 to 20.3% by 2025 (Statistics Korea 2020). By 2040, it is expected that 40% of the Korean population will be aged over 60 years (Jung et al. 2020) (Kim & Kim 2020). In the United States, it is expected that the population aged 65 and above will reach 21.6% by 2040 (Administration for Community Living 2021). However, while the population ageing increases begin in high-income countries, the fastest rate of ageing is currently occurring in middle- and low-income countries (United Nations 2019; World Health Organization 2021).

With a globally ageing population, it is important for healthcare professionals to be cognisant of the prevalence of pain in older adults; special issues related to pain perception and expression among older people; and assessment, treatment and management approaches for older persons with pain.

The epidemiology of pain across the lifespan

Determining pain prevalence across the life course is challenging, due to its subjective nature, inconsistent use

We acknowledge the important contribution of Stephen J. Gibson to the understanding of pain in older people, and his contribution to the earlier editions of this chapter.

of measurement tools and the range of sites in which it can occur (Abdulla et al. 2013). Nevertheless, reviews of the epidemiologic literature reveal a marked age-related increase in the prevalence of persistent pain (often defined as pain on most days persisting beyond 3 months) up until the seventh decade of life and then either a plateau or slight decline into very advanced age (Gibson & Lussier 2012; Helme & Gibson 2001; McBeth & Jones 2007). Further, residents of aged care facilities are found to have consistently higher prevalence of pain than community-dwelling older people (Abdulla et al. 2013). In contrast, the prevalence of acute pain in the community appears to remain relatively constant at approximately 5% regardless of age (Crook et al. 1984; Kendig et al. 1996). Absolute prevalence rates of persistent pain vary widely between different studies (7%–80%) and depend upon the time interval sampled (days, weeks, months, lifetime), the time in pain during this interval (pain every day, most days, at least weekly, any pain during the period), the severity of pain needed for inclusion as a case (mild, moderate, bothersome, activity limiting, etc.) and the sampling technique (telephone, interview, questionnaire). Nonetheless, with one exception (Crook et al. 1984), all studies show a progressive increase in pain prevalence throughout early adulthood (7%–20%), with a peak prevalence during late middle age (50–65; 20%–80%) followed by a plateau or decline in the 'old' old (75–85) and 'oldest' old (85+) adults (25%–60%) (Andersson et al. 1993; Bassols et al. 1999; Blyth et al. 2001; Brattberg et al. 1989, 1997; Herr et al. 1991; Kendig et al. 1996; Kind et al. 1998; Magni et al. 1993; Tsang et al. 2008). Patel et al. (2013) found that out of a sample of 7601 adults over 65, more than half (53%) experienced bothersome pain in the prior month.

When considering pain at specific anatomical sites, a slightly different picture emerges. Foot and leg pain have been reported to increase with advancing age well into the ninth decade of life (Benvenuti et al. 1995; Herr et al. 1991; Hill et al. 2008; Leveille et al. 1998). The prevalence of articular joint pain (particularly of weight-bearing joints) also doubles in adults over 65 years of age (Barberger-Gateau et al. 1992; Bergman et al. 2001; Harkins et al. 1994; Sternbach 1986; Von Korff et al. 1990). Conversely, the prevalence of headache (Andersson et al. 1993; D'Alessandro et al. 1988; Kay et al. 1992; Rottenberg et al. 2015; Sternbach 1986), abdominal pain (Kay et al. 1992; Lavsky-Shulan et al. 1985; Rottenberg et al. 2015) and chest pain (Andersson et al. 1993; Sternbach 1986; Tibblin et al. 1990; Von Korff et al. 1988) all peak during later middle age (45–55) and decline thereafter. Oral pain may not change in prevalence over the lifespan (Leung et al. 2008). Studies of age-specific rates of back pain are mixed, with some reports of a progressive increase over the lifespan (Dionne et al. 2006; Harkins

et al. 1994; Meucci et al. 2015; Von Korff et al. 1988) and others of a reverse trend after a peak prevalence at 40 to 50 years (Andersson et al. 1993; Borenstein 2001; Sternbach 1986; Tibblin et al. 1990). While the site of pain does seem to influence the age-related pattern of pain prevalence, with the exception of joint pain, a consensus view from these studies would still support the notion of peak pain prevalence in late middle age and then a decline in persistent pain into very advanced age. Among older adults, the back and articular joints are the most common sites of reported pain (Abdulla et al. 2013).

The very high prevalence of pain noted in older segments of the community has clear resource implications for the provision of pain management, but it is important to understand that not all persistent pain will be bothersome or of high impact. Indeed, many older persons will not seek treatment for pain and will manage pain symptoms without help. For this reason, several recent studies have started to focus on pain termed as 'clinically relevant' or 'clinically significant'. Large epidemiologic surveys show that approximately 14% of adults over 60 experience moderate-severe or significant pain, defined as continuous, needing professional treatment and occurring on most days in the past 3 months (Breivik et al. 2006; Smith et al. 2001). Adults aged 75+ have been found to be four times more likely to live with significant pain than young adults. Similarly, 15% of residents in nursing homes have moderate-severe pain, and almost half of these have been judged to have inadequate pain management (Lukas et al. 2013; Teno et al. 2003). It appears, therefore, that 'clinically relevant' pain also shows a major age-related increase in prevalence but not necessarily treated, and thus older segments of the community are in most need of state-of-the-art treatment services for the management of bothersome pain.

Age differences in pain as a presenting symptom of clinical disease

Another source of information on age-related changes in the pain experience can be derived from the patterns of symptom presentation in those clinical disease states that are known to have pain as a usual component (Gibson & Helme 2001; Pickering 2005). The majority of studies in this area have focused on somatic or visceral pain complaints and particularly myocardial pain, abdominal pain associated with acute infection and different forms of malignancy. Variations in the classic presentations of 'crushing' myocardial pain in the chest, left arm and jaw are known to be much more common in older adults. Indeed, older adults are significantly less likely to feel pain during myocardial infarction (Čulić et al. 2002; Goch et al. 2009), with approximately 35%–48% of adults over the age of 65 years experiencing apparently silent or painless heart attack (Goch et al. 2009; Konu 1977; MacDonald et al. 1983). For many persons with coronary artery disease, strenuous physical exercise will induce myocardial ischaemia as indexed by a 1 mm drop in the ST segment of the electrocardiogram. By comparing the onset and degree of exertion-induced ischaemia with subjective pain report, it is possible to provide an experimentally controlled evaluation of myocardial pain across the adult lifespan. Several studies have documented a significant age-related delay between the onset of ischaemia and the report of chest pain (Ambepitiya et al. 1993, 1994; Miller et al. 1990; Rittger et al. 2011). Adults over 70 years take almost three times as long as young adults to first report the presence of pain (Ambepitiya et al. 1993, 1994; Rittger et al. 2011). Moreover, the severity of pain report is reduced even after controlling for variations in the extent of ischaemia. Collectively, these findings provide strong support for the view that myocardial pain may be somewhat muted in adults of advanced age.

With regard to pain associated with various types of malignancy, a retrospective review of more than 1500 cases revealed a marked difference in the incidence of pain between younger adults (55% with pain), middle-aged adults (35% with pain) and older adults (26% with pain) (Cherng et al. 1991). With one exception (Vigano et al. 1998), most studies also note a significant decline in the intensity of cancer pain symptoms in adults of advanced age (70+ years) (Brescia et al. 1992; Caraceni & Portenoy 1999; Green & Hart-Johnson 2010; McMillan 1989). The presentation of clinical pain associated with abdominal complaints such as peritonitis, peptic ulcer and intestinal obstruction shows a similar pattern of age-related change. Pain symptoms become more occult after the age of 80 years and, in marked contrast to young adults, the collection of clinical symptoms (nausea, fever, tachycardia) with the highest diagnostic accuracy does not even include abdominal pain (Albano et al. 1975; Wroblewski & Mikulowski 1991). From these uncontrolled studies, it is difficult to ascertain whether the apparent decline in pain reflects some age difference in disease severity and/or the willingness to report pain as a symptom, or whether it reflects an actual age-related change in the pain experience itself.

Other reports of atypical pain presentation have been documented for pneumonia, pneumothorax and postoperative pain. For instance, several studies suggest that older adults report a lower intensity of pain in the postoperative recovery period even after matching for the type of surgical procedure and the extent of tissue damage (Morrison et al. 1998; Oberle et al. 1990; Thomas et al. 1998). This change is thought to be clinically significant and is in the order of a 10%–20% reduction per decade after the age of 60 years (Morrison et al. 1998; Thomas et al. 1998). Older men undergoing prostatectomy reported less pain on a present pain intensity scale and McGill Pain Questionnaire (but not on a visual analogue scale) in the immediate postoperative period and used less patient-controlled opioid analgesia than younger men undergoing the same procedure (Gagliese & Katz 2003).

Summary of epidemiologic studies on age differences in pain

The findings from numerous large-sample epidemiologic studies as well as retrospective case reviews of clinical pain presentation in various somatic and visceral disease states suggest that pain is most common during the late middle-aged phase of life, and that this is true regardless of the anatomical site or the pathogenic cause of pain. The one exception appears to be degenerative joint disease (e.g. osteoarthritis), which shows an exponential increase up until at least 90 years of age. Studies of clinical disease and injury would suggest a relative absence of pain, often with an atypical presentation and a reduction in the intensity of pain symptoms, with very advanced age.

Epidemiology of pain in special older populations

Persistent pain is typically more common in institutional settings such as residential care facilities and nursing homes. Almost 5% of the older adult population reside in nursing homes or long-term care settings in developed countries (Australian Bureau of Statistics 2018; Toth et al. 2020), and over half of these experience cognitive impairment or dementia (Australian Institute of Health & Welfare 2020; Gibson 2007). As a result, it is important to characterise the epidemiology of pain in these special older populations. A number of studies demonstrate an exceptionally high prevalence of pain in residential aged care facilities (Tan et al. 2015), with as many as 58–83% of residents experiencing persistent pain (Ferrell 1995; Parmelee et al. 1993; Tan et al. 2015; Weiner et al. 1998). Using the minimum data set from all nursing homes in the United States (representing almost 2.2 million residents), approximately 15% of residents had 'clinically significant' pain of moderate or severe intensity and 3.7% had excruciating pain on at least 1 day in the previous week (Teno et al. 2001, 2004). Similarly, in a study investigating clinical indicators in residential care, O'Reilly et al. (2011) found that as many as one-third of residents in a facility experienced daily pain, while up to 8% experienced severe pain.

There is some evidence to suggest a lower prevalence of pain in persons with cognitive impairment or dementia (Parmelee et al. 1993; Proctor & Hirdes 2001; Walid & Zaytseva 2009). A significant inverse relationship between pain report and cognitive impairment has been shown in nursing home residents (Cohen-Mansfield & Marx 1993; Parmelee et al. 1993). Both the prevalence and severity of pain were reduced in those with more severe cognitive impairment, and the magnitude of difference was quite large. For instance, pain was detected in just 31.5% of cognitively impaired residents, compared to 61% of cognitively intact residents, despite both groups being equally afflicted with potentially painful disease (Proctor & Hirdes 2001). Subsequent work has confirmed that the observed decrease in pain occurs when using either self-report pain assessment (Leong & Nuo 2007; Mäntyselkä et al. 2004) or, with one exception (Feldt et al. 1998), observational pain scales or proxy nurse ratings of a resident's pain (Leong & Nuo 2007; Sawyer et al. 2007; Wu et al. 2005). Given the similar findings with both self-report and observational assessments, it might be deduced that the reduced levels of pain prevalence and intensity are not simply due to deterioration in verbal communication skills with advancing dementia. There is also reduced pain report in those with dementia following acute medical procedures, including venipuncture (Porter et al. 1996) and injection (Defrin et al. 2006), as well as a possible reduction in the prevalence of post-lumbar puncture headache (Blennow et al. 1993). However, given the challenges faced with accurately assessing pain in people with dementia, it is likely these figures are an underestimate (Tan et al. 2015, 2016). People with dementia may not always communicate their pain in expected ways, often presenting with behaviours such as agitation, anxiety or refusal to move, requiring well-developed observational skills and a nuanced understanding of dementia; pain is thus often underrecognised and undertreated in people living with dementia (Rajkumar et al. 2017; Tan et al. 2015).

Explaining age differences in pain prevalence and report

The age-related increase in pain prevalence until late middle age is easy to explain given that the highest rates of surgery, injury and painful degenerative disease are found in the older segments of the population. However, the unexpected drop in pain prevalence during very advanced age is perhaps more difficult to understand, as the rates of injury and disease continue to climb over the entire adult lifespan. Indeed, several recent systematic reviews of the epidemiology of radiographic osteoarthritis demonstrate a continual and escalating rise in incident disease with advancing age (Allen & Golightly 2015; Arden & Nevitt 2006). Osteoarthritis of weight-bearing joints (hips, knees, feet) is present in the majority of individuals by age 65 years and affects more than 80% of persons over 75 years of age. This single entity could be expected to lead to a massive age-related increase in the presence of persistent pain. However, it is widely acknowledged that joints affected by osteoarthritis often remain asymptomatic (pain-free) despite the presence of radiographic change, and this apparent discordance between symptoms and disease (Hannan et al. 2000) mirrors the situation of more occult pain symptoms in many other clinical conditions (see earlier). In explaining differences in pain perception and report, one needs to consider age differences in the neurophysiological aspects underlying the experience of pain and the role of psychological and social mediators of pain in older persons.

Age differences in psychosocial aspects of pain

Modern conceptualisations of pain emphasise a biopsychosocial perspective in which biological, psychological and social factors all play a relevant role in shaping the experience and reporting of pain. As a result, changes to any one of these systems are likely to help account for the observed age-related changes in pain.

It has been suggested that older adults perceive pain as something to be expected and just a normal part of old age (Hofland 1992; Molton & Terrill 2014). With some exceptions (Gagliese & Melzack 1997; McCracken 1998), empirical studies of pain appraisals and ageing provide clear support for this view (Cornally & McCarthy 2011; Fahey et al. 2008; Liddell & Locker 1997; Ruzicka 1998; Stoller 1993; Weiner & Rudy 2002) and the idea that older adults are often more accepting of mild pain symptoms (Appelt et al. 2007; Gignac et al. 2006). For instance, when compared to arthritis patients aged 50 to 59 years, adults aged greater than 70 years were 2.3 times more likely to agree with the statement that 'arthritis is just a natural part of growing old' and 5.2 times more likely to endorse the statement that 'people should expect to have to live with pain as they grow old' (Appelt et al. 2007). This style of misattribution has important implications, as older people appear less threatened by mild pain symptoms and are less likely to seek treatment (Stoller 1993). However, this mistaken attribution of pain symptoms to normal ageing only occurs for mild-moderate aches and pains. If pain is severe, older persons are more likely to interpret the experience as a sign of serious illness and are more likely to seek rapid medical care than their younger counterparts (Leventhal & Prohaska 1986; Stoller 1993).

Attention has also started to focus on age differences in other types of pain beliefs, such as stoicism, control over pain and beliefs in finding a cure. The conviction that organic issues are important in determining the pain experience have been reported as similar between younger and older chronic pain patients (Gagliese & Melzack 1997), although older patients may be less inclined to acknowledge that pain leads to emotional disturbance (Cook et al. 1999). In addition, older adults appear to endorse a greater conviction in finding a medical cure for pain and have a lesser belief that persistent pain is disabling (Gibson 2003). The locus of control scale has been used to examine age differences in cognitive factors related to control over pain. Older people experiencing chronic pain have a greater belief in pain severity being controlled by factors of chance or fate (Gibson & Helme 2000) when compared to younger cohorts experiencing pain, who seem more likely to endorse their own behaviours and actions as the strongest determinant of pain severity. Older people with chronic pain also express more stoicism towards pain (Yong 2006; Yong et al. 2001, 2003), with higher reported stoic fortitude and a greater cautious self-doubt for pain report. This finding is consistent with other studies of stoic attitudes in older adults (Machin & Williams 1998) and provides strong empirical support for the widely held view that older cohorts are generally more stoic in response to pain (Abdulla et al. 2013; Molton & Terrill 2014).

In order to deal with the negative impacts of persistent pain on quality of life, patients often develop a variety of coping strategies. The self-perceived efficacy in being able to use coping methods to successfully manage pain does not appear to change with advancing age (Corran et al. 1994; Gagliese et al. 2000; Keefe & Williams 1990; Keefe et al. 1991; Watkins et al. 1999). The findings on age differences in coping strategies have somewhat mixed results. Studies by Keefe and colleagues have shown no age differences in the frequency of coping strategy use, although there was a strong trend for older adults to engage more with praying and hoping than young people (Keefe & Williams 1990; Keefe et al. 1991). Conversely, older people with chronic pain have been found to report fewer cognitive coping strategies and an increased use of physical methods of pain control when compared to young adults (Sorkin et al. 1990). Corran et al. (1994) examined a large sample of outpatients attending a multidisciplinary pain treatment centre and found a significantly higher prevalence of praying and hoping as well as fewer incidences of ignoring pain in adults aged greater than 60 years. Watkins et al. (1999) also reported clear age differences for patients in mild pain, with middle-aged and older adults reporting more catastrophising, praying and hoping, but

less frequent use of self-coping statements, than younger adults. Further research is needed to help document the extent and type of age differences in coping efforts and the exact circumstances under which this might occur (Chan et al. 2012; Molton & Terrill 2014).

Overall, there does appear to be some age differences in pain beliefs, coping, attributional style and attitudes towards pain. If a pain symptom is mild or transient in older adults, it is likely to be attributed to the normal ageing process, be more readily accepted and be accompanied by a different choice of strategy to cope with pain. These factors are likely to diminish the importance of mild aches and pains, and actually alter the meaning of pain symptoms. More stoic attitudes to mild pain and a stronger belief in chance factors as the major determinant of pain severity are likely to lead to the underreporting of pain symptoms by older segments of the adult population. However, many of the age differences in coping, misattribution and beliefs disappear if pain is persistent or severe.

Age-related changes in neurophysiology

Any age-related change in the function of nociceptive pathways would also be expected to alter pain sensitivity and therefore alter the perception of noxious events and the prevalence of pain complaints over the adult lifespan. Comprehensive reviews by Gibson (2003), Gibson & Farrell (2004) and Gagliese & Farrell (2005) summarise the age-related changes that occur in pain perception and the underlying neurophysiology of nociception. In general, the nervous system of older persons shows extensive alterations in structure, neurochemistry and function of both peripheral and central nervous systems, including a neurochemical deterioration of the opioid and serotonergic systems. Therefore there may be changes in nociceptive processing, including impairment of the pain inhibitory system.

Peripheral nerves show a decrease in density (both myelinated and, particularly, unmyelinated peripheral nerve fibres), and there is an increase in the number of fibres with signs of damage or degeneration. A slowing of conduction velocity and reductions in substance P, calcitonin gene-related peptide (CGRP) and somatostatin levels have been reported (Helme & McKernan 1985; Li & Duckles 1993; Ochoa & Mair 1969). Studies of the perceptual experience associated with activation of nociceptive fibres indicate a selective age-related impairment in Aδ-fibre function and a greater reliance on C-fibre information for the report of pain in older adults (Chakour et al. 1996). Given that Aδ fibres subserve the epicritic, first warning aspects of pain, while the C-fibre sensation is more prolonged, dull and diffuse, one might reasonably expect some changes in pain quality and intensity in older adults.

Consistent with these changes in peripheral nociceptive function, a number of studies using experimental pain stimuli have shown that pain threshold, or the minimum intensity of noxious stimulation required to elicit a report of just noticeable pain, is increased in older persons (i.e. they are less sensitive to faint pain). The magnitude of age-related change depends on a number of factors, including the modality of stimulation used, and, regardless of stimulus modality, the age-related change appears to be modest and somewhat inconsistent. Nonetheless, a meta-analysis of all 50+ studies of pain threshold does demonstrate a significant overall increase in pain threshold in older adults (Gibson 2003). Older people tend to have higher thresholds for thermal stimuli and a minor increase with electrical stimuli (Gibson 2003), while pressure pain thresholds may actually decrease (Lautenbacher et al. 2005). The significance of these observations in the clinical setting, where pain is a pathophysiological process, remains uncertain, although it could indicate some deficit in the early warning function of pain and contribute to a greater risk of delayed diagnosis of injury or disease (Gibson & Farrell 2004).

Similar structural and neurochemical changes have been noted in the central nervous system of older humans. There are sensory neuron degenerative changes and loss of myelin in the dorsal horn of the spinal cord, as well as reductions in substance P, CGRP and somatostatin levels. Decreases in noradrenergic and serotonergic neurons may contribute to the impairment of descending inhibitory mechanisms and may underlie the decrease in pain tolerance observed in older adults (see later). Age-related loss of neurons and dendritic connections is seen in the human brain, particularly in the cerebral cortex, including those areas involved in nociceptive processing, synthesis, and axonal transport; and receptor binding of neurotransmitters also change. Opioid receptor density is decreased in the brain but not in the spinal cord, and there may be decreases in endogenous opioids. An investigation of the cortical response to painful stimulation has documented some changes in adults over 60 years. Using the pain-related encephalographic response in order to index the central nervous system processing of noxious input, older adults were found to display a significant reduction in peak amplitude and an increased latency of response (Gibson et al. 1990). These findings might suggest an age-related slowing in the cognitive processing of noxious information and a reduced cortical activation. More recently, Cole and colleagues (2009) used neuroimaging techniques (functional magnetic resonance imaging (fMRI)) to examine the brain regions activated during noxious mechanical stimulation. Both younger and older

adults showed significant pain-related activity in a common network of areas, including the insula, cingulate, posterior parietal and somatosensory cortices. However, compared with older adults, young subjects showed significantly greater activity in the contralateral putamen and caudate, which could not be accounted for by increased age-associated atrophy in these regions. The age-related difference in pain-evoked activity was suggested to reflect a reduced functioning of striatal pain modulatory mechanisms with advancing age and a possible impairment in endogenous pain inhibitory networks (see later).

Variations in pain sensitivity depend not only on activity in the afferent nociceptive pathways but also endogenous pain inhibitory control mechanisms that descend from the cortex and midbrain onto spinal cord neurons. Two studies have reported that the analgesic efficacy of this endogenous inhibitory system may decline with advancing age (Edwards et al. 2003; Washington et al. 2000). Following activation of the endogenous analgesic system, young adults showed an increase in pain threshold of up to 150%, whereas the apparently healthy older adult group increased pain threshold by approximately 40%. Such age differences in the efficiency of endogenous analgesic modulation are consistent with many earlier animal studies (see Bodnar et al. 1988 for review) and would be expected to reduce the ability of older adults to cope with severe or strong pain. It is not surprising, therefore, that there is also convincing evidence that all 13 studies of experimental pain tolerance (or the intensity of stimulation tolerated before withdrawing from further stimulation), across several different modalities of stimulation, show a reduced pain tolerance in older adults (Gibson 2003).

Age differences in pain processing under pathophysiologic conditions

Recently there has also been research directed at developing a better understanding of age differences in pain neurophysiology under pathophysiological conditions. Such studies are needed as all clinical pain states associated with injury or disease involve some pathophysiological changes in the nociceptive system. Three studies have shown that the temporal summation of noxious input may be altered in older persons (Edwards & Fillingim 2001; Farrell & Gibson 2007; Harkins et al. 1996). Temporal summation refers to the enhancement of pain sensation associated with repeated stimulation. Using experimental pain stimuli, it can be shown that the threshold for temporal summation is lower in older persons (Edwards & Fillingim 2001; Gibson & Farrell 2004; Harkins et al. 1996). In subjects given trains of five brief electrical stimuli of varying frequency (ranging from two pulses every second through to one pulse every 5 seconds), older subjects showed temporal summation at all frequencies of stimulation, whereas summation was not seen at the slower stimulation frequencies in younger subjects (Farrell & Gibson 2007). Temporal summation of thermal stimuli was increased in older adults compared with younger subjects (Edwards & Fillingim 2001; Lautenbacher et al. 2005) and was considerably prolonged in duration (Edwards & Fillingim 2001), but temporal summation of pressure pain showed no age-related effects (Lautenbacher et al. 2005). Temporal summation is known to result from a transient sensitisation of dorsal horn neurons in the spinal cord and is thought to play a role in the development and expression of postinjury tenderness and hyperalgesia. The increased responses and prolonged duration of central sensitisation in older adults, even when stimuli are delivered further apart, may indicate that it is more difficult to reverse the pathophysiological changes in the nociceptive system once they have occurred (Farrell & Gibson 2007). Zheng et al. (2000) offer complementary findings using a different experimental model by comparing the intensity and time course of postinjury hyperalgesia in younger (20–40) and older (73–88) adults. While the intensity and area of hyperalgesia were similar in both groups, the state of mechanical tenderness persisted for a much longer duration in the older group. The mechanical tenderness was not altered by the application of local anaesthetic (Zheng et al. 2009), confirming previous research which shows that mechanical tenderness is mediated by sensitised spinal neurons. These findings may indicate a reduced capacity of the aged central nervous system to reverse the sensitisation process once it has been initiated. The clinical implication is that postinjury pain and tenderness will resolve more slowly in older persons. However, in combination with the studies of temporal summation, these findings provide strong evidence for an age-related reduction in the functional plasticity of spinal nociceptive neurons following an acute noxious event.

In summary, the evidence from numerous neurophysiologic and psychophysical studies suggests a small, but demonstrable, age-related impairment in the early warning functions of pain. The increase in pain perception threshold and the widespread change in the structure and function of peripheral and central nervous system nociceptive pathways may place the older person at greater risk of undiagnosed injury or disease. Moreover, the reduced efficacy of endogenous analgesic systems, a decreased tolerance of pain, a greater propensity to central sensitisation of the nociceptive system and the slower resolution of postinjury hyperalgesia with a heightened sensitivity to pain may make it more difficult for the older adult to cope once injury has occurred.

Pain processing in persons with dementia

Dementia may exacerbate age-related impairments in pain processing, and there is growing international debate as to whether people with dementia actually feel less pain than age-matched peers (Scherder et al. 2009), although it is far from conclusive, and may depend on the specific dementia diagnosis (Achterberg et al. 2013; Kunz et al. 2009; Molton & Terrill 2014). As discussed previously, the prevalence and severity of clinical pain appear to be reduced in persons with cognitive impairment when using self-report, observational pain scales or proxy ratings. There are blunted autonomic reactions to acute medical procedures, such as injection and venipuncture, but increased facial expression of pain and enhanced withdrawal reflexes in those with Alzheimer's disease (Defrin et al. 2006; Porter et al. 1996). Pain threshold appears to remain unchanged in persons with Alzheimer's disease, but pain tolerance may be increased (Benedetti et al. 1999; Gibson et al. 2001), suggesting a selective deterioration in the affective-motivational aspects of pain (Scherder et al. 2009). However, neuroimaging studies of central nervous system processing have revealed significantly greater pain-related activations in various regions for people with Alzheimer's disease, including regions known to be involved in the cognitive and affective components of pain processing (i.e. dorsolateral prefrontal cortex, mid-cingulate cortex and insula) (Achterberg et al. 2013; Cole et al. 2006).

It is somewhat difficult to reconcile these divergent findings of increase, decrease and no change in pain perception and associated physiological responses. It seems likely that the severity of dementia may help to explain this disparate evidence base, as most experimental studies have been conducted in those with mild disease, whereas clinical measures of pain are also taken from those with more advanced disease. At present, it appears dementia may impair pain perception at least in more severe cases, but the extent of change in pain perception with the progression of dementia remains unclear. Further research is needed in order to answer this important question.

Assessment of pain in older people

The key points regarding assessment of pain have been covered earlier in Chapter 8. As noted, chronic pain requires a multifaceted, comprehensive assessment, including due attention to pain intensity, quality and variations over time and situation; the extent of psychological disturbance; the degree of functional impairment in activities of daily life; and the social impacts of chronic pain. In older persons, it is also argued that taking a prior medical history, a full physical examination and an assessment of all comorbid disease is of particular importance (Herr 2005). Considerable work has been undertaken in this area, and documents such as the Interdisciplinary Expert Consensus Statement on Assessment of Pain in Older Persons (Hadjistavropoulos et al. 2007), the Assessment of Pain in Older People: UK National Guidelines (Schofield 2018), and the Australian Pain Society's (APS) (2019) Pain in Residential Aged Care Facilities provide important information, including recommendations for physical evaluation, recommendations for assessing pain using self-report procedures, recommendations for functional assessment and recommendations for the assessment of emotional functioning. Other consensus statements on the most suitable types of pain assessment for older adults have been published and highlight simple word descriptor scales (i.e. weak, mild, moderate, strong) and numeric rating scales (1–10) as the tools of first choice for pain assessment in older adults (American Geriatrics Society Panel on Pharmacological Management of Persistent Pain in Older Persons 2009; Goucke, 2019; Royal College of Physicians, British Geriatrics Society, British Pain Society 2007; Herr 2005). A number of other scales also have demonstrated merit (i.e. box scales, pain thermometer, faces pain scales, McGill Pain Questionnaire), but may be less preferred by some older people (Herr 2005). Visual analogue scales are generally not recommended for use in older adults as they typically have a higher failure rate (Hadjistavropoulos et al. 2007; Herr 2005). More comprehensive pain assessment tools that monitor pain intensity and the biopsychosocial impacts of pain (on mood, function, sleep, quality of life, etc.) have also been developed (Goucke, 2019; Hadjistavropoulos et al. 2007). The Brief Pain Inventory, Pain Disability Index, Multidimensional Pain Inventory and Geriatric Pain Measure have been effectively used with older adults, although there has been relatively limited testing of reliability and validity, and further studies within the clinical setting are required (Royal College of Physicians, British Geriatrics Society, British Pain Society 2007; Herr 2005). More recently, it has been suggested that assessing pain in older people should focus on movement- and function-based assessment rather than the standard self-report or observational measures (Booker et al. 2021).

Pain assessment strategies for those with cognitive impairment, sensory loss or lacking in verbal skills must seek to capitalise on the available communication repertoire of the individual. While self-report has become the de facto gold standard for pain assessment, other non-verbal methods (i.e. behavioural measures, observational tools) can provide important and clinically relevant information, and may be the preferred assessment choice in cases of moderate-severe impairment. Cognitive impairment can potentially interfere with self-report, although several recent studies have shown that such scales can remain valid and reliable in those with mild to moderate impairment (Hadjistavropoulos 2005; Herr 2005; Pautex et al. 2005; Schofield 2018). There has been a rapid proliferation of new observer-rated scales for pain assessment in those with dementia over the last two decades (Hadjistavropoulos 2005). Most scales grade the presence or absence of various behaviours that are thought to be indicative of pain. For instance, combinations of facial expressions, negative vocalisations, altered body language (e.g. rubbing, limping) and physiologic signs (e.g. blood pressure) can be scored to provide an index of likely pain intensity. More recently, there have even been some direct comparisons of the relative strengths and weaknesses of different observer-rated measures (Aubin et al. 2007; Zwakhalen et al. 2006). These measures represent an important advance in pain assessment of older adults affected by dementia or delirium, although further work is required to validate the new measures across different settings and older populations. See Schofield (2018) for a comprehensive list and evaluation of available measures.

Managing pain in older persons

Persistent pain is known to be most common in the older segments of the population, yet the vast majority of pain treatment studies and intervention trials have been conducted in young adult populations. The degree to which standard pain treatment approaches might need to be modified in order to meet the special needs of the older person has not been systematically examined, and possible age differences in treatment efficacy have rarely been considered. Nonetheless, in recent years, several useful guidelines have been developed by key organisations such as the American Geriatric Society (American Geriatrics Society Panel on Persistent Pain in Older Persons 2002; American Geriatrics Society Panel on Pharmacological Management of Persistent Pain in Older Persons 2009), the Australian Pain Society (2019), the American Medical Directors Association (2003) and the British Geriatrics Society (Abdulla et al. 2013) to guide practitioners working with older persons who may experience pain. See, for example, the American Geriatrics Society's 2009 document on Pharmacological Management of Persistent Pain in Older Persons (American Geriatrics Society Panel on Pharmacological Management of Persistent Pain in Older Persons 2009). These guidelines document a wide range of treatments and include the following broad recommendations. The selection of appropriate analgesics for the older person requires an understanding of age-related pharmacokinetic and pharmacodynamic changes and must account for the impact of comorbid disease and concurrent medication use. For this reason, simple analgesics (i.e. paracetamol) are the pharmacologic treatment of choice for the management of mild-moderate persistent pain and particularly musculoskeletal conditions. Nonsteroidal compounds (NSAIDs and COX2) should be used with caution and all medications, including opioids and adjuvant analgesics (i.e.

anticonvulsants, antidepressants), carry a balance of benefits and risks that must be weighed up for each older individual. Most guidelines emphasise that pharmacological therapy for persistent pain is always more effective when combined with nonpharmacological approaches. For certain selected patients, interventional treatments (including joint injection techniques, orthopaedic surgery, indwelling pumps for intrathecal administration of analgesic compounds or use of spinal cord stimulation techniques for the management of refractory pain) might also be considered and have been shown to play a useful role in the management of chronic pain in older persons.

Nonpharmacological approaches with evidence of efficacy in older populations include physical therapies (i.e. graded exercise programme, heat/cold, transcutaneous electrical nerve stimulation (TENS)), psychological methods (i.e. relaxation, cognitive–behavioural therapy, mindfulness), education programmes, social support interventions and certain types of complementary therapies (i.e. glucosamine, acupuncture). However, the lack of an appropriate evidence base and the urgent need for further research on most treatment modalities is universally acknowledged in all of these guidelines. Multidisciplinary pain programmes that combine several modes of pharmacological and nonpharmacological treatment have demonstrated efficacy for the management of persistent pain in older adults (Cassidy et al. 2012; Ersek et al. 2003; Joypaul et al. 2019; Katz et al. 2005; Takahashi et al. 2019), including for those in residential aged care (Cook 1998; Mimi & Ho 2013). This treatment approach is considered to be state of the art for chronic pain management but appears to be underutilised at present. Older patients are underrepresented in pain management clinics, are less likely to be offered treatment and receive fewer treatment options when attending such clinics (Kee et al. 1998). Undertreatment of pain continues to be an issue of concern for this cohort, particularly within residential care (Denny & Guido 2012; Tracy & Morrison 2013). There have been some attempts to move the essential features of a multidisciplinary pain management programme so that it can be delivered as a home-based service (Kung et al. 2000) or via mobile technologies (Parker et al. 2013). Initiatives such as these should help to improve access to multidisciplinary treatment and ultimately improve pain management options for those frail, incapacitated or institutionalised older persons who experience persistent and bothersome pain. However, they do not replace good clinical observational skills and attention to the specific needs of older adults.

Conclusion

With the rapid ageing of the world's population, there is a clear need to be fully informed about any age-related change in pain perception and report as this is likely to affect options for the best available assessment and treatment approaches. The literature shows that pain, particularly of the joints, is very common in older adults. However, there is also clear evidence for a greater proportion of atypical presentations of usually painful disease states, including a relative absence of pain symptoms and a reduced intensity of pain when it is actually reported. Older persons with dementia represent a special population of older adults and generally show an even greater magnitude of change in pain perception and report.

Evidence suggests that older persons are more accepting of mild aches and pains, have altered pain beliefs and attitudes, including increased stoicism, and are less likely to seek medical attention. There is also a demonstrable age-related decline in pain sensitivity to mild noxious stimuli and some impairment in the structure and function of nociceptive pathways (both peripheral and central nervous system). These changes may partly compromise the early warning functions of pain, leading to the underreporting of mild pain, and may place the older person at greater risk of undiagnosed disease or injury. Conversely, experimental studies show that the endogenous analgesic system (e.g. endorphins) may be less efficient in persons of advanced age, and that tolerance of strong pain is reduced. Prolonged pain and tenderness after injury and poorer repair mechanisms also indicate that the older person may be more vulnerable to the negative impacts of strong, persistent pain. Thus there are many reasons for age-related changes in pain, including physiological and psychological influences, but the current pool of knowledge in this area remains incomplete. A better understanding of age-related differences and similarities in the pain experience will ultimately contribute to a more rational and effective management of pain and suffering in older persons.

Review questions Q

1. Which conditions are common in middle-aged and older people?
2. What are some of the psychosocial factors that might affect older people's beliefs about and/or strategies for dealing with pain?
3. What are some of the physiological factors that might affect older people's experience of pain?
4. How might the experience of pain differ for an older person living with dementia?
5. What are the ways you can use to determine if an older person has pain?
6. What are some key principles about managing pain in older people?

References

Abdulla, A., Adams, N., Bone, M., Elliott, A.M., Gaffin, J., Jones, D., et al., 2013. Guidance on the management of pain in older people. Age Ageing 42, i1–i57.

Achterberg, W., Pieper, M.J.C., Van Dalen-Kok, A.H., De Waal, M.W.M., Husebo, B.S., Lautenbacher, S., et al., 2013. Pain management in patients with dementia. Clin. Interv. Aging 2013:81471—1482.

Administration for Community Living, 2021. 2020 Profile of Older Americans. US Department of Health and Human Services.

Albano, W., Zielinski, C.M., Organ, C.H., 1975. Is appendicitis in the aged really different? Geriatrics. 30, 81–88.

Allen, K.D., Golightly, Y.M., 2015. State of the evidence. Curr. Opin. Rheumatol. 27 (3), 276–283.

Ambepitiya, G.B., Iyengar, E.N., Roberts, M.E., 1993. Silent exertional myocardial ischaemia and perception of angina in elderly people. Age. Ageing. 22 (4), 302–307.

Ambepitiya, G.B., Roberts, M., Ranjadayalan, K., 1994. Silent exertional myocardial ischemia in the elderly: a quantitative analysis of anginal perceptual threshold and the influence of autonomic function. J. Am. Geriatr. Soc. 42, 732–737.

American Geriatrics Society Panel on Persistent Pain in Older Persons, 2002. Clinical practice guidelines: the management of persistent pain in older persons. J. Am. Geriatr. Soc. 50, S205–S224.

American Geriatrics Society Panel on Pharmacological Management of Persistent Pain in Older Persons, 2009. Pharmacological management of persistent pain in older persons. J. Am. Geriatr. Soc. 57 (8), 1331–1346.

American Medical Directors Association, 2003. Chronic Pain Management in the Long-Term Care Setting. AMDA, San Diego, CA.

Andersson, H., Ejlertsson, G., Leden, I., et al., 1993. Chronic pain in a geographically defined general population: studies of differences in age, gender, social class, and pain localization. Clin. J. Pain. 9 (3), 174–182.

Appelt, C.J., Burant, C.J., Siminoff, L.A., et al., Kwoh, C. K., Ibrahim, S. A. 2007. Arthritis-specific health beliefs related to aging among older male patients with knee and/or hip osteoarthritis. J. Gerontol. A. Biol. Sci. Med. Sci. 62A (2), 184–190.

Arden, N., Nevitt, M.C., 2006. Osteoarthritis: epidemiology. Clin. Rheumatol. 20 (1), 3–25.

Aubin, M., Giguère, A., Hadjistavropoulos, T., et al., 2007. The systematic evaluation of instruments designed to assess pain in persons with limited ability to communicate. Pain. Res. Manag. 12 (3), 195–203.

Australian Bureau of Statistics, 2018. Disability, Ageing and Carers, Australia: Summary of Findings. Available from https://www.abs.gov.au/statistics/health/disability/disability-ageing-and-carers-australia-summary-findings/latest-release.

Australian Institute of Health & Welfare, 2020. Australia's Health: Dementia. AIHW. Available from https://www.aihw.gov.au/reports/australias-health/dementia.

Australian Pain Society, 2019. Pain in Residential Aged Care Facilities: Management Strategies, second ed. Australian Pain Society, North Sydney.

Barberger-Gateau, P., Chaslerie, A., Dartigues, J., et al., 1992. Health measures correlates in a French elderly community population: the PAQUID study. J. Gerontol. 47 (2), S88–S95.

Bassols, A., Bosch, F., Campillo, M., et al., 1999. An epidemiologic comparison of pain complaints in the general population of Catalonia (Spain). Pain. 83 (1), 9–16.

Benedetti, F., Vighetti, S., Ricco, C., et al., 1999. Pain threshold and tolerance in Alzheimer's disease. Pain. 80 (1–2), 377–382.

Benvenuti, F., Ferrucci, L., Guralnik, J.M., et al., 1995. Foot pain and disability in older persons: an epidemiologic survey. J. Am. Geriatr. Soc. 43 (5), 479–484.

Bergman, S., Herrström, P., Högström, K., et al., 2001. Chronic musculoskeletal pain, prevalence rates, and sociodemographic associations in a Swedish population study. J. Rheumatol. 28 (6), 1369–1377.

Blennow, K., Wallin, A., Häger, O., 1993. Low frequency of post-lumbar puncture headache in demented patients. Acta. Neurol. Scand. 88 (3), 221–223.

Blyth, F.M., March, L.M., Brnabic, A.J.M., et al., 2001. Chronic pain in Australia: a prevalence study. Pain. 89 (2,3), 127–134.

Bodnar, R.J., Romero, M.T., Kramer, E., 1988. Organismic variables and pain inhibition: roles of gender and aging. Brain. Res. Bull. 21 (6), 947–953.

Booker, S.Q., Herr, K.A., Horgas, A.L., 2021. A paradigm shift for movement-based pain assessment in older adults: practice, policy and regulatory drivers. Pain. Manag. Nurs. 22 (1), 21–27.

Borenstein, D.G., 2001. Epidemiology, etiology, diagnostic evaluation, and treatment of low back pain. Curr. Opin. Rheumatol. 13 (2), 128–134.

Brattberg, G., Parker, M.G., Thorslund, M., 1997. A longitudinal study of pain: reported pain from middle age to old age. Clin. J. Pain. 13 (2), 144–149.

Brattberg, G., Thorslund, M., Wikman, A., 1989. The prevalence of pain in the general community: the results of a postal survey in a county of Sweden. Pain. 37 (1), 21–32.

Breivik, H., Collett, B., Ventafridda, V., et al., 2006. Survey of chronic pain in Europe: prevalence, impact on daily life, and treatment. Eur. J. Pain. 10 (4), 287–333.

Brescia, F.J., Portenoy, R.K., Ryan, M., et al., 1992. Pain, opioid use, and survival in hospitalized patients with advanced cancer. J. Clin. Oncol. 10 (1), 149–155.

Caraceni, A., Portenoy, R.K., 1999. An international survey of cancer pain characteristics and syndromes. Pain. 82 (3), 263–274.

Cassidy, E.L., Atherton, R.J., Robertson, N., Walsh, D.A., Gillett, R., 2012. Mindfulness, functioning and catastrophizing after multidisciplinary pain management for chronic low back pain. Pain. 153 (3), 644–650.

Chan, S., Hadjistavropoulos, T., Carleton, R. N., & Hadjistavropoulos, H. 2012. Predicting Adjustment to Chronic Pain in Older Adults. Can. J. Behav. Sci. 44 (3), 192–199. https://doi.org/10.1037/a0028370.

Chakour, M.C., Gibson, S.J., Bradbeer, M., et al., 1996. The effect of age on A-delta and C-fibre thermal pain perception. Pain. 64 (1), 143–152.

Cherng, C.H., Ho, S.T., Kao, S.J., et al., 1991. The study of cancer pain and its correlates. Ma. Zui. Xue. Za. Zhi. 29 (3), 653–657.

Cohen-Mansfield, J., Marx, M.S., 1993. Pain and depression in the nursing home: corroborating results. J. Gerontol. 48 (2), P96–P97.

Cole, L., Farrell, M.J., Egan, G., et al., 2009. Age differences in pain sensitivity and fMRI pain related brain activity. Neurobiol. Aging. 31 (3), 494–503.

Cole, L., Farrell, M.J., Tress, B., et al., 2006. Pain sensitivity and fMRI pain related brain activity in persons with Alzheimer's disease. Brain. 129 (11), 2957–2965.

Cook, A.J., 1998. Cognitive-behavioral pain management for elderly nursing home residents. J. Gerontol. B. Psychol. Sci. Soc. Sci. P51–P59.

Cook, A.J., DeGood, D.E., Chastain, D.C., 1999. Age differences in pain beliefs. In: 9th World Congress on Pain, p. 557 Vienna.

Cornally, N., McCarthy, G., 2011. Chronic pain: the help-seeking behavior, attitudes, and beliefs of older adults living in the community. Pain. Manag. Nurs. 12 (4), 206–217.

Corran, T.M., Gibson, S.J., Farrell, M.J., et al., 1994. Comparison of chronic pain experience between young and elderly patients. In: Gebhart, G.F., Hammond, D.L., Jenson, T.S. (Eds.), Proceedings of the 7th World Congress on Pain, Progress in Pain Research and Management, vol. 2. IASP Press, Seattle, pp. 895–906.

Crook, J., Rideout, E., Browne, G., 1984. The prevalence of pain complaints in a general population. Pain. 18 (3), 299–305.

Čulić, V., Eterović, D., Mirić, D., Silić, N., 2002. Symptom presentation of acute myocardial infarction: influence of sex, age, and risk factors. Am. Heart. J. 144 (6), 1012–1017.

D'Alessandro, R., Benassi, G., Lenzi, P.L., et al., 1988. Epidemiology of headache in the republic of San Marino. J. Neurol. Neurosurg. Psychiatry. 51 (1), 21–27.

Defrin, R., Lotan, M., Pick, C.G., 2006. The evaluation of acute pain in individuals with cognitive impairment: a differential effect of the level of impairment. Pain. 124 (3), 312–320.

Denny, D.L., Guido, G.W., 2012. Undertreatment of pain in older adults. Nurs. Ethics. 19 (6), 800–809.

Dionne, C.E., Dunn, K.M., Croft, P.R., 2006. Does back pain prevalence really decrease with increasing age? Age. Ageing. 35 (3), 229–234.

Edwards, R.R., Fillingim, R.B., 2001. The effects of age on temporal summation and habituation of thermal pain: clinical relevance in healthy older and younger adults. J. Pain. 6 (2), 307–317.

Edwards, R.R., Fillingim, R.B., Ness, T.J., 2003. Age-related differences in endogenous pain modulation: a comparison of diffuse noxious inhibitory controls in healthy older and younger adults. Pain. 101 (1–2), 155–165.

Ersek, M., Turner, J.A., McCurry, S.M., et al., 2003. Efficacy of a self-management group intervention for elderly persons with chronic pain. Clin. J. Pain. 19, 156–167.

Fahey, K.F., Rao, S.M., Douglas, M.K., et al., 2008. Nurse coaching to explore and modify patient attitudinal barriers interfering with effective cancer pain management. Oncol. Nurs. Forum. 35 (2), 233–240.

Farrell, M., Gibson, S.J., 2007. Age interacts with stimulus frequency in the temporal summation of pain. Pain. Med. 8 (6), 514–520.

Feldt, K.S., Warne, M.A., Ryden, M.B., 1998. Examining pain in aggressive cognitively impaired older adults. J. Gerontol. Nurs. 24 (11), 14–22.

Ferrell, B.A., 1995. Pain evaluation and management in the nursing home. Ann. Intern. Med. 123 (9), 681–695.

Gagliese, L., Farrell, M., 2005. The neurobiology of ageing, nociception and pain: an integration of animal and human experimental evidence. In: Gibson, S.J., Weiner, D. (Eds.), Progress in Pain Research and Management: Pain in the Older Person. IASP Press, Seattle, pp. 25–44.

Gagliese, L., Jackson, M., Ritvo, P., et al., 2000. Age is not an impediment to effective use of patient-controlled analgesia by surgical patients. Anesthesiology. 93 (3), 601–610.

Gagliese, L., Katz, J., 2003. Age differences in postoperative pain are scale dependent: a comparison of measures of pain intensity and quality in younger and older surgical patients. Pain. 103 (1,2), 11–20.

Gagliese, L., Melzack, R., 1997. Age differences in the quality of chronic pain: a preliminary study. Pain. Res. Manag. 2 (3), 157–162.

Gibson, S.J., Lussier, D., 2012. Prevalence and relevance of pain in older persons. Pain. Med. 13 (Suppl 2), S23–S26.

Gibson, S.J., 2003. Pain and ageing. In: Dostrovsky, J.O., Carr, D.B., Koltzenburg, M. (Eds.), Proceedings of 10th World Congress on Pain. IASP Press, Seattle, pp. 767–790.

Gibson, S.J., 2007. The IASP Global Year against Pain in Older Persons: highlighting the current status and future perspectives in geriatric pain. Expert Rev. Neurother. 7 (6), 627–635.

Gibson, S.J., Farrell, M.J., 2004. A review of age differences in the neurophysiology of nociception and the perceptual experience of pain. Clin. J. Pain. 20 (4), 227–239.

Gibson, S.J., Gorman, M.M., Helme, R.D., 1990. Assessment of pain in the elderly using event-related cerebral potentials. In: Bond, M.R., Charlton, J.E., Woolf, C. (Eds.), Proceedings of the VIth World Congress on Pain. Elsevier Science Publishers, Amsterdam, pp. 523–529.

Gibson, S.J., Helme, R.D., 2000. Cognitive factors and the experience of pain and suffering in older persons. Pain. 85 (3), 375–383.

Gibson, S.J., Helme, R.D., 2001. Age-related differences in pain perception and report. Clin. Geriatr. Med. 17 (3), 433–456.

Gibson, S.J., Voukelatos, X., Flicker, L., et al., 2001. A comparison of nociceptive cerebral event related potentials and heat pain threshold in healthy older adults and those with cognitive impairment. Pain. Res. Manag. 6 (3), 126–133.

Gignac, M.A., Davis, A.M., Hawker, G., et al., 2006. 'What do you expect? You're just getting older': a comparison of perceived osteoarthritis-related and aging-related health experiences in middle- and older-age adults. Arthritis. Rheum. 55 (6), 905–912.

Goch, A., Misiewicz, P., Rysz, J., Banach, M., 2009. The clinical manifestation of myocardial infarction in elderly patients. Clin. Cardiol. 32 (6), E45–E50.

Goucke, C.R. (Ed.), 2019. Pain in Residential Aged Care Facilities: Management Strategies, second ed. Australian Pain Society, Sydney.

Green, C.R., Hart-Johnson, T., 2010. Cancer pain: an age-based analysis. Pain. Med. 11 (10), 1525–1536.

Hadjistavropoulos, T., 2005. Assessing pain in older persons with severe limitations in ability to communicate. In: Gibson, S.J., Weiner, D.K. (Eds.), Pain in Older Persons, Progress in Pain Research and Management, vol. 35. IASP Press, Seattle, pp. 135–151.

Hadjistavropoulos, T., Herr, K., Turk, D.C., et al., 2007. An interdisciplinary expert consensus statement on assessment of pain in older persons. Clin. J. Pain. 23, S1–S43.

Hannan, M.T., Felson, D.T., Pincus, T., 2000. Analysis of the discordance between radiographic changes and knee pain in osteoarthritis of the knee. J. Rheumatol. 27 (6), 1513–1517.

Harkins, S.W., Davis, M.D., Bush, F.M., et al., 1996. Suppression of first pain and slow temporal summation of second pain in relation to age. J. Gerontol. A. Biol. Sci. Med. Sci. 51A (5), M260–M265.

Harkins, S.W., Price, D.D., Bush, F.M., 1994. Geriatric pain. In: Wall, P.D., Melzack, R. (Eds.), Textbook of Pain. Churchill Livingstone, New York, pp. 769–787.

Helme, R.D., Gibson, S.J., 2001. The epidemiology of pain in elderly people. Clin. Geriatr. Med. 17 (3), 417–431.

Helme, R.D., McKernan, S., 1985. Neurogenic flare responses following topical application of capsaicin in humans. Ann. Neurol. 18 (4), 505–511.

Herr, K., 2005. Pain assessment in the older adult with verbal communication skills. In: Gibson, S.J., Weiner, D.K. (Eds.), Pain in Older Persons, Progress in Pain Research and Management, vol 35. IASP Press, Seattle, pp. 111–133.

Herr, K.A., Mobily, P.R., Wallace, R.B., Chung, Y., 1991. Leg pain in the rural Iowa 65+ population. Prevalence, related factors, and association with functional status. Clin. J. Pain 7 (2), 114–121. https://doi.org/10.1097/00002508-199106000-00007.

Hill, C.L., Gill, T.K., Menz, H.B., Taylor, A.W., 2008. Prevalence and correlates of foot pain in a population-based study: the North West Adelaide health study. J. Foot. Ankle. Res. 1 (1), 2.

Hofland, S.L., 1992. Elder beliefs: blocks to pain management. J. Gerontol. Nurs. 18 (6), 19–23.

Joypaul, S., Kelly, F.S., King, M.A., 2019. Turning pain into gain: evaluation of a multidisciplinary chronic pain management program in primary care. Pain. Med. 20 (5), 925–933.

Jung, M., Ko, W., Muhwava, W., Choi, Y., Kim, H., Park, Y.S., et al., 2020. Mind the gaps: age and cause specific mortality and life expectancy in the older population of South Korea and Japan. BMC. Publ. Health. 20 (1), 819.

Katz, B., Scherer, S., Gibson, S.J., 2005. Multidisciplinary pain management clinics for older adults. In: Gibson, S.J., Weiner, D.K. (Eds.), Pain in Older Persons, Progress in Pain Research and Management, vol 35. IASP Press, Seattle, pp. 45–65.

Kay, L., Jorgensen, T., Schultz-Larsen, K., 1992. Abdominal pain in a 70-year-old Danish population. An epidemiological study of the prevalence and importance of abdominal pain. J. Clin. Epidemiol. 45 (12), 1377–1382.

Kee, W.G., Middaugh, S.J., Redpath, S., et al., 1998. Age as a factor in admission to chronic pain rehabilitation. Clin. J. Pain. 14, 121–128.

Keefe, F.J., Caldwell, D.S., Martinez, S., et al., 1991. Analysing pain in rheumatoid arthritis patients: pain coping strategies in patients who have had knee replacement surgery. Pain. 46 (2), 153–160.

Keefe, F.J., Williams, D.A., 1990. A comparison of coping strategies in chronic pain patients in different age groups. J. Gerontol. 45 (4), 161–165.

Kendig, H., Helme, R.D., Teshuva, K., 1996. Health Status of Older People Project: Data from a Survey of the Health and Lifestyles of Older Australians. Report to the Victorian Health Promotion Foundation. Victorian Government, Melbourne.

Kim, K.W., Kim, O.S., 2020. Super aging in South Korea unstoppable but mitigatable: a sub-national scale population projection for best policy planning. Spat. Demogr. 8 (2), 155–173.

Kind, P., Dolan, P., Gudex, C., et al., 1998. Variations in population health status: results from a United Kingdom national questionnaire survey. Br. Med. J. 316 (7133), 736–741.

Konu, V., 1977. Myocardial infarction in the elderly. Acta. Med. Scand. 604 (Suppl l), 3–68.

Kung, F., Gibson, S.J., Helme, R.D., 2000. A community-based program that provides free choice of intervention for older people with chronic pain. J. Pain. 1, 293–308.

Kunz, M., Mylius, V., Scharmann, S., Schepelman, K., Lautenbacher, S., 2009. Influence of dementia on multiple components of pain. Eur. J. Pain. 13 (3), 317–325.

Lautenbacher, S., Kunz, M., Strate, P., et al., 2005. Age effects on pain thresholds, temporal summation and spatial summation of heat and pressure pain. Pain. 115 (3), 410–418.

Lavsky-Shulan, M., Wallace, R.B., Kohout, F.J., et al., 1985. Prevalence and functional correlates of low back pain in the elderly: the Iowa 65+ rural health study. J. Am. Geriatr. Soc. 33 (1), 23–28.

Leong, I.Y., Nuo, T.H., 2007. Prevalence of pain in nursing home residents with different cognitive and communicative abilities. Clin. J. Pain. 23 (2), 119–127.

Leung, W.S., McMillan, A.S., Wong, M.C., 2008. Chronic orofacial pain in southern Chinese people: experience, associated disability, and help-seeking response. J. Orofac. Pain. 22 (4), 323–330.

Leveille, S.G., Gurlanik, J.M., Ferrucci, L., et al., 1998. Foot pain and disability in older women. Am. J. Epidemiol. 148 (7), 657–665.

Leventhal, E.A., Prohaska, T.R., 1986. Age, symptom interpretation, and health behaviour. J. Am. Geriatr. Soc. 34 (3), 185–191.

Li, Y., Duckles, S.P., 1993. Effect of age on vascular content of calcitonin gene-related peptide and mesenteric vasodilator activity in the rat. Eur. J. Pharmacol. 236 (3), 373–378.

Liddell, A., Locker, D., 1997. Gender and age differences in attitudes to dental pain and dental control. Community. Dent. Oral. Epidemiol. 25 (4), 314–318.

Lukas, A., Mayer, B., Fialová, D., Topinkova, E., Gindin, J., Onder, G., et al., 2013. Treatment of pain in European nursing homes: results from the services and health for elderly in long TERm Care (SHELTER) Study. J. Am. Med. Dir. Assoc. 14 (11), 821–831.

MacDonald, J.B., Baillie, J., Williams, B.O., 1983. Coronary care in the elderly. Age. Ageing. 12 (1), 17–20.

Machin, P., de C Williams, A.C., 1998. Stiff upper lip: coping strategies of World War II veterans with phantom limb pain. Clin. J. Pain. 14 (4), 290–294.

Magni, G., Marchetti, M., Moreschi, C., et al., 1993. Chronic musculoskeletal pain and depression in the national health and nutrition examination. Pain. 53 (2), 163–168.

Mäntyselkä, P., Hartikainen, S., Louhivuori-Laako, K., et al., 2004. Effects of dementia on perceived daily pain in home-dwelling elderly people: a population-based study. Age. Ageing. 33 (5), 496–499.

McBeth, J., Jones, K., 2007. Epidemiology of chronic musculoskeletal pain. Clin. Rheumatol. 21 (3), 403–425.

McCracken, L.M., 1998. Learning to live with the pain: acceptance of pain predicts adjustment in persons with chronic pain. Pain. 74 (1), 21–27.

McMillan, S.C., 1989. The relationship between age and intensity of cancer related symptoms. Oncol. Nurs. Forum. 16, 237–342.

Meucci, R.D., Fassa, A.G., Faria, N.M.X., 2015. Prevalence of chronic low back pain: systematic review. Rev. Saude. Publica. 49 (0), 1–10.

Miller, P.F., Sheps, D.S., Bragdon, E.E., 1990. Aging and pain perception in ischemic heart disease. Am. Heart. J. 120 (1), 22–30.

Mimi, M., Ho, S.S., 2013. Pain management for older persons living in nursing homes: a pilot study. Pain. Manag. Nurs. 14 (2), e10–e21.

Molton, I.R., Terrill, A.L., 2014. Overview of persistent pain in older adults. Am. Psychol. 69 (2), 197–207.

Morrison, R.S., Ahronheim, J.C., Morrison, G.R., et al., 1998. Pain and discomfort associated with common hospital procedures and experiences. J. Pain. Symptom. Manage. 15 (2), 91–101.

Oberle, K., Paul, P., Wry, J., 1990. Pain, anxiety and analgesics: a comparative study of elderly and younger surgical patients. Can. J. Aging. 9 (1), 13–19.

Ochoa, J., Mair, W.G.P., 1969. The normal sural nerve in man. II. Changes in the axon and Schwann cells due to ageing. Acta. Neuropathol. 13 (3), 217–253.

O'Reilly, M., Courtney, M., Edwards, H., Hassall, S., 2011. Clinical outcomes in residential care: setting benchmarks for quality. Australas. J. Ageing. 30 (2), 63–69.

Parker, S.J., Jessel, S., Richardson, J.E., Reid, M.C., 2013. Older adults are mobile too! Identifying the barriers and facilitators to older adults' use of mHealth for pain management. BMC. Geriatr. 13 (1), 43.

Parmelee, P.A., Smith, B., Katz, I.R., 1993. Pain complaints and cognitive status among elderly institution residents. J. Am. Geriatr. Soc. 41, 517–522.

Patel, K.V., Guralnik, J.M., Dansie, E.J., Turk, D.C., 2013. Prevalence and impact of pain among older adults in the United States: findings from the 2011 National Health and Aging Trends Study. Pain. 154 (12), 2649–2657.

Pautex, S., Herrmann, F., Le Lous, P., et al., 2005. Feasibility and reliability of four pain self-assessment scales and correlation with an observational rating scale in hospitalized elderly demented patients. J. Gerontol. A. Biol. Sci. Med. Sci. 60, 524–529.

Pickering, G., 2005. Age differences in clinical pain states. In: Gibson, S.J., Weiner, D.K. (Eds.), Pain in Older Persons, Progress in Pain Research and Management. IASP Press, Seattle, pp. 67–86.

Porter, F.L., Malhotra, K.M., Wolf, C.M., et al., 1996. Dementia and response to pain in the elderly. Pain. 68 (2,3), 413–421.

Proctor, W.R., Hirdes, J.P., 2001. Pain and cognitive status among nursing home residents in Canada. Pain. Res. Manag. 6 (3), 119–125.

Rajkumar, A.P., Ballard, C., Fossey, J., Orrell, M., Moniz-Cook, E., Woods, R.T., et al., 2017. Epidemiology of pain in people with dementia living in care homes: longitudinal course, prevalence, and treatment implications. J. Am. Med. Dir. Assoc. 18 (5), 453.e451–453.e456.

Rittger, H., Rieber, J., Breithardt, O.A., et al., 2011. Influence of age on pain perception in acute myocardial ischemia: a possible cause for delayed treatment in elderly patients. Int. J. Cardiol. 149 (1), 63–67.

Rottenberg, Y., Jacobs, J.M., Stessman, J., 2015. Prevalence of pain with advancing age brief report. J. Am. Med. Dir. Assoc. 16 (3), 264.e261–264.e265.

Royal College of Physicians, British Geriatrics Society, British Pain Society, 2007. Concise Guidance to Good Practice Series, No 8 the Assessment of Pain in Older People: National Guidelines. Royal College of Physicians, British Geriatrics Society and British Pain Society, London. Online. Available from https://www.britishpainsociety.org/static/uploads/resources/files/book_pain_older_people.pdf.

Ruzicka, S.A., 1998. Pain beliefs: what do elders believe? J. Holist. Nurs. 16 (3), 369–382.

Sawyer, P., Lillis, J.P., Bodner, E.V., et al., 2007. Substantial daily pain among nursing home residents. J. Am. Med. Dir. Assoc. 8 (3), 158–165.

Scherder, E., Herr, K., Pickering, G., et al., 2009. Pain in dementia. Pain. 145 (3), 276–278.

Schofield, P., 2018. The assessment of pain in older people: UK National Guidelines. Age. Ageing. 47 (Suppl 1), i1–i22.

Smith, B.H., Elliott, A.M., Chambers, W.A., et al., 2001. The impact of chronic pain in the community. Fam. Pract. 18 (3), 292–299.

Sorkin, B.A., Rudy, T.E., Hanlon, R.B., et al., 1990. Chronic pain in old and young patients: differences appear less important than similarities. J. Gerontol. A. Biol. Sci. Med. Sci. 45 (2), 64–68.

Statistics Korea, 2020. 2020 Statistics on the Aged. Available from: http://kostat.go.kr/portal/eng/pressReleases/11/3/index.board.

Sternbach, R.A., 1986. Survey of pain in the United States: the Nuprin pain report. Clin. J. Pain. 2 (1), 49–54.

Stoller, E.P., 1993. Interpretations of symptoms by older people: a health diary study of illness behaviour. J. Aging. Health. 5 (1), 58–81.

Takahashi, N., Takatsuki, K., Kasahara, S., Yabuki, S., 2019. Multidisciplinary pain management program for patients with chronic musculoskeletal pain in Japan: a cohort study. J. Pain. Res. 12, 2563–2576.

Tan, E.C., Jokanovic, N., Koponen, M., Thomas, D., Hilmer, S.N., Bell, J.S., 2015. Prevalence of analgesic use and pain in people with and without dementia or cognitive impairment in aged care facilities: a systematic review and meta-analysis. Curr. Clin. Pharmacol. 10 (3), 194–203.

Tan, E.C., Visvanathan, R., Hilmer, S.N., Vitry, A., Emery, T., Robson, L., et al., 2016. Analgesic use and pain in residents with and without dementia in aged care facilities: a cross-sectional study. Australas. J. Ageing. 35 (3), 180–187.

Teno, J., Bird, C., Mor, V., 2003. The Prevalence and Treatment of Pain in US Nursing Homes. Centre for Gerontology and Health Care Research, Brown University, Providence, RI.

Teno, J.M., Kabumoto, G., Wetle, T., et al., 2004. Daily pain that was excruciating at some time in the previous week: prevalence, characteristics, and outcomes in nursing home residents. J. Am. Geriatr. Soc. 52 (5), 762–767.

Teno, J.M., Weitzen, S., Wetle, T., et al., 2001. Persistent pain in nursing home residents. J. Am. Med. Assoc. 285 (16), 2081.

Thomas, T., Robinson, C., Champion, D., 1998. Prediction and assessment of the severity of post operative pain and of satisfaction with management. Pain. 75 (2,3), 177–185.

Tibblin, G., Bengtsson, C., Furness, B., et al., 1990. Symptoms by age and sex. Scand. J. Prim. Health. Care. 8 (1), 9–17.

Toth, M., Palmer, L.A.M., Bercaw, L.E., Johnson, R., Jones, J., Love, R., et al., 2020. Understanding the Characteristics of Older Adults in Different Residential Settings: Data Sources and Trends. U.S. Department of Health and Human Services. Available from: https://aspe.hhs.gov/reports/understanding-characteristics-older-adults-different-residential-settings-data-sources-trends.

Tracy, B., Morrison, R.S., 2013. Pain management in older adults. Clin. Therapeut. 35 (11), 1659–1668.

Tsang, A., Von Korff, M., Lee, S., et al., 2008. Common chronic pain conditions in developed and developing countries: gender and age differences and comorbidity with depression-anxiety disorders. J. Pain. 9, 883–891.

United Nations, Department of Economic and Social Affairs, Population Division, 2017. World Population Ageing 2017 - Highlights (ST/ESA/SER.A/397). Available from: https://www.un.org/en/development/desa/population/publications/pdf/ageing/WPA2017_Highlights.pdf.

United Nations, Department of Economic and Social Affairs, Population Division, 2019. World Population Ageing 2019: Highlights (ST/ESA/SER.A/430). Available from: https://www.

un.org/en/development/desa/population/publications/pdf/ageing/WorldPopulationAgeing2019-Highlights.pdf.

Vigano, A., Bruera, E., Suarex-Almazor, M.E., 1998. Age, pain intensity, and opioid dose in patients with advanced cancer. Cancer. 83 (6), 1244–1250.

Von Korff, M., Dworkin, S.F., Le Resche, L., 1990. Graded chronic pain status: an epidemiologic evaluation. Pain. 40 (3), 279–291.

Von Korff, M., Dworkin, S.F., Le Resche, L., et al., 1988. An epidemiologic comparison of pain complaints. Pain. 32 (2), 173–183.

Walid, M.S., Zaytseva, N., 2009. Pain in nursing home residents and correlation with neuropsychiatric disorders. Pain. Physician. 12 (5), 877–880.

Washington, L.L., Gibson, S.J., Helme, R.D., 2000. Age-related differences in the endogenous analgesic response to repeated cold water immersion in human volunteers. Pain. 89 (1), 89–96.

Watkins, K.W., Shifren, K., Park, D.C., et al., 1999. Age, pain, and coping with rheumatoid arthritis. Pain. 82 (3), 217–228.

Weiner, D.K., Peterson, B.L., Logue, P., et al., 1998. Predictors of pain self-report in nursing home residents. Aging. Clin. Exp. Res. 10, 411–420.

Weiner, D.K., Rudy, T.E., 2002. Attitudinal barriers to effective treatment of persistent pain in nursing home residents. J. Am. Geriatr. Soc. 50 (12), 2035–2040.

World Health Organization, 2021. Ageing and Health. Available from https://www.who.int/news-room/fact-sheets/detail/ageing-and-health.

Wroblewski, M., Mikulowski, P., 1991. Peritonitis in geriatric inpatients. Age. Ageing. 20 (2), 90–94.

Wu, N., Miller, S.C., Lapane, K., et al., 2005. Impact of cognitive function on assessments of nursing home residents' pain. Med. Care. 43 (9), 934–939.

Yong, H.H., 2006. Can attitudes of stoicism and cautiousness explain observed age-related variation in levels of self-rated pain, mood disturbance and functional interference in chronic pain patients? Eur. J. Pain. 10, 399–407.

Yong, H.H., Bell, R., Workman, B., et al., 2003. Psychometric properties of the Pain Attitudes Questionnaire (revised) in adult patients with chronic pain. Pain. 104 (3), 673–681.

Yong, H.H., Gibson, S.J., Horne, D.J., et al., 2001. Development of a pain attitudes questionnaire to assess stoicism and cautiousness for possible age differences. J. Gerontol. Psychol. Serv. 56B (5), 279–284.

Zheng, Z., Gibson, S.J., Helme, R.D., et al., 2009. The effect of local anaesthetic on age-related capsaicin- induced mechanical hyperalgesia: a randomised, controlled study. Pain. 144 (1,2), 101–109.

Zheng, Z., Gibson, S.J., Khalil, Z., et al., 2000. Age-related differences in the time course of capsaicin- induced hyperalgesia. Pain. 85 (1,2), 51–58.

Zwakhalen, S.M., Hamers, J.P., Berger, M.P., 2006. The psychometric quality and clinical usefulness of three pain assessment tools for elderly people with dementia. Pain. 126 (1–3), 210–220.

Chapter | 21 |

Cancer pain

Janet Hardy, Sally Bennett, Geoffrey Mitchell, and Jenny Strong

LEARNING OBJECTIVES

At the end of this chapter, readers will be able to:
1. Understand the magnitude of the problem of cancer pain.
2. Understand the circumstances in the cancer journey when pain may occur.
3. Describe the types of pain.
4. Understand that the experience of pain can have physical, psychological and spiritual dimensions.
5. Understand the principles of pain management.
6. Understand the barriers to good pain management.
7. Appreciate the personal issues confronted by therapists dealing with cancer pain.

Overview

Pain is one of the most common symptoms in cancer. It is also one of the most feared, and patients frequently equate cancer with intolerable pain. In the patient's mind, the onset of pain can also herald disease progression and an inexorable march towards death. Cancer pain differs from chronic noncancer pain in some ways, but in other ways, it is very similar. The basic mechanisms that generate pain responses are the same. Treatment will involve similar techniques but will also include cancer-specific therapies like radiotherapy or chemotherapy.

The management of cancer-related pain is specific in many ways. The intensity of cancer pain is not static. The location and quality of the pain are more likely to change because of the dynamic nature of the illness and the treatment. The person with cancer may have multiple pain problems and interrelated symptoms that complicate management. While opioids should be avoided in patients with chronic nonmalignant pain, if at all possible, they usually form the mainstay of pain management in cancer patients.

The meaning of a change in pain may be frightening and this fear can exacerbate the experience of pain. One of the biggest differences lies in the psychological, emotional and spiritual import that pain carries. Therapists need to be mindful of this potential and adapt their approach accordingly. If the pain a patient suffers is not controlled with what appears to be appropriate therapy, it is possible that there is an emotional component to the problem that must be addressed. Further, therapists working in this area will find their own attitudes and beliefs about pain, suffering and death challenged by the experiences and responses they encounter in their patients. It is therefore important to consider personal attitudes and to consider how to approach patients whose beliefs may differ from the therapists.

This chapter will consider the problem of pain experienced in cancer from a range of perspectives. The causes of cancer pain will be briefly described. Differentiating pain and suffering is important, and the therapist needs to recognise that all aspects of the person's pain experience must be addressed. Cancer pain management will be discussed in some detail, with an overview of medication management and consideration of nonmedication management of pain. However, this is not a text on how to manage pain. Useful resources include the Clinical Practice Guidelines, Adult Cancer Pain (v2.2019) published by the National Comprehensive Cancer Network (NCCN) (National Comprehensive Cancer Network 2019) and the European Guidelines for the management of cancer-related pain (Bennett et al. 2019).

Box 21.1 defines some key terms.

Frequency of pain in cancer

Pain in cancer is common, increasing in frequency as death approaches (Aman et al. 2021; van den Beuken-van Everdingen et al. 2007). Most studies report a frequency range, such as 54%–92% (Teunissen et al. 2007), with such differences in prevalence largely due to differences in definition, the point in the disease trajectory and the setting where the measures take place. For example, the documented prevalence of pain in palliative care and pain centres is higher than in oncology settings.

It is important to note that pain is not universal in people with cancer and that some people have no pain at all. In one study concentrating on the palliative phase of cancer, 30% of people experienced no pain, 37% had minimal-to-mild pain, 28% described moderate-to-strong pain and 5% had severe-to-extreme pain (Wilson et al. 2009).

Types of cancer pain

Symptoms can be defined as 'subjective experience[s] reflecting changes in the biopsychosocial functioning, sensations, or cognition of an individual' (Dodd et al. 2001).

The *sensation* of pain arises from stimulation of nociceptors or damage to the neural tracts that carry pain. However, the *experience* of pain is modified by a range of factors.

Cancer pain can be directly attributable to tumour growth and invasion of structures, or be associated with the treatment of cancer (e.g. chemotherapy-induced peripheral neuropathies or painful strictures from graft). Ashby was the first to demonstrate that classifying pain by its mechanistic basis influences the type of pain treatment that is offered (Ashby et al. 1992). Two broad categories of pain are recognised: nociceptive pain and nonnociceptive pain (see Chapter 7). Nociceptive pain arises from the stimulation of nociceptive receptors (see Table 21.1 for definition). The nature of this pain varies depending on the structures where those pain receptors are located (e.g. the capsule of the liver or lung). Non-nociceptive pain is either neuropathic (arising from damage to or disease of the neural tracts) or nonneurogenic (Finnerup et al. 2021).

With recent improvements in cancer treatment resulting in prolonged survival for many patients, cancer pain may be long-standing, with many chronic pain features. It can change with damage to tissues from tumour growth or treatment, and therefore has acute pain features.

Foley (1987) described five different types of cancer pain that still hold true today.

1. Acute pain associated with the cancer or the treatment. This often heralds the onset or recurrence of the illness, with associated psychological ramifications. In contrast, acute pain associated with treatment is often self-limiting and better tolerated by the patient if they are hopeful about outcome. Consequently, psychological effects may be limited. In both cases, treatment must be targeted to the cause of pain.

2. Chronic pain, either from the cancer or the therapy. Chronic pain associated with the cancer usually reflects tumour progression and psychological issues become much more important. Anxiety and feelings of hopelessness can further exacerbate the pain. Chronic pain may also be due to soft tissue, nerve or bony injury related to cancer treatment, and be unrelated to the tumour. Identifying the cause of the pain is important to reassure the patient that the pain is not caused by cancer progression. Treatment of patients with chronic pain related to treatment is aimed at the symptom rather than the cause.

3. Chronic pain from another source, generally pre-existing. The patients often already have psychological and functional limitations and require considerable support as the presence of multiple illnesses is very taxing.

4. Pain in patients actively involved with illicit drug use. These patients are very difficult to treat. It is important to differentiate any drugs used to treat the cancer pain from drugs of dependence (Hardy et al. 2020).

TABLE 21.1 Mechanistic classification of cancer pain

| | NOCICEPTIVE | | | NEUROGENIC | |
Superficial somatic	**Deep somatic**	**Visceral**			
Origin of stimulus	1. Skin, subcutaneous tissue	1. Bone, joints, ligaments, tendons, muscles	1. Within solid or hollow organs	1. Pure deafferentation	
	2. Mucosal surfaces, e.g. mouth, urethra	2. Superficial lymph nodes	2. Deep tumour masses	2. Mixed: nociceptive element due to tumour invasion or nerve compression	
		3. Organ capsules, pleura and peritoneum	3. Deep lymph nodes		
Examples	Malignant ulcers, stomatitis	Bony metastases, liver capsule distension	Gut obstruction, ureteric colic	1. Pure: postherpetic neuralgia, phantom pain 2. Mixed: brachial plexus invasion, spinal cord compression	
Description	Burning, stinging	Dull aching may be aggravated by movement (e.g. deep breath or cough in pleural involvement)Capsular involvement is not aggravated by movement	Dull, deep colicky pain	1. Abnormal sensation, e.g. tingling, burning, pins and needles 2. Allodynia 3. Lancinating, shooting 4. Phantom	
Localisation	Very well defined	Well defined	Poor	Nerve or dermatomal distribution	
Referral	No	Maybe	Maybe	Yes	
Local tenderness	Yes	Yes	Maybe	No	
Autonomic effects	No	No	Sweating, vomiting, nausea, BP and heart rate changes	Autonomic instability, e.g. warmth, cold, sweating, pallor	

BP, Blood pressure.

Modified from Ashby, M.A., Fleming, B.G., Brooksbank M, Rounsefell, B., Runciman, W.B., Jackson, K., et al., 1992. Description of a mechanistic approach to pain management in advanced cancer. Preliminary report. Pain 51 (2), 153–161.

---

5. Cancer pain in patients who are dying. The focus of treatment is on maximising comfort and providing psychological care.

Therapists need to take into account the complexity and changing nature of cancer pain. Pain management approaches vary depending on the site of pain, chronicity of pain, characteristics of the individual patient and the stage of disease. Therapists may modify their pain management approaches according to whether the patient is on active treatment with a likelihood of recovery, or is dying and receiving palliative care. There are different management procedures for treatment and palliation phases. Careful assessment and flexibility in management are vital.

Impact of and responses to cancer pain

The presence of cancer pain impacts significantly on the quality of life (QOL) of the patient and their family. Pain interacts with a range of other symptoms such as fatigue, nausea and constipation, amplifying their impact and that of the pain. Although the physical aspects of pain are commonly evident, people experiencing cancer pain also experience a range of psychological, social and spiritual challenges.

Anxiety, depression, anger and a sense of helplessness are common responses to unrelieved cancer pain. In turn, depression and anxiety related to a cancer pain and its treatment can aggravate pain. People with advanced cancer and severe pain are twice as likely to experience clinical depression and three times more likely to have an anxiety disorder as those with less severe pain (Wilson et al. 2009). Pain may also impact on a person's cognitive function, particularly placing greater demands on memory. Not surprisingly, the effect of ongoing pain is to reduce the individual's feeling of control. It is important for the therapist to acknowledge this sense of loss of control and to modify their approach accordingly, for example, letting the individual chose the preferred time for therapy, rather than the therapist scheduling treatment to suit themselves. The functional impact of cancer pain also limits peoples' ability to participate in meaningful activities, relationships and overall enjoyment of life.

An individual's experience and expression of pain is partly socioculturally determined. Their previous experience of pain within their family, and their culture's perception of pain, suffering and illness, influence the person's thoughts and coping styles with regard to pain. Many patients are cared for predominantly at home, and their pain management occurs at home. Therefore the patient and/or their family or carers are often responsible for medication and other pain-reducing procedures. It has been found that patients are often undermedicated due to beliefs held by themselves and/or their caregivers, e.g. that they should put up with pain as long as possible or until 'they really need it'. This can be compounded by fear of addiction (Darawad et al. 2019; Jho et al. 2014; Murnion et al. 2010). Responses to cancer pain therefore clearly relate in some part to the attitudes, beliefs and knowledge of patients and carers, and require appropriate education.

Cancer pain in the later phase of the disease suggests to patients that their disease is progressing. This opens questions about mortality and related spiritual issues. Spiritual distress may occur when there is conflict between the patient's experience of pain and suffering and their world view, leading to anxiety, depression, anger and withdrawal, as well as physical pain.

As in all pain situations, it is inappropriate to think of cancer pain as just physical. Dame Cicely Saunders used the phrase *total pain* to describe a person's suffering from physical, psychological, social, spiritual and practical distress. All aspects need attention and should be considered in the assessment and management of cancer pain.

Assessment and measurement of cancer pain

Readers are advised to refer to Chapter 8, which covers assessment and measurement issues. Inadequate cancer pain assessment results in poor control of pain, whereas the integration of a systematic bedside pain assessment tool into care has been shown to improve outcomes (Fallon et al. 2018). Pain assessment should involve assessment of:

- Pain intensity
- Characteristics/quality of the pain
- Pain history (sites, severity, duration, mood, previous pain experience, etc.)
- Factors that exacerbate or relieve pain
- Impact of pain on function and QoL
- Psychosocial factors (patient distress, psychiatric history, social supports, etc.)
- Cultural, spiritual and religious considerations
- Patient's goals and expectations.

In addition, a thorough physical examination, laboratory studies and imaging results need to be considered.

Assessment considerations

Assessment of cancer pain should be multidimensional and multidisciplinary. Pain involves a complexity of sensory, cognitive, behavioural and affective phenomena, requiring a coordinated assessment effort by different disciplines. The source of the pain can be identified by assessing the location, distribution, quality, intensity and duration (see Table 21.1). Comprehensive assessment of pain should also consider other symptoms that may interact with, and exacerbate, pain, such as fatigue. Awareness of suffering and other psychosocial and spiritual distress in association with cancer pain is essential for good palliative care. Hence, a multidimensional approach to assessment that encompasses evaluation of the patient's physical, social and psychological function and spiritual needs is vital.

Patients with cancer pain may have reporting biases because cancer is an anxiety-provoking condition. They may fear that a change in pain may reflect progression of disease. Therefore there is a need to assess in a way to minimise bias, either towards underreporting or overreporting. People may underreport their pain due to a concern about not being a nuisance to ward staff or family members, or due to denial of the increasing seriousness of their condition. A new pain in a patient with cancer should always be investigated thoroughly. It may signal a treatable new problem or the exacerbation of an existing problem that requires reassessment. A change in the patient's report of pain should be reported immediately to the treating physician and other members of the team.

One of the key recommendations for the assessment of cancer pain is that it is reassessed at frequent intervals (National Comprehensive Cancer Network 2019). Cancer pain should be assessed frequently to fully understand changes in the pain and underlying influences, such as the temporal relationship to the time of last medication, physical activity, anxiety or time of day. In addition, the time of day that pain is assessed is important. For example, a patient's cancer pain may be worse in the early evening and better in the early morning.

Frequency of assessment will depend to some extent on the setting and type of pain. If the patient's pain is stable and they are attending as an outpatient, pain can be monitored during appointments, or the patient can be asked to keep a diary. Patients should be given the opportunity to not only describe their pain at the consultation, but also give an overall picture of the pain at its worst and its best. In this way, the therapist is able to build up a more complete understanding of the variability in the patient's pain.

The fluctuations in pain relative to various reference points, such as the time of day, medication status, activity level or anticipation of some event, should be charted. Patients with uncontrolled pain need frequent assessment. In this situation, pain should probably be assessed at least daily and sometimes more often, particularly to determine response to treatments (National Comprehensive Cancer Network 2019). The measurement tools for this type of assessment regimen need to be accurate, brief and comprehensive to avoid overtaxing the person. They should also be appropriate for multiple evaluations and reliable and practical for use with severely ill people.

As pain is subjective, the patient's self-report should be a standard source of assessment. In order for this to be an effective policy to follow, the treatment ethic of the clinical service must encourage accuracy in patient self-report by acting on information provided by the patient. Clinicians should provide sufficient education about the aspects of illness and its treatment so that the patient is unafraid to give information about their pain. Simply asking a question such as, 'How is your pain?' does not provide enough opportunity to fully describe it. Various tools which have been shown to be sensitive and reliable should be used (see Chapter 8).

Methods for assessing pain include Numerical Rating Scales (NRS), Visual Analogue Scales (VAS) and the McGill Pain Questionnaire (MPQ) (Chapter 8). NRS and the VAS are quickly administered and easy to use with patients with cancer. Its reliability has been established with patients with cancer. The MPQ is longer but is multidimensional and also has good psychometric properties. If the patient is especially ill or fatigued, the short-form MPQ can be used.

Patients should be asked to describe the characteristics or quality of pain. Particular descriptive words can give valuable clues about the cause of the pain. For example, pain described as burning or tingling is likely to involve neural structures. Assessment of symptoms that may interact with pain may be achieved through symptom-specific measures or through measures that assess multiple prevalent cancer-related symptoms, such as the Memorial Symptom Assessment Scale (Chang et al. 2004).

There are many approaches to the measurement of function and wider patient concerns. Disease-specific QOL instruments are one way of ascertaining the interface between cancer pain, other symptoms and functioning. Several measures of QOL for the patient with cancer have been developed which have acceptable psychometric properties. The Functional Assessment of Cancer Therapy (FACT) Scale is a brief, 33-item, self-report measure of QOL over the past week. It covers physical well-being, social/family well-being, relationship with doctor and emotional and functional well-being (Overcash et al. 2001).

Another measure is the European Organization for Research and Treatment of Cancer Quality of Life Questionnaire (QLQ-C30) (Mercieca-Bebber et al. 2019). It consists of 30 items which tap 9 subscales of function (physical, role, cognitive, emotional and social) and associated cancer-related symptoms such as fatigue, pain, nausea and vomiting, global health, and QOL. A shorter 15-item version (QLQ-C15) is much more likely to be completed by easily fatigued cancer patients (Groenvold et al. 2006).

In general, in assessing a person's pain, a structured or semi-structured questionnaire format is preferable, as it is more objective and reduces the number of details that can be inadvertently forgotten. However, incorporating an interview can add valuable information and foster a good working rapport with the patient and their family.

Impact of pain on the occupations of daily life

Pain from cancer can have significant impact on an individual's occupations of daily life. Associated fatigue can also impair occupational performance. Patterns of activity, ability to perform functional activities of daily living, ability to meet desired occupational goals, QOL and coping strategies should therefore be assessed. The impact of the pain and the cancer on the person's ability to mobilise should be considered by physiotherapists. The impact on performing daily life occupations should be a particular emphasis of the occupational therapist. Specific forms of cancer (e.g. head and neck malignancies) may impact a person's ability to swallow; this should be carefully assessed by speech pathologists and speech and language therapists.

Aggravating and alleviating factors of the cancer pain should be investigated by asking the patient and by observation. A patient's attitudes towards, and beliefs about, pain and taking medication need to be taken into consideration when attempting to gather a true understanding of the patient's level of pain. Therapists should be particularly attuned to the patient's desired occupational goals and should work to enable patients to attain meaningful occupational goals that are within the capability of the patient. This might be as simple as being able to get out of bed unaided or walking short distances.

Family context

The family context is another aspect to be considered. Family members may have many fears and beliefs about cancer, about the 'horror' of cancer pain, about the potential for addiction from medication and about the ways they can best care for their loved one. This requires the careful attention of the treatment team. For example, the family may be resolute in the need to care for their family member with advanced cancer within the home environment, despite seemingly major obstacles to such management. Both conscious and unconscious interactions between patient and family are relevant to the design and implementation of a pain management plan. In the team, the professional responsibility for gathering information about family relationships and pain may vary. However, it is always necessary for the therapist to be at least aware of the details already gathered in designing their part of the intervention strategies. In summary, pain assessment for people with cancer needs to occur frequently and take into account the multidimensional nature of pain, factors which influence it and the impact it may have on both the person with cancer pain and their family (Smyth et al. 2018).

Principles of pain management

In all situations where pain management is required by patients, a collaborative team approach is the preferred method of practice. Beyond this, it has been determined that supporting active patient involvement in their therapy is important. That is, patients should be involved in decisions about treatment regimens and timing of pain interventions around their lifestyle as much as possible. Such active patient involvement is important, in part, in counteracting the feelings of loss of control.

Broadly speaking, cancer pain management can be categorised into pharmacological and nonpharmacological means.

Pharmacological means of pain control

The World Health Organization devised the WHO pain ladder (Fig. 21.1) as a means of assisting in decisions

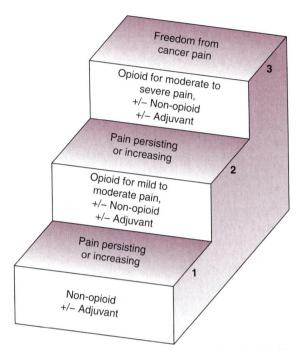

Fig. 21.1 WHO Pain Relief Ladder. (Reprinted from the World Health Organization 1986, with kind permission, http://www.who.int/cancer/palliative/painladder/en/.)

around pain management (World Health Organization 2020). The ladder contains three levels or steps: nonopioid agents, weak opioids and strong opioids, corresponding to mild, moderate and severe pain. The main function of the pain ladder was to introduce simple principles for pain management and legitimise the use of opioids for chronic pain in areas of the world where access is either severely restricted or banned altogether. Although often criticised, it has been of significant benefit for the control of pain worldwide (Yang et al. 2020).

Nonopioid medications include paracetamol, aspirin and nonsteroidal antiinflammatory agents (NSAIDs). They are effective at relieving mild pain and are the drugs of choice in cancer pain management at step 1. They are also safe when used according to guidelines, although there are side effects. Paracetamol causes liver toxicity in severe overdose but is safe when taken as directed. Long-term aspirin (rarely used nowadays for pain management) can cause gastrointestinal upset and bleeding and may be contraindicated in patients with a predisposition to stomach upsets or reflux, or who are at risk of bleeding. NSAIDS similarly can cause gastric irritation and are relatively contraindicated in patients with renal impairment or heart failure. Both analgesic aspirin and NSAIDS should be taken with caution by people already taking anticoagulants such as warfarin and covered by the concurrent use of proton pump inhibitors such as pantoprazole.

Drugs such as codeine, often in combination with paracetamol or NSAIDs, are often used at step 2. Other options at this level are agents such as tramadol and tapentadol that are not pure opioids, but have some opioid-like activity.

Opioids

Opioids are the mainstay of cancer pain treatment and are appropriate for use at low dose at step 2 of the WHO analgesic ladder for moderate pain or at higher dose at step 3 (Caraceni et al. 2012). They are very powerful analgesics that can be titrated from small doses to very large doses if needed. They are particularly effective when the pain is nociceptive in origin. They can be used for neurogenic pain, but the effect is less certain and other agents (co-analgesics or adjuvants) often need to be employed concurrently. The other major advantage of opioids is the range of formulations available and the different means of delivery. They can be taken orally in short- or long-acting preparations, transdermally via skin patches, parenterally as an injection or subcutaneously through a portable pump device. Opioids can even be administered directly to the central nervous system via the epidural or intrathecal space.

Opioids have a number of side effects. For people who have never taken them before, there may be transient nausea and mental clouding. Constipation is almost inevitable and a constant side effect for as long as the drug is taken. It is mandatory for a laxative that stimulates bowel movement to be prescribed at the same time as an opioid. Other side effects include drowsiness, dry mouth and muscle twitches (myoclonus). In overdose, opioids can cause serious respiratory depression and loss of consciousness. Overdose is entirely avoidable if the dose is started low and escalated slowly. Overdose can occur unintentionally in people with impaired renal function because some opioids, for example morphine, are excreted renally. Fentanyl, buprenorphine and methadone are not dependent on renal function for elimination.

The most common opioids used are morphine, oxycodone, fentanyl and buprenorphine. Less commonly used opioids are methadone and hydromorphone.

Adjuvants

The term 'adjuvant' refers to medicines that modify pain without being analgesics 'per se'. In nociceptive pain, they act by reducing the factors that stimulate nociceptive receptors. Hence, NSAIDs and steroids reduce the release of inflammatory mediators that cause nociceptive

stimulation. Antispasmodic agents reduce the colicky pain that accompanies a blocked hollow organ like the gut or the bile duct.

In neurogenic (or neuropathic) pain, adjuvant therapies are the mainstay of treatment. They modify neural transmission and alter the perception of stimuli once they reach the brain. Groups of medicines that work in this way include antiepileptics, anti-arrythmics and local anaesthetic agents. They work much more slowly than analgesics and must be titrated slowly upwards to avoid unwanted side effects. Many adjuvants in this class can be sedating. However, they are used widely because they can be effective and do not have the side effects of strong analgesics (Kong & Irwin 2009).

Comprehensive detail on the use of medicines is outside the scope of this chapter and has been provided in the pharmacology chapter in this textbook. For further detail, recommended reading includes the on-line Therapeutic Guidelines series (Therapeutic Guidelines: Palliative Care 2020) or the NCCN Clinical Practice Guidelines in Oncology—Adult Cancer Pain V2 (National Comprehensive Cancer Network 2019).

Therapists' understanding of pharmacological approaches to cancer pain management

While the management of medication regimens is the concern of physicians, pharmacists and nurses, knowledge of the commonly used drugs and methods of administration and mechanisms of action is important for therapists. This can help therapists to answer questions, support a patient's understanding of the role of medication and structure their therapy around the most optimal times.

A therapist may realise that the patient is not taking the medication appropriately. Fear that addiction might occur or that medication should not be taken until the pain is severe, and other misunderstandings about pain medication, may result in the patient receiving poor pain relief. Therapists should clarify and redirect the patient to their physician if required. Therapists may also be more aware of whether the patient experiences side effects, and whether the medication is improving or hindering the client's occupational performance. Possible side effects of medications such as opioids may impact upon the patient's safe performance of activities of daily living (ADLs) such as stair walking or driving. The reader is referred to Chapter 15 for a comprehensive consideration of pharmacological methods.

Nonpharmacological medical methods

Nonpharmacological medical methods may be used for patients in whom adequate relief of pain is not achieved by pharmacological methods. Common examples of these are listed in Box 21.1. Methods used include radiation therapy, surgery and neurosurgical procedures such as nerve blocks or neuroablation. Best practice guidelines for the Interventional Management of Cancer-Associated Pain have recently been published by the American Society of Pain and Neuroscience (Aman et al. 2021). An understanding of the reasons for performing these procedures, in the case of each individual patient, is the professional responsibility of the therapist.

Therapists may be involved in the postprocedural rehabilitation of the patient. Physiotherapists and occupational therapists work with such patients to maximise independence, increase safety in the activities of daily living, teach energy conservation techniques and work with clients on attaining valued occupational goals (Hesselstrand 2015).

Education

Education about pain and pain management techniques is essential for people with cancer, and their family and caregivers. Since much of the care is conducted on an outpatient basis, patients and families will assume considerable responsibility and should therefore be included in discussions about management of pain where possible. Studies attest to several misconceptions held by patients with cancer and their family members which interfere with good pain management. These include the view that pain medicines should be spared until the pain is *really* bad, the belief that they could become addicted to their medication and the fear of getting bad side effects from taking pain relief medication (Darawad et al. 2019; Rafii et al. 2021). Patients can also be reticent to report their pain to their doctors as they fear that pain could be an indicator of disease progression.

Individualised education and coaching to address misconceptions about pain and its treatment, and to encourage increased patient communication about their pain with their oncologists and healthcare team, is therefore important. Recent systematic reviews and randomised controlled trials of patient education programmes for people with cancer pain have indicated modest improvements in terms of pain reduction (Bennett et al. 2009; Lovell et al. 2014; Yates et al. 2004). A systematic review of interventions to improve patient understanding of pain compared with no intervention found improvement in knowledge and attitudes, and average and worst pain intensity by 1 point on a 10-point scale. There is evidence of a modest, but significant, improvement in pain, suggesting that education should be considered alongside other pain-relieving treatments (Bennett et al. 2009). Education in pain management in cancer patients requires repeated information, allowing time for overcoming

resistance related to dysfunctional beliefs and fear (Ekstedt & Rustøen 2019).

The following aspects are considered basic requirements in patient education programmes:

1. Information about the principles of assessing and managing cancer pain.
2. A discussion about beliefs and misconceptions about opioid use and how these can interfere with good management.
3. Information about different pain medications, dosage and scheduling.
4. Provision of tools for monitoring pain, medication and activities, such as a pain diary.

It is not completely clear what the most effective content, delivery methods and timing of such programmes are (Hoffmann 2010). Principles of effective health education and communication that use a patient-centred approach are particularly valuable. Patient-centred communication acknowledges the patients' needs, goals and expectations and tailors communication and education to the needs, abilities and preferences of the individual (Hoffmann & Tooth 2010). Multiple methods of delivery should be used, including written materials, audio-delivered information such as CDs, visual material and discussions.

Nonpharmacological physical methods

Other nonpharmacological physical methods that are noninvasive and may be applied by a therapist or supported if chosen by the patient include acupuncture, cutaneous stimulation, cold therapy, heat, exercise, careful positioning and immobilisation. The reader is referred to Chapters 11 and 14 for more detail about these techniques.

People who experience pain from cancer often protect themselves from pain by lying down or staying in certain positions for long periods of time. Gentle exercise plays an important role in reducing pain related to immobility through maximising the use of stiff joints and developing muscle strength. Further exercise can prevent painful contractures through nonuse of painful limbs. Exercise may range from a regular walking programme through to sitting out of bed in a chair or simple movements while lying in bed. Family members can encourage participation in any functional activities that also incorporate movement. Generally, some level of exercise is possible for all people with cancer throughout the varying stages of their disease, but the use of exercise should be monitored so as not to contribute to breakthrough pain, and tailored to individual needs (Cheville et al. 2019).

Exercise is also effective in the management of pain due to specific nerve or tissue damage. For example, patients with head and neck cancer who have shoulder disability and pain due to spinal accessory nerve damage have been shown to benefit from progressive resistive exercise (McNeely et al. 2008). Finally, exercise has been found to improve mood, which in turn may make it easier for people to cope with chronic pain (Dujits et al. 2011; López-Sendín et al. 2012).

Pain may be exacerbated by pressure in the region of the tumour or from being in one position for prolonged periods of time. Attention to positioning, correct body alignment and use of pillows and supports may relive pressure-related pain. Equipment that has adjustable features, such as reclining chairs, height-adjustable toilet seats and alternating pressure mattresses may assist in achieving temporary pain relief.

Cutaneous stimulation includes such methods as massage, pressure, heat, cold and transcutaneous electrical nerve stimulation (TENS, see Chapter 16). TENS units operate by producing small-intensity currents. Electrodes are applied to the skin overlying the painful area or along a nerve pathway. They appear to produce stimulation that 'overrides' or 'negates' the pain stimuli. A Cochrane review of the efficacy of TENS in chronic pain failed to identify studies of sufficient power or size to be able to recommend its routine use (Hurlow et al. 2012), although there is some evidence of benefit for the management of cancer bone pain (Searle et al. 2009). The stimulation may be applied to the painful area if the skin is not compromised.

Massage can relieve the pain of muscle spasm around a painful joint or the back and neck. It may improve pain thresholds, relax muscles and encourage lymphatic drainage. Although it may seem evident that massage is effective for relieving pain, the effects may be short term (Kutner et al. 2008). Caution is required to avoid massage directly to tumour sites or to recently irradiated tissue that may be sensitive. NCCN guidelines recommend the use of massage, but systematic reviews point to the lack of quality evidence to support this (Shin et al. 2016).

General musculoskeletal pain may respond to the use of heat or cold packs, and again, care is required not to place these over previously irradiated areas. Cutaneous stimulation and other types of counterstimulation may offer relief to a patient at various times throughout the day while providing a sense of control over the treatment for the patient. However, an increase in the use of such methods initiated by patients should be carefully monitored in case it indicates the need for further medication management. These methods are not intended to replace pharmacological methods.

Psychosocial approaches

Psychosocial approaches to the management of cancer pain encompass a range of interventions, including cognitive behavioural therapy (CBT), relaxation, guided imagery, distraction and music. These can be powerful adjuncts to physical methods of pain relief.

CBT has been found to be helpful in the management of chronic pain (Williams et al. 2012) and has been recommended in guidelines for cancer pain management (Miaskowski et al. 2005). In short, CBT targets a person's perception of cancer pain and attempts to modify behaviours and/or related cognitions. Although individualised CBT can be effective in managing cancer pain, there is no clear evidence of benefit from group delivery (Tatrow & Montgomery 2006). This approach has been covered in more detail in other parts of this book. There is value in introducing psychosocial methods early in the course of the illness when the patient's cognitive capacity is more likely to be sufficient to understand concepts. In this way, the support element of intervention is developed early enough to be well established by the time the patient may need supportive psychotherapy.

A variety of relaxation methods are available, including progressive muscle relaxation (PMR), guided imagery yoga and meditation (Charalambous et al. 2016). These are often used in conjunction with, or as part of, cognitive–behavioural approaches. Guided imagery may be used alone or in conjunction with another relaxation technique. Therapists can train patients in PMR so that they are able to use the relaxation method at any time. Ideally, patients need to be trained in PMR while they are pain free or have relatively low pain intensity and while they are able to concentrate. Sometimes it will not be possible to teach PMR if patients are concurrently taking analgesic medication that is impairing their mental functioning. The development of proficiency in muscle relaxation while undistracted by moderate-to-severe pain will increase the likelihood that the technique will be used with positive results when pain intensity increases (Kapogiannis et al. 2018).

In a similar fashion, the therapist can introduce the patient to guided imagery techniques, which patients then have in their repertoire for use as required (De Paolis et al. 2019). Three categories of visual imagery have been proposed. *Imaginative transformation of the pain context* is a method where the pain is acknowledged and then symbolically changed to another object (e.g. a bird) to leave the patient. *Imaginative inattention* refers to creating a pleasant and relaxing setting in one's mind, with multiple sensory aspects to attend to, but no pain. *Imaginative transformation* is a method where the patient recodes the pain sensation as something less noxious, such as a tingling or tickling feeling. The reader is referred to Chapter 9 for earlier coverage of some of these techniques.

Mindfulness base stress reduction (MBSR) is a type of meditation that can help to reduce anxiety and depression among people with cancer (Shennan et al. 2011). Although there is no clear evidence of benefit for reducing cancer pain from MBSR, the relaxation state and acceptance states that it achieves may help people to manage their pain (Deng 2019).

A caution must be sounded here. Although patients can become independent in using PMR and guided imagery, it is still valuable for the therapist to monitor the use of the techniques, providing retraining and support as required. If such support is not given, the techniques may become ineffective, and the client may feel abandoned and discouraged.

Distraction is an approach that moves attention away from pain stimuli or from the negative emotions accompanying pain (Bani Mohammad & Ahmad 2019). People commonly use distraction in everyday life, often without thinking. It may seem that distraction does not require any particular skill. Any patient may have some methods he or she uses for distraction, that can be supplemented by suggestions from a repertoire of techniques offered by the therapist. Introducing a cognitive component to the use of distraction may be helpful. The patient can be encouraged to develop and elaborate a personal picture of their current use of distraction, and to problem-solve about its effectiveness and methods of possible change.

Some activities that are useful for distraction include singing, rhythmic breathing, listening to music, playing games, talking with a specific focus (e.g. to describe a picture) and playing computer games. Distraction may be most effective when needed for relatively short periods (e.g. until medication works) and is particularly helpful in coping with procedural pain (Bukola & Paula 2017).

There is some evidence that music-based interventions alone can help pain intensity (Bradt et al. 2016).

Peer or self-help groups are a useful resource for patients with cancer. They can provide support, companionship and motivation. They are also invaluable in assisting the education process. Syntheses of numerous studies have shown that participation in a support group is associated with short-term improvements in a patient's psychological outcomes and improvement in pain scores (Bardia et al. 2006; Mustafa et al. 2013).

Spiritual intervention from a specialist in this area can reduce the suffering associated with the pain. This involves identifying what gives meaning and purpose for the person and facilitating the person's capacity to tap into these things (Mitchell et al. 2010). The greatest liability a life-threatening disease like cancer confers on an individual is fear—of pain, of the future and of dependence. Spiritual care provides the hope that overcomes fear by reminding the person of those things that have greater import for them. Sometimes the deepest source of spiritual support is religious beliefs and practices, but it may be something quite different—music, poetry, art or time with family and friends (Mitchell et al. 2010).

Lifestyle adjustment

There are several aspects to consider when advising about adjustments to a patient's lifestyle in response to their cancer pain. Some aspects are covered in Chapter 10. Life goals, life roles and general everyday activities may all need adjustment. Adjustment may be achieved slowly and thoughtfully in some instances or may be forced upon an individual quite suddenly by a radical change in health status.

Life goals are often redetermined by the patient, either privately or in discussion with their family, a counsellor, a spiritual advisor and the oncologist. Therapists have a responsibility to become aware of the patient's life goals and to provide the patient with support in achieving them. This may occur through identifying the life roles that are important to the achievement of these goals and helping to achieve maximum efficiency and minimum discomfort from pain in the daily activities associated with these roles.

Methods for adjusting lifestyle so that the pain is least incapacitating include the following:

- **Setting goals:** Patients can be encouraged to set realistic goals on a daily or weekly basis, and review them frequently, until a manageable number and priority of goals is determined.
- **Adjusting timing or routine:** For example, tasks that require the most energy, or may result in the most pain, might be scheduled for earlier in the day when energy levels are higher, or may closely follow medication so that the pain will be less troublesome. Activities normally completed in one session may be paced to occur over two or more sessions, and perhaps even over more than one day.
- **Adjusting methods used in task completion:** Adapting the way in which tasks are carried out can help a patient maintain participation in important life roles essential to maintaining a sense of control. Normal principles of activity analysis and task management apply. For example, activities normally carried out while standing, such as self-care, can be adapted so they can be completed in a sitting position. Activities may be scheduled to be completed when someone is available to assist.
- **Varying the amount and type of adaptive equipment needed:** If pain is limiting the range of motion, for instance, adaptive equipment for dressing may be useful. Different seating and cushioning may be chosen to relieve pressure and so on.

In summary, there is a wide range of approaches for managing cancer pain with nonpharmacological methods to complement pharmacological approaches. Because of this, cancer pain management is delivered by a multidisciplinary team and should be frequently reviewed.

Barriers to adequate pain management

While there are numerous pain-relief strategies, both pharmacologically and nonpharmacologically based, pain relief remains elusive for many. A meta-analysis demonstrated pain prevalence rates of 55% during anticancer treatment and 66% in advanced, metastatic or terminal disease, with moderate-to-severe pain reported by 38.0% of all patients (van den Beuken-van Everdingen et al. 2016).

As mentioned, there are often significant barriers impeding optimal pain management. From the patient and family perspective in cancer pain, there is a belief that suffering pain is an integral part of having cancer, and some believe that nothing can be done to treat it. Others are aware of the existence of management options such as opioids but have a fear of addiction or dependence. They also believe mistakenly that timely introduction of opioids will mean not having anything to fall back on as the disease progresses. Others believe that reporting symptoms may disqualify them from further treatment aimed at cure. Others do not follow treatment directions because of misunderstanding, cost or dislike of side effects (Darawad et al. 2019).

The therapist may not have an awareness of the existence of the patient's pain, due to time pressures impeding adequate assessment of the patient. There may be a higher priority given to curative treatment rather than addressing symptom burden. This may be compounded by an inadequate knowledge of pain management techniques and tools. Some clinicians are over-fearful of legal or regulatory sanctions relating to opioid use. There may also be regulatory barriers to access to adequate pain medication management; some countries severely restrict the use of opioid medications (Kwon 2014).

Finally, a lack of coordination of care and a lack of communication between team members and between specialists and primary care providers can impede the identification and proper management of cancer pain.

Contexts for cancer pain management

There are many settings in which therapists may encounter patients with cancer pain. If cancer is the primary diagnosis, patients are likely to be either inpatients in hospital or attending an outpatient service. They may also be in a hospice or in hospice home care. In each of these settings, the role of the occupational therapist or physiotherapist will vary according to the centre's philosophy and organisation. However, the principles of pain management for patients with cancer still apply.

Therapists will also encounter patients with cancer in settings where cancer is not the primary diagnosis of all the patients. For instance, a community-based day centre for older people is likely to have clients with a range of diagnoses, and some may have cancer. In such cases, it is important that the therapist does not assume the need to introduce a pain management programme without first checking whether this has been done within another facility already. If there is a pain management programme in existence, the therapist has a responsibility to follow and support it for as long as the client remains in that facility.

Cancer pain in children

Children with cancer may experience pain associated with the cancer itself (e.g. bone pain), the therapy (e.g. cramping abdominal pain from the side effects of chemotherapy) and/or the procedure (e.g. from injections) (Tutelman et al. 2018). A study at a major Australian children's' hospital indicated that 46% of children who died from cancer suffered 'a lot' or a 'great deal' of pain in their last month of life (Heath et al. 2010). The reader is referred to Chapter 19 for a comprehensive coverage of pain in childhood, its assessment, measurement and management.

Palliative care pain management

Palliative care is 'the active holistic care of individuals across all ages with serious health-related suffering due to severe illness and especially of those near the end of life. It aims to improve the QOL of patients, their families and their caregivers' (Radbruch et al. 2020). Palliative care involves working with the patient and their family, in hospital, at home or in a hospice, to minimise suffering, and to reduce the medicalisation of dying. It is important to facilitate communication between the patient, family and health professionals as to the goals of care. The essential features include pain and symptom control, advance care planning, terminal care and bereavement support. Pain control should be organised and anticipatory, so that QOL is enhanced for the patient and the family.

If the patient is at home or in a situation where his or her needs and wishes, and those of the close relatives and/or friends, are paramount, the health professional must often adjust his or her style of practice. One must be prepared to follow a more flexible time schedule and to accept that a patient does not wish to be involved in a particular therapy procedure.

Often palliative and hospice care involve a bereavement stage for the family and other carers after the patient has died. Therapists may be involved in this stage, following their previous close therapeutic involvement with the

CASE STUDY 21.1

Mr P

Mr P was a 63-year-old man diagnosed with prostate cancer. He was married with a 32-year-old daughter and 30-year-old son. He worked full time as an engineer, consulting on a number of building projects.

During the early stages of his illness, he underwent surgery (prostatectomy) and later received a course of radiotherapy. He experienced short-lived acute pain related to surgery which resolved within a few weeks.

After 5 years of symptom-free time, Mr P developed an intense pain in his left hip which significantly affected his mobility. His prostate cancer had recurred with metastatic spread to his left head of femur. He was started on hormone treatment in an attempt to control the disease. In addition, he was commenced on regular oral morphine until palliative radiation herapy could be arranged. He continued oral morphine for a short time until the effects of the radiation were realised, after which it was ceased.

Mr P's pain continued to increase so that he had difficulty with weight-bearing. He restarted regular oral morphine, but despite escalating dosages, his sleep was still being interrupted by pain. An X-ray revealed a lytic bone metastasis in the neck of his femur. Mr P was offered surgical stabilisation. This provided relief of pain in his left hip and he was able to mobilise more easily again.

After a few more months Mr P started developing a central aching pain in his pelvis. On examination, it was clear that he had recurrent disease at the site of the primary prostate tumour. About this time, he became increasingly fatigued. The combination of pain and fatigue severely limited his ability to walk, reduced his endurance for activities of daily living such as showering, and he found it difficult to sit comfortably. He commenced oral morphine again, using a slow release formula.

It was at this point that he was referred for physiotherapy and occupational therapy. Physiotherapy input focused on facilitating Mr P's mobilisation throughout this time and advice on positioning to relieve pressure to his groin when sitting, lying and toileting. As his fatigue increased, a walking frame was prescribed which took weight through his arms, decreasing pressure on weight-bearing.

Occupational therapy involvement was initially requested for home assessment, as Mr P expressed a desire to stay at home as long as possible. The occupational therapist assessed his occupational status (i.e. roles of importance to him, his functional status and performance components).

Adaptive equipment such as a shower chair and over toilet seat were prescribed to enable him to perform self-care independently, and ways of conserving his energy were explored. In addition, the therapist worked with Mr P and his family to find ways of adapting the environment so he could remain involved in family activities. For instance, at times when he was too uncomfortable to mobilise or sit in chairs, a bed was placed in the family room so he could participate in activities when his friends or his children visited. He also found listening to music helped to some extent to distract him from the pain. The therapist discussed other ways of maintaining a sense of control. He used the telephone and internet for some time to remain in contact with friends and workmates, following the progress of some of the building projects he had been involved with. Support and education were also provided for his family.

As his disease progressed, it became increasingly difficult for his family to care for him at home and he was transferred to a hospice unit. His pain was closely monitored and he was commenced on a subcutaneous infusion of morphine when he was no longer able to swallow. Psychosocial and spiritual support became very important to him in the last few weeks of his life.

Mr P presented as a patient with many common characteristics of cancer pain, that is, varying types and sites of pain as his disease progressed, changing intensities of pain that required constant re-evaluation and trialing of a number of different methods of pain relief. A multidisciplinary approach with good communication between health carers and family involvement was essential to optimal supportive care as his disease progressed.

patient and the family. See Case study 21.1 which illustrates many of these complex issues.

Issues facing practitioners when working with patients with cancer

When working with patients who have cancer pain, psychological aspects need to be considered. This is important from both the patient's and the therapist's point of view. Therapists working with patients who have cancer should take some time to examine and become comfortable with their own feelings and values about, and understanding of, the issues of potentially terminal illness, dying, pain and responses to severe pain. A number of factors can impact on a therapist and contribute to therapist stress:

1. Their own personal feelings and meanings about disease and death, including their personal philosophical or religious beliefs and values.
2. Their previous experiences and expectations about the medical system and what can be achieved.
3. The complexities, uncertainties and challenges that arise when caring for patients who are dying.

Coping strategies therapists may use include maintaining a personal support system, examining one's own personal and professional attitudes on death and dying, having realistic expectations about what can be done and using personal stress management techniques such as relaxation and exercise (Gillman et al. 2015).

Patients who have cancer may exhibit many defence mechanisms, which must be understood in order to understand their behaviour, and to design management and intervention. People develop a personal style of defence mechanism over their life. For example, a person may use denial or projection more than regression or rationalisation. Defence mechanisms are unconscious, and usually operate in a positive way to buffer or protect against stress. However, in some situations, the use of such defence mechanisms may inhibit communication and decision-making or may even affect treatment choices.

There are many defence mechanisms, but the two most commonly seen in major illness are *projection* and *denial*. Projection, in essence, involves attributing to others the feelings we are experiencing ourselves. For example, if someone is angry that he has cancer, he may see others, usually doctors or nurses or family members, as being angry with him. Denial means being unable to accept or believe something, despite having been told about it very clearly, and acting as though it is not true. For example, a patient may insist they have not been told the diagnosis, despite having been told a number of times. They may put off treatment decisions, insisting that there is nothing wrong with their health. Denial is a common self-protection strategy for easing distress. Therapists need to understand its complexity and exercise care when communicating with the patient. Treatment decisions need to be carefully facilitated, while allowing patients to face reality at a pace they can cope with.

Because of defence mechanisms and other types of psychological reaction, it is not uncommon for the patient with cancer, or the family, to react aggressively to members of staff with whom they come into contact. It is important that the professional staff member does not take such a reaction personally but is able to respond to what may be the underlying concern, such as a need for time to talk, a need for more information or a need to express fear and anger.

As well as the operation of defence mechanisms, there are other reasons for patients to be miserable or irritable. There may be events occurring in their private relationships that are stressful; continual coping with pain may become wearisome; or they may simply be having a bad day. All patients have the right to be irritable sometimes, and the therapist has the responsibility to respond maturely and to be able to provide intervention without always requiring pleasant sociability in return.

Conclusion

This chapter has established differences between the management of people with cancer pain and those with non-cancer pain. Cancer pain is not a static phenomenon due to only one cause. It can be multifactorial and constantly changing, especially in those with progressive disease. Cancer pain is of considerable import to those with cancer. It is important for occupational therapists and physical therapists working with clients with cancer to be well acquainted with the types of cancer pain, and methods for pain assessment, measurement and management.

While there may be special management strategies to be used with people with cancer pain, such as analgesic plans, radiotherapy and surgical procedures, therapists must also remember the value of more basic therapeutic modalities, such as energy conservation techniques. Therapists must be aware of particular issues related to working in a palliative care setting.

Review questions Q

1. What are the different types of cancer pain which patients may present with?
2. Suggest two possible reasons why cancer pain may not be adequately managed in patients.
3. How often should the pain of a person with cancer be assessed?
4. What measurement tools should be routinely used with a patient with cancer pain?
5. Identify five techniques which the physiotherapist might use to help a patient with cancer pain.
6. Identify five techniques which the occupational therapist may use to help a patient with cancer pain.

References

Aman, M.M., Mahmoud, A., Deer, T., Sayed, D., Hagedorn, J.M., Brogan, S.E., et al., 2021. The American Society of Pain and Neuroscience (ASPN) best practices and guidelines for the interventional management of cancer-associated pain. J. Pain Res. 14, 2139–2164.

Ashby, M.A., Fleming, B.G., Brooksbank, M., et al., 1992. Description of a mechanistic approach to pain management in advanced cancer. Preliminary report. Pain 51 (2), 153–161.

Bani Mohammad, E., Ahmad, M., 2019. Virtual reality as a distraction technique for pain and anxiety among patients with breast cancer: a randomized control trial. Palliat. Support. Care 17 (1), 29–34.

Bardia, A., Barton, D.L., Prokop, L.J., et al., 2006. Efficacy of Complementary and alternative medicine therapies in relieving cancer pain: a systematic review. J. Clin. Oncol. 24, 5457–5464.

Bennett, M.I., Eisenberg, E., Ahmedzai, et al., 2019. Standards for the management of cancer-related pain across europe – a position paper from the EFIC task force on cancer pain. Eur. J. Pain 23 (4), 660–668.

Bennett, M.I., Bagnall, A.M., Jose Closs, S., 2009. How effective are patient-based educational interventions in the management of cancer pain? Systematic review and meta-analysis. Pain 143 (3), 192–199.

Bradt, J., Dileo, C., Magill, L., Teague, A., 2016. Music interventions for improving psychological and physical outcomes in cancer patients. Cochrane Database Syst. Rev. 15 (8), CD006911.

Bukola, I.M., Paula, D., 2017. The effectiveness of distraction as procedural pain management technique in pediatric oncology patients: a meta-analysis and systematic review. J. Pain Symptom Manage. 54 (4), 589–600.e1.

Caraceni, A., Hanks, G., Kaasa, S., et al., 2012. Use of opioid analgesics in the treatment of cancer pain: evidence-based recommendations from the EAPC. Lancet Oncol. 13 (2), e58–e68.

Chang, V.T., Hwang, S.S., Thaler, H.T., et al., 2004. Memorial symptom assessment scale. Expert. Rev. Pharmacoecon. Outcomes Res. 4 (2), 171–178.

Charalambous, A., Giannakopoulou, M., Bozas, E., et al., 2016. Guided imagery and progressive muscle relaxation as a cluster of symptoms management intervention in patients receiving chemotherapy: a randomized control trial. PLoS One 11 (6), e0156911.

Cheville, A.L., Moynihan, T., Herrin, J., et al., 2019. Effect of collaborative telerehabilitation on functional impairment and pain among patients with advanced-stage cancer: a randomized clinical trial. JAMA Oncol. 5 (5), 644–652.

Darawad, M., Alnajar, M.K., Abdalrahim, M.S., et al., 2019. Cancer pain management at oncology units: comparing knowledge, attitudes and perceived barriers between physicians and nurses. J. Cancer Educ. 34 (2), 366–374.

Deng, G., 2019. Integrative medicine therapies for pain management in cancer patients. Cancer J. 25 (5), 343–348.

Dodd, M., Janson, S., Facione, N., et al., 2001. Advancing the science of symptom management. J. Adv. Nurs. 33 (5), 668–676.

De Paolis, G., Naccarato, A., Cibelli, F., et al., 2019. The effectiveness of progressive muscle relaxation and interactive guided imagery as a pain-reducing intervention in advanced cancer patients: a multicentre randomised controlled non-pharmacological trial. Complement. Ther. Clin. Pract. 34, 280–287.

Duijts, S.F., Faber, M.M., Oldenburg, H.S., van Beurden, M., Aaronson, N.K., 2011 Feb. Effectiveness of behavioral techniques and physical exercise on psychosocial functioning and health-related quality of life in breast cancer patients and survivors--a meta-analysis. Psycho. Oncol. 20 (2), 115–126.

Ekstedt, M., Rustøen, T., 2019. Factors that hinder and facilitate cancer patients' knowledge about pain management-a

qualitative study. J. Pain Symptom Manage. 57 (4), 753–760. e1.

Fallon, M., Walker, J., Colvin, L., Rodriguez, A., Murray, G., Sharpe, M., 2018 May 1. Edinburgh Pain Assessment and Management Tool Study Group. Pain management in cancer center inpatients: a cluster randomized trial to evaluate a systematic integrated approach-the Edinburgh pain assessment and management tool. J. Clin. Oncol. 36 (13), 1284–1290.

Finnerup, N.B., Kuner, R., Jensen, T.S., 2021 Jan 1. Neuropathic pain: from mechanisms to treatment. Physiol. Rev. 101 (1), 259–301.

Foley, K.M., 1987. Cancer pain syndromes. J. Pain Symptom. Manage. 2, S13–S17.

Gillman, L., Adams, J., Kovac, R., Kilcullen, A., House, A., Doyle, C., 2015 12. Strategies to promote coping and resilience in oncology and palliative care nurses caring for adult patients with malignancy: a comprehensive systematic review. JBI Database. System. Rev. Implement. Rep. 13 (5), 131–204.

Groenvold, M., Petersen, M.A., Aaronson, N.K., Arraras, J.I., Blazeby, J.M., Bottomley, A., et al., 2006. The development of the EORTC QLQ-C15-PAL: a shortened questionnaire for cancer patients in palliative care. Eur. J. Cancer 42 (1), 55–64.

Hardy, J., Pinkerton, C.R., Mitchell, G., 2020. Stringent control of opioids: sound public health measures, but a step too far in palliative care? Curr. Oncol. Rep. 22 (4), 34 2020;22(4):34.

Heath, J.A., Clarke, N.E., Donath, S.M., et al., 2010. Symptoms and suffering at the end of life in children with cancer: an Australian perspective. Med. J. Aust. 192, 71–75.

Hesselstrand, M., Samuelsson, K., Liedberg, G., 2015. Occupational therapy interventions in chronic pain–a systematic review. Occup. Ther. Int. 22 (4), 183–194.

Hoffmann, T., 2010. Critically appraised paper. Patient-based educational interventions for cancer pain management reduce pain intensity and improve attitudes and knowledge towards cancer pain. Aust. Occup. Ther. J. 57, 146–149.

Hoffmann, T., Tooth, L., 2010. Talking with clients about evidence. In: Hoffmann, T., Bennett, S., Del Mar, C. (Eds.), Evidence-Based Practice across the Health Professions. Elsevier, Sydney, pp. 276–299.

Hurlow, A., Bennett, M.I., Robb, K.A., et al., 2012. Transcutaneous electric nerve stimulation (TENS) for cancer pain in adults. Cochrane Database Syst. Rev. 3, CD006276.

Jho, H.J., Kim, Y., Kong, K.A., Kim, D.H., Choi, J.Y., Nam, E.J., et al., 2014. Knowledge, practices, and perceived barriers regarding cancer pain management among physicians and nurses in Korea: a nationwide multicenter survey. PLoS One 9 (8), e105900.

Kapogiannis, A., Tsoli, S., Chrousos, G., 2018. Investigating the effects of the progressive muscle relaxation-guided imagery combination on patients with cancer receiving chemotherapy treatment: a systematic review of randomized controlled trials. Explore 14 (2), 137–143.

Kong, V.K., Irwin, M.G., 2009. Adjuvant analgesics in neuropathic pain. Eur. J. Anaesthesiol. 26 (2), 96–100.

Kutner, J.S., Smith, M.C., Corbin, L., et al., 2008. Massage therapy versus simple touch to improve pain and mood in patients with advanced cancer: a randomized trial. Ann. Intern. Med. 149 (6), 369–379.

Kwon, J.H., 2014. Overcoming barriers in cancer pain management. J. Clin. Oncol. 32, 1727–1733.

López-Sendín N, Alburquerque-Sendín F, Cleland JA, Fernández-de-las-Peñas C. Effects of physical therapy on pain and mood in patients with terminal cancer: a pilot randomized clinical trial. J. Altern. Complement Med.18(5):480-486.

Lovell, M.R., Luckett, T., Boyle, F.M., Phillips, J., Agar, M., Davidson, P.M., 2014. Patient education, coaching, and self-management for cancer pain. J. Clin. Oncol. 32 (16), 1712–1720.

Mercieca–Bebber, R., Costa, D.S.J., Norman, R., et al., 2019. The EORTC Quality of Life Questionnaire for cancer patients (QLQ–C30): Australian general population reference values. Med. J. Aust. 210, 499–506.

McNeely, M.L., Parliament, M.B., Seikaly, H., et al., 2008. Effect of exercise on upper extremity pain and dysfunction in head and neck cancer survivors: a randomized controlled trial. Cancer 113 (1), 214–222.

Miaskowski, C., Cleary, J., Burney, R., et al., 2005. Guideline for the Management of Cancer Pain in Adults and Children. American Pain Society, Glenview, IL. PP. 166.

Mitchell, G., Murray, J., Wilson, P., et al., 2010. 'Diagnosing' and 'managing' spiritual distress in palliative care: creating an intellectual framework for spirituality useable in clinical practice. Australas. Med. J. 3 (6), 364–369.

Murnion, B.P., Gnjidic, D., Hilmer, S.N., 2010. Prescription and administration of opioids to hospital in-patients, and barriers to effective use. Pain Med. 11 (1), 58–66.

Mustafa, M., Carson-Stevens, A., Gillespie, D., Edwards, A.G.K., 2013. Psychological interventions for women with metastatic breast cancer. Cochrane Database Syst. Rev. (6), Art. No: CD004253. https://doi.org/10.1002/14651858.CD004253.pub4. (Accessed 21 July 2021).

National Comprehensive Cancer Network, 2019. NCCN Clinical Practice Guidelines in Oncology – Adult Cancer Pain V.2. NCCN, Washington, DC.

Overcash, J., Extermann, M., Parr, J., et al., 2001. Validity and reliability of the FACT-G scale for use in the older person with cancer. Am. J. Clin. Oncol. 24, 591–596.

Rafii, F., Taleghani, F., Khatooni, M., 2021. Barriers to effective cancer pain management in home setting: a qualitative study. Pain Manag. Nurs. 22 (4), 531–538.

Radbruch, L., De Lima, L., Knaul, F., Wenk, R., Ali, Z., Bhatnaghar, S., et al., 2020. Redefining palliative care-a new consensus-based definition. J. Pain Symptom. Manage. 60 (4), 754–764.

Searle, R.D., Bennett, M.I., Johnson, M.I., et al., 2009. Transcutaneous nerve stimulation (TENS) for cancer bone pain. J. Pain Symptom. Manage. 37 (3), 424–428.

Shennan, C., Payne, S., Fenlon, D., 2011. What is the evidence for the use of mindfulness-based interventions in cancer care: a review. Psycho. Oncol. 20 (7), 681–697.

Shin, E.S., Seo, K.H., Lee, S.H., et al., 2016. Massage with or without aromatherapy for symptom relief in people with cancer. Cochrane Database Syst. Rev. 6.

Smyth, J.A., Dempster, M., Warwick, I., Wilkinson, P., McCorry, N.K., 2018. A systematic review of the patient- and carer-related factors affecting the experience of pain for advanced cancer patients cared for at home. J. Pain Symptom. Manage. 55 (2), 496–507.

Tatrow, K., Montgomery, G.H., 2006. Cognitive behavioral therapy techniques for distress and pain in breast cancer patients: a meta-analysis. J. Behav. Med. 29 (1), 17–27.

Teunissen, S.C., Wesker, W., Kruitwagen, C., et al., 2007. Symptom prevalence in patients with incurable cancer: a systematic review. J. Pain Symptom Manage. 34 (1), 94–104.

Therapeutic Guidelines: Palliative Care, 2020. eTG. Therapeutic Guidelines, Melbourne.

Tutelman, P.R., Chambers, C.T., Stinson, J.N., et al., 2018. Pain in children with cancer: prevalence, characteristics, and parent management. Clin. J. Pain 34, 198–206.

van den Beuken-van Everdingen, M.H.J., de Rijke, J.M., Kessels, A.G., et al., 2007. Prevalence of pain in patients with cancer: a systematic review of the past 40 years. Ann. Oncol. 18, 1437–1449 2007.

van den Beuken-van Everdingen, M.H.J., Hochstenbach, L.M.J., Elbert, A.J., Joosten, A.E.J., et al., 2016. 2016 update on prevalence of pain in patients with cancer: systematic review and meta-analysis J. Pain Symptom Manage. 5, pp. 1070–1090.

Williams AC de, C., Fisher, E., Hearn, L., Eccleston, C., 2012. Psychological therapies for the management of chronic pain (excluding headache) in adults. Cochrane Database Syst. Rev. 11(11), CD007407. https://doi.org/10.1002/14651858.CD007407.pub3.

Wilson, K.G., Chochinov, H.M., Allard, P., et al., 2009. Prevalence and correlates of pain in the Canadian national palliative care survey. Pain. Res. Manage. 14 (5), 365–370.

World Health Organization, 2020. National Cancer Control Programs: Policies and Managerial Guidelines, second ed. WHO, Geneva.

Yang, J., Bauer, B.A., Wahner-Roedler, D.L., Chon, T.Y., Xiao, L., 2020. The modified WHO analgesic ladder: is it appropriate for chronic non-cancer pain? J. Pain Res. 13, 411–417.

Yates, P., Edwards, H., Nash, R., et al., 2004. A randomized controlled trial of a nurse-administered educational intervention for improving cancer pain management in ambulatory settings Patient. Educ. Couns. 53, 227–237.

Chapter 22

Inequities in pain: pain in low- and middle-income countries and among Indigenous peoples

Ivan Lin, Roger Goucke, Jonathan Bullen, Saurab Sharma, and Cheryl Barnabe

LEARNING OBJECTIVES

At the end of this chapter, readers will be able to:

1. Understand the complexities and disparities when assessing pain in low- and middle-income countries and in Indigenous populations.
2. Understand some of the determinants and risk factors for the development of persistent pain in low- and middle-income countries.
3. Describe some of the challenges to delivering effective pain care in these communities.
4. Appreciate some of the possibilities in addressing the inequities in delivering patient-centred, evidence-based, pain management to low- and middle-income countries.

Introduction

The considerable burden of persistent pain on individuals and societies internationally is well recognised. However, across and within countries, experiences and effects of this burden are not equal. Some population groups experience a disproportionately high prevalence and burden of pain, or face barriers to access high-quality pain care. Frequently the impacts are greatest on those who are already marginalised or disadvantaged. This chapter will discuss the epidemiology, determinants and risk factors, and challenges to care access for persons living with pain in low- and middle-income countries (LMICs) and who are Indigenous peoples of colonised countries.

LMICs are those classified by The World Bank with a level of Gross National Income per capita less than $12,535 (low-income: less than $1035, lower-middle income: $1036–$4045, upper-middle: $4046–$12,535) (The World Bank 2021a). Approximately 10% of the global population live in low-income countries. Middle-income countries include 75% of the world's population and 62% of the world's poor (The World Bank 2021b). People in LMICs experience a significant and increasing burden of persistent pain but may lack access to health and rehabilitation services, a skilled pain care workforce, essential pain medications and support if unable to work (Sharma et al. 2019a). Simultaneously, overuse of low-value care therapies has been increasing in LMICs, which is adversely affecting health and is an inefficient use of available healthcare resources.

Ironically, countries with highly resourced healthcare systems such as Australia, Canada, New Zealand and the United States are not meeting pain care needs of the Indigenous peoples of those colonised lands. In addition to a high prevalence of pain, there are structural barriers for Indigenous people to access healthcare for its management. This is in part related to inequities in funding of the healthcare system, the lack of willingness of Western-based providers to embrace traditional Indigenous knowledge and approaches to health maintenance, but also that culturally unsafe healthcare services result in Indigenous peoples choosing to avoid care that puts them at further risk of racism, bias and discrimination.

Although the upstream determinants of inequity, such as socioeconomic disadvantage and entrenched societal racism, may be beyond the direct influence of healthcare services and healthcare clinicians, there are actions that clinicians and members of the international pain community can take to ensure appropriate pain management for all who require it. We present several examples to illustrate possible actions. Training healthcare workers in LMICs in contemporary pain management is a simple solution, as the fundamentals of pain care do not require expensive resources. This can also avoid the pitfalls of iatrogenic care practices found in some high-resource settings. Partnering with primary care services initiated and operated by the local Indigenous communities to deliver healthcare models that integrate cultural epistemologies of health and wellness with contemporary pain knowledge is also a simple, yet effective strategy. Clinicians are often aware they need to provide culturally appropriate care, although they may not know how to do this. Adapting pain information resources so that they are appropriate and acceptable and utilising culturally appropriate communication are two strategies provided.

In this chapter, we ask readers whether, in the 21st century, these disparities are acceptable or fair. Is it acceptable that while some people within societies are oversupplied with pain care options, others miss out? This chapter calls for recognition of pain disparities and engagement by the pain community. Our case studies from practice show that there are steps that can be taken now to improve pain management in LMICs and Indigenous healthcare settings. We challenge providers, system leaders and influencers in the pain community to play their part in reducing the inequitable burden and contribute to fair and high-quality outcomes for all people who live with pain.

Epidemiology and impact of pain in LMIC and among Indigenous populations

Low- and middle-income countries

Pain is one of the most common clinical problems globally. A systematic review of 119 epidemiological studies from 28 LMICs documented that persistent pain has a prevalence of 21%–62% (Jackson et al. 2016). In the overall population, the prevalence of general chronic pain was 34%–62%; chronic musculoskeletal pain 25%–44%; and chronic low back pain 21%–28%. The prevalence of chronic low back pain increased up to 3.1 times in working populations at 79% (95% confidence interval:

60%–94%). The prevalence of chronic pain is higher in women compared to men and older adults compared to younger adults and children (Jackson et al. 2016; Louw et al. 2007).

A systematic review of prevalence studies of low back pain in Africa found that one in every two adults and one in every three adolescents reported low back pain (Morris et al. 2018). A surprising finding in this review was that low back pain was not only common in adults but also in children in LMICs in Africa. In a recent population-based study in South Africa, chronic pain prevalence was 18% (Kamerman et al. 2020), similar to high-income countries (HICs; e.g., Australia) (Blyth et al. 2001). A recent scoping review of literature of all pain research in Nepal summarised the prevalence of musculoskeletal pain conditions ranged from 44% to 71% (Sharma et al. 2019c). The prevalence of low back pain was as high as 91% in some working populations (e.g. dentists). The prevalence of chronic pain ranged from 48% to 50% and the prevalence of headache was 85% in the community.

Although the prevalence of pain is high in LMICs, the extent to which it impacts on an individual's ability to function and quality of life needs further exploration. Although Global Burden of Disease (GBD) studies highlight that musculoskeletal disorders such as low back pain are the leading cause of years lived with disability in most LMICs (Vos et al. 2017), the findings rely on the results of modelling rather than high-quality, primary data. Original high-quality epidemiological studies are required to understand the impact of pain in several LMICs. This is limited, at least partly, by unavailability of measurement instruments to assess these domains in the local languages. Furthermore, while the prevalence of pain is high in both HICs and LMICs, little information is available to describe the severity of pain. While the GBD studies report calculated Disability Adjusted Life Years (DALYs), the disability weightings used to calculate them do not readily allow for exploration of severity. For example, existing disability weightings do not account for people with back pain or headache who are unable to work because of their condition. Furthermore, in many LMIC communities, pain, such as that caused by cancer, is accepted (and expected) as a normal feature of life (Daher 2012). To what degree this is compounded by a lack of access to, or knowledge about, effective pain management strategies is unknown.

The prevalence of chronic pain in LMICs is expected to increase in the next decades as the population increases and health demography changes. These changes are a result of reduced maternal and child deaths, improvement in life-saving medical advances (e.g. surgery), population ageing and the increased prevalence of comorbidities associated with pain such as other noncommunicable diseases and mental health conditions (Institute of Medicine

Committee on Advancing Pain Research & Education 2011; Sharma et al. 2019a). Injuries as the result of trauma and disasters are also escalating, leading to increased rates of musculoskeletal pain (Cordero et al. 2020). In addition, a large proportion of people living in LMICs are involved in physically challenging occupations (e.g. heavy manual occupations such as farming), which are associated with persistent pain conditions.

Indigenous populations

Indigenous populations have an increased prevalence of pain of multiple causes globally, even though inadequate pain measurement methods potentially underestimate prevalence among Indigenous peoples (Julien et al. 2018). Variations in pain descriptions, cultural beliefs, functional impacts and management approaches (Jimenez et al. 2011) mean that the measurement of pain and its impact may be poorly understood or misconstrued in academic literature.

In a comprehensive systematic review on chronic non-cancer pain among Indigenous Peoples of Canada (First Nations, Inuit, Métis) (Julien et al. 2018), only two studies were identified that reported the prevalence of self-reported chronic pain (those answering 'no' to whether they were usually free from pain or discomfort) from two cycles of the Canadian Community Health Survey. Indigenous men and women had significantly higher prevalence of pain than non-Indigenous respondents (15.4% vs 9.3% of men and 16.5% vs 11.6% of women) in 2007 to 2008 (Ramage-Morin & Gilmour 2010), reflecting trends seen in the 2000 to 2001 survey although with lower estimates (Meana et al. 2004). In a study of physical pain indicators in youth in Atlantic Canada, those identifying as First Nations had a significantly higher proportion of pain diagnoses (93.6%), predominantly throat, ear, dental conditions and headache, relative to the non-First Nations cohort (85.5%) (Latimer et al. 2018).

Similarly, Indigenous people of America, Australia and New Zealand experience disproportionately greater prevalence of pain than non-Indigenous peoples. In a review published a decade ago, prevalence rates of painful conditions and pain were elevated for American Indian and Alaska Native populations compared to non-First Nations populations (Jimenez et al. 2011). Rates were increased for inflammatory arthritis conditions in both youth and adults, low back pain, generalised musculoskeletal pain, oral pain, recurrent headaches and neck pain, but not cancer pain. In Wave 2 of the National Epidemiology Study on Alcohol and Related Conditions, fewer American Indian and Alaskan Native respondents reported the absence of pain (52.5%) relative to other racial minority populations (Black 60.7%, Asian/Pacific Islander 67.9%, Hispanic 69.0%) and

White respondents (63.2%) (Johnson-Jennings et al. 2020). They were also most likely to report extreme pain (American Indian and Alaskan Native 6.9%, with Black 3.8%, Asian/Pacific Islander 1.7%, Hispanic 2.2% and White 2.9%) (Johnson-Jennings et al. 2020). In Australia, the prevalence of musculoskeletal pain was higher in the Aboriginal population relative to the non-Aboriginal population, with rate ratios of 1.1 for back pain, 1.2 to 1.5 for osteoarthritis and up to 2.0 for rheumatoid arthritis (Lin et al. 2018). In remote-living older Aboriginal Australians, nearly 65% reported pain in the past year, which was persistent for 20.2%, multifocal for 22.4% and rated as severe in 41.2% (Wong et al. 2020). Persistent pain in the Māori of New Zealand was 20% more frequent than non-Māori residents. However, this pattern does not seem to be universal (Eriksen et al. 2016) and requires further investigation.

The impact of pain also appears to be more significant among Indigenous populations compared to non-Indigenous populations. It is important to recognise that Indigenous patients may experience stereotyping related to risk for addictions and substance misuse when seeking care for pain, which results in unaddressed pain and potentially in misuse of prescription drugs (Health Canada 2021; Mittinty et al. 2018; Nelson et al. 2016). Indigenous patients treated for rheumatoid arthritis in Alberta, Canada reported worse scores for global evaluation, pain, sleep, quality of life, well-being and physical function, and greater likelihood of impact on daily activities when compared to non-Indigenous patients (Barnabe et al. 2018). In Australia, the overall burden of musculoskeletal pain among Aboriginal Australians, expressed as DALYs, was 1.4 times that of non-Aboriginal Australians (Australian Institute of Health and Welfare (AIHW) 2017). The exception was the burden of low back pain which was 30% lower (ibid). However, this contrasts with qualitative findings that persistent low back pain had profound impacts for Australian Aboriginal people on their daily lives, employment, sport and family participation, as well as emotional and cultural well-being (Lin et al. 2012). Similar to LMICs, these contrasting findings question the suitability of applying existing disability weightings and whether they fully capture the impact of a condition in cultural contexts different to those in which they were originally developed.

Pain care needs in Indigenous populations are further compounded by a high frequency of comorbid conditions. In an Australian study, pain among older Aboriginal people was associated with poor vision, hypertension, heart problems and higher and clinically insignificant depression scores (Wong et al. 2020). Significant functional impairments included mobility, activities of daily living, sleep and participation in enjoyable activities, with 29.4% being classified as disabled (ibid).

Pain determinants and risk factors

Pain, or the 'conscious knowledge of threat' (Moseley 2007), is a multidimensional phenomenon, influenced by biological, psychological, lifestyle and social factors. The unique interaction of these factors ultimately results in an individual person's experience of pain. There is limited research investigating risk factors for pain for people in LMICs. For Indigenous peoples, the lasting legacies of colonisation increase the risk of pain (Lin et al. 2020a). Conversely, there are cultural factors that are potentially protective (Chandler & Lalonde 2008; Oster et al. 2014), although these are yet to be examined in the context of pain.

Low- and middle-income countries

The association of pain with age and lower socioeconomic positioning appears to be a global phenomenon. Little is known about pain determinants and risk factors in LMICs, which should be prioritised as an area of future research. From what is known, persistent pain is associated with female gender, older age and geographical locations in different LMICs (Guo et al. 2019; Kamerman et al. 2020; Karunanayake et al. 2013; Sharma et al. 2018).

A recent study conducted in Northwestern China found that participants who were women, lived in rural areas compared to cities, had lower incomes, were unemployed and experienced poorer general and mental health, were more likely to report pain (Guo et al. 2019). Similarly, sociodemographic factors such as education and income not only predicted pain but also physical function in people with chronic musculoskeletal conditions in Nepal (Sharma et al. 2018). A study in Brazil found that depressive symptoms were positively associated, and satisfaction with life negatively associated, with disabling persistent knee pain, even after adjusting for sociodemographic and clinical factors, indicating the general importance of well-being above and beyond socioeconomic and clinical factors (Azevedo et al. 2021).

The association of pain and sociodemographic factors is especially problematic in LMICs because a high proportion of the population are socioeconomically disadvantaged. Similarly, ageing populations are rapidly increasing in LMICs, increasing the prevalence of pain conditions.

Understanding social determinants of pain is extremely important in order to treat pain well, particularly in LMICs. Knowledge of the association of pain with modifiable and nonmodifiable factors may help clinicians identify modifiers of treatment effects, as well as the potential limitations of their interventions. This foregrounds the fact that pain can be influenced by factors beyond the individual level and therefore beyond the scope of most pain clinicians. Systems-level strategies, such as healthcare financing, media campaigns, leadership and policy, are necessary to improve the health and pain of individuals and the overall population (Sharma et al. 2019a).

Indigenous populations

Despite improvements in some areas of health (Department of the Prime Minister Cabinet 2018), there are ongoing disparities in a range of health outcomes between Indigenous and non-Indigenous people globally (Anderson et al. 2016; Australian Institute of Health and Welfare (AIHW) 2015; Marmot et al. 2008; Vos et al. 2009). The determinants of this differentiation—including socioeconomic status, educational access, housing, transportation, behavioural factors, community capacity and support and discrimination—form part of the complex foundation upon which Indigenous health trajectories begin and are maintained (Gracey & King 2009; Marmot & Wilkinson 2005; Paradies 2018). Many Indigenous populations share similar colonial underpinnings, with loss of culture, land, family and language, factors which are fundamental determinants of well-being (King et al. 2009; Paradies 2018; Vickery et al. 2007). These common distal determinants are complemented by, and linked to, other more proximally situated determinants such as genetic, health behavioural and socioenvironmental interaction factors (Loppie Reading & Wien 2013).

This context increases the likelihood of poorer pain-related outcomes. Unfavourable socioeconomic factors are associated with an increased likelihood of persistent pain, increased pain severity and higher levels of pain-related disability (Mills et al. 2019). The history of colonisation, dispossession, cultural destruction and removal has resulted in intergenerational trauma and emotional distress. For example, Aboriginal Australians are 2.7 times more likely to report high or very high levels of psychological distress than non-Aboriginal Australians (AIHW 2015), a well-recognised risk factor for persistent pain (Blyth et al. 2001; de Heer et al. 2014).

Further consequences of colonisation and disadvantage are health behaviours that are strongly associated with pain presentations. Indigenous peoples in Australia and Canada suffer higher rates of injuries (AIHW 2019; Brussoni et al. 2016), higher rates of comorbid health conditions such as cardiovascular disease, diabetes and overweight/obesity (AIHW 2019), and adverse lifestyle behaviours including smoking and physical inactivity (AIHW 2020). These factors are associated with persistent pain and are hypothesised to share common mechanistic pathways via maladaptive stress and/or inflammatory responses (Bruggink et al. 2019; van Hecke et al. 2017). This situation is further compounded by barriers to healthcare access for Indigenous people. The cultural safety of healthcare institutions and their practitioners, strongly influences the willingness by Indigenous people to seek healthcare. Discrimination towards Indigenous people seeking healthcare and in the wider community is common (Beyond Blue 2014; Larson et al. 2007; Paradies 2018); differentiated clinical treatment is well-documented, as are the links between psychological effects of discrimination and chronic health conditions (Mellor 2004; Priest et al. 2011, 2013). Reports of racism are 25% more common among Aboriginal and Torres Strait Islander Australians compared to non-Indigenous Australians (Blair et al. 2017). Antecedent to future healthcare seeking, historical healthcare experiences of Indigenous populations (particularly those perceived as discriminatory) are strong determinants of health behaviour and barriers to seeking and accessing healthcare (Coffin 2007; Durey et al. 2011). Clearly, individual and systemic discrimination within global health systems influence the quality of, and access to, healthcare for Indigenous populations (Durey & Thompson 2012; Kelaher et al. 2014).

Each of these interrelated determinants causes and maintains Indigenous disadvantage relative to non-Indigenous populations (King et al. 2009; Marmot & Wilkinson 2005; Marrone 2007). They are complex issues to disentangle or address and many are embedded within colonising societies. Indeed, the complexity of their interrelatedness, and the continuing consequences exemplified by the high burden of disease and ongoing intergenerational disadvantage, makes them deeply challenging to change (Baum et al. 2013; Carey et al. 2014).

The legacy of colonisation has left a grim profile of health unwellness, including a higher risk of pain. In contrast, there is increasing evidence supporting the protective function of Indigenous culture. Seminal work in the area of youth suicide in the province of British Columbia in Canada demonstrated strong associations between cultural continuity, such as sovereignty of traditional lands, preservation of culture including language and self-determination, and markedly lower rates of youth suicide (Chandler & Lalonde 2008). Cultural continuity is also associated with higher levels of physical activity among First Nations and Cree/Néhiyaw First Nations adults in Canada (Ironside et al. 2020) and lower prevalence of diabetes in First Nations people in Alberta, Canada (Oster et al. 2014). In Australia, improved cardiovascular mortality in a remote community was attributed to connectedness, to culture and to primary healthcare delivered 'on country' (Rowley et al. 2008). These data highlight the protective effects of culture and the opportunity to improve pain outcomes by integrating pain management with cultural processes.

Challenges to pain care in LMICs and Indigenous communities

While the social, economic and political realities are unique to and within LMICs and Indigenous communities, challenges in providing pain care are similar. We discuss these aspects for both LMICs and Indigenous communities in this section.

Low-value care for pain conditions

Health inequities are exacerbated by low healthcare quality and negative patient experiences in healthcare interactions (Jones et al. 2020). There is a growing body of research documenting evidence of practice gaps in the management of pain conditions, highlighting the need to improve practice. This is across the spectrum of care from diagnosis to treatment, including unwarranted investigations, prescribing (Mathieson et al. 2020), pain interventions, surgeries (Abram et al. 2019; Judge et al. 2014) and physical therapy practices (Zadro et al. 2019). Conversely, some recommended practices are not occurring, including the assessment of red flags for serious conditions, psychosocial assessment and recommended surgeries such as total joint replacement in end-stage osteoarthritis management (Lin et al. 2018).

Despite a dearth of research investigating low-value pain care in LMICs and Indigenous populations, there are concerning trends. In Nepal, there is a disproportionate focus on biomedical aspects of pain care including radiological imaging, invasive diagnostic procedures, injections and surgeries (Sharma et al. 2019c). A lack of concordance between healthcare practices and guideline recommended care has also been reported for neuropathic pain in Mali (Maiga et al. 2021) and rheumatoid arthritis in the Middle East and Africa (El Zorkany et al. 2013). Better support of the pain care workforce in LMICs through enhanced education and continuing professional development to gain the knowledge and skills to better manage pain conditions has been widely recommended (El Zorkany et al. 2013; Maiga et al. 2021; Parker & Jelsma 2010; Sharma et al. 2019a).

Low-value healthcare for pain conditions in Indigenous populations widely manifests as inappropriate prescribing (Webster 2013). This has played a role in fuelling the opioid crisis and unintentional death rate in several Indigenous communities. Aboriginal Australians are twice as likely to be prescribed an opioid medication in primary care (Holliday et al. 2015) and three times as likely to die of an unintentional overdose drug-induced death, most commonly caused by an opioid (Penington Institute 2020). Unhelpful iatrogenic beliefs about low back pain have also been reported among Aboriginal Australians with disabling low back pain (Lin et al. 2013). In Canada, the First Nations Health Authority of British Columbia reported in 2017 that five times as many overdose events and three times as many overdose deaths involved First Nations peoples (First Nations Health Authority 2017), with further substantial increases prior to and following the COVID-19 pandemic (First Nations Health Authority 2021).

Lack of culturally informed pain care

For Indigenous patients, healthcare services are frequently oriented towards Western approaches and neglect the cultural needs of Indigenous peoples (Jones et al. 2020). The absence of culturally informed approaches in healthcare also mean that important aspects of Indigenous patients' experiences, including cultural safety, racism and relationships with care providers are not routinely measured (Green et al. 2021). For Indigenous patients, suboptimal experiences of care have been reported across a range of healthcare domains and specialties (Nolan-Isles et al. 2021), including pain management in cancer care (Green et al. 2021), tertiary arthritis care (Thurston et al. 2014) and substance use (Goodman et al. 2017). Inappropriate and suboptimal care also exists for culturally and linguistically diverse people and ethnic minorities (Brady et al. 2017), highlighting the importance for healthcare services to be more attendant to cultural difference overall. An additional challenge is translating this information into improvements in healthcare (Sheard et al. 2019).

Multiple factors contribute to Indigenous peoples' adverse pain care experiences. Cultural beliefs and Indigenous approaches to health and wellness are not uniformly accepted by biomedical-focused Western providers, creating conflict for location, content and nature of the healthcare interaction (Jones et al. 2020). In a survey of Canadian rheumatologists, there was a reported 'openness' to including Indigenous healing practices in rheumatology care plans, although there was significant hesitancy related to concern of risks of these practices, the potential for interactions with Western-based medications and potential reduction of patient adherence to Western-based treatment plans (Logan et al. 2020). This may be mitigated by ensuring that Indigenous health professionals are available who may bridge these belief and knowledge systems, but this relies on sufficient numbers and availability of these professionals. As it stands, the majority of Indigenous populations are served by non-Indigenous practitioners. High-value pain care requires practitioners with the skills to work successfully with Indigenous patients, including effective communication and the ability to build trust (Lin et al. 2020a). Healthcare services often seek to improve Indigenous healthcare by some form of cultural training. However, this training may result in increased practitioner knowledge rather than skills, attitudes and beliefs, and it is unclear how beneficial training alone is for improving patient health outcomes (Jongen et al. 2018).

There is inherent mistrust of the healthcare system created by legacies of colonisation, and the ability of healthcare providers to create trust varies (Jones et al. 2020). Indigenous patients expect to encounter racism and discrimination within health services (Allan & Smylie 2015; Turpel-Lafond 2021), including the explicit racist comments captured during the live-streamed death of Joyce Echaquan in Quebec, Canada, and the death of Ms Dhu in hospital under police guard in Port Hedland, Western Australia (Blue 2017). These experiences are powerfully influential in decisions to access care (King et al. 2009; Paradies 2018). For example, there is lower use of primary and tertiary care for musculoskeletal pain despite their higher prevalence, due to avoidance of harmful environments. Stigmatisation; lack of empowerment in treatment decision-making; and perceiving the clinician to not have cultural knowledge, interest or experience to understand the pain ultimately lead to lack of trust (Lin et al. 2014; Strong et al. 2015).

Ineffective communication is another significant contributor to suboptimal pain care (Lin et al. 2018). This can be related to using medical jargon or even an absence of communication all together (Lin et al. 2014; Strong et al. 2015). Further, an inherent power differential between health services, practitioners and patients leaves many Indigenous people feeling powerless, uncertain, mistrustful and intimidated (Towle et al. 2006). The consequences are typified by late presentation for healthcare, discharge against medical advice (Katzenellenbogen et al. 2013), downstream impacts upon the diagnostic and treatment stages of healthcare (Huot et al. 2019) and implications for continuity of care for individuals and communities (Strong et al. 2015; Tarlier et al. 2007). In contrast, practitioners who are known to the community, are attentive listeners and perceived as honest, and who provide space for relationship building and sharing stories, are favourably viewed (Lin et al. 2014; Strong et al. 2015).

Finally, healthcare environments are not frequently aligned with cultural norms which support a positive experience (Jones et al. 2020). The physical spaces of non-Indigenous healthcare environments are often noted as unwelcoming, with minimal markers of culture (Mbuzi et al. 2017; Smith et al. 2017) and limited opportunity for interaction with family and community members (Anderson et al. 2012). A lack of culturally relevant consumer health education and information also plays a part in the quality of preventative and public health initiatives (Jones et al. 2020).

Limited or maldistributed healthcare

In addition to cultural barriers, access to care can be limited because of an absence, limitation or maldistribution of healthcare resources.

In LMICs, the changes in healthcare needs of the population from communicable diseases to noncommunicable diseases, including chronic pain conditions (Sharma et al. 2019a), are not matched by health systems' focus and resources. This includes an inadequate number of healthcare clinicians and availability of suitable pain medications (El Zorkany et al. 2013; Nchako et al. 2018). This is compounded by the lack of health professionals' training in pain management, unhelpful pain and treatment beliefs of clinicians and patients, maladaptive coping strategies and the lack of health insurance and universal health coverage in many countries. Within countries, there is a high variation in need, with those who are more disadvantaged experiencing a greater burden, both in terms of the prevalence of pain conditions (Stewart Williams et al. 2015) and limited access to healthcare (Parker & Jelsma 2010). To better address the burden, there has been a call to improve population health and service delivery, access to essential analgesics and rehabilitation services, health information systems, financing, leadership and governance, and improvements in the health workforce (Briggs et al. 2021; Sharma et al. 2019a).

In Australia, the proportion of the population who are Indigenous increases with increasing remoteness. For many Indigenous populations, a maldistribution of healthcare resources with fewer health clinicians in rural and remote areas compared to urban areas, further reduces access to care (Lin et al. 2020a). Regional and remote areas typically have proportionally lower levels of funding for health services than metropolitan areas, and a consequent challenge of sourcing sufficient numbers of culturally capable health practitioners (Nolan-Isles et al. 2021). This is particularly important in the context of Indigenous people being able to receive healthcare 'on country', something poorly understood or disregarded in its relationship to Indigenous conceptualisations and predictors of health and well-being (Jones et al. 2020). Indigenous patients—particularly those from disparate geographic regions who must travel to receive healthcare—often experience poorly coordinated healthcare (Dwyer et al. 2020), with communication constraints and impediments between services and regions proving common (Jones et al. 2020). This is often exacerbated by a lack of language interpreter services (Amery 2017; Towle et al. 2006). Conversely, the COVID-19 pandemic has seen a rapid and dramatic increase in the use of telehealth, which has the potential to reduce geographical barriers to pain care for people living in rural and remote areas provided there is access to the internet. The accessibility,

acceptability and uptake of telehealth pain care models, with patient care provided by distant clinicians working in concert with local healthcare workers, is an area for future development.

Health system funding in Canada contributes to limited healthcare access for Treaty First Nations and Inuit in Canada, characterised by complex multilevel and multijurisdictional systems with various reporting and fiduciary responsibilities. This originated with the assimilationist policies and rules and regulations for controlling First Nations persons, which included regulations related to health practices. Regulated and limited healthcare was even linked to the detrimental legacy of the residential school system, which was never adequately resourced to provide healthcare, even though it was contracted to do so (Truth and Reconciliation Commission of Canada 2015). Subsequent healthcare acts have served to shift federal responsibility for hospital and medical care to First Nations and Inuit communities (Note: although Métis peoples are recognised as Aboriginal in the Canadian Constitution, they do not fall under the jurisdiction of federal health plans at this time). These shifts have been promoted by the government as steps towards self-governance but are also seen as reneging on treaty promises (Lavoie 2018).

A universal healthcare plan within the country was instituted through the introduction of the Canada Health Act (1984) (Government of Canada 1985). This introduced a shared model for roles and responsibilities for healthcare services between provincial/territorial and federal governments. In this act, there is no direct reference to First Nations and Inuit (or Métis) populations, leaving ambiguity about the responsibility for service provision, especially in light of the treaty agreements being between the federal government and First Nations, but with healthcare provided provincially or territorially and without direct responsibility to Indigenous communities. There have been serial federal government disinvestments in several levels of health services including medications, dental care and preventative/early intervention programmes (Lavoie 2018). This has created variations in accessibility and service provision between First Nations groups in different provincial and territorial jurisdictions and leaves local health services to negotiate funding and services for the community. At an individual level, patients are left caught between systems. One of the most prominent examples is that of Jordan River Anderson, an infant born with complex health needs. Once stabilised to leave hospital, Jordan could not be discharged as necessary in-home care costs were disputed between federal and provincial governments (First Nations Child & Family Caring Society 2021). Jordan died in hospital at the age of 5 years without ever have being discharged (ibid). Following a Canadian Human Rights Tribunal ruling, it is now a legal requirement for any public service to be made available to First Nations children without delay or denial (Government of Canada 2021). This ruling does not extend to adults though, leaving Indigenous patients without access to necessary treatments for their pain conditions.

Steps to moving forward

There are unique differences between different countries and Indigenous peoples, as there are among individuals with persistent pain. Although this chapter has presented 'broad brush strokes', we caution against drawing generalised conclusions about pain management in LMICs or Indigenous peoples. Reducing the burden of persistent pain in LMICs and among Indigenous populations is complex. For example, adequate healthcare resources to address healthcare for persistent pain may not exist in some LMICs. While people in some LMICs may lack access to simple analgesic medication, individuals in the same country may receive medications such as opioids when they are not recommended or safe (Sharma et al. 2019a). The potential for vested interests may result in inefficient use of resources at the expense of simpler more effective treatments, for instance when pharmaceutical companies market inappropriate pain treatments to LMICs (as well as to HICs) (Traeger et al. 2019). Improvements are likely to require political/economic strategies. Alternatively, local 'grass-roots' approaches may result in meaningful improvements at an individual or community level, such as simple ergonomic changes to daily manual tasks (Hoy et al. 2003). Because LMICs, Indigenous communities and individuals are heterogeneous, readers are advised to seek a deep and nuanced understanding about each particular context.

From a healthcare perspective, Briggs et al. recently identified system-level priorities at macro (health system) and meso (health service) levels to address the burden of musculoskeletal pain globally (Briggs et al. 2021). These priorities provide a useful framework for conceptualising healthcare needs for persistent pain. Eight strategic priority areas are identified:

- engaging, empowering and educating communities;
- leadership, governance and shared accountability;
- financing approaches;
- service delivery;
- equitable access to medicines and technologies;
- workforce;
- surveillance; and
- research and innovation.

The strategic priorities were developed in an international Delphi study and representatives from LMICs prioritised leadership from the World Health Organization,

establishment of essential packages of care, inclusion of musculoskeletal health in primary and secondary prevention initiatives for noncommunicable diseases, access to low-cost technologies and interventions, building capacity in the primary care workforce and educating health practitioners. Briggs et al. (2021) noted that few national health policies related to musculoskeletal pain existed in LMICs, indicating an orientation towards other health issues and reiterating the need for leadership.

For pain in Indigenous health contexts, recommendations include Indigenous leadership, improving health services recognition and commitment to culturally secure care (e.g. policies within mainstream health services that support cultural ways of working), an increased Indigenous pain workforce, and cultural training and support for the non-Indigenous pain workforce (Lin et al. 2020a). Two recent national strategies for pain management in Australia and Canada have a significant focus on improving pain management among Indigenous peoples. The Canadian Pain Task Force released its Action Plan for Pain in March 2021 (Health Canada 2021). This Action Plan prioritises Indigenous engagement and leadership, so that solutions are truly designed with community priorities, solutions and wellness at their core. Accessibility of health systems is to be addressed in a distinction-based approach (i.e. recognising and responding to the cultural distinctiveness of different Indigenous cultural groups), in addition to health provider education to reduce racism in health care. The Australian National Strategic Action Plan for Pain Management (Pain Australia 2021) has less focus on Indigenous engagement and leadership and the structural inequalities that result in persistent pain, but identifies the importance of focusing efforts on addressing specific needs of Aboriginal and Torres Strait Islander peoples in pain management strategies.

Below we present three examples of strategies aiming to improve pain management in LMICs or Indigenous healthcare settings. Each case study addresses a different aspect of improving pain outcomes in LMICs and among Indigenous peoples, and highlights lessons for those seeking to enhance pain care.

Building workforce capacity through pain education

Essential Pain Management (EPM, www.esentialpain-management.org) is a simple, low resource education programme for health and community workers that addresses up-to-date fundamentals for managing pain (Goucke et al. 2015). EPM was developed by three anaesthesiologists from Papua New Guinea, New Zealand and Australia. It is based on the awareness that pain is a common yet poorly managed condition across the globe. Education is a key component to address this issue. EPM is a 1-day programme that provides an early primer in pain. It provides a systematic approach to management of people in pain and teaching others. EPM aims to improve pain knowledge, teach healthcare workers to recognise, assess and treat (RAT) pain and train local healthcare workers to teach EPM. Participants have been primarily nurses and doctors but also physiotherapists, pharmacists and other healthcare workers. Since its launch in Papua New Guinea in 2010, EPM has been taught in over 60 countries worldwide, including Asia (Mongolia, Vietnam, Thailand, Laos) Africa (Rwanda, Kenya and South Africa) and in the Americas (Canada, Honduras, Venezuela, Argentina). It has been translated into nine languages and is a component of pain education in over 50% of medical schools in the United Kingdom. EPM has also been taught in Australian Aboriginal Community Controlled Health Care Services and Aboriginal community-based settings. Evaluation of the impact of EPM on global pain management would be complex (Marun et al. 2019), but regular participant feedback has been very positive and global uptake in low, middle and HICs is encouraging.

Another capacity-building strategy is supported by the International Association for the Study of Pain (IASP). The IASP offers its members up to 10 project grants each year to improve pain education in developing countries (International Association for the Study of Pain 2021). Grants are worth up to US $10,000. As of 2021, at least 173 grants have been offered to at least 50 different countries. These grants facilitate training of pain clinicians (physiotherapists, nurses, doctors, etc.), using contemporary knowledge and research findings. They facilitate development of written teaching materials and online learning programmes, as well as development and implementation of local and national policy changes. The IASP also offers mentorship to write applications for members who are new to grant writing.

Orienting service delivery to enhance accessibly: Indigenous community-based rheumatology care

Rheumatology practice in Canada has significant human resource limitations to meet recommended care (Barber et al. 2017). Contemporary treatment standards for rheumatological conditions include rapid access to diagnosis and treatment, and frequent re-evaluation and medication rotation to achieve remission. These standards are essential to minimise arthritis-related pain and related morbidity. They have driven several health service innovations, including centralised triage systems. These systems prioritise inflammatory conditions at the expense of osteoarthritis and other painful musculoskeletal conditions. Subspecialised clinical services have evolved but are reliant on centralised tertiary and quaternary

care providers. The drive to increase health system efficiency has resulted in onerous expectations on patients and referring providers to provide medical information and complete investigations before scheduling consultations, and has created care pathways fraught with pitfalls for those not able to navigate the system, especially Indigenous patients (Lopatina et al. 2019). Recognising this, an outreach model of care for rheumatology conditions was initiated in one First Nations community, further partnerships have since formed with several other community sites and one urban Indigenous clinic in the province of Alberta, Canada.

In these partnerships, a self-referral model was initially established as a walk-in for rheumatology care, with additional appointment time allotted for scheduled follow-ups, with the flexibility of same-day appointments (Barnabe et al. 2017; Nagaraj et al. 2018). Family physicians shadowed rheumatologists to learn history taking and physical examination skills and were given lessons in recognising and treating rheumatic diseases. The rheumatologist involved has gained skills in, and now provides education on, culturally aligned care provision for other rheumatologists (Barnabe et al. 2021). With patients, treatment courses are decided collaboratively, providing informed decision-making as formal shared decision-making is instituted (Umaefulam et al. 2021a). Responding to the need for greater health system access, holistic care and embedding peer-support and culture, an 'Arthritis Liaison' model was tested in one community, with evidence of improved patient experiences (Umaefulam et al. 2021b). Clinical relationships are strengthened by partnerships with communities, including response to service delivery needs (e.g. vaccination clinics for COVID-19) and research to address inequities in social determinants of health. Providing care as a partnership with Indigenous healthcare services has resulted in improved patient, health service and clinician outcomes, and has been recommended as a model for pain rehabilitation (Lin et al. 2020a).

Culturally informed pain care: My Back on Track, My Future

Increasing access to high-value care includes improving access to care that is culturally acceptable and meaningful for patients living with pain. Providing information to enable patients to understand their condition and management options is a central aspect of evidence-based pain management (Lin et al. 2019). Unfortunately, there are few patient information resources that are suitable for Aboriginal Australians. The My Back on Track, My Future project aimed to develop culturally appropriate information for Aboriginal people with low back pain in the Midwest area (Yamaji country) of Western Australia (Lin et al. 2017).

Key back pain messages were identified from low back pain clinical guidelines and interviews with Aboriginal people with low back pain (Lin et al. 2013). The low back pain messages were developed into scripts and filmed, as a series of short video stories, working with community actors (see: https://www.aci.health.nsw.gov.au/chronic-pain/our-mob). This aligns with Aboriginal traditions of storytelling as a way to convey information. When evaluated, the My Back on Track, My Future resources addressed language barriers found in standard low back pain information resources and were preferred by the majority of Aboriginal people (Lin et al. 2017). The project highlights the importance of culturally adapted information for Indigenous peoples and people from other nondominant cultural groups. Adapting 'traditional' pain resources and programmes to be more culturally appropriate has been reported to be acceptable and credible, and to improve outcomes for people with pain in LMICs (Mukhtar et al. 2021; Sharma et al. 2019b).

Culturally informed pain care: clinical yarning

Effective patient–clinician communication underpins high-value, person-centred pain management (Lin et al. 2020b). Unfortunately, healthcare communication with clinicians is frequently suboptimal for Indigenous people with pain (Jimenez et al. 2011; Lin et al. 2018). Miscommunication about pain, the use of medical jargon by clinicians, language differences or an absence of communication are some of the barriers faced by Indigenous people. The consequences of poor communication are a lack of trust between patients and clinicians. Indigenous patients may not be provided with an understanding of their condition or management options, and may ultimately walk away from care (Lin et al. 2018).

One approach to address this problem is the development of a guide for clinicians when communicating with Aboriginal Australian patients called clinical yarning. Clinical yarning is a person-centred communication framework that uses yarning (a conversational communication style utilised by Aboriginal people) to engage with the patient's health concerns in a friendly and culturally appropriate manner (Lin et al. 2016). Instead of a traditional practitioner-centred, question–answer approach, communication is reconceptualised as a social, diagnostic and management yarn. Clinical yarning focuses on trust and connectedness with patients and understanding their health concerns by listening to their health story. It focuses on clinicians explaining health information in ways that make sense and are culturally and contextually meaningful, e.g. through the use of storying and metaphors. The basis of the management yarn is that if patients are informed and understand their pain condition, they are able to engage in collaborative management decision-making.

Clinical yarning adopts a skills focus to train clinicians in its use. It is one way to operationalise culturally appropriate care. Similar approaches can be developed in other Indigenous cultural contexts or LMICs.

Conclusion

This chapter has aimed to increase recognition of the inequitable burden of pain in LMICs and Indigenous communities. We have also highlighted the limitations in the assessment of pain severity and a lack of comprehensive knowledge on the impact of chronic pain in these populations. Contributors to pain in these populations are complex. Recognition of these determinants by health systems and health providers is essential. Following recognition, solutions need to be implemented, some of which are relatively simple. Appropriate health provider training, novel models of care which redistribute power and control and culturally relevant pain treatment are tangible steps forward.

Although the progress in pain management in LMICs and Indigenous communities is suboptimal, international organisations have started to consider pain as an important global public health concern. The World Health Organisation is developing a Package of Interventions for Rehabilitation for two most common and burgeoning pain conditions using standard methods, osteoarthritis and low back pain (Rauch et al. 2019). This is in line with the World Health Organisation's Rehabilitation 2030 initiative (https://www.who.int/initiatives/rehabilitation-2030) to strengthen rehabilitation in health systems with specific focus on LMICs. This initiative is an important recognition of the burden of pain in resource-limited settings. Similarly, increasing recognition of pain among Indigenous populations, articulated in national pain strategies, is occurring. These are positive steps and offer optimism of increasing awareness and commitment to addressing the inequitable burden of pain.

Review questions	Q
1. Why might the prevalence of persistent pain increase in low- and middle-income countries in the next decade?	
2. Name two risk factors for pain determinants in LMICs.	
3. Identify three social determinants of health that affect outcomes in Indigenous communities.	
4. Give an example of low-value healthcare from a low- and middle-income country or an Indigenous population.	
5. Name two possible strategic priorities to address the burden of musculoskeletal pain globally.	

References

Abram, S.G.F., Judge, A., Beard, D.J., Wilson, H.A., Price, A.J., 2019. Temporal trends and regional variation in the rate of arthroscopic knee surgery in England: analysis of over 1.7 million procedures between 1997 and 2017. Has practice changed in response to new evidence? Br. J. Sports. Med. 53 (24), 1533.

AIHW, 2019. Hospitalised Injury Among Aboriginal and Torres Strait Islander People 2011–12 to 2015–16. (1760544930).

AIHW, 2022. Determinants of health for Indigenous Australians. Available from: https://www.aihw.gov.au/reports/australias-health/social-determinants-and-indigenous-health#Where%20do%20I%20go%20for%20more%20information?.

Allan, B., Smylie, J., 2015. First Peoples, Second Class Treatment: The Role of Racism in the Health and Well-Being of Indigenous Peoples in Canada, Discussion Paper. Wellesley Institute.

Amery, R., 2017. Recognising the communication gap in Indigenous health care. Med. J. Aust. 207 (1), 13–15.

Anderson, K., Cunningham, J., Devitt, J., Preece, C., Cass, A., 2012. Looking back to my family": indigenous Australian patients' experience of hemodialysis. BMC. Nephrol. 13 (1), 1–8.

Anderson, I., Robson, B., Connolly, M., Al-Yaman, F., Bjertness, E., King, A., et al., 2016. Indigenous and tribal peoples' health (The Lancet-Lowitja Institute Global Collaboration): a population study. Lancet 388 (10040), 131–157.

Australian Institute of Health and Welfare (AIHW), 2015. The Health and Welfare of Australia's Aboriginal and Torres Strait Islander Peoples 2015.

Australian Institute of Health and Welfare (AIHW), 2017. The burden of Musculoskeletal Conditions in Australia: A Detailed Analysis of the Australian Burden of Disease Study 2011.

Australian Institute of Health Welfare, 2019. Musculoskeletal Conditions and Comorbidity in Australia. AIHW, Canberra. Arthritis series no. 25. Cat. no. PHE 241.

Azevedo, D.C., Machado, L.A.C., Giatti, L., Griep, R.H., Telles, R.W., Barreto, S.M., 2021. Different components of subjective well-being are associated with chronic nondisabling and disabling knee pain: ELSA-Brasil Musculoskeletal Cohort. J. Clin. Rheumatol. 27 (6S), S301–S307.

Barber, C.E., Jewett, L., Badley, E.M., Lacaille, D., Cividino, A., Ahluwalia, V., et al., 2017. Stand up and be counted: measuring and mapping the rheumatology workforce in Canada. J. Rheumatol. 44 (2), 248–257.

Barnabe, C., Lockerbie, S., Erasmus, E., Crowshoe, L., 2017. Facilitated access to an integrated model of care for arthritis in an urban Aboriginal population. Can. Fam. Physician. 63 (9), 699.

Barnabe, C., Crane, L., White, T., Hemmelgarn, B., Kaplan, G.G., Martin, L., et al., 2018. Patient-reported outcomes, resource use, and social participation of patients with rheumatoid arthritis treated with biologics in Alberta: experience of indigenous and non-indigenous patients. J. Rheumatol. 45 (6), 760–765.

Barnabe, C., Kherani, R.B., Appleton, T., Umaefulam, V., Henderson, R., Crowshoe, L., 2021. Participant-reported effect of an Indigenous health continuing professional development initiative for specialists. BMC Med. Educ. 21 (1), 1–8.

Baum, F.E., Laris, P., Fisher, M., Newman, L., MacDougall, C., 2013. Never mind the logic, give me the numbers": former

Australian health ministers' perspectives on the social determinants of health. Soc. Sci. Med. 87, 138–146.

Blair, K., K. M. Dunn, A. Kamp and O. Alam (2017). Challenging Racism Project 2015-16 National Survey Report. Sydney, Western Sydney University.

Blue, B., 2014. Discrimination against Indigenous Australians: A Snapshot of the Views of Non-indigenous People Aged 25–44. Beyond Blue. Available from: https://www. beyondblue. org. au/docs.

Blue, E., 2017. Seeing Ms. Dhu: inquest, conquest, and (in) visibility in black women's deaths in custody. Settl. Colon. Stud. 7 (3), 299–320.

Blyth, F.M., March, L.M., Brnabic, A.J.M., Jorm, L.R., Williamson, M., Cousins, M.J., 2001. Chronic pain in Australia: a prevalence study. Pain 89 (2–3), 127–134.

Brady, B., Veljanova, I., Chipchase, L., 2017. An exploration of the experience of pain among culturally diverse migrant communities. Rheumatol. Adv. Pract. 1 (1), rkx002.

Briggs, A.M., Huckel Schneider, C., Slater, H., Jordan, J.E., Parambath, S., Young, J.J., et al., 2021. Health systems strengthening to arrest the global disability burden: empirical development of prioritised components for a global strategy for improving musculoskeletal health. BMJ Glob. Health. 6 (6), e006045.

Bruggink, L., Hayes, C., Lawrence, G., Brain, K., Holliday, S., 2019. Chronic pain: 'Overlap and specificity in multimorbidity management'. Aust. J. Gen. Pract. 48 (10), 689.

Brussoni, M., George, M.A., Jin, A., Lalonde, C.E., McCormick, R., 2016. Injuries to Aboriginal populations living on- and off-reserve in metropolitan and non-metropolitan areas in British Columbia, Canada: incidence and trends, 1986-2010. BMC Publ. Health 16 (1), 397.

Carey, G., Crammond, B., Keast, R., 2014. Creating change in government to address the social determinants of health: how can efforts be improved? BMC Publ. Health. 14 (1), 1–11.

Chandler, M.J., Lalonde, C.E., 2008. Cultural continuity as a protective factor against suicide in First Nations youth. Horizons 10 (1), 68–72.

Coffin, J., 2007. Rising to the challenge in Aboriginal health by creating cultural security. Aborig. Isl. Health. Work. J. 31 (3), 22–24.

Cordero, D.M., Miclau, T.A., Paul, A.V., Morshed, S., Miclau III, T., Martin, C., et al., 2020. The global burden of musculoskeletal injury in low and lower-middle income countries: a systematic literature review. OTA Int. 3 (2).

Daher, M., 2012. Cultural beliefs and values in cancer patients. Ann. Oncol. 23 (Suppl. 3), 66–69.

de Heer, E.W., Gerrits, M.M.J.G., Beekman, A.T.F., Dekker, J., van Marwijk, H.W.J., de Waal, M.W.M., et al., 2014. The association of depression and anxiety with pain: a study from NESDA. PLoS One. 9 (10), e106907.

Department of the Prime Minister Cabinet, 2018. Closing the Gap Prime Minister's Report 2018. Commonwealth of Australia, Canberra, Australia.

Durey, A., Thompson, S.C., 2012. Reducing the health disparities of Indigenous Australians: time to change focus. BMC Health. Serv. Res. 12 (1), 151.

Durey, A., Thompson, S.C., Wood, M., 2011. Time to bring down the twin towers in poor Aboriginal hospital care:

addressing institutional racism and misunderstandings in communication. Intern. Med. J. 42 (1), 17–22.

Dwyer, J., Kelly, J., Willis, E., Glover, J., Mackean, T., Pekarsky, B., 2020. Managing Two Worlds Together: City Hospital Care for Country Aboriginal People–Project Report. The Lowitja Institute, Melbourne.

El Zorkany, B., AlWahshi, H.A., Hammoudeh, M., Al Emadi, S., Benitha, R., Al Awadhi, A., et al., 2013. Suboptimal management of rheumatoid arthritis in the Middle East and Africa: could the EULAR recommendations be the start of a solution? Clin. Rheumatol. 32 (2), 151–159.

Eriksen, A.M., Schei, B., Hansen, K.L., Sørlie, T., Fleten, N., Javo, C., 2016. Childhood violence and adult chronic pain among indigenous Sami and non-Sami populations in Norway: a SAMINOR 2 questionnaire study. Int. J. Circumpolar. Health. 75 (1), 32798.

First Nations Child & Family Caring Society, 2021. Jordan's Principle. First Nations Child & Family Caring Society. Available from: https://fncaringsociety.com/jordans-principle.

First Nations Health Authority, 2017. Overdose Data and First Nations in BC: Preliminary Findings. Available from https://www.fnha.ca/AboutSite/NewsAndEventsSite/NewsSite/Documents/FNHA_OverdoseDataAndFirstNationsInBC_PreliminaryFindings_FinalWeb_July2017.pdf.

First Nations Health Authority, 2021. First Nations Toxic Drug Deaths Doubled during the Pandemic in 2020. First Nations Health Authority. Available from: https://www.fnha.ca/about/news-and-events/news/first-nations-toxic-drug-deaths-doubled-during-the-pandemic-in-2020.

Goodman, A., Fleming, K., Markwick, N., Morrison, T., Lagimodiere, L., Kerr, T., et al., 2017. They treated me like crap and I know it was because I was Native": the healthcare experiences of Aboriginal peoples living in Vancouver's inner city. Soc. Sci. Med. 178, 87–94.

Goucke, C.R., Jackson, T., Morriss, W., Royle, J., 2015. Essential pain management: an educational program for health care workers. World. J. Surg. 39 (4), 865–870.

Government of Canada, 1985. Canada Health Act. (R.S.C., 1985, c. C-6).

Government of Canada, 2021. Jordan's Principle. Government of Canada. Available from: https://www.sac-isc.gc.ca/eng/1568396042341/1568396159824.

Gracey, M., King, M., 2009. Indigenous health part 1: determinants and disease patterns. Lancet 374 (9683), 65–75.

Green, M., Cunningham, J., Anderson, K., Griffiths, K., Garvey, G., 2021. Measuring health care experiences that matter to Indigenous people in Australia with cancer: identifying critical gaps in existing tools. Int. J. Equity. Health. 20 (1), 1–10.

Guo, J., Fu, M., Qu, Z., Wang, X., Zhang, X., 2019. Risk factors associated with pain among community adults in Northwest China. J. Pain Res. 12, 1957.

Health Canada, 2021. An Action Plan for Pain in Canada (H134-19/2021e-PDF). Available from: https://www.canada.ca/content/dam/hc-sc/documents/corporate/about-health-canada/public-engagement/external-advisory-bodies/canadian-pain-task-force/report-2021-rapport/report-rapport-2021-eng.pdf.

Holliday, S., Morgan, S., Tapley, A., Dunlop, A., Henderson, K., van Driel, M., et al., 2015. The pattern of opioid management by Australian general practice trainees. Pain Med 16 (9), 1720–1731.

Hoy, D., Toole, M.J., Morgan, D., Morgan, C., 2003. Low back pain in rural Tibet. Lancet 361 (9353), 225–226.

Huot, S., Ho, H., Ko, A., Lam, S., Tactay, P., MacLachlan, J., et al., 2019. Identifying barriers to healthcare delivery and access in the Circumpolar North: important insights for health professionals. Int. J. Circumpolar. Health. 78 (1), 1571385.

Institute of Medicine Committee on Advancing Pain Research & Education, 2011. The National Academies Collection: Reports Funded by National Institutes of Health. In Relieving Pain in America: A Blueprint for Transforming Prevention, Care, Education, and Research. National Academies Press, Washington, D.C.

International Association for the Study of Pain, 2021. IASP Developing Countries Project: Initiative for Improving Pain Education. International Association for the Study of Pain. Available from: https://www.iasp-pain.org/resources/grants-awards/iasp-developing-countries-project-initiative-for-improving-pain-education/.

Ironside, A., Ferguson, L.J., Katapally, T.R., Foulds, H.J., 2020. Cultural connectedness as a determinant of physical activity among Indigenous adults in Saskatchewan. Appl. Physiol. Nutr. Metabol. 45 (9), 937–947.

Jackson, T., Thomas, S., Stabile, V., Shotwell, M., Han, X., McQueen, K., 2016. A systematic review and meta-analysis of the global burden of chronic pain without clear etiology in low-and middle-income countries: trends in heterogeneous data and a proposal for new assessment methods. Anesth. Analg. 123 (3), 739–748.

Jimenez, N., Garroutte, E., Kundu, A., Morales, L., Buchwald, D., 2011. A review of the experience, epidemiology, and management of pain among American Indian, Alaska Native, and Aboriginal Canadian Peoples. J. Pain. 12 (5), 511–522.

Johnson-Jennings, M., Duran, B., Hakes, J., Paffrath, A., Little, M.M., 2020. The influence of undertreated chronic pain in a national survey: prescription medication misuse among American Indians, Asian Pacific Islanders, Blacks, Hispanics and Whites. SSM-Popul. Health. 11, 100563.

Jones, B., Heslop, D., Harrison, R., 2020. Seldom heard voices: a meta-narrative systematic review of Aboriginal and Torres Strait Islander peoples healthcare experiences. Int. J. Equity. Health. 19 (1), 1–11.

Jongen, C., McCalman, J., Bainbridge, R., 2018. Health workforce cultural competency interventions: a systematic scoping review. BMC Health. Serv. Res. 18 (1), 1–15.

Judge, A., Murphy, R.J., Maxwell, R., Arden, N.K., Carr, A.J., 2014. Temporal trends and geographical variation in the use of subacromial decompression and rotator cuff repair of the shoulder in England. Bone. Joint. J. 96-B (1), 70.

Julien, N., Lacasse, A., Labra, O., Asselin, H., 2018. Review of chronic non-cancer pain research among Aboriginal people in Canada. Int. J. Qual. Health. Care. 30 (3), 178–185.

Kamerman, P.R., Bradshaw, D., Laubscher, R., Pillay-van Wyk, V., Gray, G.E., Mitchell, D., et al., 2020. Almost 1 in 5 South African adults have chronic pain: a prevalence study conducted in a large nationally representative sample. Pain 161 (7), 1629–1635.

Karunanayake, A.L., Pathmeswaran, A., Kasturiratne, A., Wijeyaratne, L.S., 2013. Risk factors for chronic low back pain in a sample of suburban Sri Lankan adult males. Int. J. Rheum. Dis. 16 (2), 203–210.

Katzenellenbogen, J.M., Sanfilippo, F.M., Hobbs, M.S., Knuiman, M.W., Bessarab, D., Durey, A., et al., 2013. Voting with their feet-predictors of discharge against medical advice in Aboriginal and non-Aboriginal ischaemic heart disease inpatients in Western Australia: an analytic study using data linkage. BMC Health. Serv. Res. 13 (1), 1–10.

Kelaher, M.A., Ferdinand, A.S., Paradies, Y., 2014. Experiencing racism in health care: the mental health impacts for Victorian Aboriginal communities. Med. J. Aust. 201 (1), 44–47.

King, M., Smith, A., Gracey, M., 2009. Indigenous health part 2: the underlying causes of the health gap. Lancet 374, 76–85.

Larson, A., Gilles, M., Howard, P., Coffin, P., 2007. It's enough to make you sick: the impact of racism on the health of Aboriginal Australians. Aust. N. Z. J. Publ. Health. 31 (4), 322–329.

Latimer, M., Rudderham, S., Lethbridge, L., MacLeod, E., Harman, K., Sylliboy, J.R., et al., 2018. Occurrence of and referral to specialists for pain-related diagnoses in First Nations and non–First Nations children and youth. Can. Med. Assoc. J. 190 (49), E1434–E1440.

Lavoie, J.G., 2018. Medicare and the care of First Nations, Métis and Inuit. Health. Econ. Pol. Law. 13 (3–4), 280–298.

Lin, I.B., O'Sullivan, P.B., Coffin, J.A., Mak, D.B., Toussaint, S., Straker, L.M., 2012. 'I am absolutely shattered': the impact of chronic low back pain on Australian Aboriginal people. Eur. J. Pain. 16 (9), 1331–1341.

Lin, I.B., O'Sullivan, P.B., Coffin, J.A., Mak, D.B., Toussaint, S., Straker, L.M., 2013. Disabling chronic low back pain as an iatrogenic disorder: a qualitative study in Aboriginal Australians. BMJ Open. 3 (4), e002654.

Lin, I., O'Sullivan, P., Coffin, J., Mak, D., Toussaint, S., Straker, L., 2014. 'I can sit and talk to her': Aboriginal people, chronic low back pain and healthcare practitioner communication. Aust. Fam. Physician. 43 (5), 320–324.

Lin, I., Green, C., Bessarab, D., 2016. 'Yarn with me': applying clinical yarning to improve clinician–patient communication in Aboriginal health care. Aust. J. Prim. Health. 22 (5), 377–382.

Lin, I.B., Ryder, K., Coffin, J., Green, C., Dalgety, E., Scott, B., et al., 2017. Addressing disparities in low back pain care by developing culturally appropriate information for Aboriginal Australians: "My Back on Track, My Future". Pain. Med. 18 (11), 2070–2080.

Lin, I.B., Bunzli, S., Mak, D.B., Green, C., Goucke, R., Coffin, J., et al., 2018. Unmet needs of Aboriginal Australians with musculoskeletal pain: a mixed–method systematic review. Arthritis. Care. Res. 70 (9), 1335–1347.

Lin, I., Wiles, L., Waller, R., Goucke, R., Nagree, Y., Gibberd, M., et al., 2019. What does best practice care for musculoskeletal pain look like? Eleven consistent recommendations from high-quality clinical practice guidelines: systematic review. Br. J. Sports. Med. 54, 79–86.

Lin, I., Coffin, J., Bullen, J., Barnabe, C., 2020a. Opportunities and challenges for physical rehabilitation with indigenous populations. Pain. Rep. 5 (5), e838.

Lin, I., Wiles, L., Waller, R., Caneiro, J.P., Nagree, Y., Straker, L., et al., 2020b. Patient-centred care: the cornerstone for high-value musculoskeletal pain management. Br. J. Sports. Med. 54, 1240–1242.

Logan, L., McNairn, J., Wiart, S., Crowshoe, L., Henderson, R., Barnabe, C., 2020. Creating space for Indigenous healing practices in patient care plans. Can. Med. Educ. J. 11 (1), e5.

Lopatina, E., Miller, J.L., Teare, S.R., Marlett, N.J., Patel, J., Barber, C.E., et al., 2019. The voice of patients in system redesign: a case study of redesigning a centralized system for intake of referrals from primary care to rheumatologists for patients with suspected rheumatoid arthritis. Health. Expect. 22 (3), 348–363.

Loppie Reading, C., Wien, F., 2013. Health Inequalities and the Social Determinants of Aboriginal Peoples' Health. Prince George. National Collaborating Centre for Aboriginal Health, British Columbia, Canada.

Louw, Q.A., Morris, L.D., Grimmer-Somers, K., 2007. The prevalence of low back pain in Africa: a systematic review. BMC Muscoskel. Disord. 8, 105.

Maiga, Y., Sangho, O., Konipo, F., Diallo, S., Coulibaly, S.D.P., Sangare, M., et al., 2021. Neuropathic pain in Mali: the current situation, comprehensive hypothesis, which therapeutic strategy for Africa? eNeurologicalSci 22, 100312.

Marmot, M., Wilkinson, R., 2005. Social Determinants of Health. OUP, Oxford.

Marmot, M., Friel, S., Bell, R., Houweling, T.A., Taylor, S., on behalf of the Commission on Social Determinants of Health, 2008. Closing the gap in a generation: health equity through action on the social determinants of health. Lancet 372 (9650), 1661–1669.

Marrone, S., 2007. Understanding barriers to health care: a review of disparities in health care services among indigenous populations. Int. J. Circumpolar. Health. 66 (3), 188–198.

Marun, G.N., Morriss, W.W., Lim, J.S., Morriss, J.L., Goucke, C.R., 2019. Addressing the challenge of pain education in low-resource countries: essential pain management in Papua New Guinea. Anesth. Analg. 130 (6), 1608–1615.

Mathieson, S., Wertheimer, G., Maher, C.G., Christine Lin, C.-W., McLachlan, A.J., Buchbinder, R., et al., 2020. What proportion of patients with chronic noncancer pain are prescribed an opioid medicine? Systematic review and meta-regression of observational studies. J. Intern. Med. 287 (5), 458–474.

Mbuzi, V., Fulbrook, P., Jessup, M., 2017. Indigenous cardiac patients' and relatives' experiences of hospitalisation: a narrative inquiry. J. Clin. Nurs. 26 (23–24), 5052–5064.

Meana, M., Cho, R., DesMeules, M., 2004. Chronic pain: the extra burden on Canadian women. BMC Wom. Health. 4 (1), 1–11.

Mellor, D., 2004. Responses to racism: a taxonomy of coping styles used by Aboriginal Australians. Am. J. Orthopsychiatry. 74 (1), 56–71.

Mills, S.E.E., Nicolson, K.P., Smith, B.H., 2019. Chronic pain: a review of its epidemiology and associated factors in population-based studies. Br. J. Anaesth. 123 (2), e273–e283.

Mittinty, M.M., McNeil, D.W., Jamieson, L.M., 2018. Limited evidence to measure the impact of chronic pain on health outcomes of Indigenous people. J. Psychosom. Res. 107, 53–54.

Morris, L.D., Daniels, K.J., Ganguli, B., Louw, Q.A., 2018. An update on the prevalence of low back pain in Africa: a systematic review and meta-analyses. BMC Muscoskel. Disord. 19 (1), 1–15.

Moseley, G.L., 2007. Reconceptualising pain according to modern pain science. Phys. Ther. Rev. 12 (3), 169–178.

Mukhtar, N.B., Meeus, M., Gursen, C., Mohammed, J., Dewitte, V., Cagnie, B., 2021. Development of culturally sensitive pain neuroscience education materials for Hausa-speaking patients with chronic spinal pain: a modified Delphi study. PLoS One. 16 (7), e0253757.

Nagaraj, S., Barnabe, C., Schieir, O., Pope, J., Bartlett, S.J., Boire, G., et al., 2018. Early rheumatoid arthritis presentation, treatment, and outcomes in aboriginal patients in Canada: a Canadian early arthritis cohort study analysis. Arthritis. Care. Res. 70 (8), 1245–1250.

Nchako, E., Bussell, S., Nesbeth, C., Odoh, C., 2018. Barriers to the availability and accessibility of controlled medicines for chronic pain in Africa. Int. Health. 10 (2), 71–77.

Nelson, S.E., Browne, A.J., Lavoie, J.G., 2016. Representations of Indigenous peoples and use of pain medication in Canadian news media. Int. Indig. Policy. J. 7 (1).

Nolan-Isles, D., Macniven, R., Hunter, K., Gwynn, J., Lincoln, M., Moir, R., et al., 2021. Enablers and barriers to accessing healthcare services for Aboriginal people in New South Wales, Australia. Int. J. Environ. Res. Publ. Health. 18 (6), 3014.

Oster, R.T., Grier, A., Lightning, R., Mayan, M.J., Toth, E.L., 2014. Cultural continuity, traditional Indigenous language, and diabetes in Alberta First Nations: a mixed methods study. Int. J. Equity. Health. 13 (1), 1–11.

Pain Australia, 2021. The National Strategic Action Plan for Pain Management. Australian Government Department of Health. Available from: https://www.health.gov.au/resources/publicati ons/the-national-strategic-action-plan-for-pain-management.

Paradies, Y., 2018. Racism and Indigenous Health. In Oxford Research Encyclopedia of Global Public Health. Oxford University Press.

Parker, R., Jelsma, J., 2010. The prevalence and functional impact of musculoskeletal conditions amongst clients of a primary health care facility in an under-resourced area of Cape Town. BMC Muscoskel. Disord. 11 (1), 2.

Penington Institute, 2020. Australia's Annual Overdose Report 2020.

Priest, N., Paradies, Y., Stewart, P., Luke, J., 2011. Racism and health among urban Aboriginal young people. BMC Publ. Health. 11 (1), 1–9.

Priest, N., Paradies, Y., Trenerry, B., Truong, M., Karlsen, S., Kelly, Y., 2013. A systematic review of studies examining the relationship between reported racism and health and wellbeing for children and young people. Soc. Sci. Med. 95, 115–127.

Ramage-Morin, P.L., Gilmour, H.L., 2010. Chronic Pain at Ages 12 to 44. Statistics Canada.

Rauch, A., Negrini, S., Cieza, A., 2019. Toward strengthening rehabilitation in health systems: methods used to develop a WHO package of rehabilitation interventions. Arch. Phys. Med. Rehabil. 100 (11), 2205–2211.

Rowley, K.G., O'Dea, K., Anderson, I., McDermott, R., Saraswati, K., Tilmouth, R., et al., 2008. Lower than expected morbidity and mortality for an Australian Aboriginal population: 10-year follow-up in a decentralised community. Med. J. Aust. 188 (5), 283–287.

Sharma, S., Pathak, A., Jha, J., Jensen, M.P., 2018. Socioeconomic factors, psychological factors, and function in adults with chronic musculoskeletal pain from rural Nepal. J. Pain Res. 11, 2385–2396.

Sharma, S., Blyth, F.M., Mishra, S.R., Briggs, A.M., 2019a. Health system strengthening is needed to respond to the burden of pain in low- and middle-income countries and to support healthy ageing. J. Glob. Health. 9 (2) 020317-020317.

Sharma, S., Jensen, M.P., Moseley, G.L., Abbott, J.H., 2019b. Results of a feasibility randomised clinical trial on pain education for low back pain in Nepal: the Pain Education in Nepal-Low Back Pain (PEN-LBP) feasibility trial. BMJ Open. 9 (3), e026874.

Sharma, S., Jensen, M.P., Pathak, A., Sharma, S., Pokharel, M., Abbott, J.H., 2019c. State of clinical pain research in Nepal: a systematic scoping review. Pain Rep 4 (6).

Sheard, L., Peacock, R., Marsh, C., Lawton, R., 2019. What's the problem with patient experience feedback? A macro and micro understanding, based on findings from a three–site UK qualitative study. Health. Expect. 22 (1), 46–53.

Smith, K., Fatima, Y., Knight, S., 2017. Are primary healthcare services culturally appropriate for Aboriginal people? Findings from a remote community. Aust. J. Prim. Health. 23 (3), 236–242.

Stewart Williams, J., Ng, N., Peltzer, K., Yawson, A., Biritwum, R., Maximova, T., et al., 2015. Risk factors and disability associated with low back pain in older adults in low-and middle-income countries. Results from the WHO Study on Global AGEing and Adult Health (SAGE). PLoS One 10 (6), e0127880.

Strong, J., Nielsen, M., Williams, M., Huggins, J., Sussex, R., 2015. Quiet about pain: experiences of Aboriginal people in two rural communities. Aust. J. Rural. Health. 23 (3), 181–184.

Tarlier, D.S., Browne, A.J., Johnson, J., 2007. The influence of geographical and social distance on nursing practice and continuity of care in a remote First Nations community. Can. J. Nurs. Res 126–149.

Thurston, W.E., Coupal, S., Jones, C.A., Crowshoe, L.F.J., Marshall, D.A., Homik, J., et al., 2014. Discordant indigenous and provider frames explain challenges in improving access to arthritis care: a qualitative study using constructivist grounded theory. Int. J. Equity. Health. 13 (1), 46.

Towle, A., Godolphin, W., Alexander, T., 2006. Doctor-patient communications in the Aboriginal community: towards the development of educational programs. Patient. Educ. Couns. 62 (3), 340–346.

Traeger, A.C., Buchbinder, R., Elshaug, A.G., Croft, P.R., Maher, C.G., 2019. Care for low back pain: can health systems deliver? Bull. World. Health. Organ. 97 (6), 423.

Truth and Reconciliation Commission of Canada, 2015. Honouring the Truth, Reconciling for the Future: Summary of the Final Report of the Truth and Reconciliation Commission of Canada. Truth and Reconciliation Commission of Canada.

Turpel-Lafond, M.E., 2021. Summary Report, November 2020. Addressing Racism Review. In: In plain Sight: Addressing Indigenous-specific Racism and Discrimination in BC Health Care.

Umaefulam, V., T. L. Fox and C. Barnabe (2021). Decision Needs and Preferred Strategies for Shared Decision Making in Rheumatoid Arthritis: Perspectives of Canadian Urban Indigenous Women. Arthritis Care Res. (Hoboken). 74(8): 1325–1331.

Umaefulam, V., A. Loyola-Sanchez, V. B. Chief, A. Rame, L. Crane, T. Kleissen, L. Crowshoe, T. White, D. Lacaille and C. Barnabe (2021). At-a-glance-Arthritis liaison: a First Nations community-based patient care facilitator. Health Promot. Chronic Dis. Prev. Can. 41(6): 194–198.

van Hecke, O., Hocking, L.J., Torrance, N., Campbell, A., Padmanabhan, S., Porteous, D.J., et al., 2017. Chronic pain, depression and cardiovascular disease linked through a shared genetic predisposition: analysis of a family-based cohort and twin study. PLoS One 12 (2), e0170653.

Vickery, J., Faulkhead, S., Adams, K., Clarke, A., 2007. Indigenous insights into oral history, social determinants and decolonisation. In: Ian Anderson, Fran Baum and Michael

Bentley (eds) Beyond Bandaids: Exploring the Underlying Social Determinants of Aboriginal Health. Co-operative Research Centre for Aboriginal Health, Darwin. vol. 19, p. 36.

Vos, T., Barker, B., Begg, S., Stanley, L., Lopez, A.D., 2009. Burden of disease and injury in aboriginal and Torres Strait islander peoples: the indigenous health gap. Int. J. Epidemiol. 38 (2), 470–477.

Vos, T., Abajobir, A.A., Abate, K.H., Abbafati, C., Abbas, K.M., Abd-Allah, F., et al., 2017. Global, regional, and national incidence, prevalence, and years lived with disability for 328 diseases and injuries for 195 countries, 1990–2016: a systematic analysis for the Global Burden of Disease Study 2016. Lancet 390 (10100), 1211–1259.

Webster, P.C., 2013. Indigenous Canadians confront prescription opioid misuse. Lancet 381 (9876), 1447–1448.

Wong, A., Hyde, Z., Smith, K., Flicker, L., Atkinson, D., Skeaf, L., et al., 2020. Prevalence and sites of pain in remote-living older Aboriginal Australians, and associations with depressive symptoms and disability. Intern. Med. J. 51 (7), 1092–1100.

T. World Bank, 2021a. World Bank Country and Lending Groups. The World Bank. Available from: https://datahelpdesk.worldbank.org/knowledgebase/articles/906519.

T. World Bank, 2021b. The World Bank in Middle Income Countries. The World Bank. Available from: https://www.worldbank.org/en/country/mic/overview.

Zadro, J., O'Keeffe, M., Maher, C., 2019. Do physical therapists follow evidence-based guidelines when managing musculoskeletal conditions? Systematic review. BMJ. Open. 9 (10), e032329.

Chapter | 23 |

Chronic pain and psychiatric problems

George Ikkos, Paul St John Smith, Awais Aftab, and Parashar Ramanuj

LEARNING OBJECTIVES

At the end of this chapter, readers will be able to:
1. Understand the nature and practice of psychiatric expertise.
2. Summarise the pluralist philosophical and evolutionary medical perspectives on psychiatry and pain.
3. Learn about the prevalence and clinical significance of comorbidity of psychiatric syndromes and chronic pain.
4. Identify features and treatment of psychiatric syndromes commonly comorbid with chronic pain.
5. Understand risk and its relevance to decisions regarding referral from pain medicine to psychiatry.
6. Learn what to expect and how to prepare a patient when referring to a psychiatrist.

Introduction

Neuropsychiatric disorders contribute approximately 25% of the total burden of disease in men and 30% in women in Europe (Wittchen et al. 2011). A UK study found that chronic pain was the most common long-term condition in people with depression and/or anxiety, especially in disadvantaged populations (Hodgson et al. 2020). High prevalence, common psychosocial determinants (Marmot et al. 2020; Patel et al. 2018) and overlapping psychobiological mechanisms (Ikkos & Ramanuj 2020) explain this frequent co-occurrence (Beckman & Tobin 2018). A Swiss study of adolescents with chronic pain and mental comorbidity found that 'The most substantial temporal associations were those with onset of mental disorders preceding onset of chronic pain' (Tegethoff et al. 2015). Frontal-limbic cortical connections are likely to play a major part in this (Vachon-Presseau et al. 2016). It is necessary, therefore to integrate psychiatry and pain medicine. To achieve this, understanding of the complexity of psychiatric problems is essential (Ikkos et al. 2011).

Affect, not the brain, is the primary object of psychiatrists' specialist medical expertise (Ikkos 2015). Affect is conceptualised as feelings, emotions and agitations. The ability to bring an integrated view from neuroscience, other biomedical research and psychosocial perspectives to the understanding of these phenomena places psychiatrists in a strong position to contribute to the care of some of the most complex patients that pain clinicians see.

Commonly referred to as emotion (Bennett & Hacker 2006; Thompson 2010), affect is a complex biopsychosocial phenomenon. It coordinates responses to biological and interpersonal needs by giving valence to thoughts and feelings, and manifesting in perception, imagination, behaviour and social relationships. It depends on factors such as social and family setting; genetic and personal history; metabolic and other biological phenomena; personal attitudes and habits; or simply chance. Mental disorders are therefore complex biopsychosocial phenomena too. A clinical psychiatric formulation extends beyond diagnosis to integrate available information and plan an effective therapeutic response jointly with patients, in the light of their values and preferences. It requires a pluralist approach.

In this chapter, we summarise pluralist, enactive and evolutionary perspectives in psychiatry. Using the evolutionary perspective as a bridge between biomedical and psychosocial understandings, we illustrate its relevance to clinical phenomena in pain medicine, including attachment, placebo, dependent substance use and depression. We then discuss specific mental disorders. Reference to mental or psychiatric 'disorder' has become controversial over the years. This is because, as the sections below should make clear, there are different ways of looking at the same phenomena. Moreover, some patients find the word 'disorder' stigmatising or undermining. Arguably the term 'syndrome' or 'constellation' would be more appropriate. We use the term 'disorder' as it remains prevalent in use, including in textbooks, official classification and research systems, and is recognised in law, for example in personal injury claims. It should be understood within a pluralist perspective, not narrowly biomedical, and the language used in consultations and reports should be mindful of patients' sensitivities. We conclude with reference to the importance of a holistic assessment of people with persistent pain and suspected mental health problems.

Points of view: pluralist perspective on psychiatry and pain

There are multiple methods/levels of analyses/perspectives on psychiatric disorders. Pluralism refers to multiple perspectives in our explanation and understanding of phenomena, while acknowledging that each offers only partial knowledge about an aspect of a phenomenon (Campaner 2014). Explanatory pluralism is often complemented by a form of pragmatism, which gives different explanatory perspectives differential weight in the context of specific explanatory interests and practical aims (Maung 2020).

The philosophical roots of modern pluralistic thinking in psychiatry are often traced back to the early 20th-century German psychiatrist and philosopher Karl Jaspers. He identified causal explanation (*erklären*) and meaningful understanding (*verstehen*) as two methods to understand psychopathology. When applied to the relationship between pain and depressed mood, for example, one can study this connection in terms of inflammatory markers and activity of brain circuits (*erklären*), and one can also comprehend the depressed mood experientially because of living with constant pain (*verstehen*).

Pluralism allows for a more holistic and integrated understanding of not only how pain and psychiatric disorder influence each other, but the way they interact with personality factors, generate adaptive/maladaptive coping behaviours (e.g. excessive use of alcohol or analgesics) and alter the trajectory of one's life story. One framework for such a pluralistic formulation, referred to as the *Perspectives* approach, utilises the four perspectives of diseases, dimensions of personality, goal-directed behaviours and life stories (McHugh & Slavney 1998).

In de Haan's *enactive framework*, psychopathology has four integrated main dimensions: *physiological, experiential, sociocultural* and *existential* (de Haan 2020a). Existential in this context refers to aspects of mind in which we are aware of being aware (e.g. being anxious about being anxious). Fig. 23.1 depicts an example of how select variables relevant to the comorbidity of pain and depressed mood can interact in the space of the dimensions of enactivism. Such interactions apply to most, if not all, relationships between pain and psychiatric disorder.

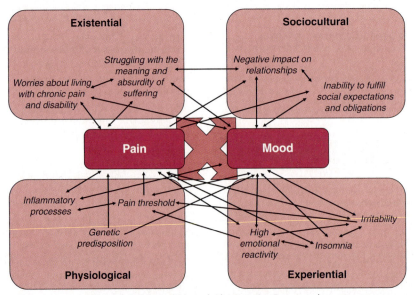

Fig. 23.1 Pain and Moood: The Enactive Framework

The enactive framework also interfaces with, and integrates, two other conceptual approaches in psychiatry: network theory of mental disorders and complex, dynamic systems. Network theory posits that psychiatric symptoms, rather than being the result of an undiscovered underlying and determining cause, exist in networks of relationships in which they cause each other through mutually reinforcing, self-sustaining feedback loops (Borsboom 2017; Borsboom & Cramer 2013). Within an enactive framework, the self-sustaining causal loops involve relevant causal factors across the four dimensions. Pertinently, pain becomes a part of the causal network, where it can directly activate other symptoms, such as insomnia, anxiety, irritability, low mood and poor concentration. These in turn can activate other symptoms (including pain).

Within a *complex, dynamic system*, the influence of any causal factor depends on the presence of other causal factors, as well as the overall context. 'Causes are only causes in specific contexts', de Haan writes (2020b, p. 241). For instance, an individual with chronic back pain who is otherwise physically healthy and has robust psychological coping mechanisms and adequate social support, may experience minimal negative psychiatric sequelae. In contrast, in another person with obsessional traits, employment difficulties, marital conflict and a habit of drinking alcohol excessively, the same chronic back pain can tip the symptom network into a major depressive episode. Network theory and complex dynamic systems recognise that the interaction of a variety of factors can create critical tipping points with rapid transitions from one to a different state of mind and health. Coninx and Stilwell (2021) offer a detailed application of the enactive approach to understanding and helping in chronic pain.

A point of view: evolutionary perspective

Emotions as protection

Evolutionary medicine is another perspective in psychiatry. It distinguishes between *defence* and *disease* (Nesse & Williams 1996). Defences are Darwinian-evolved mechanisms that operate outside conscious awareness and protect organisms from harm. They are a key constituent of affect and find expression in feelings and thoughts too. Some symptoms arise from the activation of these defences, which have been shaped by natural selection to protect us from danger. Examples include pain, cough, nausea, vomiting, diarrhoea, fatigue, alarm and low or irritable mood. The distress caused by these defences can lead to them being mistaken for disease (Nesse 2019a). However, even though they may not be a disease in the narrow

sense, their highly aversive nature makes them a legitimate target for therapeutic attention in pain medicine, psychiatry and other branches of medicine.

A hypothetical system for health maintenance, shaped by evolution, has been referred to as a 'health governor' (Humphrey & Skoyles 2012). Aspects of this 'governor' are shared across many species, but it is most developed in humans and operates entirely outside conscious awareness. Natural selection has shaped emotional mechanisms to build on defence mechanisms. Emotions depend on an individual's appraisal of the meaning of events to facilitate the achievement of biosocial goals (Nesse 2019c). They adjust multiple psychobiological response parameters, thus increasing the organism's fitness to adapt to challenging scenarios. Emotions can be experienced as positive or negative. In situations that threaten health or survival, negative emotions are useful and positive emotions harmful. Deficits in negative affect and excesses of positive affect are both problematic. Clinicians often come across the denial of illness, an example of preservation of positive affect, which can be harmful because of failure to engage with appropriate treatment. Therefore despite the associated suffering, aversive emotions are not necessarily bad for organisms. Furthermore, unlike other sensory systems, nociceptive systems may undergo long-lasting, even permanent, enhancement of function following sufficiently intense activation (Chapter 7). This feature may have had evolutionary advantages in protecting organisms from repeated traumas and has been assumed to contribute to chronic pain conditions (Walters & Williams 2019).

An evolutionary approach considers the functional benefits of psychological processes, acknowledging that they have evolved to maximise safety (fitness/survival) in our species' history rather than to indiscriminately produce a feeling of well-being. The immediate causes of distressing emotions can then be attributed to several categories:

- The regulation mechanism is normal, e.g. pain or anxiety in the face of injury or threat. When these lead to withdrawal or other successful defence, they may prevent further exposure and risk of injury. The links between pain and normal but distressing anxiety are discussed in Chapters 5 and 12.
- Mechanisms that have been useful in the environment of evolutionary adaptiveness (EEA) are hijacked in novel circumstances, including modern societies (see the 'hijack hypothesis' in the addictions section later).
- The regulation mechanism is normal but is useless or excessive in this instance (Nesse 2019b). Common mental disorders such as anxiety and mood disorders are often of this kind (see the immune theory of depression later). Long-term mental health problems secondary to psychological trauma or abuse are of this kind too.

- The regulation mechanism and symptoms are clearly abnormal, e.g. pain in erythromelalgia which is due to sodium channelopathy and possibly other biological abnormalities. Though there is legitimate active debate, most psychiatrists consider schizophrenia, bipolar and some other mental disorders to be broadly of this kind.

Emotional attachment as protection and relevance to pain

Humans develop through a prolonged period of gestation in utero, followed by profound material and emotional dependency after birth. The main attachment figure, often the mother, serves as a secure base on which the child can rely during early years (Bowlby 1979). The carer has the role of soothing distress during this period. Biological attachment systems have evolved both in parents and children to serve this protective and comforting interpersonal process. The fear system is activated to produce signs of 'painful' distress such as crying in response to separation from the attachment figure. If the separation persists, the child becomes quiet and withdrawn. This second-phase withdrawal response probably emerged in evolution to ensure quiet avoidance of predators if the carer fails to respond to crying. It is important to realise that pain, fear and mood are not served by separate biological systems but by overlapping pathways shaped during evolution (Ikkos & Ramanuj 2020; Solms 2018). This explains why endogenous opioids play a role not only in pain but also in fear and attachment (Ballantyne 2018; Kozlowska et al. 2015).

Through exploration of the environment and relationships, the growing child can differentiate gradually from the attachment figure for greater social integration. Adaptive advantages result from the evolution of human abilities to modify our internal environment in the light of positive and negative evaluations of external environments. When the child has enjoyed consistently sensitive and supportive parental input, they will internalise this experience and grow into an emotionally secure and socially confident adolescent and adult. As a result, they will be able to reassure themself in the face of pain, threat or loss and continue to problem-solve in conflictual or other difficult situations. In contrast, if the child has experienced insensitivity, neglect, abuse or indulgence, they will often grow to be insecure, as if living constantly under threat or being denied entitlements. In such a case, because of chronic activation of psychobiological defence mechanisms which were meant to be helpful in acute situations, they will have lower thresholds for suffering chronic pain, including fibromyalgia or irritable bowel symptoms (Burke et al. 2017), anxiety, depression and even paranoia. However, probably less than a quarter of patients with chronic pain have mental ill health (Von Korff 2009).

Finally, the goal of the attachment system is to maintain proximity to caregivers who provide safety from danger. Thus at times of threat, the attachment system becomes activated. Manifestations of attachment behaviour change with the stage of the life cycle and attachment style. At times of subjectively perceived threat, which includes illness, proximity and caring are sought from attachment figures. Such figures may come to include trusted professional carers in adult life and childhood. The placebo response may be an emergent property of this attachment.

From emotion and attachment to placebo

Placebo effects may be considered explanations for how interpersonal clinical and other relationships and caring contribute to healing, and the converse, i.e. nocebo. The universality of these responses suggests a likely evolutionary basis for underlying mechanisms (McQueen et al. 2013). Nesse stresses that placebo responses primarily modify the body's defences rather than altering disease processes (Nesse & Schulkin 2019). Evolution has selected mechanisms that defend against injury, infection or poisoning. The regulation of these defences is influenced by appraisals of the environment. However, many defences appear to generate excessive responses, e.g. chronic pain and anxiety.

A signal detection analysis can explain this apparent paradox. When the cost of expressing a defence is low compared with the potential harm it protects against, the optimal system will allow for false alarms. This has been dubbed 'the smoke detector principle' (Nesse 2005). Overexpression of many defences allows that they can be dampened without compromising adaptation or health. The regulation of defences allows deactivation of protective defences in situations of extreme danger, to facilitate escape. They may also be turned off in situations favourable for recovery, where they may no longer be necessary for protection. This may explain pain reduction both when facing immediate threat and when being cared for.

When protection is hijacked: substance use and dependence

Plants produce neurotoxic phytochemicals (e.g. nicotine, morphine, cocaine) as a defence against insects and herbivores (St John-Smith et al. 2013). Many plants are known to have analgesic, narcotic or hallucinogenic effects. Early humans may have made use of them as a pharmacological manipulation of defences to achieve desirable results ('pharmacophagy'), e.g. to produce analgesia. They may also have ingested phytochemicals for social reasons, e.g.

to produce hallucinations for religious experiences and social bonding.

Psychoactive substances would have been scarce in the environments encountered in the pre-Neolithic EEA in which humans evolved. Chemical rewards were limited. Therefore the internal biological systems shaped in this environment did not require, nor acquired, natural brakes to pharmacophagy for analgesia. Now such substances are plentiful because of cultivation and selective breeding, or significantly more concentrated because of purification or other chemical modification. They may be administered via routes leading to greater bioavailability too. Therefore pharmacophagy, which conferred reproductive benefit in the EEA, may lead to severe impairment in the modern social environment.

The 'hijack hypothesis' implies that, because of evolutionary mismatch between the EEA and our contemporary environment, a range of drugs of abuse effectively commandeer the normal neural pleasure-and-reward brain circuitry in the dopaminergic mesolimbic pathway, thus producing positive reinforcement of drug taking behaviour (Nesse 2019d). People who experience high levels of negative affect or low levels of positive affect in response to adverse circumstances may use pharmacological means to overcome their aversive state. Consequently, some individuals continue to consume the drug despite mounting harm because of the natural weakness of evolved protective mechanisms and failure to differentiate excess from success.

When protection fails or misfires: depression

Depression has a range of highly variable clinical features including feeling low, irritable, sad, listless, even pain, or behaviour such as self-neglect, social withdrawal, self-harm etc. It can be caused by a range of events including loss, trauma, infection, pain, long-term stress, interpersonal conflict, grief, loneliness, postpartum events, romantic rejection, the season, chemicals, physical disease, starvation and other mental disorders. Evolutionary hypotheses attempt to identify a benefit of depression outweighing its costs in such circumstances during the EEA. Such hypotheses are not necessarily incompatible with one another and may explain different aspects and causes of the diverse symptoms of depression (Rantala et al. 2018).

At least 11 different evolutionary hypotheses have been proposed for putative different types of depression. For example, Miller and Raison's 'The role of inflammation in depression: from evolutionary imperative to modern treatment target' (Miller & Raison 2016) suggests that inflammatory responses, depressive mood and behaviour evolved together as an integrated response to 'stress', irrespective of the origin of stress, be that infectious, interpersonal or other. This is supported by brain imaging which has demonstrated similar responses to 'physical pain' following physical injury and 'emotional pain' following separation or loss (Lieberman 2013). In the EEA, this integrated response helped organisms avoid exposure to infectious pathogens and facilitated recovery from infection and injury. Miller and Raison argue therefore that infectious threats have been less active in modern society (until the recent Covid19 pandemic) but psychosocial and environmental stresses have been more so, and depression-generating changes are often provoked by social environmental factors, including human relationships. There is clinical and research evidence confirming that inflammation triggers depression and, conversely, that depression is commonly associated with inflammatory changes (Bullmore 2018). Similar inflammatory mechanisms are implicated in chronic pain (Chapters 6 and 7), underlining the potential for common pathways in chronic pain and psychiatric disorders, and specifically the role of social and environmental factors modulating both.

Clinical psychiatric disorders

The complex nature of psychiatric disorders makes the identification of single specific causes unlikely, indeed mostly inappropriate. Psychiatric diagnosis has therefore primarily been based on clinical symptoms, rather than causation. It is best to think of each diagnosis as an 'ideal type' that gives some guidance about prognosis and possible interventions, rather than a discrete disease. Patients do not fit neatly into diagnostic categories, may have overlapping symptoms and move from one symptom constellation to another over time. For more information see the *Shorter Oxford Textbook of Psychiatry* (Harrison et al. 2018)

Substance use disorders

Whether dependent or not, and although the pattern varies from country to country, recreational use of alcohol, cannabis, opioids, benzodiazepines, psychedelics, stimulants and other illicit drugs continues worldwide (Tran et al. 2019). Gabapentinoids also cause concern (Piskorska et al. 2013). Although details of consumption and effects vary, they share psychobiological mechanisms that allow us to consider them as a group. Opioids and gabapentinoids are of special significance in chronic pain; they are discussed in Chapter 15 and will not be considered here.

There is frequent comorbidity of psychoactive substance-related and mental disorders. Because of their analgesic effects, use of cannabis, opioids, cocaine, etc.

may be high in some people with chronic pain (Gunderson et al. 2009). Where there is pre-existing alcohol or opioid misuse, higher quantities of these substances may be required because of liver enzyme induction. When intoxication, cognitive impairment, disruption of the sleep–wake cycle or other factors lead to irregular intake of analgesics or lower activity participation, they may interfere with effectiveness of treatment and rehabilitation. Specialist assessment may be required to disentangle the relative contribution of medical prescription, recreational drug use, withdrawal states and primary psychiatric symptoms to the patient's clinical condition.

Alcohol, cannabis, opioids, stimulants (amphetamine, cocaine) and benzodiazepines are associated with withdrawal symptoms, although the pattern and intensity may vary. Positive reinforcement, in the sense of a reward or 'a high', is important in habit formation and induction of dependence (Robbins & Everitt 2020). However, dependence is maintained by negative reinforcement: each time a user experiences withdrawal symptoms, the probability of discontinuing use of the substance in the future is lowered. Over time, the strength of positive reinforcement diminishes while that of negative reinforcement increases. The environment in which substances are consumed can also acquire reinforcement properties. Contemporary neuroscience has provided evidence of the specific neurobiological and psychobiological changes associated with positive and negative reinforcement (ibid). Sadly, despite neuroscientific evidence of the profound long-term neurobiological changes associated with dependency-forming drugs, users continue suffering the burden of criminalisation, in addition to the stigma of psychiatric patients. Current levels of legal controls and sanctions do not necessarily correlate with the harm that different substances cause (Crome & Nutt 2021).

Clinicians must be sensitive to the complex medical and social burden shouldered by dependent drug users, including preventable burden added by clinicians' own preconceptions. They should enquire in a straightforward manner about recreational alcohol and drug use. As a way of underlining respect for the patient, it may be helpful to preface the enquiry by an explanation that this is routine. The 4-item CAGE questionnaire (Mitchel et al. 2014) and the 10-item AUDIT questionnaire (The Alcohol Use Disorders Identification Test: Guidelines for Use in Primary Care; WHO 2001) can be useful in screening specifically for alcohol. The UK official advice is not to drink daily, not more than 14 alcohol units per week and to spread intake over 3 days or more. A 5.5% AbV (alcohol by volume) beer pint approximates 4 units, a glass of 10 to 14 AbV table wine 1.5 units and a measure of 30%–40% spirits 1 to 1.5 units. Other recreational drug use is discouraged altogether and any such use should be noted.

Dependence on psychoactive substances is signalled by regular use and clock watching; decreasing variety and increased strength of preferred substances; adverse social and occupational impact; and withdrawal symptoms if access to the substance is delayed or terminated. Formal diagnostic criteria for dependence vary per classification system, but those in the recently developed International Classification of Diseases 11th revision (ICD-11) identify as essential: impaired control over substance use often accompanied by craving; substance becomes increasing priority in life and relegates other areas of life to periphery; continued use despite problems; and physiological features, including tolerance, withdrawal and continued use to prevent or alleviate withdrawal symptoms (Poznyak 2016).

Although prescription of medication must always be consistent with regulatory standards, detoxification and treatment plans must be developed on a consensual basis wherever possible. Where users are reluctant or ambivalent in engaging appropriately, motivational enhancement therapy (MET) may be helpful (DiClemente et al. 2017). Admission to specialist inpatient units may or may not be required for detoxification for alcohol-, opioid- and stimulant-related conditions. Whether in community or inpatient settings, alcohol withdrawal must be managed under clinical supervision to avoid severe risks such as seizures, hallucinosis, delirium tremens and long-term cognitive impairment associated with Wernicke–Korsakoff Syndrome. Reducing doses of chlordiazepoxide are used to prevent these, normally with intravenous vitamin B complex to reverse dietary deficiencies.

Psychological treatments in aid of alcohol relapse prevention include MET, cognitive behaviour therapy (CBT), 12-Step Facilitation and Alcoholics Anonymous attendance. Pharmacological treatments aiming at abstinence include naltrexone and acamprosate. Those aiming at reduced consumption are nalmefene and naltrexone. Disulfiram (Antabuse) is little used now because of adverse effects. Topiramate, gabapentin, sodium oxybate, varenicline, doxazosin, modafinil and baclofen are sometimes prescribed off licence (van den Brink & Kiefer 2020).

Opioid dependence is reviewed in Chapters 15 and 25. Management of withdrawal of cannabis and psychostimulants is supportive. There are no specific pharmacological interventions. Where evidence of another comorbid psychiatric disorder emerges, it should be treated as usual. Dependent psychoactive use is often a long-term, recurrent problem associated with neurobiological changes. Therefore long-term follow-up which acknowledges vulnerability to relapse and focuses on contingency management strategies and harm minimisation should be provided.

Common mental disorders

The most prevalent mental disorders are those characterised by primary anxiety and mood-related symptoms.

They are often referred to as common mental disorders. Comorbidity of chronic pain and common mental disorders may affect adversely the prognosis of both. Patients at risk of any of these conditions may partly share certain psychological vulnerabilities, although this does not apply to all cases (Di Tella & Castelli 2016; Naylor et al. 2017). Taking our cue from ICD-11, we consider the following groups: *Mood Disorders; Disorders Specifically Associated with Stress; Anxiety and Fear-related Disorders;* and *Obsessive–Compulsive and Related Disorders* (World Health Organization 2018, *The ICD-11 Classification of Mental and Behavioural Disorders* 2018).

Mood disorders

Mood disorders include *depression* and *bipolar disorder*. Depression may be minor or major. Even in minor depression (the presence of depressive symptoms insufficient to meet threshold for major depression), we find reduction of quality of life and worse health outcomes (Ramanuj et al. 2019).

In the main diagnostic classifications, major depression is defined by the number and severity of relevant symptoms and the impairment they cause. Characteristic symptoms include low mood, lack of energy and diminished pleasure; loss of confidence, self-blame and social withdrawal; irritability, inappropriate feelings of guilt and hopelessness about the future; and deliberate self-harm or completed suicide. In relation to chronic pain, these may disrupt routines, leading to self-neglect and irregular intake of medication; lack of motivation and inconsistent engagement in rehabilitation; amplified perception of bodily sensations; and gloomy rumination and excessive fear of illness or death.

Major depression is classified as mild, moderate or severe. When severe, particularly when associated with biological symptoms such as impaired sleep, early morning wakening, diurnal mood variation (worse mood in the morning), fatigue, loss of appetite and libido, it may be referred to as *melancholia*. Severe depression may manifest psychotic symptoms which betray a marked loss of touch with reality, e.g. auditory hallucinations denigrating the patient or instructing them to self-harm. Delusions are impervious to evidence to the contrary. They are mood congruent, i.e. the patient may falsely but unshakably believe against all evidence to the contrary that they have caused harm or catastrophe, are destitute and poor or have some terminal illness.

Mild or moderately severe depression is best managed by psychological treatment (e.g. CBT, interpersonal therapy (IPT) or psychodynamic psychotherapy). However, antidepressant medication may be necessary in moderately severe depression and is the treatment of choice in severe depression. Where there are psychotic features, antipsychotic medication will be required too (Cowen 2020).

Bipolar disorder is associated with alternating cycles of morbid mood elevation and depression. On different occasions, the same patient may present in highly variable mental states, whether manic, depressed or euthymic (normal mood). Mixed states may occur too. Bipolar disorder is more likely to present with melancholia or psychosis than unipolar depression. The psychosis may be depressive with delusions of guilt, poverty, etc., or manic with delusions of grandeur or persecution. Patients with bipolar disorders appear at higher risk of experiencing pain, especially chronic pain, and migraine (Stubbs et al. 2015). Antidepressants risk precipitating morbid mood elevation and associated behaviour. Pain clinicians need to consider this before prescribing antidepressants to patients with comorbid pain and bipolar disorder! The treatment of bipolar disorder is with mood stabilisers, e.g. lithium, antipsychotics (e.g. quetiapine) and antiepileptics (e.g. lamotrigine) (Vieta et al. 2020).

Disorders specifically associated with stress

The diagnosis of prolonged grief disorder, adjustment disorder, posttraumatic stress disorder (PTSD) and complex posttraumatic stress disorder (complex PTSD) is predicated on a specific association between one or more seriously adverse events and the onset of the disorder.

Bereavement, and challenging events and circumstances, may be expected to provoke emotional responses and behavioural adjustments. Such loss may be of important relationships but also important personal resources, e.g. employment, housing, physical ability. The boundary between normal and pathological reaction is obscure and contested (Zisook et al. 2012). The diagnoses of prolonged grief disorder and adjustment disorder aim to demarcate the latter. Injury and chronic pain may precipitate adjustment disorder, i.e. emotional and/or behavioural changes associated with impaired quality of life or harm. Both prolonged grief and adjustment disorder may undermine response to pain. This may be through challenge to the sense of self, disruption of life plans, feelings of loss, social isolation, rumination and lack of confidence. Peer support, employment guidance, relationship counselling, problem-solving therapy and supportive psychotherapy have potential to help, the choice depending on the individual and their circumstances.

PTSD is a response to sudden direct exposure to an event threatening severe injury or loss of life. The threat may have been to the patient or another person in their proximity. As a result, a permanent state of tension and alarm develops, the incident may be reexperienced vividly in nightmares or flashbacks, and there may be avoidance of the location of the traumatic incident and other reminders, i.e. the triad of hypervigilance, reexperiencing and avoidance. During flashbacks, the patient feels as if they are reliving the original traumatic event. Patients with pre-existing psychiatric disorder or current psychosocial stress may be more vulnerable to developing PTSD. For others, the perceived severity of the physical or psychological trauma will be the determining factor. High anxiety and the development of PTSD following serious physical injury are risk factors for the development of chronic pain (Rosenbloom et al. 2016). It must be emphasised however that where mental health problems arise following emotional and/or physical trauma, PTSD is not the inevitable outcome, risk of depression also being increased (Beaglehole et al. 2018). In populations living in conflict zones, rates for a wide range of mental health problems are elevated (Charlson et al. 2019).

A common but not invariable feature of PTSD is the clinical phenomenon of dissociation. During day-to-day life, it is impossible to attend consciously to all stimuli and matters that may have a significant impact. To do so would be paralysing. Rather we rely on force of habit and paying attention to the priorities of the moment. In this sense, we 'dissociate' ourselves partially from our environment, a normal psychological phenomenon. Perhaps readers have experienced driving to a destination lost in thoughts and having little recall of the journey. In circumstances of acute and severe threat such as life-threatening incidents, extreme dissociative mechanisms may kick in quickly. To protect us from the enormity of the threat and fear, we may lose partial or full memory of the event, even when we have not lost consciousness.

The treatments of choice for PTSD are psychological in the form of trauma-focused CBT (TF-CBT) or eye movement desensitisation reprocessing (EMDR). Other probably effective approaches include psychodynamic therapy and IPT. As they involve deliberate recollection of the index event, these therapies risk retraumatising the patient and there is a significant rate of dropping out of treatment. Selective serotonin reuptake inhibitor antidepressants (SSRIs) and antipsychotics have some modest efficacy. The use of antipsychotics is particularly limited by side effects but can sometimes be helpful (van den Heuvel & Seedat 2020).

In complex PTSD, survivors of adverse childhood experiences (ACEs), in addition to the core symptoms of PTSD, may present with long-standing feelings of shame or guilt and self-blame, difficulty in regulating emotions, fluctuating self-image, unstable relationships and recurrent self-harm. Complex PTSD is only one of the many possible mental and physical effects of ACEs, i.e. neglect or abuse, whether emotional, physical or sexual (Kelly-Irving 2019). ACEs are associated with an array of serious adverse health outcomes, including but not limited to chronic pain and related conditions like back pain, arthritis, fibromyalgia

syndrome (FMS), chronic fatigue syndrome (CFS) and irritable bowel syndrome (IBS) (Von Korff 2009). There is frequent comorbidity between complex PTSD and such syndromes, and there is no doubt about the need to enquire about relevant history and impact (Edwards et al. 2007).

A recent meta-analysis found that complex PTSD responds poorly to treatments that are effective in PTSD (Karatzias et al. 2019). Therefore the sensitive approach to complex PTSD requires staff who are both trained and clinically experienced in its recognition and management. Diagnosis and differentiation from certain personality disorders remains uncertain, the label of personality disorder itself being controversial. In terms of emotional dysregulation, self-harm, relationship difficulties, comorbidity with anxiety and mood disorders, there is overlap between complex PTSD and emotionally unstable personality disorder (EUPD). There is interest therefore in utilising dialectical behaviour therapy (DBT), the most studied psychological treatment for EUPD (Bohus et al. 2020).

Anxiety and fear-related disorders

This diagnostic grouping is characterised by subjective suffering or psychosocial impairment caused by the morbid overexpression of the fear mechanisms discussed in the section on evolution earlier. There may be genetic predisposition, insecure attachment history and past or current psychosocial adversity or abuse. Specific diagnoses include *phobias, generalised anxiety disorder* (GAD) and *panic disorder.*

Phobias may focus on fear of needles or animals, fear of embarrassment or humiliation in social situations (*social anxiety disorder* or social phobia) or fear of open spaces and situations from where escape might be difficult, or help would not be immediately available if things go wrong (agoraphobia). In *GAD*, the patient may worry about anything or everything and be unable to contain such anxiety despite insight into its excess. There are associated physical symptoms such as generalised muscular tension, chest tightness or pain, abdominal discomfort, sweating or tremor. Panic attacks are characterised by marked physical symptoms, e.g. blurred vision, shortness of breath, palpitations of the heart, or sensations like butterflies in the stomach, which come in acute waves and are associated with an overpowering fear of death or serious harm, e.g. suffering a heart attack. When these become associated with anticipatory anxiety, i.e. anxiety of panic attacks recurring, the diagnosis of *panic disorder* applies. The experience of panic attacks in public may lead to *agoraphobia*. Agoraphobia may also develop due to falls because of musculoskeletal problems and postural and motor instability.

The above presentations can be dramatic, yet many highly anxious people are adept in presenting a calm front. Therefore enquiry about symptoms as a matter of routine is important. Simple clinical management, including simple reassurance and education about the nature and psychology of pain will often not suffice in the management of comorbid anxiety and stress-related disorder. These should therefore be identified and treated by an appropriately trained specialist therapist. As in mild and moderately severe depression, psychological treatment is preferred, the range of such treatments being broadly those for depression though tailored towards anxiety rather than mood symptoms. A significant proportion requires medication. Effective medication in these and OCD and related disorders (see immediately below) consists of SSRIs (Baldwin & Huneke 2020).

Obsessive–compulsive and related disorders

In contrast to anxiety and fear-related disorders where the sense of danger and alarm dominate the clinical picture, the dominant features of *obsessive–compulsive disorders* (OCD) and related disorders are repetitive thoughts or behaviours. In OCD, these thoughts and behaviours may be understood as responses to underlying anxiety, fear and tension. While these may relieve such states in the short term, they often complicate and burden daily functioning and are recognised by the patient as inappropriate. Obsessions are recurrent intrusive and unsuccessfully resisted thoughts, images or memories, which the patient recognises as arising from their own mind yet consider irrational and cause distress. Thoughts may consist of fear of contamination or losing control of aggressive or sexual impulses. Images may consist of vividly imagined scenes of oneself or a loved one coming to harm. Memories may be associated with obsessional self-doubt about the correctness of the patient's behaviour or rumination about what its impact has been on others on the scene.

Compulsions may be mental or physical. Some feel compelled to count or repeat an action a fixed number of times to prevent imagined harm. Another common problem is compulsive checking regarding safety, e.g. having locked the door when leaving the house. Compulsions may be covert (internal compulsions) or external. Fear of contamination may lead to excessive hand washing, complex toileting routines or compulsive avoidance of public transport or toilets. Consequences may include damage to the skin, lateness for work or markedly restricted lifestyle.

Mehraban et al. (2014) found increased rates of OCD in their chronic pain clinic, although the absence of a control group and the very high rates they report raise questions. There is no doubt, however, that this comorbidity occurs. Clinical experience confirms that the effective treatment of OCD when present can lead to marked reduction of pain, although this is not always guaranteed. The treatment of choice for OCD is behavioural in the form of exposure and response prevention (ERP), whereby the patient is exposed to the feared stimulus but helped to develop methods to avoid compulsive responses. Medication in the form of the antidepressants clomipramine or SSRIs may be helpful and sometimes necessary. Adjunctive antipsychotics may be required too. The effectiveness of other methods, especially neuromodulation, remains to be established (Fineberg et al. 2020).

Also classified in this group is *body dysmorphic disorder* (BDD), the obsessional preoccupation with some imagined bodily defect or excessive preoccupation with some objective difference in appearance. The focus of concern is usually the nose, lips, breasts or genitals. Like OCD, BDD responds to treatment with CBT and SSRIs, and associated pain may improve too (Wilhelm et al. 2014).

BDD should be distinguished from the body dysmorphia found in CRPS (Lewis et al. 2007), which refers to bizarre perceptions of the affected limb, often associated with neglect, desire for amputation or both (Ikkos et al. 2019). Desire for amputation in CRPS needs to be differentiated from body integrity dysphoria (BID). The main feature in BID is a wish for amputation even in the absence of any injury or objective deformity. Some neurophysiological correlates have been observed recently (Saetta et al. 2020).

Functional somatic disorders

Discussion of BDD, dysmorphia and BID brings us to issues of body and mind. As enactive and evolutionary theories in psychiatry and the frequency of physical–mental comorbidity underline, the Cartesian dichotomy between body and mind is not tenable. However, it persists due to the highly developed human capability for self-consciousness. This is the existential dimension in enactive theory or what philosopher Helmuth Plessner terms human 'excentricity', i.e. the ability to look at ourselves as if from outside (Bernstein 2019). *Excentricity* leads to the false body–mind division, as if we were standing outside our body looking in. The next step in this misunderstanding is to take only the concrete body as real and the mental as imagined, 'all in the mind'. It is no surprise that some patients feel blamed when psychological factors are mentioned. Where emotions take over in such situations, they may lead to numerous controversies over the nature, meaning and significance of psychological factors in chronic pain, including *chronic widespread pain* (CWP) and *FMS*. The same holds true for numerous other syndromes where physical symptoms prevail without a gross anatomical abnormality. Hence, these are referred to as functional disorders and include *migraine*, trigeminal neuralgia, *functional neurological disorders* (FNDs), *IBS*, *CFS* and *FMS*.

The psychiatric sections of current diagnostic classifications include several syndromes which straddle the imagined body–mind divide: dissociative neurological disorders and somatoform and related disorders in ICD-10; somatic symptom and related disorders in DSM5; and bodily distress disorders in ICD-11. Unsurprisingly, given the false dichotomy, these overlap with disorders included in the same classifications under other medical specialties, e.g. CWP/fibromyalgia in rheumatology and pain medicine, migraine and FND in neurology and IBS in gastroenterology. In truth, these psychiatric and other syndromes are not separate conditions. There are moves afoot to rectify the confusing situation. These are most advanced in the interface of neurology and psychiatry, where it has been acknowledged that both specialties are relevant in FNDs and what is routinely required is a joint approach. Taking their cue from this development and their own conceptual and epidemiological work, Burton et al. (2020) propose a broader diagnostic category of *functional somatic disorders* (FSDs) which includes FNDs and other syndromes listed earlier. The proposed diagnosis depends on the presence of symptoms from three clusters for at least 3 months. The clusters are musculoskeletal, gastrointestinal, cardiorespiratory, genitourinary, nervous system and fatigue related. The presence of symptoms across different clusters strengthens diagnostic certainty. Burton et al. specify that no general assumption is made about the significance of psychological vs physical factors, the relative weight of which differs from patient to patient. Where psychological factors are important, they may or may not be attributable to psychiatric problems.

FSDs are common and account for one-third of consultations across primary and specialist medical practice (Burton et al. 2020). They may be comorbid with related medical conditions with known anatomical basis, e.g. CWP/fibromyalgia with rheumatoid arthritis or non-epileptic seizures with epilepsy. They may or may not be comorbid with the psychiatric syndromes discussed earlier. Significantly, Burton et al. adopt a pluralist approach towards aetiology: immune, nervous, hormonal, behavioural and psychological. They adduce evidence supporting the involvement of multiple processes thought to be shared across syndromes, even though specific processes involved may differ between individuals and syndromes. Their formulation is strongly supportive of the need for integrated multidisciplinary approaches across a wide range of medical specialities including pain medicine (Creed et al. 2011).

Personality disorders

This category is as important as it is controversial (Lewis & Appleby 1988; Tyrer 2001, 2020). Important because it is commonly encountered in chronic pain populations and possibly more common in chronic pain than psychiatric outpatient clinics (Weisberg 2000). Controversial because some argue that the label is unreliable and stigmatises people who have survived years of trauma and abuse. ICD-11 specifies the core features as: persistent disturbance in thinking, feeling, relating and behaving for more than 2 years; not due to another mental disorder; associated with substantial distress to self or others; or significant impairment across a range of intimate, family, work and other social circumstances. They may be particularly evoked by certain circumstances but are manifested across a range of settings and situations (Bach & First 2018).

ICD-11 defines three levels of severity (mild, moderate or severe) and specifies five dimensions along which personality traits must be assessed: *negative affectivity, detachment, disinhibition, dissociality* and *anankastia*. Dissociality refers to antisocial features; anankastia to obsessionality leading to rigid thinking, rule adherence and difficulty coping with change. ICD-11 allows for an additional *borderline pattern*. This is important because not only are those so labelled distressed, but their relations with clinicians may be troubled too. Patients may suffer chronic feelings of emptiness, inadequacy and emotional instability, leading to episodes of self-harm, other self-defeating behaviour or inappropriate anger. These and other features often lead to unstable interpersonal relationships, sometimes including with attending clinicians. They may idealise or denigrate clinicians, sometimes the same clinician on different occasions. This reflects a tendency to see relationships in black and white. Clinicians need to be careful to not be enticed into their idealisation by the patient, nor should they unreflectively collude in denigration of colleagues, both of which can override appropriate professional boundaries.

Research, mostly carried out on the borderline type, offers some evidence in support of the efficacy of some psychological treatments (Newton-Howes & Mulde 2020). Treatments may target individual features, e.g. self-harm, rather than the disorder as such. Specific interventions include DBT, mentalisation-based therapy (MBT), psychodynamic/transference-based therapy, cognitive analytic therapy (CAT), IPT, Systems Training for Emotional Predictability and Problem Solving (STEPPS), day hospital intervention (including group therapy and partial hospitalisation), therapeutic community and nidotherapy. During an emergency, some may require acute inpatient psychiatric admission.

Other clinical syndromes

Space does not allow us to discuss important conditions like autism spectrum disorder (ASD) and attention deficit hyperactivity disorder (ADHD), eating disorders, schizophrenia and other nonaffective psychoses in detail. They are a diverse group of disorders which develop early: during childhood in the case of ASD and ADHD, and adolescence or early adulthood in eating disorders, personality disorders and schizophrenia.

Rates of ASD and ADHD have been found to be elevated among children with chronic pain (Lipsker et al. 2018). Intuitively one can recognise why the combination of joint hypermobility and hyperactivity may lead to recurrent injury and chronic pain as seen in clinics. Bou Khalil et al. (2018) offer a model integrating early traumatic events, physiological abnormalities and emotional dysregulation to explain a reported association between fibromyalgia and adult ADHD. This model may be applied more widely when considering chronic pain and mental disorder comorbidity. Patients with both chronic pain and eating disorders may share a common central sensitisation mechanism (Sim et al. 2021). In contrast, there is an inverse association between schizophrenia and clinically significant pain (Engels et al. 2014). It should be noted however that when patients with schizophrenia present to pain clinics, they may describe rather bizarre bodily experiences, usually accompanied by delusional interpretations.

Psychiatric risk

We still do not know 'whether chronic pain is a dysfunction of the pain system, a sustained false alarm, or an artefact of modern life, or some combination' (Williams 2019). A variety of perspectives is required. In contemporary clinical practice, we risk interpreting the patient's difficulties, including emotional difficulties, as being simply responses to history and circumstances while failing to recognise impairment and disability attributable to mental disorders. This unhelpful 'normalisation' is not restricted to pain medicine (Hickox 2020, 2021). Such risk may unnecessarily disadvantage the patient, including, for example through the interpersonal dynamics associated with complex PTSD, or personality or FSD. These may erect barriers to a therapeutic alliance between pain clinician and patient. They may also expose patients to iatrogenic harm through inappropriate escalation of analgesic medication and other physical treatments. Crucially, as indicated, such disorders are often treatable. Psychiatric expertise can help evaluate the potential of physical and psychological interventions, as well as their relative merit in specific cases. In line with enactive and evolutionary approaches, we are not suggesting that psychiatric diagnosis and treatment should command priority in the support and management of all patients with chronic pain, but rather that they are judiciously included as part a range of potentially useful clinical approaches for individual patients. The criteria for referral should be considered carefully on a case-by-case basis rather than some arbitrary and poorly evidenced general rule. The key question is 'might a psychiatric assessment help this patient'?

It is not surprising that many patients with chronic pain entertain thoughts of self-injury. Both self-harm and suicide rates are elevated (Racine 2018). When self-harm or suicide occur, they may do through overdose on prescribed medication (Cheatle 2011). The association of chronic pain with ACEs, history of domestic violence and other abuse, current adversity and mental health problems means that, where such thoughts are entertained or actions carried out, the aetiology is likely to be multifactorial rather than simply pain-related. Considering the strong association between major depression and suicide, a diagnostic and risk assessment which addresses psychiatric factors is often indicated from the psychiatric point of view. It is not suggested that all thoughts of self-injury arise from mental disorder. Arguably, sometimes suicidal thoughts are the end result of rational choice rather than a mental disorder. In such cases, the psychiatrist can offer reassurance that psychiatric intervention is not required. There will be other cases where risk due to mental disorder may persist, but no further psychiatric interventions is possible. In such a case, the psychiatrist can ensure that a full assessment and exploration of options has taken place.

Conclusion

Because of stigma and fear of the potential intrusiveness of a psychiatric interview, it is important that members of the multidisciplinary pain team are aware of the essentials of psychiatric practice and have regular contact and communication with psychiatrists, including for the benefit of mutual education. Ideally, along with psychologists, the psychiatrist will be a member of the multidisciplinary pain team. If not, regular scheduled face-to-face meetings with the team will help.

With such secure foundations, the clinician referring to a psychiatrist will be able to discuss the patient's concerns about the referral and, where appropriate, offer relevant reassurance. It is essential to explain to the patient, in a level-headed and transparent manner, the purpose of and expectations from referral to the psychiatrist. There should be no hidden agendas. It is not the role of the psychiatrist to interrogate and expose suspected deliberate exaggeration or malingering, though she might be able to contribute to constructive assessment and treatment where the referrer has already raised specific concerns with the patient. The reason for referring to a psychiatrist should be the better medical and psychological understanding of the patient, including but not limited to mental disorder, for the purpose of achieving better clinical outcomes.

The only surprise should be the patient's experience of the psychiatric interview as more helpful than they may have feared.

In conclusion, we have highlighted the risk of inappropriate 'normalisation' of patients' distress. Conversely, in line with the above, if the role of the psychiatrist is to help facilitate the holistic understanding and treatment of patients, especially bridge any relevant gaps between medical and psychosocial understandings, she should not be expected, nor limit herself, to diagnostic assessment and prescribing but aim at a clinical formulation reflecting the full complexity of the patient. Otherwise, she risks obscuring rather than illuminating suffering and contributing to stigma and iatrogenic harm.

Acknowledgements

We are grateful to the following colleagues in Pain Medicine and Allied Health at the Royal National Orthopaedic Hospital NHS Trust for their helpful comments on an earlier draft of this chapter: Dr Rebecca Berman (Anaesthesia and Hypnosis), John Doyle (Physiotherapy and Allied Health), Dr Tacson Fernandez (Anaesthesia and Neuromodulation), Chloe Kitto (Occupational Therapy and Staff Wellbeing), Dr Andrew Lucas (Clinical Health Psychology), Gill Thurlow (Specialist Nurse), Dr Roxaneh Zarnegar (Anaesthesia and Pain Management).

Review questions

Q

1. When adolescents suffer with chronic pain and common mental health problems which comes first usually?
2. What is affect?
3. How can the relationship between pain and psychopathology be understood through the integration of physiological, experiential, sociocultural and existential dimensions?
4. How does evolutionary theory explain how pain mechanisms can usually be switched off without much danger?
5. In what types of way may evolutionary adaptations go wrong in modern environments?
6. What are considered safe levels of alcohol consumption?
7. Can you name four anxiety- and fear-related psychiatric syndromes?
8. Can you name three FSDs with pain as a symptom?
9. What is the most important question when considering whether to refer to a psychiatrist?
10. When referring a patient to a psychiatrist, what should you tell them to expect?

References

Bach, B., First, M.B., 2018. Application of the ICD-11 classification of personality disorders. BMC Psychiatr. 18, 351.

Baldwin, D.S., Huneke, N.T.M., 2020. Chapter 92: treatment of anxiety disorders. In: Geddes, J.R., Andreasen, N.C., Goodwin, G.M. (Eds.), New Oxford Textbook of Psychiatry, third ed. Oxford University Press, Oxford.

Ballantyne, J.C., 2018. The brain on opioids. Pain 159 (Suppl. 1), S24–S30. 2018.

Beaglehole, B., Mulder, R., Frampton, C., Boden, J., Newton-Howes, G., Bell, C., 2018. Psychological distress and psychiatric disorder after natural disasters: systematic review and meta-analysis. Br. J. Psychiatry. 213 (6), 716–722. 2018.

Beckman, N.J., Tobin, M.B., 2018. Psychiatric comorbidities in chronic pain syndromes Chapter 23. In: Anitescu, M. (Ed.), Pain Management: A Problem-Based Learning Approach. Oxford University Press, Oxford.

Bennett, M.R., Hacker, P.M.S., 2006. Emotion, Ch.7. In: Philosophical Foundations of Neuroscience. Blackwell Publishing, Oxford.

Bernstein, J.,M., 2019. Introduction. In: Plessner, H. (Ed.), Levels of Organic Life and the Human: An Introduction to Human Anthropology. Fordham University Press, NY. 2019.

Bohus, M., Kleindienst, N., Hahn, C., Müller-Engelmann, M., Ludäscher, P., Steil, R., et al., 2020. Dialectical behavior therapy for posttraumatic stress disorder (DBT-PTSD) compared with cognitive processing therapy (CPT) in complex presentations of PTSD in women survivors of childhood abuse: a randomized clinical trial. JAMA Psychiatr. 77 (12), 1235–1245. 2020.

Borsboom, D., 2017. A network theory of mental disorders. World Psychiatr. 16 (1), 5–13.

Borsboom, D., Cramer, A.O., 2013. Network analysis: an integrative approach to the structure of psychopathology. Annu. Rev. Clin. Psychol. 9, 91–121. 2013.

Bou Khalil, R., Khoury, E., Richa, S., 2018. The comorbidity of fibromyalgia syndrome and attention deficit and hyperactivity disorder from a pathogenic perspective. Pain Med. 19 (9), 1705–1709. 2018.

Bowlby, J., 1979. The Making & Breaking of Affectional Bonds. Tavistock Publications, London, UK.

Bullmore, E., 2018. The Inflamed Brain: A Radical New Approach to Depression. Short Books Ltd, London.

Burke, N.N., Finn, D.P., McGuire, B.E., Roche, M., 2017. Psychological stress in early life as a predisposing factor for the development of chronic pain: clinical and preclinical evidence and neurobiological mechanisms. J. Neurosci. Res. 95 (6), 1257–1270. 2017.

Burton, C., Fink, P., Henningsen, P., et al., 2020. Functional somatic disorders: discussion paper for a new common classification for research and clinical use. BMC Med. 18, 34. (2020).

Campaner, R., 2014. Explanatory pluralism in psychiatry: what are we pluralists about, and why? In: Galavotti, M.C., Dieks, D., Gonzalez, W.J., Hartmann, S., Uebel, T., Weber, M. (Eds.), New Directions in the Philosophy of Science. Springer, pp. 87–103.

Charlson, F., van Ommeren, M., Flaxman, A., Cornett, J., Whiteford, H., Saxena, S., 2019. New WHO prevalence estimates of mental disorders in conflict settings: a systematic review and meta-analysis. Lancet 394 (10194), P240–P248.

Cheatle, M.D., 2011. Depression, chronic pain, and suicide by overdose: on the edge pain medicine. Pain Med. 12 (Suppl. 2), S43–S48 June 2011.

Coninx, S., Stilwell, P., 2021. Pain and the field of affordances: an enactive approach to acute and chronic pain. Synthese. 199, 7835–7863.

Cowen, P.J., 2020. Management and treatment of depressive disorders Ch77. In: Geddes, R., Andreasen, N.C., Goodwin, G.M.m (Eds.), New Oxford Textbook of Psychiatry, third ed. Oxford University Press, Oxford.

Creed, F., Henningsen, P., Byng, R., 2011. Achieving optimal treatment organisation in different countries: suggestions for service development applicable across different healthcare systems, Ch.10. In: Creed, F., Henningsen, R., Fink, P. (Eds.), Medically Unexplained Symptoms, Somatisation and Bodily Distress: Developing Better Clinical Services. Cambridge University Press, Cambridge.

Crome, I., Nutt, D., 2021. Drugs, drug harms and drug laws in the UK – lessons from history, Ch 25. In: Ikkos, G., Bouras, N. (Eds.), Mind State and Society: Social History of Psychiatry and Mental Health in Britain 1960-2010. Cambridge University Press, Cambridge.

de Haan, S., 2020a. Enactive Psychiatry. Cambridge University Press, Cambridge, UK; New York, NY.

de Haan, S., 2020b. Enactivism as a new framework for psychiatry. Philos. Psychiatr. Psychol. 27 (1), 1–2. 2020.

Di Tella, M., Castelli, L., 2016. Alexithymia in chronic pain disorders. Curr. Rheumatol. Rep. 18 (7), 41 2016.

DiClemente, C.C., Corno, C.M., Graydon, M.M., Wiprovnick, A.E., Knoblach, D.J., 2017. Motivational interviewing, enhancement, and brief interventions over the last decade: a review of reviews of efficacy and effectiveness. Psychol. Addict. Behav. 31 (8), 862–887. 2017.

Edwards, V.J., Dube, S.R., Felitti, V.J., Anda, R.F., 2007. It's ok to ask about past abuse. Am. Psychol. 62 (4), 327–328 discussion 330-332.

Engels, G., Francke, A.L., van Meijel, B., Douma, J.G., de Kam, H., et al., 2014. Clinical pain in schizophrenia: a systematic review. J. Pain. 15 (5), 457–467. 2014.

Fineberg, N.,A., Drummond, L.,M., Reid, J., et al., 2020. Management and treatment of obsessive compulsive disorder. In: Geddes, J.R., Andreasen, N.C., Goodwin, G.M. (Eds.), New Oxford Textbook of Psychiatry, third edn. Oxford University Press, Oxford. Chapter 98.

Gunderson, E.W., Coffin, P.O., Chang, N., Polydorou, S., Frances, et al. 2009. The interface between substance abuse and chronic pain management in primary care: a curriculum for medical residents. Substance. Abuse. 30 (3), 253–260.

Harrison, P., Cowen, P., Burns, T., Fazel, M. (Eds.), 2018. Oxford Textbook of Psychiatry, seventh ed. Oxford University Press, Oxford.

Hickox, A., 2020. Are you OK? Psychol. 33, 56–63.

Hickox, A., 2021. The threat is coming from inside the house. Psychol 34, 28–31.

Hodgson, K., Stafford, M., Fisher, R., et al., 2020. Inequalities in Health Care for People with Depression And/or Anxiety. The Health Foundation. Available from: https://www.health.org.uk/publications/long-reads/inequalities-in-health-care-for-people-with-depression-and-anxiety.

Humphrey, N., Skoyles, J., 2012. The evolutionary psychology of healing: a human success story. Current Biology. 22 (17 Special), R695–R698.

Ikkos, G., 2015. Psychiatric expertise. Br. J. Psychiatry. 207 (5), 399. 2015.

Ikkos, G., Ramanuj, P., 2020. Brain and pain: old assumptions and new science about chronic pain. BJPsych. Adv. 26 (3), 156–158.

Ikkos, G., Cohen, H., Lucas, A., 2019. An integrated medical, psychiatric and behavioural perspective on CRPS: reflections on publication of 'Complex Regional Pain Syndrome in Adults in the UK: Guidelines for diagnosis, referral and management in primary and secondary care'. Pain. News. 17 (2), 78–85. 2019.

Ikkos, G., McQueen, D., St. Smith, P., 2011. Psychiatry's contract with society; what is expected? Acta Psychiatr. Scand. 124, 1–3. 2011.

Karatzias, T., Murphy, P., Cloitre, M., et al., 2019. Psychological interventions for ICD-11 complex PTSD symptoms: systematic review and meta-analysis. Psychol. Med. 49 (11), 1761–1775 2019.

Kelly-Irving, M., 2019. Allostatic Load: How Stress in Childhood Affects Life-Course Health Outcomes. Health Foundation. Available from https://www.health.org.uk/publications/allostatic-load.

Kozlowska, K., Walker, P., McLean, L., Carrive, P., 2015. Fear and the defense cascade: clinical implications and management. Harv. Rev. Psychiatry. 23 (4), 263–287. 2015.

Lewis, G., Appleby, L., 1988. Personality disorder: the patients psychiatrists dislike. Br. J. Psychiatry. 153:44–9. doi: 10.1192/bjp.153.1.44.

Lewis, J.S., Kersten, P., McCabe, C.S., Blake, D.R., 2007. Body perception disturbance: a contribution to pain in complex regional pain syndrome (CRPS). Pain. 133 (1–3), 111–119. 2007.

Lieberman, M.D., 2013. Broken hearts and broken legs, Ch.3. In: Lieberman, M.,D. (Ed.), Social: Why Our Brains Are Wired to Connect. Oxford University Press, Oxford.

Lipsker, W.C., Bölte, S., Hirvikoski, T., Lekander, M., Holmström, L., Wicksell, R.K., 2018. Prevalence of autism traits and attention-deficit hyperactivity disorder symptoms in a clinical sample of children and adolescents with chronic pain. J. Pain. Res. 11, 2827–2836. 2018.

Marmot, M., Allen, J., Boyce, T., et al., 2020. Health equity in England: the marmot review 10 years on. Available from www.instituteofhealthequity.org/the-marmot-review-10-years-on.

Maung, H.H., 2020. Pluralism and incommensurability in suicide research. Stud. Hist. Philos. Biol. Biomed. Sci. 80, 101247. 2020.

McHugh, P.R., Slavney, P.R., 1998. The Perspectives of Psychiatry. JHU Press, Baltimore.

McQueen, D., Cohen, S., St John-Smith, P., et al., 2013. Rethinking placebo in psychiatry: how and why placebo effects occur. Adv. Psychiatr. Treat. 19 (3), 171–180.

Mehraban, A., Shams, J., Moamenzade, S., Samimi, S.M., Rafiee, S., Zademohamadi, F., 2014. The high prevalence of obsessive-compulsive disorder in patients with chronic pain. Iran. J. Psychiatry. 9 (4), 203–208. 2014.

Miller, A.H., Raison, C.L., 2016. The role of inflammation in depression: from evolutionary imperative to modern treatment target. Nat. Rev. Immunol. 16 (1), 22–34. 2016.

Mitchel, A.J., Bird, V., Rizzo, M., Hussain, S., Meader, N., 2014. Accuracy of one or two simple questions to identify alcohol-use disorder in primary care: a meta-analysis. British. J. Gen. Pract. 64 (624), e408–e418. 2014.

Naylor, B., Boag, S., Gustin, S.M., 2017. New evidence for a pain personality? A critical review of the last 120 years of pain and personality. Scand J Pain. 17, 58–67. 2017.

Nesse, R.M., 2005. Natural selection and the regulation of defenses: a signal detection analysis of the smoke detector principle. Evol. Hum. Behav. 26 (1), 88–105.

Nesse, R.M., 2019a. Why Are Mental Disorders So Confusing? Chapter 2 in Good Reasons for Bad Feelings: Insights from the Frontier of Evolutionary Psychiatry. Dutton Books, New York, NY.

Nesse, R.M., 2019b. Reasons for Bad Feelings Part 2. In Good Reasons for Bad Feelings: Insights from the Frontier of Evolutionary Psychiatry. Dutton Books, New York, NY.

Nesse, R.M., 2019c. Good reasons for bad feelings. Chapter 4 in Good Reasons for Bad Feelings: Insights from the Frontier of Evolutionary Psychiatry. Dutton Books, New York, NY.

Nesse, R.M., 2019d. Good Feelings for Bad Reasons Chapter 13 in Good Reasons for Bad Feelings: Insights from the Frontier of Evolutionary Psychiatry. Dutton Books, New York, NY.

Nesse, R.M., Schulkin, J., 2019. An evolutionary medicine perspective on pain and its disorders, Philosophical Transactions of the Royal Society B Volume 374, Issue 1785.

Nesse, R.M., Williams, G., 1996. Why We Get Sick: The New Science of Darwinian Medicine, second ed. J.M. Dent & Sons Ltd.

Newton-Howes, G., Mulde, R., 2020. Treatment and management of personality disorder, Chapter 122. In: Geddes, J.R., Andreasen, N.C., Goodwin, G.M. (Eds.), New Oxford Textbook of Psychiatry, third ed. Oxford University Press, Oxford.

Patel, V., Saxena, S., Lund, C., Thornicroft, G., Baingana, F., Bolton, P., et al., 2018. Commission on global mental health and sustainable development. Lancet. 392 (10157), 1553–1598. 2018.

Piskorska, B., Miziak, B., Czuczwar, S.J., Borowicz, K.K., 2013. Safety issues around misuse of antiepileptics. Expert. Opin. Drug. Saf. 12 (5), 647–657. 2013.

Poznyak, V., 2016. An Update on ICD-11 Taxonomy of Disorders Due to Psychoactive Substance Use and Related Health Conditions. International Society of Research on Alcoholism (ISBRA). World Health Organization.

Racine, M., 2018. Chronic pain and suicide risk: a comprehensive review. Prog. Neuro-Psychopharmacol. Biol. Psychiatry. 87 (Pt B), 269–280. 2018.

Ramanuj, P., Ferenchik, E., Pincus, H.A., 2019. Depression in primary care. BMJ. 365, l835. 2019.

Rantala, M.J., Luoto, S., Krams, I., Karlsson, H., 2018. Depression subtyping based on evolutionary psychiatry: proximate mechanisms and ultimate functions. Brain Behav. Immun. 69, 603–617.

Robbins, T., Everitt, B.,J., 2020. Substance use disorders and the mechanisms of drug addiction Chapter 48. In: Geddes, J.R., Andreasen, N.C., Goodwin, G.M. (Eds.), New Oxford Textbook of Psychiatry, third ed. Oxford University Press, Oxford.

Rosenbloom, B.N., Katz, J., Chin, K.Y.W., Haslam, L., et al., 2016. Predicting pain outcomes after traumatic musculoskeletal injury. Pain. 157 (8), 1733–1743. 2016.

Saetta, G., Hänggi, J., Gandola, M., Zapparoli, L., Gerardo Salvato, G., et al., 2020. Neural correlates of body integrity dysphoria. Curr. Biol. 30 (Issue 11), 2191–2195.e3. 2020.

Sim, L., Harbeck Weber, C., Harrison, T., Peterson, C., 2021. Central sensitization in chronic pain and eating disorders: a potential shared pathogenesis. J. Clin. Psychol. Med. Settings. 28 (1), 40–52.

Solms, M.,L., 2018. The neurobiological underpinnings of psychoanalytic theory and therapy. Front. Behav. Neurosci. 12.

St John-Smith, P., McQueen, D., Edwards, L., Schifano, F., 2013. Classical and novel psychoactive substances: rethinking drug misuse from an evolutionary psychiatric perspective. Hum. Psychopharmacol. 28 (4), 394–401.

St John-Smith, P., McQueen, D., Edwards, L., Schifano, F., 2013. Classical and novel psychoactive substances: rethinking drug misuse from an evolutionary psychiatric perspective. Hum. Psychopharmacol. 28 (4), 394–401. 2013.

Stubbs, B., Eggermont, L., Mitchell, A.J., et al., 2015. The prevalence of pain in bipolar disorder: a systematic review and large-scale meta-analysis. Acta Psychiatr. Scand. 131 (2), 75–88. 2015.

Tegethoff, M., Belardi, A., Stalujanis, E., Meinlschmidt, G., 2015. Comorbidity of mental disorders and chronic pain: chronology of onset in adolescents of a national representative cohort. J. Pain. 16 (10), 1054–1064.

Thompson, E., 2010. Primordial dynamism: emotion and valence, Chapter12. In: Mind in Life. Harvard University Press.

Tran, B.X., Moir, M., Latkin, C.A., et al., 2019. Global research mapping of substance use disorder and treatment 1971–2017: implications for priority setting. Subst. Abuse. Treat. Prev. Policy. 14, 21. (2019).

Tyrer, P., 2001. Personality disorder. Br. J. Psychiatry. 179 (1), 81–84.

Tyrer, P., 2020. Why we need to take personality disorder out of the doghouse. Br. J. Psychiatr. 216 (2), 65–66.

Vachon-Presseau, E., Tétreault, P., Petre, B., Huang, L., Berger, S.E., Torbey, S., et al., 2016. Corticolimbic anatomical characteristics predetermine risk for chronic pain. Brain. 139 (Pt 7), 1958–1970. 2016.

van den Brink, W., Kiefer, F., 2020. Alcohol use disorder. Chapter 50 Geddes, J.R. In: Andreasen, N.C., Goodwin, G.M. (Eds.), New Oxford Textbook of Psychiatry, third ed. Oxford University Press, Oxford.

van den Heuvel, L., Seedat, S., 2020. Management and treatment of stress related disorders, Chapter 83. In: Geddes, R., Andreasen, N.C., Goodwin, G.M. (Eds.), New Oxford Textbook of Psychiatry, third ed. Oxford University Press, Oxford.

Vieta, E., Pachiarotti, I., Miklowitz, D.J., 2020. Management and treatment of bipolar disorder. Chapter 72. In: Geddes, R., Andreasen, N.C., Goodwin, G.M. (Eds.), New Oxford Textbook of Psychiatry, third ed. Oxford University Press, Oxford.

Von Korff, M.R., 2009. Global perspectives on mental-physical comorbidity. Chapter 1. In: Von Korff, M.R., Scott, K.M., Gureje, O. (Eds.), Global Perspectives on Mental-Physical Comorbidity in the WHO World Mental Health Surveys. Cambridge University Press, Cambridge.

Walters, E.T., Williams, A, C. de C., 2019. Evolution of Mechanisms and Behaviour Important for Pain. Philosophical Transactions of the Royal Society B, p. 374.

Weisberg, J.N., 2000. Personality and personality disorders in chronic pain. Curr. Rev. Pain. 4 (1), 60–70. 2000.

Wilhelm, S., Phillips, K.A., Didie, E., Buhlmann, U., Greenberg, J.L., Fama, J.M., et al., 2014. Modular cognitive-behavioral therapy for body dysmorphic disorder: a randomized controlled trial. Behav. Ther. 45 (3), 314–327. 2014.

Williams, A.C. de C., 2019. Persistence of pain in humans and other mammals. Phil. Trans. R. Soc. B. 374.

Wittchen, H.U., Jacobi, F., Rehm, J., Gustavsson, A., Svensson, M., Jönsson, B., et al., 2011. The size and burden of mental disorders and other disorders of the brain in Europe 2010. Eur. Neuropsychopharmacol. 21 (9), 655–679. 2011.

World Health Organization, 2001. The Alcohol Use Disorders Identification Test: Guidelines for Use in Primary Care. World Health Organization.

World Health Organization, 2018. The ICD-11 classification of mental and behavioural disorders, world health organization. Available from https://www.who.int/standards/classifications/classification-of-diseases.

Zisook, S., Pies, P., Corruble, E., 2012. When is grief a disease? Lancet. 379 (issue) 9826, P1590.

Acute pain

Stephan A. Schug

LEARNING OBJECTIVES

At the end of this chapter, readers will understand the:
1. Principles underlying acute pain management for postoperative patients, including multimodal and procedure-specific analgesia and the prevention of the progression of acute to chronic pain.
2. Various pharmacological options for pain management, including the use of systemic opioid and nonopioid analgesics.
3. Principles, benefits and potential problems relating to patient-controlled analgesia.
4. Regional techniques for analgesia.
5. Nonpharmacological options for pain management, including physical and cognitive treatment techniques.
6. Role of an acute pain service in dealing with postoperative pain.

Overview

Acute pain is seen in a multitude of clinical situations: in the postoperative and posttrauma setting (including burns), in acute medical diseases (e.g. pancreatitis, myocardial infarction) and as obstetric pain. Postoperative pain is the most common form of acute pain (and of major relevance for therapists); therefore this chapter will focus on management of postoperative patients.

There is widespread agreement in the literature on the inadequacy of acute pain management. There is also a wide body of evidence which suggests that relief of acute pain can also have profound effects on patient outcomes. Only over the last 20 years has considerable scientific and clinical effort been invested in providing patients in acute pain with the best quality analgesia, while ensuring safety from potentially life-threatening adverse events for each analgesic modality (Pogatzki-Zahn et al. 2017).

This chapter focuses on the importance of effective management of acute pain. It incorporates the most important pharmacological and nonpharmacological modalities of analgesia (for definitions see Box 24.1). Reference will be made to the efficacy, benefits and adverse effects of these modalities. Newer techniques have accumulated substantial evidence demonstrating an improvement, not only in quality of analgesia and patient satisfaction but also in rehabilitation, short- and long-term morbidity, and potentially, even length of hospital stay and mortality (Schug et al. 2020). Provision of appropriate analgesia in the postoperative period is one component of concepts of 'fast-track surgery' (Beverly et al. 2017). There is also increasing evidence of an association between the experience of acute pain and the development of chronic pain (Schug & Bruce 2017), so adequate acute pain management plays a role in the prevention of chronic pain.

Despite the theoretical availability of a range of appropriate agents and techniques, their insufficient, inappropriate or unsupervised application often leads to poor acute pain management. Therefore this chapter would be incomplete without a discussion of appropriate organisational structures to provide acute pain relief, that is, the concept of and the role of the APS.

Principles of acute pain management

In a large survey of postoperative patients, the median worst pain score was reported as 5/10 (Gerbershagen et al. 2013). Up to 80% of patients report moderate-to-severe pain in the days after surgery (Meissner & Zaslansky 2019). These studies are in line with many others reporting insufficient relief of postoperative pain. Psychological factors such as preoperative anxiety, depression, catastrophising, expectation of pain, fear of death and associated sleep deprivation influence postoperative pain control, so attention must be given to individual patient differences to improve outcomes (Schug et al. 2020).

Traditionally, postoperative pain has been managed using fixed doses of intramuscularly (IM) administered opioids on an as-needed basis. This approach led to unrelieved pain in more than 50% of postoperative patients (Oden 1989). The major problem with this approach is the interindividual variation in dose requirements, which can vary more than 10-fold for patients of similar age and weight having the same operation. Furthermore, opioid concentrations following IM bolus doses exhibit a pronounced peak and trough pattern, with periods of inadequate analgesia and a risk of delayed overdose (Cashman & Dolin 2004). Furthermore, opioids by any route increase the risk of respiratory depression, as well as delay postoperative recovery and rehabilitation, through adverse effects such as nausea and vomiting, constipation and sedation (Oderda et al. 2013). Last, not least, postoperative opioids can contribute to the current widespread overuse of opioids in the community with associated significant risks, now known as the 'opioid-epidemic' (Levy et al. 2020).

A more appropriate approach to acute pain management should therefore combine a wider array of techniques, commonly called *multimodal analgesia*. This approach has been studied extensively over the last 20 years. When used appropriately, it improves pain relief, and reduces consumption and therefore adverse effects of opioids (Schug et al. 2020). Multimodal analgesia may include the following pharmacological options:

- Nonopioid analgesics, such as paracetamol, nonsteroidal antiinflammatory drugs (NSAIDs) and cyclooxygenase-2 (COX-2) inhibitors;
- other systemic agents for particular settings, such as nitrous oxide (Entonox), ketamine, adrenergic drugs, antidepressants and anticonvulsants;
- administration of systemic opioids (intravenously (IV), subcutaneously (SC), orally (PO), transmucosally or transdermally) on a regular and/or as-required basis or via patient-controlled analgesia (PCA);
- intermittent or continuous peripheral neural blockade with local anaesthetic drugs;
- neuraxial analgesia (epidural or intrathecal administration of opioids and/or local anaesthetic drugs).

There are also many nonpharmacological options, which are often underutilised despite their simplicity (Schug et al. 2020):

- explanation, reassurance and discussion of analgesic options;
- various physical interventions such as splints, massage, application of heat or cold, acupuncture and transcutaneous electrical nerve stimulation (TENS);
- cognitive–behavioural interventions such as relaxation, distraction and imagery, which can be taught preoperatively.

The majority of this chapter focuses on the pharmacological options, discussing their efficacy, benefits, side effect profiles and combined efficacy with other analgesic agents.

The choice of pain relief in the postoperative period should be procedure-specific, as different surgical interventions cause different acute pain states of different intensity in different areas of the body, so a defined analgesic modality may be more effective in one setting compared to another (Lee et al. 2018). For a large range of operations, procedure-specific evidence-based recommendations for postoperative analgesia are accessible on https://esraeurope.org/prospect/.

Systemic pharmacological modalities

Systemic pharmacological modalities include nonopioid analgesics, other pharmaceuticals and opioids.

Systemic nonopioid analgesics

Paracetamol/acetaminophen

Paracetamol (acetaminophen in the United States) has analgesic and antipyretic effects, but is not antiinflammatory (see Chapter 15). It is an effective analgesic in its own right, but not as effective as the other nonopioids. As a component of multimodal analgesia, it reduces opioid requirements by 30% (Tzortzopoulou et al. 2011). With short-term use in appropriate doses, there is a side effect profile comparable to placebo. Therefore many of the contraindications to NSAIDs, in particular renal impairment, do not relate to the use of paracetamol. Combining paracetamol with NSAIDs improves analgesia and increases opioid-sparing effects and patient satisfaction in comparison to the sole use of paracetamol (Martinez et al. 2017a).

Nonsteroidal antiinflammatory drugs

Nonselective NSAIDs and COX-2 selective inhibitors, so-called coxibs, are effective analgesics in the management of mild and moderate acute pain, and also the most useful components of multimodal analgesia (see Chapter 15). These drugs reduce the level of inflammatory mediators generated at the site of tissue injury. They have this effect by inhibiting the enzyme cyclooxygenase. Nonselective NSAIDs inhibit both isoenzymes COX-1 and COX-2, while coxibs selectively inhibit COX-2.

Efficacy is similar for both groups of drugs. As components of multimodal analgesia, they are opioid-sparing, improve analgesia and reduce the incidence of opioid-related adverse effects such as nausea, vomiting and sedation (Maund et al. 2011). Because of their selectivity for the isoenzyme COX-2, coxibs have a better adverse effect profile than nonselective NSAIDs (Schug et al. 2020). In short-term use, they result in gastric ulceration rates similar to those of a placebo, even in higher-risk populations. They do not impair platelet function, leading to reduced perioperative blood loss in comparison with nonselective NSAIDs. They also do not appear to induce bronchospasm in patients with aspirin-exacerbated asthma. They might have similar but reduced adverse effects

on renal function (Schug et al. 2017). Nevertheless, they should be used with care and consideration in situations of preexisting renal impairment, hypovolemia or hypotension, and when used together with other nephrotoxic agents and angiotensin-converting enzyme (ACE) inhibitors. Although there has been an ongoing debate about the risk of cardiovascular adverse events with the long-term use of coxibs, this could not be proven for short-term use of parecoxib and/or valdecoxib used after noncardiac surgery (Schug et al. 2017). However, coxibs as well as nonselective NSAIDs should not be used after coronary artery bypass surgery and possibly any cardiac surgery, due to an increased incidence of cardiovascular events. There is a theoretical concern that these compounds impair wound and bone healing, but this has not been shown conclusively to date (Schug 2021).

Overall, these compounds play an important role in the management of postoperative pain, particularly as a component of multimodal analgesia, as they do not cause typical opioid adverse effects such as sedation, respiratory depression or impaired bowel recovery. They are particularly effective in the treatment of pain with a major inflammatory component and pain on movement (Schug & Manopas 2007).

Other systemic agents

Entonox

Entonox is a mixture of 50% oxygen and 50% nitrous oxide. It provides a safe way to administer the analgesic inhalational anaesthetic nitrous oxide in a subanaesthetic concentration (Buhre et al. 2019). The agent is usually given by self-administration via a face mask or mouthpiece. Self-administration enhances safety, as the patient will stop usage in the unlikely case of loss of consciousness. Entonox is particularly useful as a safe short-term analgesic with a rapid onset of action; therefore it is commonly used for painful procedures such as dressing changes or passive mobilisation and during labour (Macintyre & Schug 2021).

Clonidine and dexmedetomidine

Clonidine and dexmedetomidine are α2-receptor agonists and thus potentiate the descending inhibitory pathways within the spinal cord that act on pain transmission at the dorsal horn. Their use reduces pain intensity and opioid requirements and therefore the incidence of opioid-induced nausea and vomiting. They do not cause respiratory depression per se. Dexmedetomidine now has better supportive data than clonidine in this setting, but is not yet widely used (Schug et al. 2020). Potential problems resulting from the use of clonidine are sedation and hypotension. Their administration in neuraxial analgesia techniques and peripheral nerve blocks is also effective.

Ketamine

Ketamine is an antagonist at the N-methyl-D-aspartate (NMDA) receptor within the central nervous system. This receptor is involved in the production of wind-up during excitation of the dorsal horn with repetitive pain impulses (Kreutzwiser & Tawfic 2019); see Chapter 7. Ketamine, in combination with PCA, has been shown to reduce opioid consumption, improve pain control and reduce nausea and vomiting (Brinck et al. 2018). It has a specific role in the management of procedural and neuropathic pain, pain that is poorly responsive to opioids and pain in opioid-tolerant patients (Schwenk et al. 2018). Its perioperative use may reduce the risk of chronic postsurgical pain (Ning et al. 2018).

Tricyclic antidepressants and anticonvulsants

These drugs are commonly used in chronic pain management, in particular in the treatment of neuropathic pain (see Chapters 13 and 15). They also play a role in the management of acute and subacute neuropathic pain such as sciatica, pain caused by nerve or spinal cord injury and stroke. For the acute emergency treatment of neuropathic pain, IV ketamine in low subanaesthetic doses, or IV lidocaine in antiarrhythmic doses or by continuous infusion can be used (Macintyre & Schug 2021). The anticonvulsants gabapentin and pregabalin, which inhibit the release of excitatory amino acids, have recently gained an increasing role in the management of acute pain. As premedication, they improve analgesia and reduce opioid requirements and opioid-related adverse effects (Schug et al. 2020). However, ideal doses and duration of treatment to achieve maximum benefit, without untoward side effects like sedation, are unknown. Given for longer periods perioperatively, they may prevent the development of chronic postsurgical neuropathic pain (Martinez et al. 2017b).

Systemic opioid analgesics

Systemic opioids are the treatment of choice in the management of moderate-to-severe acute pain. They include 'gold-standard' morphine as well as other opioids such as fentanyl, oxycodone, hydromorphone and methadone. All bind to opioid receptors within and outside the central nervous system. The activation of the μ-receptor in particular is intrinsically linked to their analgesic effect, but explains also most of the adverse effects of opioids (Schug et al. 1992).

Systemic opioids can be given by a wide variety of routes. The choice of route depends on the individual situation of the patient, the intensity of the pain and the infrastructure of the hospital. The traditional routes of opioid administration are PO, SC and IM. There is an increasing trend towards IV administration, in particular following opioid protocols or via PCA devices. Other routes of administration, for example transmucosal, intranasal and transdermal, are increasingly utilised.

The most common side effects are nausea and vomiting, sedation, pruritus, slowing of gastrointestinal function (constipation), urinary retention and sometimes—surprisingly—dysphoria (see Chapter 15 for more details). The most serious, but rare, complication of opioid usage is respiratory depression and subsequent hypoxia, which is potentially life-threatening. There are also increasing concerns about the potential of postoperative opioid use to generate long-term opioid use in some patients (Levy et al. 2020). Widespread use of opioids for chronic pain has resulted in considerable rates of opioid abuse, diversion of prescribed opioids into illegal use and overdose toxicity. *Opioid stewardship* is advocated in acute pain management to reduce this risk (Macintyre et al. 2014).

Oral opioids

Oral opioids are an option only after return of gastric motility, i.e. once the patient is able to tolerate fluids freely. Evidence suggests that oral opioids are as effective as parenteral opioids in appropriate doses and should be used as soon as oral medication is tolerated. Oral administration is the route of choice for acute pain management (Macintyre & Schug 2021).

Codeine is used widely, but its efficacy is limited, and some patients (ca. 10%) lack the enzyme needed to generate its active metabolite morphine. Moreover, subjects carrying a gene duplication are predisposed to life-threatening opioid intoxication; this is in particular relevant in children (Schug et al. 2020).

A useful alternative to codeine is the compound tramadol, a centrally acting analgesic with a mixed mechanism of action (opioid, noradrenergic, serotonergic) (Miotto et al. 2017). This mechanism of action explains its adverse effect profile, which is different from conventional opioids. Specifically; there is a reduced risk of respiratory depression, constipation and sedation. Furthermore, the abuse potential is lower than for classic opioids. However, similar to codeine, polymorphisms of the cytochrome P450 enzymes influence the analgesic efficacy of tramadol.

Morphine itself can be used, initially often in immediate (ca. 20 minutes from onset)- and short-acting preparations such as morphine elixir or immediate-release tablets. There is an increasing trend to avoid morphine because of some of its untoward effects, in particular its active metabolites which can complicate treatment, particularly in patients with renal impairment. Strong opioid alternatives in this case are oxycodone and hydromorphone, which lack such metabolites and are available in a wide range of preparations.

All opioids mentioned above are available in sustained-release formulations, which, given at defined time intervals, can provide long-term analgesia. These preparations should be avoided in the acute setting as they are difficult to titrate and carry an increased risk of overdose toxicity (ANZCA 2018). They may, however, be useful once ongoing need for opioid analgesia in the postoperative and, more commonly, the posttrauma rehabilitation period is established.

The use of pethidine (meperidine) should be discouraged in acute and chronic pain settings, as it has a high abuse potential and a neurotoxic metabolite that may induce seizures (Latta et al. 2002).

Intramuscular opioids

As mentioned earlier, IM opioids were the mainstay of postoperative pain management using opioids until recently. Traditionally, standard doses (commonly '10 mg for everyone') were administered by intermittent IM injections, usually no more frequently than every 4 hours, hence the infamous prescription: '10 mg morphine IM, PRN (as required) 4 hourly'. Such a 'one-dose-fits-all' approach leads to some patients being left in extreme pain and others at risk of major side effects. The incidence of respiratory depression using this route has been found to range from 0.8% to 37% depending on its definition (Cashman & Dolin 2004). In addition, IM injections are painful and carry the risk of tissue damage (e.g. to nerves) and infection (e.g. abscesses). Finally, absorption from an IM injection site is slow, unpredictable and delayed by physical factors such as hypothermia, hypovolaemia and immobility, commonly encountered in the early postoperative period.

The current recommendation and standard practice is to avoid this route if at all possible (Macintyre & Schug 2021). If, for organisational, political or training (better: lack of training) reasons, IM injections are the only parenteral route of administration permitted or—inappropriately—deemed safe in a certain environment, then the dose used should be based on age and medical condition, and the administration interval should be shortened to 2 hourly PRN, to increase flexibility.

Subcutaneous (SC) opioids

Opioids can be given intermittently or as a low-volume continuous infusion via the SC route. The absorption profile is similar to that of IM administration, and both routes have similar analgesic and side effect profiles (Cooper 1996). However, patients prefer the SC route, particularly if used via an indwelling SC cannula, for obvious reasons. The approach has been shown to be beneficial as a continuous infusion (volumes <1–2 mL/h) in severe cancer pain and in postoperative patients in whom IV access is not, or not easily, available (Macintyre & Schug 2021). Morphine and hydromorphone are used preferentially as they are low irritants to the SC tissue; treatment algorithms in this area have been published. For patients with an indwelling IV line (i.e. most early postoperative patients), there are no advantages but some disadvantages (delayed onset of analgesia, second access) of SC in comparison to IV.

Intravenous opioids

Opioids can be given as boluses (e.g. 0.5–4 mg morphine every 3–5 minutes as directed by a formal IV protocol) (Macintyre & Schug 2021), as a continuous infusion or via PCA devices through the IV route. IV is the route of choice in the early postoperative period after major surgery, but there is a risk of respiratory depression with inappropriate dosing, so close monitoring and safety precautions are required.

Intermittent IV boluses

Intermittent IV boluses provide a rapid, predictable and observable response compared to other parenteral routes (Schug et al. 2020). This is also the rationale behind the use of IV PCA. The IV route is particularly useful for:

- obtaining initial and rapid pain relief such as in the immediate postoperative period and in acute trauma;
- patients who are hypovolaemic and/or hypotensive and who absorb IM/SC opioids in a delayed and unpredictable fashion; and
- treating *incident pain* caused by events such as dressing changes, mobilisation and physiotherapy.

Intermittent boluses are also an ideal path to titrated pain relief in the recovery room and bridge times of severe pain until medical review and/or more appropriate analgesic methods become accessible. Most commonly, nurse-administered bolus doses, prescribed according to a protocol or algorithm, are used. Such protocols specify (or permit some flexibility with regard to) bolus size, assessments and 'lock-out' time (Macintyre & Schug 2021).

Continuous IV infusion

This form of infusion avoids the peaks and troughs in blood concentrations associated with intermittent administration, but it is difficult to predict the required individual blood concentration for optimal analgesia. A continuous infusion requires reliable devices, with frequent assessment and monitoring by staff trained to monitor patients on level of sedation and authorised to adjust the infusion rate and give bolus doses. Adequate analgesic blood concentrations can take up to 20 hours (five half-lives) to establish; consequently, if analgesia is inadequate, a bolus is given as well as the rate of infusion being increased.

The risk of respiratory depression using a continuous morphine infusion (up to 1.65%) is the highest of all parenteral routes (Schug & Torrie 1993). This needs to be considered carefully, as fatal outcomes are reported, in particular in sleeping or sedated patients (Macintyre et al. 2011).

Patient-controlled analgesia

PCA was introduced to overcome variability in individual morphine dose requirements, problems associated with insufficient analgesia and potentially serious adverse outcomes. PCA grants a patient control of his/her pain relief. It can be utilised by various routes of systemic and regional drug administration, but is commonly associated with IV drug administration.

A PCA device is a sophisticated, programmable infusion instrument that can be activated by the patient to self-administer small bolus doses of IV opioid on demand, separated by a lock-out period, during which the device does not respond to further activation. As such, the PCA concept overcomes the interindividual variation in opioid requirements and allows the patient to adjust the level of analgesia to their own desired level of comfort, balanced to an individually acceptable severity of side effects. Intravenous opioids administered by PCA improve analgesia and patient satisfaction (McNicol et al. 2015). It has been demonstrated that, for morphine, a bolus dose of 1 mg with a 5-minute lock-out period is ideal for most patients; other regimes are associated with either inadequate analgesia or sedation and increased respiratory compromise (Owen et al. 1989). However, some patients might need different regimes, depending on age, comorbidity, pain intensity and previous opioid exposure. Therefore regular review of all patients using PCA devices by experienced personnel is mandatory for a good outcome. Other opioids such as fentanyl, hydromorphone or tramadol can also be used (Schug et al. 2020).

Following surgery, the average patient will require PCA until reliable oral intake has been reestablished. Drug consumption is maximal within the first 24 hours and rapidly declines thereafter (Schug et al. 2020). Age is the best predictor of postoperative opioid requirements, but there is little correlation between patient weight and levels of consumption. The technique provides effective, steady analgesia and is popular with patients. However, about 40% of patients using PCA have a pain score >3/10 at rest on day 1 postoperatively. It requires special infusion pumps and staff education. In addition, patients require instructions preoperatively regarding the principles and operation of PCA (Chumbley et al. 2002).

Although PCA is the safest method of administering systemic opioids, there remains a small risk of respiratory depression (incidence in the range 0.1%–0.8%) (Macintyre 2001). This risk is much smaller than that associated with continuous IV infusion or intermittent IM injection. This advantage with regard to safety is due to the fact that acute pain causes stimulation of respiratory centres in the brain. As patients use the PCA device by titrating opioids to effect, there is less likelihood of respiratory depression, especially because the sedated patient will stop using the device. In the rare cases of respiratory depression, the causes are mostly (Schug et al. 2020):

- operator error (e.g. inappropriate prescription, incorrect programming of PCA device, incorrect dilution of medication);
- patient-related error (e.g. relatives using PCA button instead of the patient);
- equipment failure (e.g. cracked syringes with gravity siphoning of opioid solution (rare)).

Other side effects associated with PCA administration of opioids are nausea and vomiting as well as sedation. These problems occur with similar incidence to other methods of opioid administration and are not reduced by the PCA approach (McNicol et al. 2015).

Continuous low-dose IV infusion, when given together with PCA, has been shown to increase the risk of side effects without significantly improving analgesia (Macintyre & Schug 2021); the incidence of respiratory depression is five to eight times higher than in the case of PCA alone, as the inherent safety concept of PCA is violated. Hence, the only patients who should be prescribed a background opioid infusion are those already receiving opioids. These patients already have some degree of opioid tolerance as well as increased requirements (e.g. chronic pain, recreational abuse, methadone substitution).

All routes of opioid administration, especially parenteral routes, need to be carefully monitored for side effects, notably respiratory depression. Specific protocols are written for each route of administration so that patients receive optimal analgesia while always being safeguarded against respiratory depression and monitored for other side effects of opioids. Safe and appropriate use of the PCA method requires frequent and informed monitoring by nurses who have undergone relevant education and accreditation in the management of these devices. Standard orders and drug dilutions are suggested to maximise the effectiveness of the PCA and minimise complications.

The risk of opioid addiction is often cited as a reason for provision of inadequate analgesia. However, addiction to opioids is rare when used in the treatment of acute pain. Patients choose not to fully relieve their pain, despite free access to drugs, and demands tend to be conservative, with patients opting to remain alert and in a small amount of discomfort (Macintyre 2001).

In conclusion, opioids delivered via a PCA device provide better analgesia and higher levels of patient satisfaction, with less risk of respiratory depression than conventional routes of opioid administration. Patients' preference for PCA is possibly associated with the degree of control it affords them over their own pain management. However, PCA offers no reduction of opioid-related adverse effects and no difference in duration of hospital stay.

To improve the analgesia provided by IV PCA, the technique should be integrated into a concept of multimodal analgesia using other appropriate techniques and medications.

Regional techniques

Peripheral neural blockade

Techniques of peripheral neural blockade are commonly used to improve analgesia with minimal adverse effects. They also reduce the requirements for opioid analgesia and thus the incidence of opioid side effects, in particular when catheters are placed to permit infusions and thereby extend the effect into the later postoperative period (Ilfeld 2017). In view of these benefits, their use in the postoperative setting is increasing (Albrecht & Chin 2020). Neural blockades are now commonly performed under ultrasound guidance, which increases success rate and reduces risks of adverse effects (Schnabel et al. 2013).

Wound infiltration

This is an extremely simple technique, usually performed by the surgeon at the end of the operation. Use of long-acting local anaesthetics such as bupivacaine and ropivacaine can provide good analgesia, lasting for many hours after surgery. It is a particularly useful technique following minor operations such as hernia repair, paediatric surgery or trauma surgery. High-volume infiltration after knee replacement has also proved to be very successful (Andersen & Kehlet 2014). Leaving a catheter in the wound area to perform continuous infusion with local anaesthetics results in improved analgesia, reduced opioid consumption and other beneficial outcomes (Raines et al. 2014).

Femoral nerve blocks

These can be performed as a single-shot technique with a long-acting local anaesthetic. Alternatively, a catheter can be placed in the fascial sheath of the femoral nerve and analgesia can be provided by bolus injections or continuous infusion of local anaesthetics. This technique is useful for relief of pain and muscle spasm following knee surgery (specifically arthroplasty) and fractures of the femur neck (Ilfeld 2017). After knee replacement, increasingly a more distal femoral nerve block (adductor canal block) is used as it reduces motor block and thereby facilitates mobilisation (Kuang et al. 2017).

Brachial plexus blocks

For these, a single-shot injection can be delivered or a catheter can be placed near the brachial plexus. Access is possible through the axilla, around the clavicle or via an interscalene approach by a variety of techniques. Depending on access and catheter position, analgesia covers nearly the entire upper limb, while also providing sympathetic blockade with resulting vasodilatation. The latter is desired in plastic surgery (skin flaps, retransplantations, etc.) and in vascular surgery (e.g. shunt formation). The block is also useful for orthopaedic surgery to the arm and the shoulder, particularly when early mobilisation is required (Ilfeld 2017).

Truncal blocks

Intercostal, interpleural and paravertebral blocks can be used to treat pain due to rib fractures, thoracotomies, breast surgery and upper abdominal surgery. Continuous paravertebral analgesia via a catheter is as effective as thoracic epidural analgesia for thoracotomies, with a better adverse effect profile (Yeung et al. 2016). A large number of new techniques for truncal blocks are currently being developed and the debate on the best technique continues (Schug et al. 2020). The most established technique is possibly the transversus abdominis plane (TAB) block, which is widely used after abdominal surgery, either by single-shot or continuous infusion via a catheter (Lissauer et al. 2014).

Neuraxial analgesia

The two types of neuraxial analgesia used in acute care are:
- **intrathecal** analgesia: drugs administered into the intrathecal space
- **epidural** (extradural) analgesia: drugs administered into the epidural space.

The intrathecal space lies inside the spinal meninges, which hold the cerebrospinal fluid (CSF), while the epidural space lies outside the meninges (dura mater). The spinal nerve roots traverse both spaces; as they pass through the epidural space, they are surrounded by a cuff of dura. The neuraxial route provides access to nerve roots supplying the thorax, abdomen, pelvic organs, perineum and lower limbs. Drugs administered by this route can affect transmission in the dorsal horn of the spinal cord, the somatic afferent (sensory) and efferent (motor) nerve roots and the sympathetic efferent nerves.

Intrathecal analgesia

Intrathecal (i.e. spinal) anaesthesia involves insertion of a spinal needle through a lumbar intervertebral space and injection of local anaesthetic ± opioid. It is usually given preoperatively as a 'single-shot' technique, which provides good surgical anaesthesia for up to 4 hours, while a long-acting opioid can provide ongoing postoperative analgesia for 12 to 24 hours or more (Popping et al. 2012). The technique is often used for urological and orthopaedic operations, as it primarily covers the pelvis and lower limbs. The use of continuous intrathecal techniques is an option in cancer pain management, which is rarely used in the postoperative setting.

Epidural analgesia

If analgesia is required for a prolonged period postoperatively, notably following upper abdominal surgery or thoracic surgery, continuous infusion is the technique of choice (Wheatley et al. 2001). A needle is inserted into the epidural space and a catheter is fed into the space, allowing longer-term infusion or repeated bolus doses of analgesic agents.

Drugs that are commonly given by the spinal route are:
- local anaesthetics (e.g. bupivacaine, ropivacaine)
- opioids (e.g. morphine, fentanyl, sufentanil, pethidine, diamorphine).

Medications used for regional blockade

Local anaesthetics

Local anaesthetics block axonal conduction and hence prevent transmission of nociceptive (pain) impulses into the dorsal horn of the spinal cord (see Chapters 6 and 15). They preferentially block those dermatomes closer to the spinal level of catheter insertion. Hence, epidural catheters are inserted lumbosacrally for lower limb surgery, at low thoracic levels for lower abdominal surgery and at mid-thoracic levels for upper abdominal and thoracic surgery.

Most side effects are related to the fact that local anaesthetic agents block axonal conduction in all nerves to some extent:
- Inadvertent overdose or injection into an epidural vessel can lead to local anaesthetic toxicity, the most serious consequences being central nervous system toxicity (convulsions and coma) and cardiovascular toxicity (fatal arrhythmias).
- Urinary retention

- *Total spinal anaesthesia* as a result of an excess of local anaesthetic inadvertently administered directly into the CSF (i.e. intrathecally), rather than the epidural space. This blocks the sympathetic outflow from the spinal cord and constitutes an emergency situation. The patient rapidly develops total body paralysis and is unable to breathe, followed by cardiovascular collapse, loss of consciousness and, if untreated, death.
- Variable haemodynamic effects of sympathetic blockade, commonly resulting in hypotension as a result of vasodilatation. This often requires treatment with vasoconstrictors and/or increased volumes of IV fluid.

Motor blockade, which can impair mobilisation, and, in combination with sensory blockade, may contribute to the development of pressure areas if nursing care is inadequate.

Opioids

Opioids administered neuraxially block opioid receptors in the dorsal horn of the spinal cord (Bujedo et al. 2012). This requires lower doses than systemic analgesia for neuraxial analgesia and therefore may reduce opioid side effects. Epidural opioids can cause analgesia by:
- diffusion through the dural membrane of the spinal root cuffs into the CSF, affecting opioid receptors in the dorsal horn and the brain (cephalad spread);
- direct transfer from the epidural space to the spinal cord via spinal arteries; and
- vascular uptake into the bloodstream, thus providing systemic analgesia.

Morphine or other hydrophilic (water-soluble) opioids stay in the CSF for longer and are more commonly associated with cephalad migration. The advantages of a single dose providing analgesia for 12 to 24 hours are offset by the potential for delayed respiratory depression for 12 to 24 hours after administration due to cephalad migration to the respiratory centre in the brain. Conversely, fentanyl and other lipophilic (fat-soluble) opioids do not stay in the CSF as long, so they provide a shorter duration of analgesia with lower risk of respiratory depression. As such, epidural fentanyl or sufentanil can and should be given as an infusion. Other side effects of neuraxial opioids, particularly morphine, are pruritus, nausea and urinary retention.

Epidural opioids are rarely given as the sole analgesic agent, as there is no clear advantage of using spinal opioids over IV opioids (Schug et al. 2020). Both provide the same quality of analgesia with the same risk of side effects. However, it has been demonstrated that use of local anaesthetic drugs in combination with opioids in the epidural space reduces the requirement for opioids and therefore the risk of opioid side effects (i.e. they are opioid-sparing) (Curatolo et al. 1998). They may in fact improve the quality of analgesia and reduce the incidence of patchy/unilateral blocks. Such a combination allows low concentrations of local anaesthetic to be used, providing good-quality analgesia with minimal motor blockade (seen as limb weakness and inability to mobilise) and reduced sympathetic blockade. Continuous infusions of these combinations, often amalgamated with a patient-controlled bolus dose as patient-controlled epidural analgesia (PCEA), are currently the most common way to provide epidural analgesia (Golster 2014).

Benefits of epidural techniques

Epidural analgesia is used after a wide variety of surgical operations, ranging from thoracic surgery to vascular surgery on the lower limbs. It can also be used for acute pain secondary to medical disease, such as angina or pancreatitis.

Local anaesthetics supplied via epidural catheters provide better analgesia than systemic opioids after abdominal surgery, in particular for mobilisation and coughing (Salicath et al. 2018).

In contrast to systemic opioid administration, there is increasing evidence that epidural analgesia offers potentially improved outcomes in terms of reduced morbidity and mortality (Popping et al. 2014). The following benefits have been shown (Schug et al. 2020):

- *Preservation of gastrointestinal function*: epidurals significantly reduce the incidence of ileus (reduced gut motility), allowing early oral feeding, and decrease the incidence of breakdown of surgical bowel anastomoses. They also reduce breakdown of body protein and energy sources (catabolism), thus preventing protein loss.
- *Preservation of pulmonary function*: epidurals significantly reduce the incidence of pulmonary infections, atelectasis and hypoxaemia.
- *Reduced incidence of thromboembolic complications*: epidurals reduce the incidence of deep venous thrombosis (DVT), pulmonary embolism (PE) and graft thrombosis after vascular reconstruction.
- *Reduced neuroendocrine response (stress response) to surgery*: this physiological response to surgery is caused by the release of catecholamines and cytokines during surgical trauma. This forces the body into a catabolic state (increased metabolic rate), depleting the body's nutritional state and leads to blood clots more readily, increasing the risk of DVT and PE. This may contribute to immunosuppression and increased risk of infection. Epidural analgesia reduces this stress response.
- *Increased protection of the heart*: epidurals reduce the oxygen requirement of the heart and increase its blood supply. Epidural analgesia may reduce the incidence of fatal arrhythmias and myocardial ischaemic events, and prevent myocardial infarction following upper abdominal surgery.

Modification of surgical and nursing protocols to ensure early oral feeding, improved nutrition and active mobilisation are required to maximise the effects of neural blockade on pain, the stress response and organ dysfunction. A multidisciplinary approach ('fast-track surgery', 'enhanced recovery after surgery' (ERAS)), which incorporates all aspects of perioperative rehabilitation, is likely to offer improved outcomes, reducing the length of hospital stays and offering cost benefits (Beverly et al. 2017).

Complications of neuraxial techniques

Neuraxial techniques have potential complications related to the insertion of an epidural needle and subsequent presence of an epidural catheter (Schug et al. 2020):

- Dural puncture is the inadvertent puncturing of the dural membrane during insertion of an epidural catheter, allowing leakage of CSF into the epidural space. This occurs during ~1% of epidural catheter insertions. There is a high chance of developing a postdural puncture headache following this, particularly if the patient is young and mobilising soon after epidural insertion.
- Neurological deficit with regional numbness as a consequence of nerve injury by needle or catheter occurs in 0.013%–0.023% of cases. This is usually temporary and complete recovery occurs at least within 3 months.
- Epidural haematoma may result in neurological deficit due to compression of the spinal cord. Unless surgical decompression takes place within hours of onset of symptoms, permanent neurological injury in the form of paraplegia can result. Fortunately, this complication is an extremely rare event, with an estimated incidence in the range of 1/6000–12,000.
- Epidural abscess or meningitis can be the result of contamination on insertion or haematogenic colonisation of the indwelling catheter. This is another extremely rare complication requiring antibiotic treatment and possibly surgical intervention. Incidence can be reduced by maintenance of appropriate asepsis during catheter placement and handling, as well as careful consideration of risks and benefits in septic patients (Hebl & Niesen 2011).
- Many different drugs have been mistakenly administered into epidural catheters, commonly due to nursing error or system failure. Consequences depend on the type of drug injected and can be severe.

Nonpharmacological modalities

Nonpharmacological techniques are used to *supplement* pharmacological modalities, but can sometimes be sufficient on their own (see Chapters 10, 11, 12, 14 and 16 for a more complete description of these therapies):

- Physical modalities
  - exercise
  - manual and massage therapies
  - warming and cooling
- Electroanalgesia (e.g. TENS) and acupuncture
- Psychological modalities
  - provision of information
  - stress and tension reduction (relaxation, mindfulness, hypnosis)
  - attentional techniques (music, virtual reality)
  - cognitive–behavioural interventions

While the evidence for the efficacy of nonpharmacological modalities in acute pain management is variable, patients may derive benefit from them in certain settings. Reasons for the limited evidence base of these interventions are the wide heterogeneity of interventions and conditions in which they have been studied, studies limited by small sample size and the risk of bias, in particular with regard to blinding (Schug et al. 2020).

Physical therapies

These techniques may provide comfort, correct physical dysfunction, alter physiological responses and reduce fears associated with pain-related immobility or activity restriction. There is limited evidence for their effectiveness in acute pain (Schug et al. 2020).

Active exercise-based therapies have shown effects on pain and function after a number of orthopaedic operations such as joint replacements (Umehara & Tanaka 2018) and spinal surgery. There may also be a role for exercise therapy before some of these operations ('prehabilitation') (Moyer et al. 2017). Exercise, activation and early mobilisation are important components of management in the postoperative period, aimed at achieving a rapid return to normal function and life after surgery, with as little deconditioning of physical function as possible and are an essential component of 'fast-track surgery' strategies (Beverly et al. 2017). The aim is the establishment of a normal routine for postoperative patients, allowing pain relief prior to intervention and scheduled rest, but with a consistent approach encouraging restoration of function and clear guidelines as to how to mobilise out of bed, how far to mobilise and how frequently to mobilise.

Massage in the treatment of acute pain shows some benefits in the early postoperative period (Kukimoto et al. 2017).

Postoperative local cooling has shown some benefit in selected postoperative states such knee arthroplasty, in particular when combined with compression (Song et al. 2016). Heat packs may reduce labour pain (Smith et al. 2018).

Electroanalgesia (e.g. TENS) and acupuncture

TENS compared to sham stimulation has shown analgesic effects in postoperative pain states (Johnson et al. 2015). In labour pain, the findings are contradictory.

Acupuncture reduces postoperative pain and opioid consumption in the postoperative setting after a number of operations (Wu et al. 2016), but has also effects in labour pain (Smith et al. 2020) and in the emergency department setting (Jan et al. 2017).

Also refer to Chapter 16.

Psychological interventions

With regard to psychological interventions, providing procedure-related information reduces postoperative pain and pre- and postoperative anxiety, e.g. in orthopaedic surgery (Szeverenyi et al. 2018).

The evidence for relaxation techniques in acute pain settings is contradictory. They may provide only limited benefit. Similarly, there is only limited evidence on mindfulness-based interventions and hypnosis, but for the latter, there are some studies showing acute pain reduction after surgery (Kekecs et al. 2014) and in labour (Madden et al. 2016).

Attentional techniques such as playing music reduce acute and procedural pain and have other beneficial effects on patients (Lee 2016). Virtual reality techniques are widely used in procedural pain, e.g. in burns patients and children (Schug et al. 2020).

Progression from acute to chronic pain

The risk of chronic pain as a consequence of surgery is underestimated, as it can occur quite often and represents a significant source of ongoing disability (chronic postsurgical pain; CPSP) (Schug et al. 2019). Estimates of chronic pain after certain surgeries such as amputation, thoracotomy and mastectomy range between 5% and 80%, with an estimated incidence of chronic severe pain in the range of 5%–10% (Schug & Bruce 2017). Even inguinal hernia repair carries a 2%–4% risk of developing chronic severe pain. This pain may be neuropathic in nature. A number of risk factors have been identified. These include preoperative moderate-to-severe pain, particularly with longer duration, as well as female gender, psychological vulnerability (e.g. catastrophising) and preoperative anxiety, and possibly also genetic predisposition. A surgical approach with danger of nerve damage increases the risk, as does moderate-to-severe postoperative pain, the psychological factors mentioned previously and, possibly, radiation therapy. Current research is focusing on attempts to reduce the incidence of chronic pain after surgery; some specific anaesthetic and/or analgesic interventions may reduce the incidence (Ning et al. 2018). Here, in particular, the use of regional anaesthesia techniques and the use of antihyperalgesic medications (such as ketamine and possibly lidocaine) look promising (Schug et al. 2020). These approaches seem to be most effective if administered during surgery and for a certain time thereafter (preventive analgesia). There is, however, no evidence-based recommendation possible for how long the treatment should last. Hopefully, future studies may lead to drugs and treatment protocols able to successfully prevent chronic pain after surgery.

The acute pain service (APS)

Acute pain is an area of growing interest in all specialties involved with inpatient care. As shown, the benefits the patient receives from effective analgesia extend beyond patient comfort.

An increasing body of knowledge covering the mechanism of acute pain and its effects on the dorsal horn of the spinal cord has emerged. This has resulted in an increased availability of better and more sophisticated techniques to treat acute pain, such as regional blockade and PCA. However, until recently, provision of optimal analgesia for acute pain has been moving at a much slower pace. A major reason for inadequate provision of analgesia was that, although more sophisticated methods of providing analgesia were being introduced, there was a lack of appropriate organisational structures for their safe and effective use. This led to the introduction of APS.

In 1986, Ready set up the first 'anaesthesiology-based postoperative pain management service' in Seattle, USA (Ready et al. 1988), with the rapid subsequent development of other similar services worldwide (Stamer et al. 2020).

Safe and effective acute pain relief requires a coordinated, organised team approach. The team should include anaesthetists, surgeons, nurses and pharmacists, not to mention a multitude of other specialists such as physiotherapists, occupational therapists, infection control specialists and psychologists. Recommendations are that acute pain teams should be established in all major hospitals and that there should be a formal, team approach to the management of acute pain with clear lines of responsibility. In summary, the role of an APS is to (Macintyre & Schug 2021):

- provide education about pain management, as well as more specialised analgesic techniques to medical and allied health staff as well as patients;
- introduce more advanced methods of pain relief (epidural and PCA);
- provide guidance to improve the more traditional analgesic techniques;
- provide and standardise orders, guidelines, procedures and methods of pain assessment for all pain-relief strategies, and carry out ongoing improvement to these based on the results of audit activity;
- provide daily supervision and 24-hour cover for patients under the care of the APS, as well as for patients with any other acute pain management problems;
- collaborate and communicate with many other disciplines in developing fast-track surgery protocols, opioid stewardship programmes; and
- undertake audit and clinical research activity.

Thus the management of acute pain has really only been fully addressed over the last 20 years. As further scientific evidence emerges outlining the benefits and safety of the more recently introduced analgesic techniques, together with the establishment of the APS, inadequate relief of acute pain should become less frequent.

APS have now been introduced into many hospitals worldwide. They have quite diverse structures, with no clear agreement on what constitutes the best model or the definition of the service. The organisational structures range from low-cost nurse-based services, via anaesthesia-led but primarily nurse-run services, to comprehensive and multidisciplinary services with 24-hour cover by an anaesthetist and supervising nurses, with involvement of other staff such as pharmacists. Many APS have moved on to become comprehensive pain services dealing with all pain-management issues in a hospital from the acute to the subacute to the chronic. Overall, some data suggest that APS have benefits in achieving reduced pain intensity scores and side effects of analgesia in a hospital (Schug et al. 2020). This aligns with other data that suggest that the development of an APS in a hospital is accompanied by significant improvement in postoperative pain management. Other potential beneficial outcomes are the reduction of postoperative morbidity or even mortality, and the reduction of the incidence of persistent pain after surgery. In this context, it is important that comprehensive pain services are able to diagnose early-onset neuropathic pain and deal with it appropriately, but that they can also manage patients with complex issues, such as opioid-tolerant or opioid-abusing patients, in the framework of a multidisciplinary setting. Detailed recommendations for the running of an APS have been published by the Royal College of Anaesthetists in the United Kingdom (RCoA 2020).

A more recent development in this area are APS outpatient clinics (Tiippana et al. 2016), now increasingly called *transitional pain services* (Mikhaeil et al. 2020). This approach aims to identify patients at risk of developing chronic postsurgical pain or requiring high opioid doses early, and to follow up these patients early as outpatients to prevent or reduce chronic pain development and address ongoing opioid requirements appropriately.

Conclusion

Acute pain caused in particular by surgery (postoperative pain), but also after trauma and due to medical diseases, continues to be undertreated. This not only causes unnecessary suffering of the patients affected, but also increases complications and impairs recovery and rehabilitation. Treatment could be dramatically improved as there is a sufficient evidence base to support therapeutic decisions without increasing risks. Recommended approaches need to be multimodal and procedure-specific. Multimodal analgesia should be governed by the principles of increasing use of appropriate nonopioids and regional techniques while minimising use of opioids. Pharmacological methods should be supported by nonpharmacological techniques including physical and psychological therapies. Utilising the organisational structure of APCs to provide acute pain relief will improve outcomes and safety. Last, not least, as the progression of acute to chronic pain has severe long-term consequences, preventive analgesia will become an important future requirement here.

Acknowledgements

This chapter is based on Chapter 26 of the previous edition of this textbook, which was co-authored by Deborah Watson and Esther Pogatzki-Zahn. Their contributions to the current chapter are hereby thankfully acknowledged.

Review questions — Q

1. How can systemic opioids be administered and what are the arguments for and against each method?
2. What are the potential benefits and dangers of patient-controlled analgesia?
3. What alternatives to systemic opioid use exist and what are the features of each treatment type?
4. By what methods can neuraxial analgesia be achieved and how do these methods compare and contrast?
5. By what methods can peripheral neural blockade be achieved and how do these methods compare and contrast?
6. What evidence exists for and against the use of nonpharmacological treatment modalities?
7. What is the function of an acute pain service?

References

Albrecht, E., Chin, K.J., 2020. Advances in regional anaesthesia and acute pain management: a narrative review. Anaesthesia 75 (Suppl. 1), e101–e110.

Andersen, L.O., Kehlet, H., 2014. Analgesic efficacy of local infiltration analgesia in hip and knee arthroplasty: a systematic review. Br. J. Anaesth. 113 (3), 360–374.

ANZCA, 2018. Position Statement on the Use of Slow-Release Opioid Preparations in the Treatment of Acute Pain. ANZCA. Available from http://www.anzca.edu.au/resources/endorsed-guidelines/position-statement-on-the-use-of-slow-release-opio.

Beverly, A., Kaye, A.D., Ljungqvist, O., Urman, R.D., 2017. Essential elements of multimodal analgesia in enhanced recovery after surgery (ERAS) guidelines. Anesthesiol. Clin. 35 (2), e115–e143.

Brinck, E.C., Tiippana, E., Heesen, M., Bell, R.F., Straube, S., Moore, R.A., et al., 2018. Perioperative intravenous ketamine for acute postoperative pain in adults. Cochrane Database Syst. Rev. 12, CD012033.

Buhre, W., Disma, N., Hendrickx, J., DeHert, S., Hollmann, M.W., Huhn, R., et al., 2019. European society of anaesthesiology task force on nitrous oxide: a narrative review of its role in clinical practice. Br. J. Anaesth. 122 (5), 587–604.

Bujedo, B.M., Santos, S.G., Azpiazu, A.U., 2012. A review of epidural and intrathecal opioids used in the management of postoperative pain. J. Opioid. Manag. 8 (3), 177–192.

Cashman, J.N., Dolin, S.J., 2004. Respiratory and haemodynamic effects of acute postoperative pain management: evidence from published data. Br. J. Anaesth. 93 (2), 212–223.

Chumbley, G.M., Hall, G.M., Salmon, P., 2002. Patient-controlled analgesia: what information does the patient want? J. Adv. Nurs. 39 (5), 459–471.

Cooper, I.M., 1996. Morphine for postoperative analgesia. A comparison of intramuscular and subcutaneous routes of administration. Anaesth. Intensive. Care. 24 (5), 574–578.

Curatolo, M., Petersen-Felix, S., Scaramozzino, P., Zbinden, A.M., 1998. Epidural fentanyl, adrenaline and clonidine as adjuvants to local anaesthetics for surgical analgesia: meta-analyses of analgesia and side-effects. Acta. Anaesthesiol. Scand. 42 (8), 910–920.

Gerbershagen, H.J., Aduckathil, S., van Wijck, A.J., Peelen, L.M., Kalkman, C.J., Meissner, W., 2013. Pain intensity on the first day after surgery: a prospective cohort study comparing 179 surgical procedures. Anesthesiology. 118 (4), 934–944.

Golster, M., 2014. Seven years of patient-controlled epidural analgesia in a Swedish hospital: a prospective survey. Eur. J. Anaesthesiol. 31 (11), 589–596.

Hebl, J.R., Niesen, A.D., 2011. Infectious complications of regional anesthesia. Curr. Opin. Anaesthesiol. 24 (5), 573–580.

Ilfeld, B.M., 2017. Continuous peripheral nerve blocks: an update of the published evidence and comparison with novel, alternative analgesic modalities. Anesth. Analg. 124 (1), 308–335.

Jan, A. L., Aldridge, E. S., Rogers, I. R., Visser, E. J., Bulsara, M. K., Niemtzow, R. C. (20171). Does ear acupuncture have a role for pain relief in the emergency setting? A systematic review and meta-analysis. Med. Acupunct, 29(5), 276-289.

Johnson, M.I., Paley, C.A., Howe, T.E., Sluka, K.A., 2015. Transcutaneous electrical nerve stimulation for acute pain. Cochrane. Database. Syst. Rev. 6, CD006142.

Kekecs, Z., Nagy, T., Varga, K., 2014. The effectiveness of suggestive techniques in reducing postoperative side-effects: a meta-analysis of randomized controlled trials. Anesth. Analg. 119 (6), 1407–1419.

Kreutzwiser, D., Tawfic, Q.A., 2019. Expanding role of NMDA receptor antagonists in the management of pain. CNS Drugs. 33 (4), 347–374.

Kuang, M.J., Ma, J.X., Fu, L., He, W.W., Zhao, J., Ma, X.L., 2017. Is adductor canal block better than femoral nerve block in primary total knee arthroplasty? A GRADE analysis of the evidence through a systematic review and meta-analysis. J. Arthroplasty. 32 (10), 3238–3248 e3233.

Kukimoto, Y., Ooe, N., Ideguchi, N., 2017. The effects of massage therapy on pain and anxiety after surgery: a systematic review and meta-analysis. Pain Manag. Nurs. 18 (6), 378–390.

Latta, K.S., Ginsberg, B., Barkin, R.L., 2002. Meperidine: a critical review. Am. J. Ther. 9 (1), 53–68.

Lee, B., Schug, S.A., Joshi, G.P., Kehlet, H., Group, P.W., 2018. Procedure-specific pain management (PROSPECT) - an update. Best. Pract. Res. Clin. Anaesthesiol. 32 (2), 101–111.

Lee, J.H., 2016. The effects of music on pain: a meta-analysis. J. Music. Ther. 53 (4), 430–477.

Levy, N., Quinlan, J., El-Boghdadly, K., Fawcett, W.J., Agarwal, V., Bastable, R.B., et al., 2020. An international multidisciplinary consensus statement on the prevention of opioid-related harm in adult surgical patients. Anaesthesia. 76 (4), 520–536.

Lissauer, J., Mancuso, K., Merritt, C., Prabhakar, A., Kaye, A.D., Urman, R.D., 2014. Evolution of the transversus abdominis plane block and its role in postoperative analgesia. Best. Pract. Res. Clin. Anaesthesiol. 28 (2), 117–126.

Macintyre, P.E., 2001. Safety and efficacy of patient-controlled analgesia. Br. J. Anaesth. 87 (1), 36–46.

Macintyre, P.E., Huxtable, C.A., Flint, S.L., Dobbin, M.D., 2014. Costs and consequences: a review of discharge opioid prescribing for ongoing management of acute pain. Anaesth. Intensive. Care. 42 (5), 558–574.

Macintyre, P.E., Loadsman, J.A., Scott, D.A., 2011. Opioids, ventilation and acute pain management. Anaesth. Intensive. Care. 39 (4), 545–558.

Macintyre, P.E., Schug, S.A., 2021. Acute Pain Management - A Practical Guide, fifth ed. CRC Press, Abingdon.

Madden, K., Middleton, P., Cyna, A.M., Matthewson, M., Jones, L., 2016. Hypnosis for pain management during labour and childbirth. Cochrane. Database. Syst. Rev. 5, CD009356.

Martinez, V., Beloeil, H., Marret, E., Fletcher, D., Ravaud, P., Trinquart, L., 2017a. Non-opioid analgesics in adults after major surgery: systematic review with network meta-analysis of randomized trials. Br. J. Anaesth. 118 (1), 22–231.

Martinez, V., Pichard, X., Fletcher, D., 2017b. Perioperative pregabalin administration does not prevent chronic postoperative pain: systematic review with a meta-analysis of randomized trials. Pain. 158 (5), 775–783.

Maund, E., McDaid, C., Rice, S., Wright, K., Jenkins, B., Woolacott, N., 2011. Paracetamol and selective and non-selective non-steroidal anti-inflammatory drugs for the reduction in morphine-related side-effects after major surgery: a systematic review. Br. J. Anaesth. 106 (3), 292–297.

McNicol, E.D., Ferguson, M.C., Hudcova, J., 2015. Patient controlled opioid analgesia versus non-patient controlled opioid analgesia for postoperative pain. Cochrane. Database. Syst. Rev. 6, CD003348.

Meissner, W., Zaslansky, R., 2019. A survey of postoperative pain treatments and unmet needs. Best. Pract. Res. Clin. Anaesthesiol. 33 (3), 269–286.

Mikhaeil, J., Ayoo, K., Clarke, H., Wasowicz, M., Huang, A., 2020. Review of the Transitional Pain Service as a method of postoperative opioid weaning and a service aimed at minimizing the risk of chronic post-surgical pain. Anaesthesiol. Intensive. Ther. 52 (2), 148–153.

Miotto, K., Cho, A.K., Khalil, M.A., Blanco, K., Sasaki, J.D., Rawson, R., 2017. Trends in tramadol: pharmacology, metabolism, and misuse. Anesth. Analg. 124 (1), 44–51.

Moyer, R., Ikert, K., Long, K., Marsh, J., 2017. The value of preoperative exercise and education for patients undergoing total hip and knee arthroplasty: a systematic review and meta-analysis. JBJS Rev. 5 (12), e2.

Ning, J., Luo, J., Meng, Z., Luo, C., Wan, G., Liu, J., et al., 2018. The efficacy and safety of first-line therapies for preventing chronic post-surgical pain: a network meta-analysis. Oncotarget. 9 (62), 32081–32095.

Oden, R., 1989. Acute postoperative pain: incidence, severity and etiology of inadequate treatment. Anesth. Clin. N. Am. 7, 1–5.

Oderda, G.M., Gan, T.J., Johnson, B.H., Robinson, S.B., 2013. Effect of opioid-related adverse events on outcomes in selected surgical patients. J. Pain. Palliat. Care. Pharmacother. 27 (1), 62–70.

Owen, H., Plummer, J.L., Armstrong, I., Mather, L.E., Cousins, M.J., 1989. Variables of patient-controlled analgesia. 1. Bolus size. Anaesthesia. 44 (1), 7–10.

Pogatzki-Zahn, E.M., Segelcke, D., Schug, S.A., 2017, Postoperative pain-from mechanisms to treatment. Pain. Rep. 2 (2). 3.

Popping, D.M., Elia, N., Marret, E., Wenk, M., Tramer, M.R., 2012. Opioids added to local anesthetics for single-shot intrathecal anesthesia in patients undergoing minor surgery: a meta-analysis of randomized trials. Pain. 153 (4), 784–793.

Popping, D.M., Elia, N., Van Aken, H.K., Marret, E., Schug, S.A., Kranke, P., et al., 2014. Impact of epidural analgesia on mortality and morbidity after surgery: systematic review and meta-analysis of randomized controlled trials. Ann. Surg. 259 (6), 1056–1067.

Raines, S., Hedlund, C., Franzon, M., Lillieborg, S., Kelleher, G., Ahlen, K., 2014. Ropivacaine for continuous wound infusion for postoperative pain management: a systematic review and meta-analysis of randomized controlled trials. Eur. Surg. Res. 53 (1–4), 43–60.

RCoA, 2020. Guidelines for the Provision of Anaesthesia Services for Inpatient Pain Management 2020. Available from: https://www.rcoa.ac.uk/gpas/chapter-11.

Ready, L.B., Oden, R., Chadwick, H.S., Benedetti, C., Rooke, G.A., Caplan, R., et al., 1988. Development of an anesthesiology-based postoperative pain management service. Anesthesiology. 68 (1), 100–106.

Salicath, J.H., Yeoh, E.C., Bennett, M.H., 2018. Epidural analgesia versus patient-controlled intravenous analgesia for pain following intra-abdominal surgery in adults. Cochrane. Database. Syst. Rev. 8, CD010434.

Schnabel, A., Meyer-Friessem, C.H., Zahn, P.K., Pogatzki-Zahn, E.M., 2013. Ultrasound compared with nerve stimulation guidance for peripheral nerve catheter placement: a meta-analysis of randomized controlled trials. Br. J. Anaesth. 111 (4), 564–572.

Schug, S.A., 2021. Do NSAIDs really interfere with healing after surgery? J. Clin. Med. 10 (11).

Schug, S.A., Bruce, J., 2017. Risk stratification for development of chronic post-surgical pain. Pain. Rev. 2 (e627).

Schug, S.A., Lavand'homme, P., Barke, A., Korwisi, B., Rief, W., Treede, R.D., The IASP Taskforce for the Classification of Chronic Pain, 2019. The IASP classification of chronic pain for ICD-11: chronic postsurgical or posttraumatic pain. Pain. 160 (1), 45–52.

Schug, S.A., Manopas, A., 2007. Updated on the role of non-opioids for postoperative pain treatment. Best. Pract. Res. Clin. Anaesthesiol. 21 (1), 15–30.

Schug, S.A., Palmer, G.M., Scott, D.A., Halliwell, R., Alcock, M., Mott, J., APM:SE Working Group of the Australian and New Zealand College of Anaesthetists and Faculty of Pain Medicine, 2020. Acute Pain Management: Scientific Evidence. Australian and New Zealand College of Anaesthetists and Faculty of Pain Medicine. .

Schug, S.A., Parsons, B., Li, C., Xia, F., 2017. The safety profile of parecoxib for the treatment of postoperative pain: a pooled analysis of 28 randomized, double-blind, placebo-controlled clinical trials and a review of over 10 years of postauthorization data. J. Pain. Res. 10, 2451–2459.

Schug, S.A., Torrie, J.J., 1993. Safety assessment of postoperative pain management by an acute pain service. Pain. 55 (3), 387–391.

Schug, S.A., Zech, D., Grond, S., 1992, May-Jun. Adverse effects of systemic opioid analgesics. Drug. Saf. 7 (3), 200–213.

Schwenk, E.S., Viscusi, E.R., Buvanendran, A., Hurley, R.W., Wasan, A.D., Narouze, S., et al., 2018. Consensus guidelines on the use of intravenous ketamine infusions for acute pain management from the American society of regional anesthesia and pain medicine, the American academy of pain medicine, and the American society of anesthesiologists. Reg. Anesth. Pain. Med. 43 (5), 456–466.

Smith, C.A., Collins, C.T., Levett, K.M., Armour, M., Dahlen, H.G., Tan, A.L., et al., 2020. Acupuncture or acupressure for pain management during labour. Cochrane. Database. Syst. Rev. 2, Cd009232.

Smith, C.A., Levett, K.M., Collins, C.T., Dahlen, H.G., Ee, C.C., Suganuma, M., 2018. Massage, reflexology and other manual methods for pain management in labour. Cochrane. Database. Syst. Rev. 3, Cd009290.

Song, M., Sun, X., Tian, X., Zhang, X., Shi, T., Sun, R., et al., 2016. Compressive cryotherapy versus cryotherapy alone in patients undergoing knee surgery: a meta-analysis. SpringerPlus. 5 (1), 1074.

Stamer, U.M., Liguori, G.A., Rawal, N., 2020. Thirty-five years of acute pain services: where do we go from here? Anesth. Analg. 131 (2), 650–656.

Szeverenyi, C., Kekecs, Z., Johnson, A., Elkins, G., Csernatony, Z., Varga, K., 2018. The use of adjunct psychosocial interventions can decrease postoperative pain and improve the quality of clinical care in orthopedic surgery: a systematic review and meta-analysis of randomized controlled trials. J. Pain. 19 (11), 1231–1252.

Tiippana, E., Hamunen, K., Heiskanen, T., Nieminen, T., Kalso, E., Kontinen, V.K., 2016. New approach for treatment of prolonged postoperative pain: APS Out-Patient Clinic. Scand. J. Pain. 12, 19–24.

Tzortzopoulou, A., McNicol, E.D., Cepeda, M.S., Francia, M.B., Farhat, T., Schumann, R., 2011. Single dose intravenous propacetamol or intravenous paracetamol for postoperative pain. Cochrane. Database. Syst. Rev. 10, CD007126.

Umehara, T., Tanaka, R., 2018. Effective exercise intervention period for improving body function or activity in patients with knee osteoarthritis undergoing total knee arthroplasty: a systematic review and meta-analysis. Braz. J. Phys. Ther. 22 (4), 265–275.

Wheatley, R.G., Schug, S.A., Watson, D., 2001. Safety and efficacy of postoperative epidural analgesia. Br. J. Anaesth. 87 (1), 47–61.

Wu, M.S., Chen, K.H., Chen, I.F., Huang, S.K., Tzeng, P.C., Yeh, M.L., et al., 2016. The Efficacy of acupuncture in post-operative pain management: a systematic review and meta-analysis. PLoS. One. 11 (3), e0150367.

Yeung, J.H., Gates, S., Naidu, B.V., Wilson, M.J., Gao Smith, F., 2016. Paravertebral block versus thoracic epidural for patients undergoing thoracotomy. Cochrane. Database. Syst. Rev. 2, CD009121.

Chapter | 25 |

Persistent pain and the law: legal aspects of persistent pain management

Marc Walden

LEARNING OBJECTIVES

At the end of this chapter, readers will understand:
1. The importance of the legal system in patient safety.
2. The relationship between public health policy, statutory developments and clinical practice.
3. How healthcare professionals can inform legal decision-making by providing their expert opinion.

Introduction

The rule of law can be best considered as a system of predictably enforced rules and regulations that govern how different members of a society are expected to relate and behave towards one another. Those societies not bound together by predictably enforceable laws are generally less successful and its members enjoy a lower overall standard of living. The rule of law is therefore important because it creates a stable society that supports innovation and economic activity among its members, ultimately benefiting all members of that society through higher standards of living through the provision of better state-provided services such as health or education.

Throughout their careers, healthcare professionals are likely to interact with many different areas of law. They will interact with public health law that governs licensing, regulation and discipline, therapeutic goods law when administering treatment and common law (sometimes referred to as tort or 'civil wrongs' law) if the actions of the health professional are seen to infringe patient autonomy or fall below a reasonable standard of care. This chapter will explore those established and emerging areas of law that, in the view of the author, are of particular relevance to health professionals practising in the field of pain medicine.

The chapter begins with the widespread changes in licensing and regulation of health professionals and the increasing recognition of patients' rights to autonomy and self-determination. Factors that may have contributed to the rise in prescription narcotic use now seen in the developed world health systems will then be discussed.

Whether it be appearing as an expert witness in Court or completing a *fitness to work* form, it is likely that at some time in their careers, practitioners will be asked to provide their opinion for other than therapeutic services. This chapter will discuss the different rules and regulations governing the duties practitioners must adhere to when providing their expert opinions for matters other than patient care. The chapter will conclude with how the common law that governs standards of consent and standards of care may relate to multidisciplinary team care of patients with persistent pain.

While much of the chapter's specific content draws upon examples from Australian law, the issues that the chapter seeks to highlight have relevance to other Anglo-American nations whose legal systems share similar legal foundations.

Regulation of healthcare practitioners

Healthcare practitioners are aware of the increasingly regulated nature of their clinical practice and that they are now held to account for their decisions and outcomes in a way that was unimaginable 20 years ago. While this section specifically examines changes that occurred in Australia with the passage of the *Health Professionals Regulation National Law Act 2010* (Cth) (National Law), similar public policy shifts towards a co-regulatory model characterised by an increased public interest in how health practitioners are regulated have occurred in other Anglo-American countries.[1]

One of the aims of the National Law was to encourage individual professions to be more flexible in adopting new workplace roles and practices that were needed to respond to an ageing population with chronic disease. These reforms are of interest to those who treat persistent pain, where the accepted biopsychosocial model of interdisciplinary care has already led to a blurring of traditionally distinct professional roles and responsibilities, with moves towards interdisciplinary and team-based care.

Because of notable failures of self-regulation by the healthcare professions[2], another aim of the regulatory reform was to establish a so called co-regulatory framework with increased public oversight and involvement in managing complaints made against healthcare practitioners.

Australia's path to healthcare workforce reform

In 2002, Australian Health Ministers identified that the State- and Territory-based systems of health workforce regulation then in force had certain deficiencies, including limiting the mobility of practitioners across State and Territory Borders and entrenching strict siloing of working practices between different professions. They also identified that inconsistencies in the regulation of healthcare professionals across different States and Territories were diminishing public confidence in the peer review model of disciplinary action. To overcome this problem, the

---

BOX 25.1 Regulated health practitioners in Australia

Chiropractor
Dental practitioner
Medical practitioner
Nursing and Midwifery
Osteopath
Optometrist
Pharmacist
Podiatrist
Physiotherapist
Psychologist
Occupational therapist
Aboriginal Torres Strait Islander health practitioner * since 30 June 2014
Chinese medicine practitioner *since 1 July 2012
Paramedicine *since 30 November 2018
Medical radiation practitioner *since 1 July 2012

Productivity Commission recommended the establishment of a single national accreditation board for registration, regulation and accreditation of training of all healthcare professionals. The overarching aim of the new legislation articulates that the health and safety of the public were to be paramount in how the law was applied and interpreted, and that any sanctions imposed upon a healthcare professional were not to be punitive but were to serve both general and specific deterrent purposes. It stated:

> the national consistency in registration and accreditation arrangements in this bill will help to improve the availability and flexibility of the provision of health services and will also protect the public by using the highest possible registration and accreditation standards nationwide, from potentially harmful health outcomes.[3]

The National Law established a single national body, the Australian Health Practitioner Regulation Agency (AHPRA) that was to be responsible for registration, regulation and training of 11 health professions initially subject to the act. Since then, four further health professions have joined the scheme. These professions are listed in Box 25.1. A key principle of the legislation was that all registered professions were to be subject to the same complaints handling processes, professional standards and disciplinary sanctions.

Health professions not regulated by AHPRA such as naturopaths, acupuncturists, dieticians and massage therapists are mostly unable to be sanctioned by

---

[1] The United Kingdom has nine separate bodies who oversee the regulation of 32 different health professions and there is an overarching 'super regulator', The Professional Standards Authority for Health and Social Care, that oversees the regulating council. In 2021, the UK government commenced public consultation to streamline and simplify the current UK health professional's regulation system. In latter part of the 20th century, Canada and the United States moved to a coregulatory system with increased public and state interest that restricted the autonomy previously enjoyed by health professions.
[2] In the last decades of the 20th century, The Bristol Paediatric Cardiac Surgery scandal was one of several highly publicised examples in which failure of self-regulation of the profession by the profession lead to the loss of public trust.

[3] Lucas P, Minister of Health Introducing the Bill into Parliament, 2009. Queensland, *Parliamentary Debates*, 6 October.

AHPRA and are not subject to the same complaints processes and disciplinary sanctions as the registered professions. Other areas of consumer law and trade practice law can be used to regulate those trades not registered under the National Law.

While there is a public safety argument for increasing the number of health professions subject to the National Law, registering a health trade under the National Law may be seen as an official endorsement of emerging fields of expertise not yet subject to the same rigorous education, training and examination requirements that apply to the traditional healthcare professions.

Disciplinary breaches and sanctions against registered health practitioners

The Australian National Regulator (AHPRA), in conjunction with profession specific boards, has considerable powers to investigate complaints made about individual healthcare practitioners including the right to enter a practitioner's premises and to seize records, but has no jurisdiction to investigate complaints about other healthcare organisations such as hospitals or clinics. If it is determined that a health practitioner has performed or behaved in a manner that breaches standards that could affect public safety, the practitioner can be found to have breached one of three professional standards: unsatisfactory professional performance, unprofessional conduct or professional misconduct.

Unsatisfactory professional performance relates to an unsatisfactory standard of a practitioner's clinical practice, whereas the latter two findings are considered to be breaches of a practitioner's standard of professional and private behaviour. A finding of either unprofessional conduct or professional misconduct is likely to result in a public reprimand.[4] A finding that a practitioner's behaviour has constituted professional misconduct is more serious, and is likely to result in a period of suspension or removal (erasure) from the register, thereby rendering the offending practitioner unable to practise.

Unsatisfactory professional performance means the knowledge, skill or judgement possessed or care exercised by the practitioner in the practice of the health profession is below the standard reasonably expected of a health practitioner of an equivalent training or experience. Poor record keeping not resulting in patient harm would be an example of unsatisfactory professional performance.

Unprofessional conduct means professional conduct and behaviour that is of a *lesser standard* that which might reasonably be expected of the health practitioner by the public or the practitioner's profession. Breaches of confidentiality would be an example of unprofessional conduct.

Professional misconduct means unprofessional conduct or behaviour by the practitioner that amounts to conduct that is *substantially below* the standard reasonably expected of a registered health practitioner of an equivalent level of training and experience *or* more than one instance of unprofessional conduct or conduct of the practitioner, whether occurring in connection with the practice of their profession or not that is inconsistent with the practitioner being a 'fit and proper' person to hold registration in the profession. Importantly a practitioner's behaviours that can be considered in a finding of professional misconduct include professional practice behaviours *and* also private behaviours not in connection with professional practice.

Defining a 'fit and proper' person' is a throwback to earlier centuries when the professions were mostly self-regulated. In the modern era of co-regulation, the interpretation of 'fit and proper' includes both the private behaviours of a practitioner as well as the professional behaviours of a practitioner. Being found guilty of a crime, even if that crime was not healthcare related and even when no complaint was made, would usually be found to have breached the standard of being 'fit and proper' and would result in some form of regulatory sanction. The severity and nature of the sanction would depend upon the proximity of the practitioner's unsatisfactory conduct to their clinical practice; for example, a drink drive penalty when not working would be seen as a lesser breech then that of a drink drive penalty while working. Similarly, making a fraudulent personal financial declaration would be seen as a lesser breach of professional standard than making fraudulent financial claims in the course of their clinical practice.

Trends in notifications and complaints

While there will be differences in specific complaints statistics in different jurisdictions, trends in complaint statistics across the developed world reflect changing societal expectations of professional behaviours seen not only in the healthcare professions but also in other fields of professional endeavour such as law and education.

In Australia, complaints (often referred to as notifications) about registered practitioners remain fairly constant, at 1%–2% of all practitioners per annum, and over 70% of all complaints are dismissed and result in no further action being taken.[5]

---

[4] A notation is made against the practitioners name on the national register of healthcare practitioners.

[5] AHPRA 2019/20 AHPRA and National Boards Annual Report Melbourne 2020.

A little over half of all complaints are made by patients, family members or members of the public, with the remaining complaints being brought by a health complaint entity, employers or colleagues. Medical practitioners receive the highest percentage of complaint notifications, followed by dental practitioners, and then nurses and midwives. Among the allied health professions, psychologists receive the highest percentage of notifications, followed by physiotherapists and then occupational therapists.

The subject matter of notifications relates to clinical care (44%,) medication (10%), then behaviour and communication (7%). Psychologists are overrepresented in sexual misconduct violations compared to the other professions. Cultural factors would seem to be important factors in the decision to complain, because notifications are greater when the practitioner is male, more than 50 years old and if their native language is other than English.

Five percent of all notifications were judged to be of sufficient threat to public safety and resulted in immediate suspension of the practitioner from the register. Mandatory notifications (compulsory notifications by a colleague or employer about a practitioner) were greatest for nurses followed by medical practitioners then psychologists.

Clinicians will often complain about the disparity in the burdensome nature of having to provide detailed and timely responses to complaints made against them compared to the relative ease by which a patient, family member or member of the public can initiate a complaint. It may be of some comfort to know that regulators are becoming increasingly aware of the negative impact a notification (even if subsequently dismissed and no further action taken) has upon the practitioner's mental health and their remaining years in clinical practice. Realising that the practitioner may be the 'second victim' of a notification and the impact of the complaints handling process upon the practitioner has resulted in regulators and indemnity organisations providing funding of health and support services for practitioners subject to disciplinary proceedings.

The following are examples of disciplinary cases involving health professionals (Box 25.2).

Opioid misuse

The last decades of the 20th century saw several factors converge in developed countries, creating a perfect storm which led to the liberalisation of opioid prescribing. This allowed a class of medications, that were at one time restricted for short-term administration and relief of acute pain while in hospital and for end-of-life care,

BOX 25.2 Case law

Psychology Board of Australia v Cameron (2015) QCAT

A psychologist was found to have engaged in unprofessional conduct by failing to disclose being convicted of serious driving offences for which they had been punished by 12 month's imprisonment. The practitioner had not been aware of their duty to disclose the offences because they considered the offences to be traffic offences rather than serious criminal offences. Because the practitioner had demonstrated insight and their actions were not deliberate, it was determined that the practitioner had engaged in unprofessional conduct rather than professional misconduct. The practitioner was reprimanded and ordered to pay the Psychology Boards costs.

Physiotherapy Board v Soo (2017) SAHPT

A physiotherapist was found to have engaged in professional misconduct because of making fraudulent Medicare claims on multiple occasions and a lack of genuine remorse. The practitioner was also found to have engaged in unprofessional conduct because of poor record keeping. The practitioner was sanctioned with an 18-month suspension of their registration.

to become the third most frequently prescribed class of medication in Australia, and the most commonly prescribed class of medication in the United States. International comparison (Fig. 25.1) reveals there is a vast difference to be seen in opioid prescribing practices between developed and developing nations (International Narcotics Control Board 2013).

The scale and rise of the opioid harms and premature deaths is astounding. Australia has seen a steady rise in opioid prescribing from 10 million prescriptions for opioids issued in 2009 to 14 million in 2018. Between 2009 and 2014, there has been a doubling in daily opioid utilisation. In Australia, between 2011 and 2015, there were 2145 accidental deaths associated with oxycodone, codeine or morphine use that represents a 60% increase over the previous period. In the same time period in the United States, there has been a doubling of deaths associated with fentanyl.

Developed nations are now recognising the unintended harms and accidental deaths that have resulted from a widening of the indications of opioid supply. Different jurisdictions have adopted a wide range of differing responses to reduce the over prescribing of opioids that include specific changes in statute law to increasing oversight and reporting and mandating further education for prescribers. This variation in response suggests a one-size-fits-all approach does not exist, with different regulatory 'levers' needed in different countries to reduce opioid consumption.

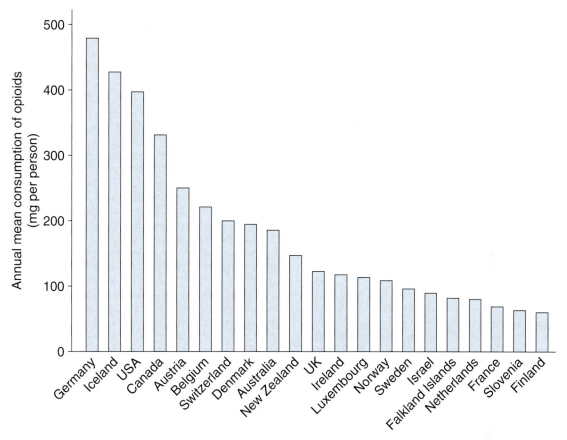

Fig. 25.1 Nations with Greatest Annual Mean Consumption of Opioids. Countries in the top decile for controlled opioid consumption (mg per person) for 2015 to 2017. It is calculated by determining the 3-year mean for 2015 to 2017 and dividing this by the 2016 population for each country. Richards, 2021 (under public licence)

Indication creep: a perfect storm

In 1986, Portenoy and Foley published a paper in which they argued that the benefits opioids provided to palliative care and cancer patients should not be denied to those suffering from other causes of persistent pain. Their paper concluded, saying: 'opioid maintenance therapy can be a safe salutary and more humane alternative … in those patients with intractable non-malignant pain and no history of drug abuse' (Portenoy & Foley 1986). The publication of this paper coincided with a number of other important developments that together created a perfect storm that allowed a widening in the previously narrow prescribing indications for this opioid class of medications.

Other developments that contributed to the perfect storm included the 1996 initiative declaring pain as the fifth vital sign, and in 2010, the publication of The

Declaration of Montreal[6] that directed governments and healthcare institutions to: 'Establish laws policies and systems that would help to promote the access of people in pain to fully adequate pain management'. The consequences of the Declaration of Montreal that pain relief was to be recognised as a basic human right resulted in a proliferation of specialist pain clinics and services specifically to treat pain. This in turn led to an increasing demand for health practitioners from multiple disciplines skilled in pain management to work in these clinics. In 1999, the Australian and New Zealand College of Anaesthetists was among the first international institutions to establish formalised training and examinations in the speciality of pain medicine, with similar developments later occurring in the United Kingdom, Europe and the United States.

---

[6] International Association for the Study of Pain, Declaration of Montreal, First International Pain Summit, Montreal, 3 September 2010.

The response of governments and of professional training bodies to the Declaration of Montreal was not the only mechanism by which the prescribing indications for narcotics changed. Prior to the 1990s, there were relatively few formulations of opioids that could be administered at home. As a consequence, this meant that, previously, the vast majority of opioid pain-reliving medications were administered in hospitals by health professionals skilled in the assessment of pain. All of this changed in the 1990s, when pharmaceutical companies began manufacturing new opioid compounds in formulations that, because of their chemical compositions, had improved bioavailability without needing to be parenterally administered. These changes whereby opioids could be reliably administered by oral, nasal, transdermal or buccal routes removed the requirement for patients who were prescribed opioid analgesics to be hospitalised for their treatment and placed the responsibility for correct administration of opioids in the hands of the patients themselves.

In addition to developing narcotic molecules capable of being self-administered and with durations of action that enabled infrequent and therefore convenient dosing, manufacturers were active in promoting the benefits of these new opioid molecules to those with prescribing authority, while downplaying emerging adverse effects to pharmaceutical regulating authorities[7] leading to contraventions of the *Therapeutic Goods Act 1989* (CTH).

Recognition of the opioid crisis

Despite the rapid rise in the supply of prescribed opioids in developed healthcare systems, it was several years before governmental safety of medicine- and poison-regulating agencies (who monitor the safety of pharmaceutical products upon population health) began to realise the harmful effects these medications were having. The reasons for the delayed recognition of opioid associated harms are difficult to ascertain, but if such a similar threat to public safety is to be prevented from happening again, it is necessary to consider why epidemiological surveillance of opioid harms and side effects upon population health went unrecognised for so long.

Unlike the harmful side effects that result from most pharmaceutical agents that occur within a relatively short time of commencing treatment, we now recognise that the morbidity and mortality associated with long-term opioid misuse is gradual and insidious. Harmful effects usually occur weeks to months after commencing therapy, by which time the patient may be seen in a different sector of the health service than that which initiated the opioid treatment.

Furthermore, the harms caused by opioids are often contingent upon interactions between the opioid and other drugs with sedative and cognitive side effects, such as benzodiazepines or alcohol, being consumed by the patient.

Case law

Prescribers of opioids now find themselves caught between the public, which has an expectation of cure, and increasingly watchful medicine safety agencies. The situation is such that a practitioner may become the subject of disciplinary sanction if they prescribe too generously, Yet, paradoxically, they may also face sanctions under both statute and common law if they are seen to be opiophobic and withholding pain-relieving treatment which results in undue pain and suffering. A useful discussion of the dilemma that faces opioid prescribers can be found in 'Between a Rock and a Hard Place; Can physicians prescribe Opioids to Treat Pain Adequately without Avoiding Legal Sanction' (Dineen & Dubois 2016).

The case law that has addressed the issue of opioid prescribing is mostly from the United States, where the harms associated with opioids first began to be recognised a decade or so before other nations, and where there have been more instances of sanctions (both professional sanctions and common law determinations) for overprescribing of opioids than for opiophobia (opioids being unreasonably being withheld). While determinations of a foreign Court do not set binding precedent[8] to Courts in other nations, the legal principle of persuasive precedent[9] does mean that such decisions can be used to guide the determinations of Courts in other jurisdictions when considering similar cases.

Judgements of disciplinary boards and Civil Court judgements for opiophobia are few and far between, in contrast to the number of actions against practitioners subject to professional sanctions, medical negligence[10] and even criminal[11] judgements when seen to have over prescribed opioids to patients. The author is aware of only one instance of a practitioner being subject to medical board sanction for underprescription of opioids (Hockman 2010).[12] In *Bergman v Chin*,[13] a clinician was successfully sued for committing the common law tort (or wrongs) of Elder Abuse for $1.5m by the family of a

---

[7] Therapeutic Goods Administration, 'Mundipharma fined for misleading advertising of opioids to health professionals' (Media release, TGA, Canberra, 20 December 2019).

[8] Binding precedent is a legal principle by which decisions of a superior Court have to be followed when similar facts are being considered by lower Courts within the same hierarchy. Biding precedent is an important element of common law systems because it provides for a greater degree of consistency in Court's decision-making.
[9] Persuasive precedent as the title would suggest is the legal principle by which a Court can choose and look to the decisions and reasonings of different Court systems in arriving at a determination.
[10] *Koon v Walden*, US 539 SW 3d 752 (2017).
[11] *United States v Mackay*, US 20 F Supp 3d 1287, 1297 (D Utah, 2014).
[12] Hockman JS A Dose of Truth About the Consequences of Opiophobia 18 January 2010 HCPlive.com
[13] *Bergman v Chin*, No H205732-1 Almeda Co. Ct CA 2001.

deceased patient for unreasonably withholding pain relief in end-of-life care.

In Australia, there is a growing interest by plaintiff lawyers in commencing proceedings against physicians for overprescribing of opioids. For the most part, deaths from opioid misuse have come under legal scrutiny in Coronial proceedings, and sanctions for possible irresponsible prescribing dealt with under health practitioner regulations rather than by common law claims for negligence or personal injury. However, because of the principle of binding precedent, it will not be until a civil law case involving opioid overprescribing has been decided by a Court that the societal view of what is appropriate and inappropriate opioid prescribing will be known. Given the recent Court mandated trends in civil justice to precourt settlements and mandatory mediations, which reduces the number of civil cases that proceed to trial (Ipp 2002; Woolf 1996), it is likely to be some considerable time before a publicly available Court determination on what constitutes appropriate opioid prescribing is made. Until that occurs, practitioners are best guided as to what constitutes appropriate and responsible opioid prescribing by peer published guidelines and recommendations.

Pharmacy Board of Australia v Ramsey (2021) SACAT (7 April 2021) concerned a practitioner who had misappropriated returned oxycodone tablets for their own personal use. After seeking assistance from their GP, the practitioner voluntarily disclosed their conduct to the regulator who took immediate action to subject the practitioner to random drug screening and ordered they seek assistance from a psychologist and psychiatrist. After a full investigation, the tribunal found the practitioner had acted in a way that constituted professional misconduct and ordered a suspension period of 4 months.

U.S. v Purdue Pharma, L P 600 F 3d 319 (4th Cir, 2010) and associated cases.

In October 2020 in the Federal Court, Purdue Pharma (the opioid manufacturer) pleaded guilty to charges of marketing its opioid products between 2007 and 2017 to healthcare providers even though Purdue had reason to believe their products were being misused and diverted. Purdue agreed an $8.2 billion dollar settlement for civil and legal wrongs that forced the company into bankruptcy. Individuals harmed by the actions of the Purdue Pharma will each be eligible for up to $48,000 by way of compensation for damages.

Australian regulatory responses to the opioid crisis

Within Australia, the availability and legal supply of opioids by prescription is governed by two separate statutes. The *Therapeutic Goods Act 1989* (Cth) is a federal law that establishes a register of therapeutic goods that categorises pharmaceuticals and poisons according to the level of control required to ensure public safety. State-based statutes, for example, the *Health Act 1937* (Qld) then determine how opioids and other pharmaceuticals are supplied, prescribed, dispensed and accounted for. These statutes already provide a mechanism for a number of regulatory reforms to reduce the potential misuse and harms associated with opioids, such as by changing available standard pack sizes of the medicines, and by altering the wording on labels attached to opioid medications when they are being dispensed. Changes such as these would not stigmatise opioid use or limit accessibility to opioids for therapeutic use.

It is also recognised that additional measures to changes in regulations are needed to increase the safety of opioid prescribing, such as changes in prescriber's behaviour and real-time prescription monitoring that will need statutory changes to be made.[14] Box 25.3 lists a number of strategies that can be used to improve the safety of opioid prescribing, but perhaps the real challenge that healthcare professionals face that cannot be achieved by changing regulations or statutes is how to alter patient expectation of pain relief from heavy reliance upon medication use to an expectation that effective pain management should include a combination of pharmaceutical and nonpharmaceutical treatments and interventions. Many of these other nonpharmacological interventions have been described in other chapters in this textbook, including psychological interventions (Chapter 12), exercise therapy (Chapter 11), self-management (Chapter 10), manual therapy (Chapter 14) and workplace rehabilitation (Chapter 17).

US regulatory response to the opioid crisis

In the United States, the Federal Drugs Administration (FDA) authority is the chief pharmaceutical body established under the *Federal Food, Drug and Cosmetic Act (1938)* responsible for the approval of pharmaceuticals, whereas the monitoring and enforcement of drug prescribing practices is regulated by individual State laws. This has resulted in different responses to suppress the supply of opioids being adopted by different States using the levers of changes in regulation and statutes legislation rather than changes in opioid governance, prescriber education or oversight of supply. Quoting the Centre of Disease Control (CDC) figures for harms and deaths when higher opioid doses were prescribed, a number of US states, led by public health officials and physicians, petitioned the

---

[14] Health (Drugs and Poisons) Amendments Regulation No. 3 (2020) to the *Health Act 1937* (Qld) was required to provide for real-time sharing of pharmacy dispensing information for controlled drugs to enable sharing in real time of that data with healthcare practitioners.

BOX 25.3 **Potential Australian responses to improve the safety of opioid prescribing**

- Real-time prescription monitoring
- Medication labelling reforms
- Improving access to treatments for opioid dependence
- Reconsideration of pack sizes for strong opioids
- Reviewing and standardising the prescribing indications for strong opioids
- Restricting the listing of high dose opioid products (>90 MME) on the register of therapeutic goods
- Restricting the prescribing of high-dose opioids (>90 MME) to specialists or authority prescribers only
- Improving the availability of newer products for pain relief and opioid antidotes through expedited review and listing processes for new and novel analgesic agents
- Abuse deterrent formulations
- Changes to box labelling such as pharmacist added labelling or consumer medicine information
- Mandatory training for professionals licensed to prescribe opioids with increased awareness among health professionals about alternatives to opioids including better education at undergraduate and postgraduate level, improved clinical pathways

MME, Morphine milligram equivalents.

FDA to remove all pharmaceutical products containing >90 MME (milligram morphine equivalent) from the US market. This proposal prompted the FDA to amend the prescribing guidelines for opioids so as to require the prescriber to justify when opioid products >90 MME were required on a case-by-case basis. Florida now has among the most restrictive laws,[15] which limits opioid prescription to 3 days for acute pain and up to 7 days in certain specified situations.

Adopting a different risk management approach to suppressing opioid prescription, the New York State Department of Health has introduced mandatory training requirement for prescribers of strong opioids to undergo 3 hours of course work on pain management, palliative care and addiction every 3 years in order to be able to prescribe these medications.[16] Because of the variability in the restrictions imposed by these laws and the recency in implementation, their effectiveness in reducing opioid related harms and deaths is yet to be fully evaluated. Paradoxically, where individual States have legislated restrictions in opioid supply that have been in place for a number of years,[17] there has been a shift in

opioid-related deaths. Deaths from prescription opioid-related deaths have fallen to a quarter of their previous level, while deaths from illegally produced heroin (less expensive and more available than legally prescribed opioids) and more recently, from fentanyl, have skyrocketed (Hadland 2018).

Canadian regulatory response to the opioid crisis

In Canada, a range of regulatory levers have been employed which aim to reduce the harm of opioid misuse through measures that reduce the availability of opioids while at the same time reducing the harm associated with opioid supply to patients already dependent upon opioid compounds (Box 25.4).

UK response to the opioid crisis

The United Kingdom, which currently ranks 12th in the table of national opioid prescription alongside Scandinavian nations, and behind North America, Western Europe and Australasia, has not seen the magnitude of opioid harms that have been seen in other Anglo-American nations. There are several factors that have contributed to this. First, the same level of government has responsibility for both the registration of pharmaceuticals and for their therapeutic use [18]. Second, the primary care system in the United Kingdom, in which patients access the majority of their medical care through a single practitioner or practice, reduces the risk of inadvertent opioid misuse or diversion. Third, the UK National Health Service (NHS), through the widespread availability of pain management clinics, has long adopted a treatment goal of *managing pain* rather than *removing pain.* Such a focus has led to a different community expectation and a lower demand for pharmaceutical pain relief than in other countries.

Rather than changing the unwieldy levers of increased regulation adopted by the United States that has unfortunately restricted opioid supply to those who need access, the UK response has been to provide better oversight of opioid prescribing across all healthcare facilities (an approach that has also been successfully employed in the Australian State of Tasmania). The Controlled Drugs (Supervision of Management and Use) Regulations 2013 (UK) requires all hospitals and healthcare facilities to appoint a Controlled Drug Accountable Officer (CDAO—a senior manager or clinical lead) responsible

---

[15] Florida State Senate. Florida statutes § 456.44(1).

[16] Cuomo A, Mandatory Prescriber Education Guidance, New York State Department of Health, 22 July 2016.

[17] New York State, Massachusetts and Connecticut first introduced opioid prescribing suppression laws in 2010.

[18] In the United Kingdom, medication licencing and supply are controlled through two laws which have nationwide application: *Misuse of Drugs Act 1971* and *The Controlled Drugs (Supervision of Management and Use) Regulations 2013* (UK).

Box 25.4 Canadian regulatory responses to improve the safety of opioid prescribing

- Improving access to medications that can be used in the treatment of opioid use disorders.
- Rescheduling of naloxone including naloxone nasal spray to be available without prescription.
- Instituting expedited approval processes for nonopioid analgesic medications that includes removing the requirement for such medications already approved by the European Union, the United States or Switzerland to be immediately available in Canada.
- Reducing the risk of drug diversion by providing specific guidance on the return of unused medication and encouraging unused opioids' return to pharmacies for destruction.
- Powers to make it mandatory for pharmaceutical companies to manage community risk associated with opioid use by postmarketing surveillance.

for overseeing all aspects of controlled drug policy including oversight of supply storage and that safe prescribing practices are instituted within their organisations. Each CDAO submits quarterly reports to a regional CDAO who then submits reports to the NHS Quality and Complaints Commission. This system of increased oversight and governance is aimed to provide an early recognition of emerging trends, so as to enable appropriate action to be put in place to detect and report on all causes of adverse drug effects early.

The pain practitioner as an expert witness

Persistent pain, as well as being a condition in its own right, is also a prevalent symptom of many other conditions. It is therefore almost inevitable that a clinician practising in the field of pain management will at some time in their careers be asked to communicate, either in writing or verbally, regarding the health and treatment of a patient to persons or organisations outside of the patient's treating team. Such requests cover a wide range of situations, from certifying an individual as unable to attend work, to more complex situations that enable a patient to access income protection or superannuation benefits. It may also include the requirement to assist a Judge or Court to better understand the effect that a health condition is having on an individual's functional capacity, so as to inform whether there has been negligence or personal injury. When acting in these capacities, the clinician must realise that they are no longer acting as a treating clinician, and that their normal duty of care to their patients is supplanted by an overarching duty to justice and to the rule of law.

Acting in an expert capacity

Without the assistance of expert witnesses, Courts and Judges would struggle to understand the specialised and scientific knowledge required to arrive at properly informed decisions concerning personal injury and negligence. The role of the expert witness is to bridge that gap between healthcare knowledge held by an average lay person and the healthcare knowledge held by a health professional. While individual practitioners may not consider themselves to be an expert in comparison to their professional peers, Courts have determined that an expert is an individual who possesses a field of knowledge not generally held by the general public. As fields of scientific and technical knowledge and expertise have expanded throughout history, Courts have had to grapple with deciding when new and emerging fields of knowledge require the assistance of an expert's opinion. One of the most significant pieces of legislation here, is the Daubert Standard, which is a rule of expert evidence based on a series of three North American Supreme Court cases[19] which have been used to decide when an emerging field of expert scientific or technical knowledge and opinion is sufficiently robust to be considered as admissible expert evidence and therefore taken into consideration in determining a matter by a Court.

Advances in civil litigation

Courts and Tribunals administer justice through a process of presenting evidence (evidence in chief), testing that evidence by cross-examination, and then considering only those parts of presented evidence that are deemed admissible into the Court's determinations. When acting as an expert to the Court, a health professional's expert evidence is usually in the form of a written report or by oral testimony and is unique among evidence provided by other witnesses. Because, unlike nonexpert witnesses whose admissible evidence has to be limited to the *facts* of a case, an *opinion* from an expert who is within their field of expertise is seen to comprise admissible evidence. Judges and other fact finders have long been frustrated about the expert opinions that are proffered in legal cases. There has been a view, that rather than the expert's evidence being truly independent, that expert evidence is often partisan and favouring the party retaining and remunerating the expert as a

---

[19] Daubert v Merrell Dow Pharmaceuticals, 509 US 579 (1993), General Electric Company v Joiner, 522 US 136 (1997), Kumho Tire Company v Carmichael, 526 US 137 (1999).

'Hired Gun,'[20] rather than being truly independent. Courts have therefore developed rules of expert evidence and codes of conduct that experts must acknowledge and agree to before their written opinion (medicolegal report), or oral testimony can be admitted into evidence so as to encourage expert opinions to be truly impartial. By signing a Court's code of conduct, an expert is acknowledging the supremacy of the expert's duty is to the Court and to no other party, and acknowledges their willingness to follow any directions given to them by the Court.

The rise in the number and complexity of healthcare disputes has made Courts and Tribunals increasingly reliant upon health professionals providing expert evidence. This has led to an escalation in the costs and length of healthcare civil litigation, thereby restricting access to civil justice to all but well financially resourced parties. This often leads to significant proportions of any eventual financial settlement being consumed by legal fees, disbursements and Court costs. In an effort to reign in the time and costs of healthcare litigation and to increase the public's access to justice in matters involving healthcare disputes, Courts in many common law jurisdictions have introduced a number of procedural reforms which seek to reduce the number of cases proceeding to trial by encouraging precourt mediation, limit the numbers of experts called to give evidence and mandating precourt disclosure of documents between disputing parties.

Conclave and conjoint evidence

An interesting development in the provision of expert opinion evidence that first originated in the Land Court of New South Wales Australia has been the development of conjoint and conclave evidence (colloquially known as 'hot tubbing' because of the simultaneous appearance of experts in the witness box). Conjoint evidence refers to a process in which experts retained by all parties to provide opinion on the same issue appear in Court simultaneously to answer questions put to them by all parties and by the Judge. Conclave evidence refers to a process by which experts retained by different parties but with similar expertise are instructed to meet outside of Court in order to narrow down the matters upon which they disagree. Experts ordered to participate in conjoint or conclave evidence are not required or expected to mediate, negotiate or decide the matters in dispute among those participating in the conclave. Their purpose is to advise the Court upon which matters they do not agree and why they do not agree, and in so doing narrow down the list of disputes brought before the Court to determine. Given the

success of conjoint and conclave evidence in Australia, other countries, such as the United Kingdom, South Africa and Canada have either adopted similar processes or are conducting evaluations of conjoint and conclave evidence in their own Court processes.[21] Experts who have participated in conjoint and conclave evidence also support its introduction, finding the conjoint and conclave processes less adversarial, more collegiate, and more likely to arrive at a just decision than traditional adversarial cross-examination of expert witnesses (Stone 2018 and Mahler & Shardley 2021).

Experts' scope of opinion

What constitutes health experts' scope of opinion will depend not only upon their professional qualifications but also upon their workplace experience. Healthcare professionals who regularly work in multidisciplinary teams with other disciplines would rightly be able to opine on matters that boundary upon those of other disciplines. For example, a physiotherapist working in a multidisciplinary pain clinic would be able to provide expert opinion upon certain psychological matters, as could a psychiatrist working within a multidisciplinary pain clinic provide opinion upon appropriate use of interventional pain-relieving procedures.

Courts have been known to be somewhat scathing[22] when experts use pseudoscience and scientific language to cover a shortfall in their field of knowledge. Experts should restrict their opinion to matters within or substantially within their field of knowledge and expertise. When faced with situations where there is scientific uncertainty or debate, for example, the pathophysiology of complex regional pain syndrome or aetiology of central sensitisation, a far better approach for an expert to take would be to explain in their report (or in their oral testimony) the limitations of their knowledge in the particular case in question.

Negligence and consent in multidisciplinary pain management

Whatever their profession, every health practitioner who provides treatment may at some time find themselves the subject of an allegation of professional negligence. In common law, for an allegation of negligence to succeed, the plaintiff (the party initiating the claim) bears the burden of proof that on the balance of probability ($P > 50\%$) that the clinician has breached their duty of care by providing treatment of a lesser than acceptable standard, and that resulting from that breach the plaintiff has suffered loss (or damages).

---

[20] Cochrane W, Expert Evidence the View from The Bench Queensland Courts, November 2015, p. 8.

[21] Stone S, Farthing S, Concurrent Evidence Kordamentha, 1 November 2018.
[22] *Branagan v Robinson* (2006) ACTSC 66, [240] (Harper J).

Duty of care from multidisciplinary teams

When care is provided by an individual practitioner, establishing that the healthcare practitioner owes a duty of care is straightforward, and unlikely to be disputed. Establishing what constitutes an acceptable standard of care is not so straightforward, but it can be guided by expert opinion and professional guidelines. However, because a multidisciplinary team is not a single legal entity, the common law does not recognise the existence of a collective duty of care. Therefore, when a patient is subject to care by multiple practitioners acting as a single team, it becomes unclear as to whether a duty of care exists and who in the multidisciplinary team owes that duty of care to the patient. Unless an adverse outcome is traceable to the action of a single individual, the existence of duty of care when patients are collectively managed by networks of individual practitioners remains unclear. This is likely to result in all members of a multidisciplinary team being joined as parties in an allegation of breach of duty. The situation is changed if a single hospital employs all members of a multidisciplinary team, because it can then be logically argued that a duty of care exists between the institution and the patient.

Pain management from multidisciplinary teams is promoted as being an ideal standard of care for individuals with persistent pain as it produces better outcomes and improved patient satisfactions and functional restoration. Does it thus follow that, should a patient not be referred to a multidisciplinary pain management team, that an acceptable standard of care has not been delivered? Further, should a patient not be provided with multidisciplinary team care, and not achieve a sufficient treatment response, is there a collective breach of duty of care? These are complex questions that give pause for thought.

Consent and privacy in multidisciplinary care

In tort law, assault and battery are committed when any treatment is administered in the absence of an individual's consent. Whereas assault does not require any physical contact with the patient, battery involves actual bodily contact. Obtaining consent to receive treatment is therefore necessary for all pain management treatment, not just procedural interventions. Joint health records sharing in which members of the multidisciplinary teams are allowed to access information provided to other team members may give rise to

consent actions and invoke privacy concerns because patients receiving multidisciplinary pain management might not, in the ordinary course of events, expect there to be a sharing of information between different members of the treating team. Because a multidisciplinary team has no legal basis, it is unclear in law whether treatment dissent among members of multidisciplinary teams should be communicated to the patient or whether the lead clinician should simply convey the majority view.

Case law

To the author's knowledge, a Court in any common law jurisdiction has yet to make a decision addressing whether not providing a multidisciplinary approach for persistent pain management would be determinative of breach of duty. Case law does exist in other multidisciplinary fields of healthcare, notably in management of obesity and of cancer care, where multidisciplinary care from surgeons, oncologists, radiotherapists, psychologists and other allied health professionals are increasingly seen as providing best outcomes. In *Varipatis v Almiro* 2013 NSWCA 76 there was an acceptance that multidisciplinary care is the preferred model and standard of cancer care.

The issue of managing concerns over maintaining patient privacy of medical records in the setting of multidisciplinary care has been explored in *KJ v Wentworth Area Health Service* 2004 NSWADT 84. The issue in this case was that psychiatrists and psychologists' notes were placed in the general medical record of a patient undergoing multidisciplinary cancer care without the express consent of the patient, leading to a complaint. In judgement there were seen to be two broad categories to consenting. The first was consent to a particular course of treatment or a procedure, while the second was consenting to have personal information shared between different members of a multidisciplinary team, which required an additional specific consent to be obtained.

Conclusion and emerging areas of law and pain medicine

This chapter has highlighted the effects of recent legislative changes upon registration and regulation of health professionals, where there is an emerging body of case law that supports the principle of maintaining public confidence and safety is being achieved using a coregulatory system. Changes to opioid prescribing legislation and guidelines that have been introduced to curb opioid-related misuse and harms have been less successful and would suggest that other measures such as better education and training might be more successful than using somewhat blunt and arbitrary legislative changes. Further areas of law reform that are as yet so recent in their introduction as to be unable to accurately predict the effect upon clinical practice are the easing of access to cannabinoid products to treat persistent pain conditions and the legalisation of euthanasia and physician assisted dying as an alternative to unrelieved pain and suffering. Healthcare practitioners should not be afraid to use their expertise to guide and assist how Courts and Tribunals will apply and interpreted these latter legislative changes by provision of expert opinion and evidence.

Review questions | Q

1. What areas of law affect the clinical practice of multidisciplinary teams of health professionals working with patients with chronic pain?
2. With respect to the opioid crisis, what are the factors that prescribing health professionals must consider?
3. How are health professionals working with patients with persistent pain likely to be affected by emerging changes to laws and regulations?
4. What are the key points a health professional should remember when providing expert witness testimony?

References

Dineen, K., 2016. Dubois between a rock and a hard place: can physicians prescribe opioids to treat pain adequately without avoiding legal sanction? Am. J. Law. Med. 42 (1), 7–52.

Hadland, S., 2018. Tighter regulation drives illicit opioid sales. BMJ 361, k2480.

Hockman, J.S., 2010. A Dose of Truth about the Consequences of Opiophobia. HCPlive.com.

International Narcotics Control Board, 2013. Narcotics Drugs; Estimated World Requirements for 2013. United Nations, New York, NY.

Ipp, D.A., 2002. Review of the Law of Negligence Commonwealth of Australia.

Mahler, B., Shardley, J., 2021. Concurrent Evidence Practices Survey. KordaMentha.com.

Portenoy, R., Foley, M., 1986. Chronic use of opioid analgesics in non malignant pain: report of 38 cases. Pain Mat. 25 (2), 171–186.

Richards, G., Aronson, J., Mahtani, R., May 4 2021. Global, regional and national consumption of controlled opioids: a cross-sectional study of 214 countries and non metropolitan territories. Br. J. Pain 16 (1), 34–40.

Woolf, L., 1996. Access to Justice. HM Government.

Chapter | 26 |

Conclusions: the future

Jenny Strong and Hubert van Griensven

The second edition of the *Pain: A Textbook for Health Professionals* was published in 2014, 12 years after the first edition. In the ensuing years, many things have improved, while other things have stayed the same.

With respect to what has improved, there has been a continued growth in understanding of the neuroscience of pain. Some of the important advances in this field have been illuminated in several chapters, specifically those about neuroanatomy and neurophysiology. Another important advance has been the swell of understanding of the critical need for health professionals to work *in partnership* with people in pain. This textbook makes a contribution to this important aspect of clinical practice. Our chapter entitled 'The patient's voice' sets the scene in this third edition of the textbook, along with new chapters on communication and pain education.

The past 10 years have seen the publication of a plethora of clinical guidelines and consensus statements, to help clinicians make decisions based on the best available evidence. For example, the Australian Government Department of Health published the *National Strategic Action Plan for Pain Management* in 2021. The Australian and New Zealand College of Anaesthetists and Faculty of Pain Medicine published the fourth edition of its *Acute Pain Management: Scientific Evidence* guidelines in 2015 (Schug et al. 2020), while the Australian Pain Society published its *Guiding Principles for Pain Management* statement in 2017. The British Pain Society published the second edition of its Core Standards for Pain Management Services in 2021. It was also involved in producing a set of validated outcome measures in 2019, in collaboration with the Faculty of Pain Medicine and the Royal College of Anaesthetists. The UK's National Institute for Health and Clinical Excellence (NICE) continues to produce guidance for treatment based on current evidence, such as Guideline NG193 for the assessment and management of chronic pain. Consensus statements abound, such as *The Assessment of Pain in Older People: UK National Guidelines* (Schofield et al. 2018) and the Australian Pain Society's second edition of the

Pain in Residential Aged Care Facilities: Management Strategies in 2019. There is a wealth of knowledge available to clinicians and patients alike.

Since the previous edition of this textbook, the tragedy of the worldwide opioid crisis has befallen us. As discussed in Chapter 25, opioid compounds, advocated and marketed to provide relief to patients with chronic noncancer pain, have led to harm for many. The other crisis has been the SARS-CoV-2 virus that caused the COVID-19 pandemic. Although initially it seemed to manifest as a respiratory condition, it is now clear that COVID-19 can be associated with widespread and varied symptoms including persistent pain (see, for example, Carvalho Soares et al. 2021). The disease has put pressure on resources for health and social care worldwide. This has sadly brought to light the gap between privileged populations and those who are not well off. However, it has also shown the remarkable resilience of professionals, patients, carers and families. The availability of digital technologies has played an important part in this.

Now perhaps more than when we published the previous edition of this book, we believe that there is a critical need for health professionals to be conversant with the most appropriate and up-to-date evidence-based therapeutic tools to support the many individuals who suffer from acute or persistent pain. We therefore feel that this new edition of our textbook is necessary and important.

We urge therapists and health professionals to utilise the knowledge in this book and to use its resources as a basis for further learning. It will help them to aid the prevention of chronic pain, participate in the rehabilitation of those who have persistent pain and advocate for people who have pain. This is particularly important for those who are unable or unwilling to speak for themselves, or are vulnerable in other ways, such as children, older people, those who have cognitive deficits, and people who have linguistic and cultural differences from the dominant culture. Health professionals have an ethical, moral and professional imperative to assist in the relief of suffering for all.

References

Australian Government Department of Health, 2021. National Strategic Action Plan for Pain Management. Commonwealth Government, Canberra. Creative Commons Attribution 4.0 International Public License.

Australian Pain Society, 2017. Guiding Principles for Pain Management. Available from https://www.apsoc.au/position-papers.

Australian Pain Society, 2019. Pain in Residential Aged Care Facilities: Management Strategies, second ed. Australian Pain Society, Sydney.

Carvalho Soares, F.H., Kubota, G.T., Fernandes, A.M., Hojo, B., Couras, C., Costa, B.V., et al., 2021. Prevalence and characteristics of new-onset pain in COVID-19 survivors, a controlled study. Eur. J. Pain 25, 1342–1354.

Schofield, P. (Ed.), 2018. The assessment of pain in older people: UK National Guidelines. Age Ageing 47, i1–i22.

Schug, S.A., Palmer, G.M., Scott, D.A., Alcock, M., Halliwell, R., Mott, J.F., et al., 2020. Australian and New Zealand College of Anaesthetists and Faculty of Pain Medicine. Acute Pain Management: Scientific Evidence, fifth ed. ANZCA & FPM, Melbourne.

Index